Aging Mechanisms: Brain Networks and Pathology

Aging Mechanisms: Brain Networks and Pathology

Editor: Adler Brown

AMERICAN
MEDICAL PUBLISHERS
www.americanmedicalpublishers.com

AMERICAN
MEDICAL PUBLISHERS
www.americanmedicalpublishers.com

Cataloging-in-Publication Data

Aging mechanisms : brain networks and pathology / edited by Adler Brown.
p. cm.
Includes bibliographical references and index.
ISBN 978-1-63927-863-3
1. Geriatric neurology. 2. Geriatric pathology. 3. Communicative disorders in old age.
4. Geriatrics. 5. Older people--Health and hygiene. 6. Aging. I. Brown, Adler.
RC346 .A35 2023
616.8--dc23

American Medical Publishers,
41 Flatbush Avenue,
1st Floor, New York,
NY 11217, USA

ISBN 978-1-63927-863-3 (Hardback)

Contents

Preface

Aging is the process of growing older. It is a risk factor for most prevalent neurodegenerative diseases, such as mild cognitive impairment, dementias involving Alzheimer's disease, cerebrovascular disease, Parkinson's disease, and Lou Gehrig's disease. The brain is a complicated organ that is made up of many different types of tissue and matter. The function of various tissues in brain may be more or less susceptible to age- induced changes. The structure of brain's network is formed through anatomical connection of the neurons. The aging of brain is a complex process that begins early in life and accelerates with age, affecting everything from the subcellular to the organ level. Brain volume loss, cortical thinning, white matter degradation, loss of gyrification, and ventricular enlargement are morphological symptoms of brain aging. Neuron cell shrinking, dendritic degeneration, demyelination, small vessel disease, metabolic slowing, microglial activation, and the formation of white matter lesions are pathophysiological symptoms of brain aging. This book explores all the important aspects of ageing in the present day scenario. It will provide comprehensive knowledge to the readers.

The information contained in this book is the result of intensive hard work done by researchers in this field. All due efforts have been made to make this book serve as a complete guiding source for students and researchers. The topics in this book have been comprehensively explained to help readers understand the growing trends in the field.

I would like to thank the entire group of writers who made sincere efforts in this book and my family who supported me in my efforts of working on this book. I take this opportunity to thank all those who have been a guiding force throughout my life.

Editor

1

Melatonin Supplementation, a Strategy to Prevent Neurological Diseases through Maintaining Integrity of Blood Brain Barrier in Old People

Wen-Cao Liu[1], Xiaona Wang[2,3], Xinyu Zhang[2,3], Xi Chen[4] and Xinchun Jin[2,3]**

[1]Department of Emergency, Shanxi Provincial People's Hospital, Taiyuan, China, [2]Jiangsu Key Laboratory of Translational Research and Therapy for Neuro-Psycho-Diseases and Institute of Neuroscience, Department of Neurology, the Second Affiliated Hospital of Soochow University, Suzhou, China, [3]School of Pharmacy, Key Laboratory of Molecular Pharmacology and Drug Evaluation (Yantai University), Ministry of Education, Yantai University, Yantai, China, [4]Department of Core Facility, the People's Hospital of Baoan Shenzhen, Shenzhen, China

***Correspondence:**
Xi Chen
beating_u5@hotmail.com
Xinchun Jin
xinchunjin@gmail.com

Blood brain barrier (BBB) plays a crucial role in maintaining homeostasis of microenvironment that is essential to neural function of the central nervous system (CNS). When facing various extrinsic or intrinsic stimuli, BBB is damaged which is an early event in pathogenesis of a variety of neurological diseases in old patients including acute and chronic cerebral ischemia, Alzheimer's disease and etc. Treatments that could maintain the integrity of BBB may prevent neurological diseases following various stimuli. Old people often face a common stress of sepsis, during which lipopolysaccharide (LPS) is released into circulation and the integrity of BBB is damaged. Of note, there is a significant decrease of melatonin level in old people and animal. Melatonin has been shown to preserves BBB integrity and permeability via a variety of pathways: inhibition of matrix metalloproteinase-9 (MMP-9), inhibition of NADPH oxidase-2, and impact on silent information regulator 1 (SIRT1) and nucleotide-binding oligomerization domain-like receptor family pyrin domain-containing 3 (NLRP3) inflammasome. More important, a recent study showed that melatonin supplementation alleviates LPS-induced BBB damage in old mice through activating AMP-activated protein kinase (AMPK) and inhibiting gp91^{phox}, suggesting that melatonin supplementation may help prevent neurological diseases through maintaining the integrity of BBB in old people.

Keywords: melatonin, blood brain barrier, neurological diseases, old people, lipopolysaccharide

---

Abbreviations: AMPK, AMP-activated protein kinase; BBB, blood brain barrier; CNS, central nervous system; iNOS, inducible nitric oxide synthase; LPS, lipopolysaccharide; MMP-9, matrix metalloproteinase-9; nNOS, neuronal nitric oxide synthase; NADPH, nicotinamide adenine dinucleotide phosphate; NF-κB, nuclear factor kappa-light-chain-enhancer of activated B cells; NLRP3, nucleotide-binding oligomerization domain-like receptor family pyrin domain-containing 3; ROS, reactive oxygen species; SIRT1, silent information regulator 1; TBI, traumatic brain injury; TJPs, tight junction proteins; TLR4, toll like receptor 4.

INTRODUCTION

The Blood Brain Barrier Damage and Neurological Diseases

The blood brain barrier (BBB) is a regulated interface between the peripheral circulation and the central nervous system (CNS; Jin et al., 2014). BBB, which is composed of cerebral microvascular endothelial cells, neurons, astrocytes, pericytes and the extracellular matrix, plays a key role in maintaining homeostasis of microenvironment that is essential to neural function of the CNS (Hawkins and Davis, 2005). When facing various extrinsic or intrinsic stimuli (Weiss et al., 2009), BBB is damaged and BBB dysfunction is an early event in pathogenesis of a variety of neurological diseases in old patients including vascular cognitive impairment, amyotrophic lateral sclerosis, Alzheimer's disease, neuropathic pain, brain trauma, acute and chronic cerebral ischemia, multiple sclerosis, and brain infections (Rosenberg, 2012; please see **Figure 1**). Treatments that could maintain the integrity of BBB will have important roles in preventing stimuli-produced neurological diseases.

The tight junction proteins (TJPs), composed of occludin, claudin and zo-1, are key components of the BBB (Hawkins and Davis, 2005). It seals the interendothelial cleft forming a continuous blood vessel, leads to high endothelial electrical resistance, and allows low paracellular permeability of water-soluble substances from the blood into brain parenchyma (Stamatovic et al., 2008). Free radicals of oxygen and nitrogen and the proteases, matrix metalloproteinases (MMPs) and cyclooxgyenases, play key roles in the early and delayed BBB disruption as the neuroinflammatory response progresses (Liu and Rosenberg, 2005). During an injury, free radicals and proteases attacked the cell membranes and degraded the TJPs between endothelial cells and the integrity of BBB is damaged (Jin et al., 2013; Liu et al., 2016; Wang et al., 2016). It is worth of note, death of endothelial cells of microvessels is also a major contributor to the disruption of BBB integrity (Simard et al., 2007). Therefore, protective effect on intergrity of BBB should consider both death of endothelial cells of microvessels and degradation of TJPS.

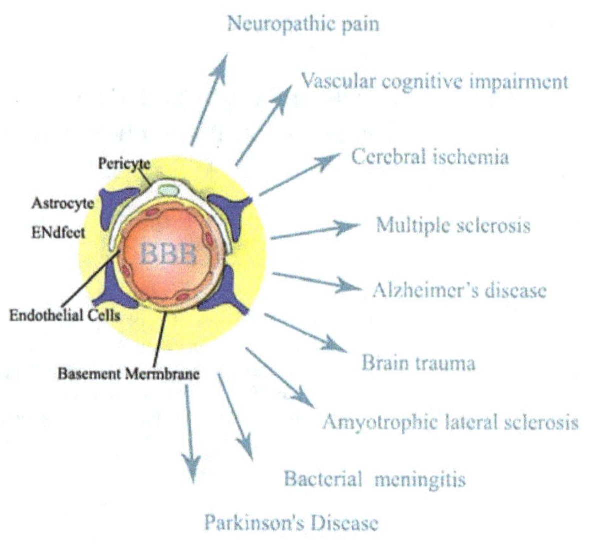

FIGURE 1 | Structure of blood brain barrier (BBB) which is related to neurological diseases.

BBB Disruption Induced by Lipopolysaccharide (LPS)

Lipopolysaccharide (LPS) could produce neuroinflammation (Shi, 2015), promoting the generation of reactive oxygen species (ROS) in cerebral microvascular endothelial cells and BBB disruption (Seok et al., 2013). Worth of note, LPS has been shown to increase BBB permeability *in vitro* (Nonaka et al., 2004) and compromise BBB integrity in young (Ruiz-Valdepeñas et al., 2011; Zhou T. et al., 2014) and old mice (Wang et al., 2017). More interesting, LPS has been shown to induce BBB dysfunction via nicotinamide adenine dinucleotide phosphate (NADPH) oxidase-derived ROS (Liu et al., 2012; Zhao et al., 2014). NADPH oxidases, a major source of ROS generation in the brain, critically contributes to BBB disruption under various neurological disorders (Kahles et al., 2007). Of note, $gp91^{phox}$ is the catalytic subunit of NADPH oxidase and BBB disruption is significantly reduced in $gp91^{phox}$ knockout mice compared to wild-type mice after stroke (Kahles et al., 2007) and reduction of $gp91^{phox}$ expression has shown protective effect against ischemia-induced brain injury and BBB damage (Liu et al., 2008, 2011). More importantly, Wang et al. (2017) showed that LPS increased $gp91^{phox}$ expression in both endothelial cells and in old mice, suggesting that $gp91^{phox}$ up-regulation may be an important mechanism responsible for LPS-induced BBB permeability increase in old mice.

Relationship between Melatonin and Aging

Melatonin, which is produced mainly in the pineal gland, retina and the gastrointestinal tract, plays important roles in many physiological and biochemical functions (Bubenik and Konturek, 2011), such as acting as an anti-inflammatory and immunoregulating molecule as well as a circadian rhythm regulator (Manchester et al., 2015). Melatonin is a potent free radical scavenger, lack of melatonin may result in decreased antioxidant function in the old people which have significant influence not only on aging *per se* but also on the incidence or severity of age-related diseases (Karasek, 2004). In addition, oxygen radical detoxification processes was significantly decreased during aging and there was a obvious downregualtion in pineal biosynthetic activity in aging hamster (Bubenik and Konturek, 2011). More interesting, melatonin levels in serum and brain decline as a result of aging (Bubenik and Konturek, 2011; Hill et al., 2013). In addition, melatonin has been reported to regulate aging and neurodegeneration through energy metabolism, epigenetics, autophagy and circadian rhythm pathways (Jenwitheesuk et al., 2014).

Beneficial Role of Melatonin in Sepsis

Sepsis is a systemic inflammatory response to infection that causes severe neurological complications (Zhao et al., 2015) and it is a common stress that old people often face (Martin et al., 2006), in which LPS is released into circulation (Shukla et al., 2014).

Melatonin has been shown to restore the mitochondrial production of ATP in septic mice (López et al., 2006a), block the septic response by disrupting connection of the nuclear factor kappa-light-chain-enhancer of activated B cells (NF-κB) with nucleotide-binding oligomerization domain-like receptor family pyrin domain-containing 3 (NLRP3) in mice (El Frargy et al., 2015) and improve survival in a zymosan A-induced rat model of sepsis/shock (Reynolds et al., 2003). In addition, melatonin has been shown to protect organs against sepis-inuduced injury. For example, melatonin improved cardiac mitochondria and survival rate in rat septic heart injury (Zhang et al., 2013) through inhibition of inducible nitric oxide synthase (iNOS) and preservation of neuronal nitric oxide synthase (nNOS; Ortiz et al., 2014) and attenuated sepsis-induced cardiac dysfunction via a PI3K/Akt-dependent mechanism (An et al., 2016). Furthermore, melatonin protected liver bioenergetics from sepsis-induced damage (Basile et al., 2004), modified cellular stress in the liver of septic mice by reducing ROS and increasing the unfolded protein response (Kleber et al., 2014), protected against sepsis-induced functional and biochemical changes in rat ileum and urinary bladder (Paskaloglu et al., 2004), improved colonic anastomotic healing in a rat experimental sepsis model (Ersoy et al., 2016) and counteracted inducible mitochondrial nitric oxide synthase-dependent mitochondrial dysfunction in skeletal muscle (Escames et al., 2006) and diaphragm (López et al., 2006b) in septic mice.

Melatonin's Effect on LPS-Induced Injury

Melatonin has been shown to ameliorate LPS-induced brain injury in neonatal rats (Wong et al., 2014), alleviate LPS-induced placental cellular stress response in mice (Wang et al., 2011) as well as LPS-induced hepatic SREBP-1c activation and lipid accumulation in mice (Chen et al., 2011). Of note, melatonin shown protective effect against BBB damage induced by various stimuli, including transient focal cerebral ischemia in mice (Chen et al., 2006), excitotoxic injury in neonatal rats (Moretti et al., 2015) and methamphetamine-induced inflammation (Jumnongprakhon et al., 2016). Therefore, decreased levels of melatonin in old mice may contribute to the BBB disruption when facing various extrinsic or intrinsic stimuli because melatonin has demonstrated its protective effects against LPS-induced injury to the heart (Lu et al., 2015), brain (Carloni et al., 2016), lung (Lee et al., 2009) and liver (Wang et al., 2007) by scavenging a variety of free radicals (Manchester et al., 2015). Interestingly, chronic melatonin treatment has also shown reduction of age-dependent inflammatory process in senescence-accelerated mice (Rodríguez et al., 2007). In a recent study, Wang et al. (2017) showed that 1 week melatonin treatment significantly alleviated LPS-induced BBB damage accompanied by reduction of occludin and claudin-5 degradation, suggesting that melatonin supplementation is important in decreasing sepsis and neuroinflammation-induced TJPs degradation as well as BBB damage.

Possible Molecular Mechanism Underlying Melatonin's Effect on LPS-Induced BBB Damage in Old Mice

Melatonin has shown protective effect on BBB integrity via a variety of pathways: inhibition of the toll like receptor 4 (TLR4)/NF-κB signaling pathway in neonatal rats (Hu et al., 2017), inhibition of NADPH oxidase-2 (Jumnongprakhon et al., 2016), inhibition of MMP-9 (Alluri et al., 2016), inhibiton of AMP-activated protein kinase (AMPK) activation (Wang et al., 2017) and impact on silent information regulator 1 (SIRT1; Zhao et al., 2015) and NLRP3 inflammasome (Rahim et al., 2017).

AMPK Activation

AMPK activation has been shown to play important role in maintaining the integrity of BBB (Liu et al., 2012) and it is also reported that LPS inhibits the activation of AMPK, a serine/threonine protein kinase regulating cellular and organismal metabolism (Wang et al., 2017). Interestingly, AMPK activation has been shown to alleviate LPS-induced BBB disruption in both *in vitro* cell model (Zhao et al., 2014) and *in vivo* mice model (Zhou X. et al., 2014; Wang et al., 2017). Activation of AMPK also demonstrated protective effect against diabetes-induced BBB damage by inhibiting NADPH oxidase expression upregulation in brain capillary endothelial cells (Liu et al., 2012). In a recent study, Wang et al. (2017) showed that AMPK activation by melatonin reduced LPS-induced BBB damage in old mice and AMPK activation by metformin decreased LPS-induced gp91^{phox} up-regulation in brain capillary endothelial cells (**Figure 2**). AMPK activation might be important in maintaining the integrity of BBB in old patients and AMPK dysfunction might play a key role in the initiation and progression of neurological disorders in old people. Therefore, activation of AMPK may be a strategy to reduce neurological disorders following sepsis and neuroinflamation-induced BBB damage in old people.

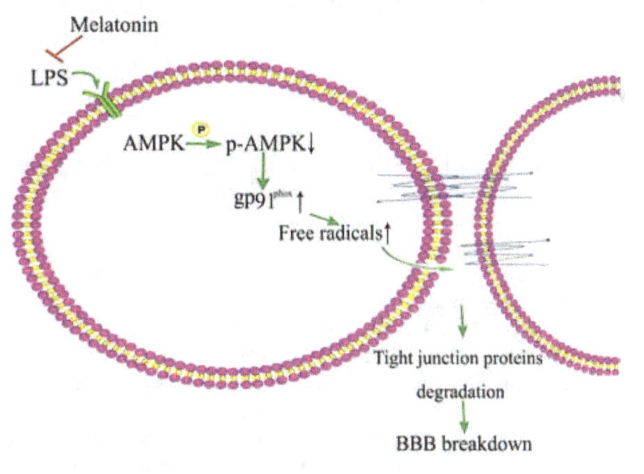

FIGURE 2 | Schematic illustration of melation's protective effect on lipopolysaccharide (LPS)-induced damage of BBB integrity.

Matrix Metalloproteinase-9 (MMP-9)

MMP-9 has been shown to play important role in BBB damage (Jin et al., 2013, 2015; Cai et al., 2015) and melatonin has been shown to bind to MMP-9 to act as its endogenous inhibitor. Melatonin treatment provided protection against traumatic brain injury (TBI)-induced BBB hyperpermeability via MMP-9 inhibition (Alluri et al., 2016), indicating its potential as a therapeutic agent for BBB damage.

Silent Information Regulator 1 (SIRT1)

SIRT1 was reported to be beneficial in sepsis. Using EX527, a SIRT1 inhibitor, the authors figured out that melatonin alleviated BBB damage in mice which subjected to cecal ligation and puncture via SIRT1 to inhibit inflammation, apoptosis and oxidative stress (Zhao et al., 2015).

NLRP3 Inflammasome

Aging and sepsis triggered NLRP3 inflammasome activation (Volt et al., 2016), which has been shown to be involved in the innate immune response during inflammation (Rahim et al., 2017). Furthermore, NLRP3 inflammasome activation was showed to be associated with the upregulation of apoptotic signaling pathway in various inflammatory diseases (Volt et al., 2016) and melatonin attenuated subarachnoid hemorrhage-induced BBB damage via attenuating the expressions of NLRP3 (Dong et al., 2016).

Dark Side/Downsides of Melatonin Supplementation

Although acute toxicity of melatonin is extremely low in both animal and human studies, melatonin may still cause minor adverse effects, such as headache, insomnia and nightmares (Malhotra et al., 2004). Based on previous studies, melatonin could be used as a daily supplement to delay or prevent changes associated with age. However, long-term side effect of melatonin has to be tested, because melatonin has been used as a contraceptive for women which could have reproduction alterations by consumption of melatonin (Voordouw et al., 1992). In addition, there was a decrease in sperm motility in male rats (Gwayi and Bernard, 2002), and long-term administration of melatonin inhibited testicular aromatase levels (Luboshitzky et al., 2002). It does not matter to provide old people with daily melatonin to prevent neurological diseases even if these two side effects may happen as they would not have reproduction anymore. Other side effects should be considered, for example, melatonin may accelerate the development of autoimmune conditions (Mattsson et al., 1994), increase atherosclerosis in the aorta in hypercholesterolemic rats (Tailleux et al., 2002) and produce opposite effects in cancer treatment with poorly timed administration (Bartsch and Bartsch, 1981).

Conclusion

In conclusion, decreased melatonin levels may account for the BBB damage in old people who often face the common stress of sepsis and neuroinflammation. Melation supplementation treatment significantly inhibits such events. Therefore, continuous daily melatonin supplementation may help prevent sepsis and neuroinflammation-related neurological diseases through maintaining the integrity of BBB in old people. Since melatonin has low toxicity profile and high efficacy in many pathophysiological states, it should be more commonly tested/used in the medical and veterinary arenas. Further studies are needed to verify the important significance of daily melatonin supplementation in old people.

AUTHOR CONTRIBUTIONS

W-CL, XW, XZ, XC and XJ wrote the manuscript and XC, XJ obtained the funding. XW drew the figures. All authors have approved the final version of this review article.

ACKNOWLEDGMENTS

This work was supported by National Natural Science Foundation of China (81671145), by Natural Science Foundation of Jiangsu Province of China (L221506415) and by grants from Shenzhen Science and Technology Innovation Commission (JCYJ20150402152005623). This work was also partly supported by Priority Academic Program Development of Jiangsu Higher Education Institutions of China.

REFERENCES

Alluri, H., Wilson, R. L., Anasooya Shaji, C., Wiggins-Dohlvik, K., Patel, S., Liu, Y., et al. (2016). Melatonin preserves blood-brain barrier integrity and permeability via matrix metalloproteinase-9 inhibition. *PLoS One* 11:e0154427. doi: 10.1371/journal.pone.0154427

An, R., Zhao, L., Xi, C., Li, H., Shen, G., Liu, H., et al. (2016). Melatonin attenuates sepsis-induced cardiac dysfunction via a PI3K/Akt-dependent mechanism. *Basic Res. Cardiol.* 111:8. doi: 10.1007/s00395-015-0526-1

Bartsch, H., and Bartsch, C. (1981). Effect of melatonin on experimental tumors under different photoperiods and times of administration. *J. Neural Transm.* 52, 269–279. doi: 10.1007/bf01256752

Basile, M., Romeo, C., Gitto, E., Spitz, L., Pierro, A., and Eaton, S. (2004). Melatonin protects from, but does not reverse, the effects of mediators of sepsis on liver bioenergetics. *Pediatr. Surg. Int.* 20, 263–266. doi: 10.1007/s00383-003-1123-1

Bubenik, G. A., and Konturek, S. J. (2011). Melatonin and aging: prospects for human treatment. *J. Physiol. Pharmacol.* 62, 13–19.

Cai, H., Mu, Z., Jiang, Z., Wang, Y., Yang, G. Y., and Zhang, Z. (2015). Hypoxia-controlled matrix metalloproteinase-9 hyperexpression promotes behavioral recovery after ischemia. *Neurosci. Bull.* 31, 550–560. doi: 10.1007/s12264-015-1533-1

Carloni, S., Favrais, G., Saliba, E., Albertini, M. C., Chalon, S., Longini, M., et al. (2016). Melatonin modulates neonatal brain inflammation through endoplasmic reticulum stress, autophagy, and miR-34a/silent information regulator 1 pathway. *J. Pineal Res.* 61, 370–380. doi: 10.1111/jpi.12354

Chen, T. Y., Lee, M. Y., Chen, H. Y., Kuo, Y. L., Lin, S. C., Wu, T. S., et al. (2006). Melatonin attenuates the postischemic increase in blood-brain barrier permeability and decreases hemorrhagic transformation of tissue-plasminogen activator therapy following ischemic stroke in mice. *J. Pineal Res.* 40, 242–250. doi: 10.1111/j.1600-079x.2005.00307.x

Chen, X., Zhang, C., Zhao, M., Shi, C.-E., Zhu, R.-M., Wang, H., et al. (2011). Melatonin alleviates lipopolysaccharide-induced hepatic SREBP-1c activation and lipid accumulation in mice. *J. Pineal Res.* 51, 416–425. doi: 10.1111/j.1600-079x.2011.00905.x

Dong, Y., Fan, C., Hu, W., Jiang, S., Ma, Z., Yan, X., et al. (2016). Melatonin attenuated early brain injury induced by subarachnoid hemorrhage via regulating NLRP3 inflammasome and apoptosis signaling. *J. Pineal Res.* 60, 253–262. doi: 10.1111/jpi.12300

El Frargy, M., El-Sharkawy, H. M., and Attia, G. F. (2015). Use of melatonin as an adjuvant therapy in neonatal sepsis. *J. Neonatal Perinatal Med.* 8, 227–232. doi: 10.3233/NPM-15814072

Ersoy, O. F., Özkan, N., Özsoy, Z., Kayaoglu, H. A., Yenidogan, E., Çelik, A., et al. (2016). Effects of melatonin on cytokine release and healing of colonic anastomoses in an experimental sepsis model. *Ulus. Travma Acil Cerrahi Derg.* 22, 315–321. doi: 10.5505/tjtes.2015.49465

Escames, G., López, L. C., Tapias, V., Utrilla, P., Reiter, R. J., Hitos, A. B., et al. (2006). Melatonin counteracts inducible mitochondrial nitric oxide synthase-dependent mitochondrial dysfunction in skeletal muscle of septic mice. *J. Pineal Res.* 40, 71–78. doi: 10.1111/j.1600-079x.2005.00281.x

Gwayi, N., and Bernard, R. T. (2002). The effects of melatonin on sperm motility *in vitro* in Wistar rats. *Andrologia* 34, 391–396. doi: 10.1046/j.1439-0272.2002.00522.x

Hawkins, B. T., and Davis, T. P. (2005). The blood-brain barrier/neurovascular unit in health and disease. *Pharmacol. Rev.* 57, 173–185. doi: 10.1124/pr.57.2.4

Hill, S. M., Cheng, C., Yuan, L., Mao, L., Jockers, R., Dauchy, B., et al. (2013). Age-related decline in melatonin and its MT1 receptor are associated with decreased sensitivity to melatonin and enhanced mammary tumor growth. *Curr. Aging Sci.* 6, 125–133. doi: 10.2174/1874609811306010016

Hu, Y., Wang, Z., Pan, S., Zhang, H., Fang, M., Jiang, H., et al. (2017). Melatonin protects against blood-brain barrier damage by inhibiting the TLR4/NF-κB signaling pathway after LPS treatment in neonatal rats. *Oncotarget* 8, 31638–31654. doi: 10.18632/oncotarget.15780

Jenwitheesuk, A., Nopparat, C., Mukda, S., Wongchitrat, P., and Govitrapong, P. (2014). Melatonin regulates aging and neurodegeneration through energy metabolism, epigenetics, autophagy and circadian rhythm pathways. *Int. J. Mol. Sci.* 15, 16848–16884. doi: 10.3390/ijms150916848

Jin, X., Liu, J., and Liu, W. (2014). Early ischemic blood brain barrier damage: a potential indicator for hemorrhagic transformation following tissue plasminogen activator (tPA) thrombolysis? *Curr. Neurovasc. Res.* 11, 254–262. doi: 10.2174/1567202611666140530145643

Jin, X., Liu, J., Liu, K. J., Rosenberg, G. A., Yang, Y., and Liu, W. (2013). Normobaric hyperoxia combined with minocycline provides greater neuroprotection than either alone in transient focal cerebral ischemia. *Exp. Neurol.* 240, 9–16. doi: 10.1016/j.expneurol.2012.11.018

Jin, X., Sun, Y., Xu, J., and Liu, W. (2015). Caveolin-1 mediates tissue plasminogen activator-induced MMP-9 up-regulation in cultured brain microvascular endothelial cells. *J. Neurochem.* 132, 724–730. doi: 10.1111/jnc.13065

Jumnongprakhon, P., Govitrapong, P., Tocharus, C., and Tocharus, J. (2016). Melatonin promotes blood-brain barrier integrity in methamphetamine-induced inflammation in primary rat brain microvascular endothelial cells. *Brain Res.* 1646, 182–192. doi: 10.1016/j.brainres.2016.05.049

Kahles, T., Luedike, P., Endres, M., Galla, H. J., Steinmetz, H., Busse, R., et al. (2007). NADPH oxidase plays a central role in blood-brain barrier damage in experimental stroke. *Stroke* 38, 3000–3006. doi: 10.1161/STROKEAHA.107.489765

Karasek, M. (2004). Melatonin, human aging, and age-related diseases. *Exp. Gerontol.* 39, 1723–1729. doi: 10.1016/j.exger.2004.04.012

Kleber, A., Kubulus, D., Rössler, D., Wolf, B., Volk, T., Speer, T., et al. (2014). Melatonin modifies cellular stress in the liver of septic mice by reducing reactive oxygen species and increasing the unfolded protein response. *Exp. Mol. Pathol.* 97, 565–571. doi: 10.1016/j.yexmp.2014.10.009

Lee, Y. D., Kim, J. Y., Lee, K. H., Kwak, Y. J., Lee, S. K., Kim, O. S., et al. (2009). Melatonin attenuates lipopolysaccharide-induced acute lung inflammation in sleep-deprived mice. *J. Pineal Res.* 46, 53–57. doi: 10.1111/J.1600-079X.2008.00621.x

Liu, W., Chen, Q., Liu, J., and Liu, K. J. (2011). Normobaric hyperoxia protects the blood brain barrier through inhibiting Nox2 containing NADPH oxidase in ischemic stroke. *Med. Gas Res.* 1:22. doi: 10.1186/2045-9912-1-22

Liu, K. J., and Rosenberg, G. A. (2005). Matrix metalloproteinases and free radicals in cerebral ischemia. *Free Radic. Biol. Med.* 39, 71–80. doi: 10.1016/j.freeradbiomed.2005.03.033

Liu, W., Sood, R., Chen, Q., Sakoglu, U., Hendren, J., Cetin, O., et al. (2008). Normobaric hyperoxia inhibits NADPH oxidase-mediated matrix metalloproteinase-9 induction in cerebral microvessels in experimental stroke. *J. Neurochem.* 107, 1196–1205. doi: 10.1111/j.1471-4159.2008.05664.x

Liu, J., Weaver, J., Jin, X., Zhang, Y., Xu, J., Liu, K. J., et al. (2016). Nitric oxide interacts with caveolin-1 to facilitate autophagy-lysosome-mediated claudin-5 degradation in oxygen-glucose deprivation-treated endothelial cells. *Mol. Neurobiol.* 53, 5935–5947. doi: 10.1007/s12035-015-9504-8

Liu, C., Wu, J., and Zou, M. H. (2012). Activation of AMP-activated protein kinase alleviates high-glucose-induced dysfunction of brain microvascular endothelial cell tight-junction dynamics. *Free Radic. Biol. Med.* 53, 1213–1221. doi: 10.1016/j.freeradbiomed.2012.07.003

López, L. C., Escames, G., Ortiz, F., Ros, E., and Acuña-Castroviejo, D. (2006a). Melatonin restores the mitochondrial production of ATP in septic mice. *Neuro. Endocrinol. Lett.* 27, 623–630.

López, L. C., Escames, G., Tapias, V., Utrilla, P., Leon, J., and Acuña-Castroviejo, D. (2006b). Identification of an inducible nitric oxide synthase in diaphragm mitochondria from septic mice: its relation with mitochondrial dysfunction and prevention by melatonin. *Int. J. Biochem. Cell Biol.* 38, 267–278. doi: 10.1016/j.biocel.2005.09.008

Lu, Q., Yi, X., Cheng, X., Sun, X., and Yang, X. (2015). Melatonin protects against myocardial hypertrophy induced by lipopolysaccharide. *In Vitro Cell. Dev. Biol. Anim.* 51, 353–360. doi: 10.1007/s11626-014-9844-0

Luboshitzky, R., Shen-Orr, Z., Nave, R., Lavi, S., and Lavie, P. (2002). Melatonin administration alters semen quality in healthy men. *J. Androl.* 23, 572–578. doi: 10.1002/j.1939-4640.2002.tb02281.x

Malhotra, S., Sawhney, G., and Pandhi, P. (2004). The therapeutic potential of melatonin: a review of the science. *MedGenMed* 6:46.

Manchester, L. C., Coto-Montes, A., Boga, J. A., Andersen, L. P., Zhou, Z., Galano, A., et al. (2015). Melatonin: an ancient molecule that makes oxygen metabolically tolerable. *J. Pineal Res.* 59, 403–419. doi: 10.1111/jpi.12267

Martin, G. S., Mannino, D. M., and Moss, M. (2006). The effect of age on the development and outcome of adult sepsis. *Crit. Care Med.* 34, 15–21. doi: 10.1097/01.ccm.0000194535.82812.ba

Mattsson, R., Hannsson, I., and Holmdahl, R. (1994). Pineal gland in autoimmunity: melatonin-dependent exaggeration of collagen-induced arthritis in mice. *Autoimmunity* 17, 83–86. doi: 10.3109/08916939409014661

Moretti, R., Zanin, A., Pansiot, J., Spiri, D., Manganozzi, L., Kratzer, I., et al. (2015). Melatonin reduces excitotoxic blood-brain barrier breakdown in neonatal rats. *Neuroscience* 311, 382–397. doi: 10.1016/j.neuroscience.2015.10.044

Nonaka, N., Hileman, S. M., Shioda, S., Vo, T. Q., and Banks, W. A. (2004). Effects of lipopolysaccharide on leptin transport across the blood-brain barrier. *Brain Res.* 1016, 58–65. doi: 10.1016/j.brainres.2004.04.066

Ortiz, F., García, J. A., Acuña-Castroviejo, D., Doerrier, C., López, A., Venegas, C., et al. (2014). The beneficial effects of melatonin against heart mitochondrial impairment during sepsis: inhibition of iNOS and preservation of nNOS. *J. Pineal Res.* 56, 71–81. doi: 10.1111/jpi.12099

Paskaloğlu, K., Sener, G., Kapucu, C., and Ayanoğlu-Dülger, G. (2004). Melatonin treatment protects against sepsis-induced functional and biochemical changes in rat ileum and urinary bladder. *Life Sci.* 74, 1093–1104. doi: 10.1016/j.lfs.2003.07.038

Rahim, I., Djerdjouri, B., Sayed, R. K., Fernández-Ortiz, M., Fernández-Gil, B., Hidalgo-Gutiérrez, A., et al. (2017). Melatonin administration to wild-type mice and non-treated NLRP3 mutant mice share similar inhibition of the inflammatory response during sepsis. *J. Pineal Res.* doi: 10.1111/jpi.12410 [Epub ahead of print].

Reynolds, F. D., Dauchy, R., Blask, D., Dietz, P. A., Lynch, D., and Zuckerman, R. (2003). The pineal gland hormone melatonin improves survival in a rat model of sepsis/shock induced by zymosan A. *Surgery* 134, 474–479. doi: 10.1067/s0039-6060(03)00253-8

Rodríguez, M. I., Escames, G., Löpez, L. C., Löpez, A., García, J. A., Ortiz, F., et al. (2007). Chronic melatonin treatment reduces the age-dependent inflammatory process in senescence-accelerated mice. *J. Pineal Res.* 42, 272–279. doi: 10.1111/j.1600-079x.2006.00416.x

Rosenberg, G. A. (2012). Neurological diseases in relation to the blood-brain barrier. *J. Cereb. Blood Flow Metab.* 32, 1139–1151. doi: 10.1038/jcbfm.2011.197

Ruiz-Valdepeñas, L., Martínez-Orgado, J. A., Benito, C., Millán, A., Tolón, R. M., and Romero, J. (2011). Cannabidiol reduces lipopolysaccharide-induced vascular changes and inflammation in the mouse brain: an intravital microscopy study. *J. Neuroinflammation* 8:5. doi: 10.1186/1742-2094-8-5

Seok, S. M., Kim, J. M., Park, T. Y., Baik, E. J., and Lee, S. H. (2013). Fructose-1,6-bisphosphate ameliorates lipopolysaccharide-induced dysfunction of blood-brain barrier. *Arch. Pharm. Res.* 36, 1149–1159. doi: 10.1007/s12272-013-0129-z

Shi, F. D. (2015). Neuroinflammation. *Neurosci. Bull.* 31, 714–716. doi: 10.1007/s12264-015-1568-y

Shukla, P., Rao, G. M., Pandey, G., Sharma, S., Mittapelly, N., Shegokar, R., et al. (2014). Therapeutic interventions in sepsis: current and anticipated pharmacological agents. *Br. J. Pharmacol.* 171, 5011–5031. doi: 10.1111/bph.12829

Simard, J. M., Kent, T. A., Chen, M., Tarasov, K. V., and Gerzanich, V. (2007). Brain oedema in focal ischemeia: molecular pathophysiology and theoretical implications. *Lancet Neurol.* 6, 258–268. doi: 10.1016/s1474-4422(07)70055-8

Stamatovic, S. M., Keep, R. F., and Andjelkovic, A. V. (2008). Brain endothelial cell-cell junctions: how to "open" the blood brain barrier. *Curr. Neuropharmacol.* 6, 179–192. doi: 10.2174/157015908785777210

Tailleux, A., Torpier, G., Bonnefont-Rousselot, D., Lestavel, S., Lemdani, M., Caudeville, B., et al. (2002). Daily melatonin supplementation in mice increases atherosclerosis in proximal aorta. *Biochem. Biophys. Res. Commun.* 293, 1114–1123. doi: 10.1016/s0006-291x(02)00336-4

Volt, H., Garcia, J. A., Doerrier, C., Diaz-Casado, M. E., Guerra-Librero, A., Lopez, L. C., et al. (2016). Same molecule but different expression: aging and sepsis trigger NLRP3 inflammasome activation, a target of melatonin. *J. Pineal Res.* 60, 193–205. doi: 10.1111/jpi.12303

Voordouw, B. C., Euser, R., Verdonk, R. E., Alberda, B. T., de Jong, F. H., Drogendijk, A. C., et al. (1992). Melatonin and melatonin-progestin combinations alter pituitary-ovarian function in women and can inhibit ovulation. *J. Clin. Endocrinol. Metab.* 74, 108–117. doi: 10.1210/jc.74.1.108

Wang, X., Liu, Y., Sun, Y., Liu, W., and Jin, X. (2016). Blood brain barrier breakdown was found in non-infarcted area after 2-h MCAO. *J. Neurol. Sci.* 363, 63–68. doi: 10.1016/j.jns.2016.02.035

Wang, H., Li, L., Zhao, M., Chen, Y. H., Zhang, Z. H., Zhang, C., et al. (2011). Melatonin alleviates lipopolysaccharide-induced placental cellular stress response in mice. *J. Pineal Res.* 50, 418–426. doi: 10.1111/j.1600-079x.2011.00860.x

Wang, X., Xue, G. X., Liu, W. C., Shu, H., Wang, M., Sun, Y., et al. (2017). Melatonin alleviates lipopolysaccharide-compromised integrity of blood-brain barrier through activating AMP-activated protein kinase in old mice. *Aging Cell* 16, 414–421. doi: 10.1111/acel.12572

Wang, H., Xu, D. X., Lv, J. W., Ning, H., and Wei, W. (2007). Melatonin attenuates lipopolysaccharide (LPS)-induced apoptotic liver damage in D-galactosamine-sensitized mice. *Toxicology* 237, 49–57. doi: 10.1016/j.tox.2007.04.021

Weiss, N., Miller, F., Cazaubon, S., and Couraud, P. O. (2009). The blood-brain barrier in brain homeostasis and neurological diseases. *Biochim. Biophys. Acta* 1788, 842–857. doi: 10.1016/j.bbamem.2008.10.022

Wong, C. S., Jow, G. M., Kaizaki, A., Fan, L. W., and Tien, L. T. (2014). Melatonin ameliorates brain injury induced by systemic lipopolysaccharide in neonatal rats. *Neuroscience* 267, 147–156. doi: 10.1016/j.neuroscience.2014.02.032

Zhang, H., Liu, D., Wang, X., Chen, X., Long, Y., Chai, W., et al. (2013). Melatonin improved rat cardiac mitochondria and survival rate in septic heart injury. *J. Pineal Res.* 55, 1–6. doi: 10.1111/jpi.12033

Zhao, L., An, R., Yang, Y., Yang, X., Liu, H., Yue, L., et al. (2015). Melatonin alleviates brain injury in mice subjected to cecal ligation and puncture via attenuating inflammation, apoptosis, and oxidative stress: the role of SIRT1 signaling. *J. Pineal Res.* 59, 230–239. doi: 10.1111/jpi.12254

Zhao, Z., Hu, J., Gao, X., Liang, H., and Liu, Z. (2014). Activation of AMPK attenuates lipopolysaccharide-impaired integrity and function of blood-brain barrier in human brain microvascular endothelial cells. *Exp. Mol. Pathol.* 97, 386–392. doi: 10.1016/j.yexmp.2014.09.006

Zhou, X., Cao, Y., Ao, G., Hu, L., Liu, H., Wu, J., et al. (2014). CaMKKbeta-dependent activation of AMP-activated protein kinase is critical to suppressive effects of hydrogen sulfide on neuroinflammation. *Antioxid. Redox Signal.* 21, 1741–1758. doi: 10.1089/ars.2013.5587

Zhou, T., Zhao, L., Zhan, R., He, Q., Tong, Y., Tian, X., et al. (2014). Blood-brain barrier dysfunction in mice induced by lipopolysaccharide is attenuated by dapsone. *Biochem. Biophys. Res. Commun.* 453, 419–424. doi: 10.1016/j.bbrc.2014.09.093

2

Neuroanatomical and Neuropsychological Markers of Amnestic MCI: A Three-Year Longitudinal Study in Individuals Unaware of Cognitive Decline

Katharina S. Goerlich[1†], Mikhail Votinov[1,2,3†], Ellen Dicks[1,4], Sinika Ellendt[1], Gábor Csukly[5] and Ute Habel[1,2]*

[1] Department of Psychiatry, Psychotherapy and Psychosomatics, Medical Faculty, RWTH Aachen University, Aachen, Germany, [2] Jülich Aachen Research Alliance (JARA) – Translational Brain Medicine, Aachen, Germany, [3] Institute of Neuroscience and Medicine (INM-10), Research Centre Jülich, Jülich, Germany, [4] Alzheimer Center and Department of Neurology, Neuroscience Campus Amsterdam, VU University Medical Center, Amsterdam, Netherlands, [5] Department of Psychiatry and Psychotherapy, Semmelweis University, Budapest, Hungary

***Correspondence:**
Katharina S. Goerlich
kgoerlich@ukaachen.de

† Shared first authorship

Structural brain changes underlying mild cognitive impairment (MCI) have been well-researched, but most previous studies required subjective cognitive complaints (SCC) as a diagnostic criterion, diagnosed MCI based on a single screening test or lacked analyses in relation to neuropsychological impairment. This longitudinal voxel-based morphometry study aimed to overcome these limitations: The relationship between regional gray matter (GM) atrophy and behavioral performance was investigated over the course of 3 years in individuals unaware of cognitive decline, identified as amnestic MCI based on an extensive neuropsychological test battery. Region of interest analyses revealed GM atrophy in the left amygdala, hippocampus, and parahippocampus in MCI individuals compared to normally aging participants, which was specifically related to verbal memory impairment and evident already at the first measurement point. These findings demonstrate that GM atrophy is detectable in individuals with amnestic MCI despite unawareness of beginning cognitive decline. Thus, individuals with GM atrophy in regions associated with verbal memory impairment do not necessarily need to experience SCC before meeting neuropsychological criteria for MCI. These results have important implications for future research and diagnostic procedures of MCI.

Keywords: mild cognitive impairment, voxel-based morphometry, subjective cognitive complaints, gray matter atrophy, amygdala, hippocampus, longitudinal

INTRODUCTION

Age-related neurodegenerative diseases such as Alzheimer's disease (AD) impose a high social and financial burden for society that will increase in the following decades, given predictions of a 9% increase of people above 60% in 2050 (United Nations, Department of Economic and Social Affairs, 2013). Along with population aging, the prevalence of AD (currently 4.7%) is predicted to increase by approximately 225% by 2050 (Prince et al., 2013).

Memory disturbances constitute early symptoms of AD, and with progressing impairment, other domains become affected, including language, problem-solving, and visuospatial perception (for a review, see Dubois et al., 2016). The neuropathological hallmarks of AD are brain atrophy, extracellular amyloid plaques, and neurofibrillary tangles (Kandel et al., 2013), yet its underlying cause remains unidentified (Zetterberg and Mattsson, 2014). Early diagnosis is in dire need for disease prevention and the development of new treatment strategies. Detecting AD at an early time point would enable early intervention and a timely start of treatment, possibly preventing disease progression.

A promising endeavor to provide such early diagnosis lies in the identification of the transitional state between normal aging and pathological cognitive decline. Since 1997, the term mild cognitive impairment (MCI) is used to mark the difference between continuous levels of cognitive impairment in normally aging controls compared to AD patients (Petersen et al., 1997). The concept of MCI is now widely accepted and continues to receive great attention in the literature as it represents a possible treatment target for AD. Its predictive power is reflected in annual conversion rates of up to 15% from MCI to AD (DeCarli, 2003) compared to conversion rates of 1–2% from normal aging to AD (Petersen et al., 1999).

Currently, MCI is diagnosed by: (a) abnormal cognitive function adjusted for age and education level, (b) self-reported cognitive complaints, (c) normal activities of daily living, and (d) absence of a dementia diagnosis (Winblad et al., 2004). Impairment severity is commonly assessed on the basis of general cognitive screening tests, such as the Mini-Mental State Examination (MMSE). However, such tests have been criticized for being not sufficiently specific regarding the subtle nature of MCI (Nickl-Jockschat et al., 2012; Forlenza et al., 2013). Even if specific neuropsychological tests for MCI diagnosis are used, studies often rely on only one diagnostic test (Bondi et al., 2014). Moreover, there is great variation in how the criteria for aberrant cognitive function are implemented. Thus, there is no standardized approach for diagnosing MCI, and prevalence rates are therefore highly dependent on the classification scheme used (Chapman et al., 2016; Clark et al., 2016). Furthermore, MCI was originally conceptualized as a prodromal stage for AD and thus focused on memory impairment (Petersen et al., 1999). However, MCI has been revealed to be a much broader construct affecting several cognitive domains (Winblad et al., 2004). Thus, extensive neuropsychological testing is required to identify early-stage MCI.

Critically, doubts have arisen regarding subjective cognitive complaints (SCC), which are currently implemented in the diagnosis of MCI. While these may be a marker of MCI (Clark et al., 2016), including SCC may lead to false omission of possible MCI candidates who are misdiagnosed as healthily aging individuals because they are not yet aware of beginning cognitive impairment (Edmonds et al., 2014). Such a lack of awareness has indeed been identified by several studies (e.g., Purser et al., 2006; Lenehan et al., 2012; Fragkiadaki et al., 2016; for a review, see Roberts et al., 2009), and the inclusion of SCC resulted in increased rates of false negative and false positive diagnoses (Lenehan et al., 2012). Moreover, subjective complaints are strongly related to individual differences in depression and neuroticism, casting further doubt on their reliability as a diagnostic marker of MCI (Reid and MacLullich, 2006). Taken together, the drawbacks of including SCC in the diagnosis of MCI seem to outweigh its benefits. Thus, the present study took a novel approach by investigating MCI in elderly individuals unaware of any cognitive impairment.

In addition to more thorough neuropsychological testing, the need for neuroanatomical biomarkers of MCI has been recognized (Ruan et al., 2016). For AD, the most widely studied biomarkers are: decreased cerebrospinal fluid amyloid beta (CSF Aβ), increased CSF tau, decreased fluorodeoxyglucose uptake on positron-emission tomography (FDG-PET), PET amyloid imaging, and structural MRI measures of cerebral atrophy. Importantly, strong evidence suggests that MRI, FDG-PET, and CSF tau biomarkers are already abnormal in the MCI phase of AD (Ewers et al., 2007; Sluimer et al., 2008; Shaw et al., 2009), and while both CSF tau and MRI are predictive of conversion from MCI to AD, the predictive power of structural MRI is greater. Moreover, cognitive measures correlate strongly with structural MRI, but not with CSF tau in patients with MCI (Vemuri et al., 2009). Structural MRI studies using longitudinal voxel-based morphometry (VBM) identified the medial temporal lobe (MTL) as a core region for progression of MCI to AD (Ferreira et al., 2011; Nickl-Jockschat et al., 2012; Yang et al., 2012). This is not surprising given that the MTL contains essential structures for memory consolidation (Kandel et al., 2013). The identification of progressing MCI patients can be made apparent already 4 years prior to conversion to AD on the basis of hippocampal atrophy patterns (Adaszewski et al., 2013). Comparing rates of hippocampal atrophy between healthy controls, MCI individuals and AD patients, annual atrophy rates of 1.9–2.8% were observed for the controls, 2.6–3.7% for MCI individuals, and 3.5% for AD patients (Jack et al., 2000). Moreover, meta-analyses indicate that a consistent atrophy pattern underlies MCI, comprising the amygdala, hippocampus, precuneus, and posterior cingulate gyrus (Nickl-Jockschat et al., 2012; Yang et al., 2012).

Although gray matter (GM) changes accompanying MCI have been well-researched, most of the previous studies identified MCI on the basis of general cognitive screening tests such as the MMSE, which may be insufficient to capture the subtle nature of MCI and presumably identifies MCI at a rather late stage, missing the beginning of cognitive decline. Even if the MMSE was not used for MCI diagnosis, previous VBM studies correlated GM atrophy with cognitive decline based on the MMSE and thus lack analyses in relation to specific behavioral impairment (e.g., Jack et al., 2000; Whitwell et al., 2007; Sluimer et al., 2008; Weiner et al., 2013).

The present study aimed to overcome these limitations by taking a novel, more sensitive approach: Elderly volunteers (minimum age: 50 years) from a community sample were included who had no subjective complaints, i.e., were not aware of potential cognitive impairment. MCI was then identified on the basis of a thorough neuropsychological test battery assessing memory, intelligence, executive functions, psychomotor speed, visuo-construction and visuo-spatial skills, attention, and language. To our knowledge, this is the first VBM study investigating the longitudinal trajectory of morphological changes underlying early-stage MCI in individuals still unaware of beginning cognitive impairment. We predicted more pronounced region of interest (ROI) GM atrophy in individuals classified as MCI compared to HCs even without subjective awareness of cognitive deficits, and hypothesized faster atrophy rates in the MCI compared to the HC group. Moreover, we hypothesized ROI GM atrophy to be related to specific behavioral impairment in the MCI group only.

MATERIALS AND METHODS

Participants

Participants for the Helmholtz Alliance for Mental Health in an Aging Society (HelMA) study (Drexler et al., 2013; Chechko et al., 2014; Ellendt et al., 2016) were recruited through visitations to social facilities for elderly people (charity organizations and citizen centers) and advertisements in local newspapers. From 81 volunteers initially participating in the first measurement time point (T_1), 43 participants (27 women, aged 50–83 years) eventually completed all three measurement time points (T_1, T_2, and T_3) with a mean follow-up interval of 1.12 years, *SD* 0.38 years. Reasons for dropping out varied from refusing to further participate for time reasons or a lack of interest (13 participants), moving to another city (four participants), newly acquired MR contraindications following surgery during the course of the study (six participants), to illness (11 participants) and death (four participants).

Participants were included if they were 50 years or older, had sufficient German language and adequate visual performance abilities. Exclusion criteria comprised a diagnosis of dementia, neurological or psychiatric disorders according to DSM-IV axis I as assessed by the German version of Structured Clinical Interview (SKID; Wittchen et al., 1997), physical disease that could interfere with cognitive performance, lifetime or current drug addiction, seriously reduced vision, inability to follow the protocol, and medication use with possible cognitive side effects. The study was approved by the ethics committee of the medical faculty, RWTH Aachen University. All participants gave written informed consent and were paid for participation.

Neuropsychological Data Analysis

In addition to several dementia screening tests applied with the objective of eliminating dementia rather than diagnosing MCI, all participants underwent an extensive neuropsychological test battery evaluating memory, intelligence, executive functions, psychomotor speed, visuo-construction and visuo-spatial skills, attention, and language at each time point. **Table 1** provides an overview of all neuropsychological tests used for MCI assessment and diagnosis (for further details, see Drexler et al., 2013; Ellendt et al., 2016). The testing procedure was accomplished by trained psychologists. To counteract learning effects, tests were presented in counterbalanced order. Sessions took place in the mornings and lasted approximately 3 h. Short breaks were offered and if necessary, a second appointment was arranged.

TABLE 1 | Neuropsychological test battery used for the assessment and diagnosis of mild cognitive impairment (MCI).

Domain	Test
Memory	Benton Visual Retention Test (BRVT) Wechsler Memory Scale – digit span (WMS-R) California Verbal Learning Test, German version (VLMT)
Intelligence	Premorbid intelligence; Multiple-choice word test, German version (MWT-B)
Executive functions	Cognitive flexibility, divided attention, psychomotor speed: Trail-Making-Test A and B (TMT A/B) Planning and problem-solving: Tower of London (TL-D) Lexical and semantic fluency: Regensburger Wortflüssigkeitstest (RWT)
Dementia screening	Mini-Mental-State-Examination, German version (MMSE) Syndrom Kurz Test (SKT) Test zur Früherkennung von Demenzen (TFDD) Consortium to Establish a Registry for Alzheimer's Disease (CERAD-PLUS) including language, object naming abilities (Boston Naming Test), verbal learning, visuospatial functions, delayed recall, memory consolidation, recognition, executive functions

The classification criteria for MCI were based on those described by Winblad et al. (2004). That is, (1) greater memory impairment than expected for age, (2) preserved activities of the daily living, and (3) absence of dementia. The criterion of memory impairment greater than expected for age was identified by an impaired score of at least 1.5 standard deviations (SD) below the mean according to normative datasets in at least one test assessing memory functioning (i.e., VLMT, Benton, WMS, memory assessing subtests of the CERAD-Plus battery). If the neuropsychological test comprised multiple subtests (as in VLMT and CERAD), at least two subtests had to indicate impairment, i.e., 1.5 *SD* below normative data, which is considered a conservative method for identifying MCI (Jak et al., 2009). The decision to classify subjects solely on their performance in tests regarding memory functioning can be accounted on the fact that amnestic MCI patients show a higher prevalence to develop AD compared to non-amnestic MCI patients, who have an increased risk of developing other types of dementia (Petersen and Morris, 2005). Note that impairment in cognitive domains other than memory was not observed in this sample. Thus, all MCI participants identified here can be classified as belonging to the single-domain amnestic MCI subtype. Correspondingly, the present results are of relevance specifically to amnestic MCI.

The original classification criteria proposed by Winblad et al. (2004) also include SCC but because the requirement of SCCs could lead to omitting subjects which would otherwise be classified as MCI (Edmonds et al., 2014), this criterion was not applied. In fact, all participants reported not to have experienced any difficulties regarding memory or any other cognitive domain beyond expected for their respective age. Thus, none of the participants were aware of any cognitive impairment.

The neuropsychological data were analyzed in SPSS 20 by means of multivariate analyses of covariance (MANCOVA) comparing performance between the MCI group and the HC group at each time point, corrected for age, gender, and education. The initial significance threshold was $p < 0.05$, and all results were Bonferroni corrected for multiple comparisons.

VBM Data Analysis

T1 anatomical images (TE: 3.03; TR: 2300 ms; FOV = 256 mm × 256 mm; number of sagittal slices = 176; voxel size: 1 mm × 1 mm × 1 mm) from the 43 study participants were acquired on a 3 Tesla Siemens® Trio MR scanner. Differences in GM volume between the MCI and HC group were assessed using longitudinal VBM (Ashburner and Friston, 2000; Ashburner and Ridgway, 2013) implemented in SPM12 (Wellcome Trust Centre for Neuroimaging, University College London, London, UK). The following preprocessing steps were applied: First, serial longitudinal registration, which produces one midpoint file and Jacobian determinants for each subject at each of the three time points. Next, each subject's midpoint average was segmented into GM, white matter (WM), and CSF. Then, GM images were computed for each subject at each time point using the respective Jacobian determinants. These images were spatially normalized by creating a customized group-specific template using the DARTEL approach and warping each of the individual GM segmentations onto this template. The warped GM segmentations were modulated to reflect the volume and smoothed using a Gaussian kernel of 8 mm at full width at half-maximum (FWHM). Data quality was ensured by visually checking each T1 image for abnormalities before preprocessing, checking volume orientation before smoothing during preprocessing, and by means of a sample homogeneity check after preprocessing, revealing no outliers.

Region of interest analyses were performed on GM volumes of eight anatomically defined *a priori* ROIs based on MCI meta-analyses (Nickl-Jockschat et al., 2012; Weiner et al., 2013): Left and right amygdala, hippocampus, parahippocampus, and precuneus. Anatomical ROIs for these regions were created using the automatic anatomic labeling (AAL) atlas templates (Tzourio-Mazoyer et al., 2002) provided by the WFU Pickatlas toolbox (Wake Forest School of Medicine, Winston Salem, NC, USA). Mean parameter estimates from these ROIs were extracted using MarsBaR[1] and analyzed by means of a Linear Mixed Model (LMM) Analysis in SAS 9.2. The factor group (MCI versus HC) was included in the LMM as a between-subjects fixed effect, and the model controlled for age, gender, education, and mean total intracranial volume (TIV, i.e., GM + WM + CSF). An unstructured covariance matrix was used, which was estimated by means of the null model estimation method.

Relationships between mean neuropsychological performance and mean GM volumes of the eight ROIs across the whole sample and within the HC and the MCI group were examined by means of partial correlations controlling for age, gender, education, and TIV. To this end, the residuals of each neuropsychological test as well as the residuals of the GM volumes of each ROI at each measurement point were calculated, controlling for age, gender, education, and TIV, and partial correlations were then performed between the neuropsychological test residuals and the ROI GM volume residuals. The Holm–Bonferroni correction was applied to control for multiple comparisons, resulting in an initial significance threshold of $p < 0.006$ ($p = 0.05/n = 8$ ROIs). Moreover, whole-brain analyses comparing GM volumes between the MCI and HC group at each time point were conducted at an uncorrected threshold $p < 0.001$.

RESULTS

Neuropsychological Performance

Based on the neuropsychological test battery, 16 participants were classified as MCI (6 male, mean age 66.13, *SD* 8.46 years, mean years of education 9.43, *SD* 1.59), and 27 participants were classified as HC (10 male, mean age 66.15, *SD* 6.15 years, mean years of education 10.5, *SD* 1.88). Groups did not differ in age ($p > 0.05$), but the HC group had more years of education ($p < 0.05$). The results on the neuropsychological tests for the HC and the MCI group are presented in **Table 2**, revealing significantly worse performance of the MCI group compared to the HC group on the total immediate recall and delayed recall subtests of the VLMT and the CERAD. At a lower significance threshold ($p < 0.05$ uncorrected), worse performance was additionally observed in the Benton test (correct drawings and number of mistakes) and the WMS-R subtests digit span forward and backward. The MMSE could not distinguish between the MCI and the HC group, as opposed to the TFDD, which indicated lower performance in MCI compared to HC participants (see **Table 2**). Note that none of the study participants converted to dementia during the course of the investigation.

ROI GM Volumes

The LMM analyses on each ROI demonstrated a linear decrease in all ROI GM volumes in both groups over the course of the 3 years of observation. A group analysis between the MCI and HC group revealed significantly lower GM volume in the left amygdala, left hippocampus, and left parahippocampus in MCI participants compared to HCs at all three time points (see **Table 3**). Thus, MCI participants had significantly lower GM volume than controls in these areas already at the first time point, which then continued to decrease over the course of the following 2 years (effect of time in these ROIs: $p < 0.001$; see **Figure 1A**). However, there was no significant interaction between group and time point ($p > 0.05$), suggesting that atrophy rates were comparable between groups. Whole-brain analyses additionally indicated smaller left amygdala and left hippocampal volumes in the MCI compared to the HC group at each time point (see **Figure 1B**). No further activation outside of the ROIs was observed at $p < 0.001$. For visualization, **Figure 2** shows the decrease of ROI GM volumes across the age range of 50–83 years at T_1 in MCI and HC participants.

Associations between ROI GM Volumes and Neuropsychological Performance

Relating mean neuropsychological performance with mean ROI GM volumes across all 3 years within the whole sample showed

[1] http://marsbar.sourceforge.net/

TABLE 2 | Neuropsychological test results for the MCI group compared to the HC group.

	MCI			HC			MCI vs. HC
		T_{1-3}Mean ± SEM			T_{1-3} Mean ± SEM		T_{1-3}Mean
	T_1	T_2	T_3	T_1	T_2	T_3	*p*-value
VLMT							
Total immediate recall		45.56 ± 7.05			54.85 ± 5.75		0.0002**
	43.69	45.75	47.25	52.89	54.30	57.37	
Delayed recall		8.83 ± 2.06			11.82 ± 1.99		0.0001**
	8.56	8.63	9.31	11.15	11.67	12.63	
Lost words		2.98 ± 1.79			1.59 ± 1.33		0.09
	2.75	3.06	3.13	1.85	1.63	1.30	
Correct recognition		13.31 ± 0.92			14.37 ± 0.7		0.01*
	13.5	12.81	13.63	14.11	14.48	14.52	
Recognition residuals		10.63 ± 2.15			12.96 ± 1.63		0.01*
	11.5	9.5	10.88	12.85	12.70	13.33	
WMS-R							
Digit span forward		6.94 ± 1.64			7.89 ± 1.17		0.051
	6.94	7.38	6.5	8.26	7.63	7.78	
Digit span backward		5.69 ± 1.39			6.72 ± 1.13		0.09
	5.63	5.88	5.56	6.67	6.48	7.00	
Benton							
Correct drawings		6.02 ± 1.59			7.21 ± 1.21		0.049*
	5.19	6.31	6.56	6.52	7.56	7.56	
Number of mistakes		6.27 ± 2.97			3.76 ± 1.96		0.15
	7.25	6.19	5.38	4.78	3.30	3.22	
CERAD							
Total immediate recall		20.23 ± 3.13			23.41 ± 2.14		0.001**
	19.94	19.06	21.69	23.19	22.96	24.07	
Delayed recall		6.48 ± 1.36			8.41 ± 1.08		0.00003**
	6.31	5.81	7.31	8.41	8.04	8.78	
Percent recognition		96.88 ± 3.49			99.38 ± 1.24		0.007*
	97.19	96.88	96.56	98.89	99.63	99.63	
Intrusions		0.46 ± 0.64			0.31 ± 0.43		0.75
	0.56	0.25	0.56	0.41	0.19	0.37	
Recall drawings		8.73 ± 1.89			10.59 ± 1.69		0.05
	7.88	8.25	10.06	9.85	10.48	11.44	
General screening tests							
MMSE		28.91 ± 0.65			29.27 ± 0.59		0.32
	28.81	28.88	29.06	29.22	29.33	29.26	
SKT		2.17 ± 2.11			1.09 ± 1.19		0.074
	2.0	2.06	2.44	1.33	0.74	1.22	
TFDD		42.63 ± 2.12			45.84 ± 1.76		0.0001**
	42.44	42.44	43.00	45.48	45.22	46.82	

***p < 0.006 Bonferroni-corrected, *p < 0.05 uncorrected.*

that the association between CERAD total immediate recall performance and larger GM volume in the left amygdala (partial $r = 0.49$, $p < 0.002$), left hippocampus (partial $r = 0.51$, $p < 0.001$), and left parahippocampus (partial $r = 0.52$, $p < 0.001$) remained, indicating a robust relationship between CERAD total immediate recall performance and GM volume in these regions. In addition, WMS-R digit span forward performance was linked to larger left parahippocampal volume (partial $r = 0.44$, $p < 0.006$).

Partial correlations between neuropsychological performance and ROI GM volumes within each group revealed that the abovementioned associations were solely driven by the MCI group as there were no significant correlations between neuropsychological performance and ROI GM volume in the HC group (all $p > 0.05$). In the MCI group, CERAD total immediate recall performance was highly correlated with GM volume in the left amygdala (partial $r = 0.83$, $p < 0.001$), left hippocampus (partial $r = 0.72$, $p < 0.006$), and left parahippocampus (partial

TABLE 3 | Results of the linear mixed model (LMM) analysis comparing mean region of interest (ROI) volumes between the MCI and HC group.

ROI		MCI			HC			MCI vs. HC
		T_{1-3} Mean ± SEM			T_{1-3} Mean ± SEM			T_{1-3} Mean
		T_1	T_2	T_3	T_1	T_2	T_3	*p*-value
Amygdala	Left		0.557 ± 0.01			0.597 ± 0.01		0.006**
		0.559	0.557	0.553	0.600	0.597	0.594	
	Right		0.575 ± 0.01			0.595 ± 0.01		0.454
		0.578	0.575	0.572	0.598	0.595	0.592	
Hippocampus	Left		0.357 ± 0.01			0.379 ± 0.01		0.012*
		0.357	0.356	0.355	0.380	0.380	0.379	
	Right		0.345 ± 0.01			0.359 ± 0.01		0.217
		0.346	0.345	0.344	0.359	0.359	0.358	
Parahippocampus	Left		0.471 ± 0.01			0.493 ± 0.01		0.048*
		0.473	0.472	0.369	0.495	0.493	0.491	
	Right		0.546 ± 0.01			0.566 ± 0.01		0.342
		0.548	0.546	0.543	0.568	0.566	0.564	
Precuneus	Left		0.303 ± 0.01			0.307 ± 0.01		0.982
		0.304	0.303	0.302	0.307	0.306	0.305	
	Right		0.324 ± 0.01			0.328 ± 0.01		0.859
		0.325	0.325	0.323	0.329	0.328	0.327	

***p < 0.006 Bonferroni-corrected, *p < 0.05 uncorrected.*

$r = 0.80$, $p < 0.002$), implying a robust relationship between verbal memory impairment and GM volume reduction in these regions. MMSE scores showed no correlation with ROI GM volumes (all $p > 0.05$). **Figure 3** visualizes the relationship between mean CERAD total immediate recall performance and mean GM volumes of the left amygdala, hippocampus, and parahippocampus in the MCI and HC group across the three time points.

To find out to what extent GM atrophy in these ROIs significantly predicted verbal memory impairment in MCI participants already at the first measurement point, a stepwise linear regression was performed with the residuals (i.e., controlling for age, gender, education, and TIV) of CERAD total immediate recall performance at T_1 as dependent variable and the residuals of GM volumes of the left amygdala, hippocampus, and parahippocampus at T_1 as predictors. From this analysis, a significant model emerged [$F(1,24) = 5.79$, $p < 0.05$, $R^2 = 0.29$], revealing that GM atrophy specifically in the left parahippocampus accounted for 29% of the variance in CERAD total immediate recall performance ($\beta = 0.54, p < 0.05$). Thus, left parahippocampal atrophy significantly predicted verbal memory impairment in the MCI group already at the first measurement point.

DISCUSSION

The aim of this longitudinal imaging study was to identify the relationship between neuropsychological and neuroanatomical changes associated with early stages of MCI identified by means of a thorough neuropsychological test battery in individuals unaware of cognitive impairment. Although several previous studies investigated the longitudinal trajectory of neuroanatomical alterations underlying MCI, these studies diagnosed MCI on the basis of a single general screening tests, lacked an analysis of these changes in relation to neuropsychological performance (e.g., Besson et al., 2015; Callahan et al., 2015; Dugger et al., 2015; Fellhauer et al., 2015; Granziera et al., 2015), or included subjective complaints as a diagnostic criterion. The present study aimed to overcome these limitations. Individuals classified as MCI who were unaware of beginning cognitive impairment exhibited verbal memory deficits (indicative of amnestic MCI) and GM atrophy in the left amygdala, hippocampus, and parahippocampus, compared to controls. Atrophy rates were comparable between groups, in contrast to our hypothesis of faster atrophy rates in MCI individuals than in controls. In line with our prediction of a specific relationship between GM atrophy and behavioral impairment in MCI individuals only, GM atrophy in the MCI group, but not the control group, was highly correlated with impaired verbal memory (CERAD total immediate recall). Moreover, GM atrophy in the left parahippocampus significantly predicted verbal memory impairment in MCI individuals already at T_1, even without subjective awareness of cognitive impairment. This confirms our prediction of GM atrophy being evident in MCI individuals before they become aware of cognitive decline.

Lower GM volumes in the left amygdala, hippocampus, and parahippocampus are in accordance with previous studies reporting GM atrophy in the left MTL in MCI patients compared to controls (Ferreira et al., 2011; Nickl-Jockschat et al., 2012; Weiner et al., 2013; Csukly et al., 2016). Here, GM volume reduction in these regions was significantly linked to impaired total immediate recall performance (CERAD) in the MCI group, suggesting that GM atrophy in the MTL is specifically associated

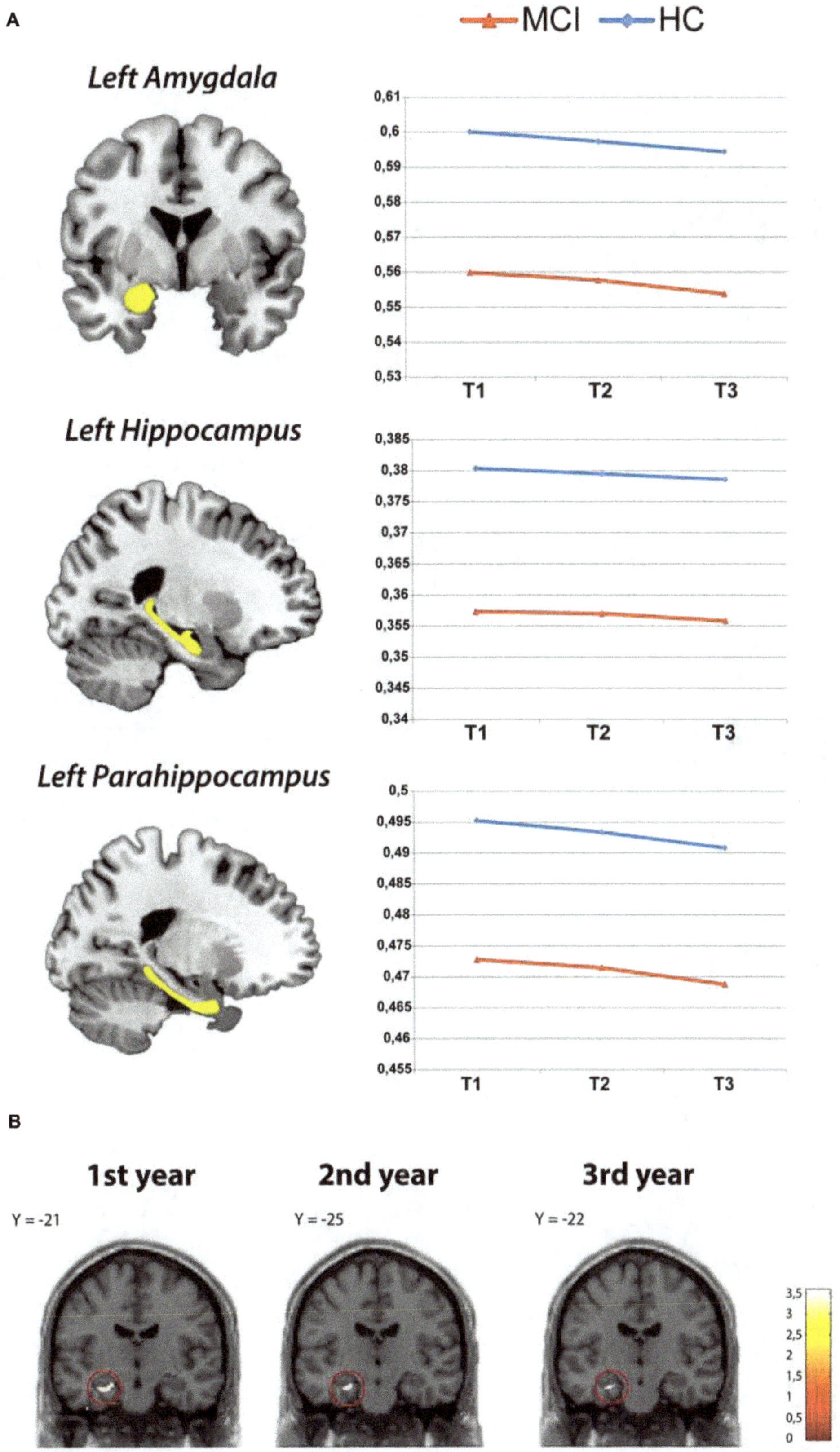

FIGURE 1 | (A) Decline of region of interest (ROI) gray matter (GM) volume in the HC and mild cognitive impairment (MCI) group. **(B)** Whole-brain analysis: GM volume reduction in the amygdala and hippocampus (MCI > HC).

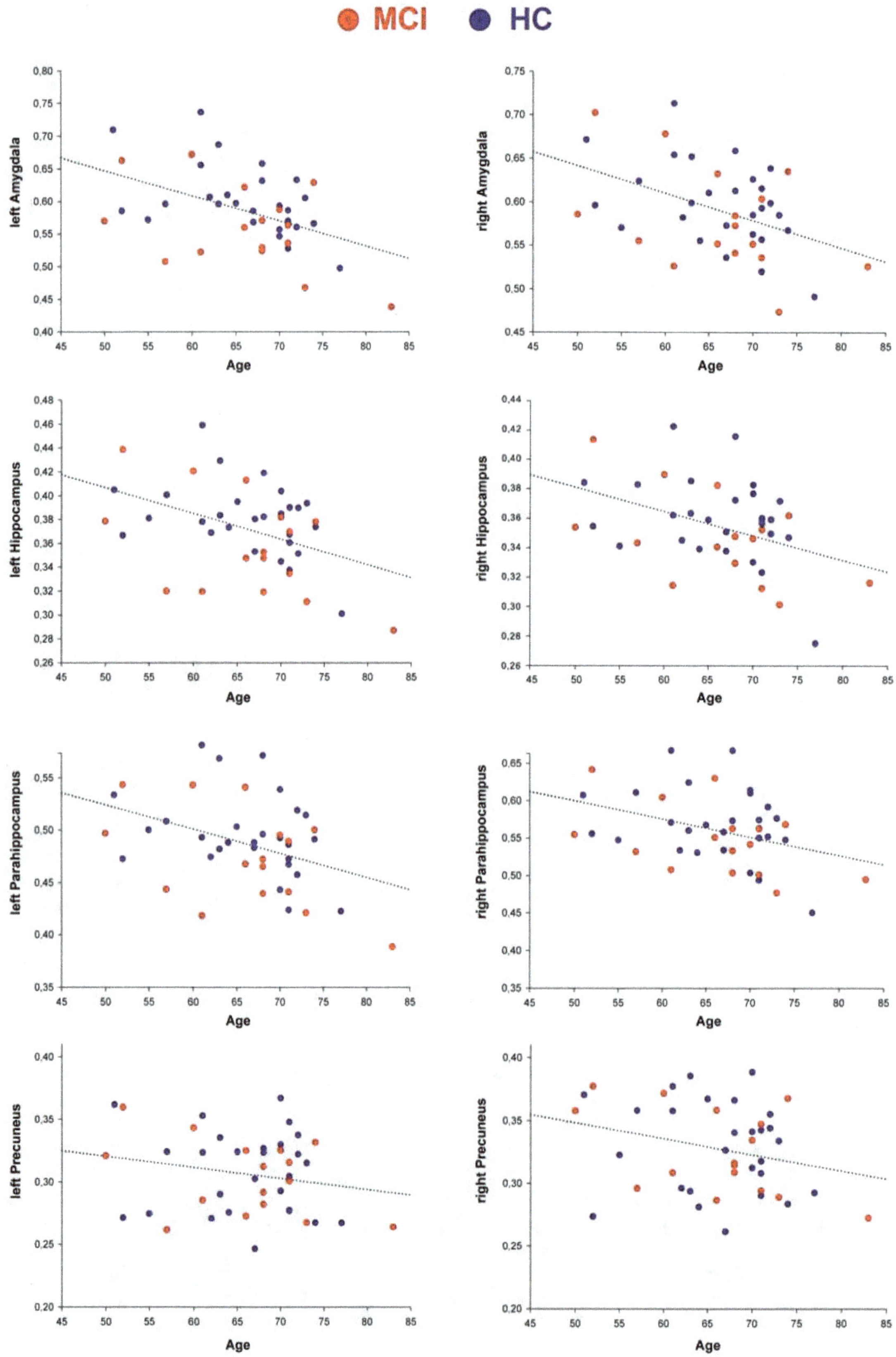

FIGURE 2 | Region of interest GM volume decrease across age in MCI and HC participants at T_1.

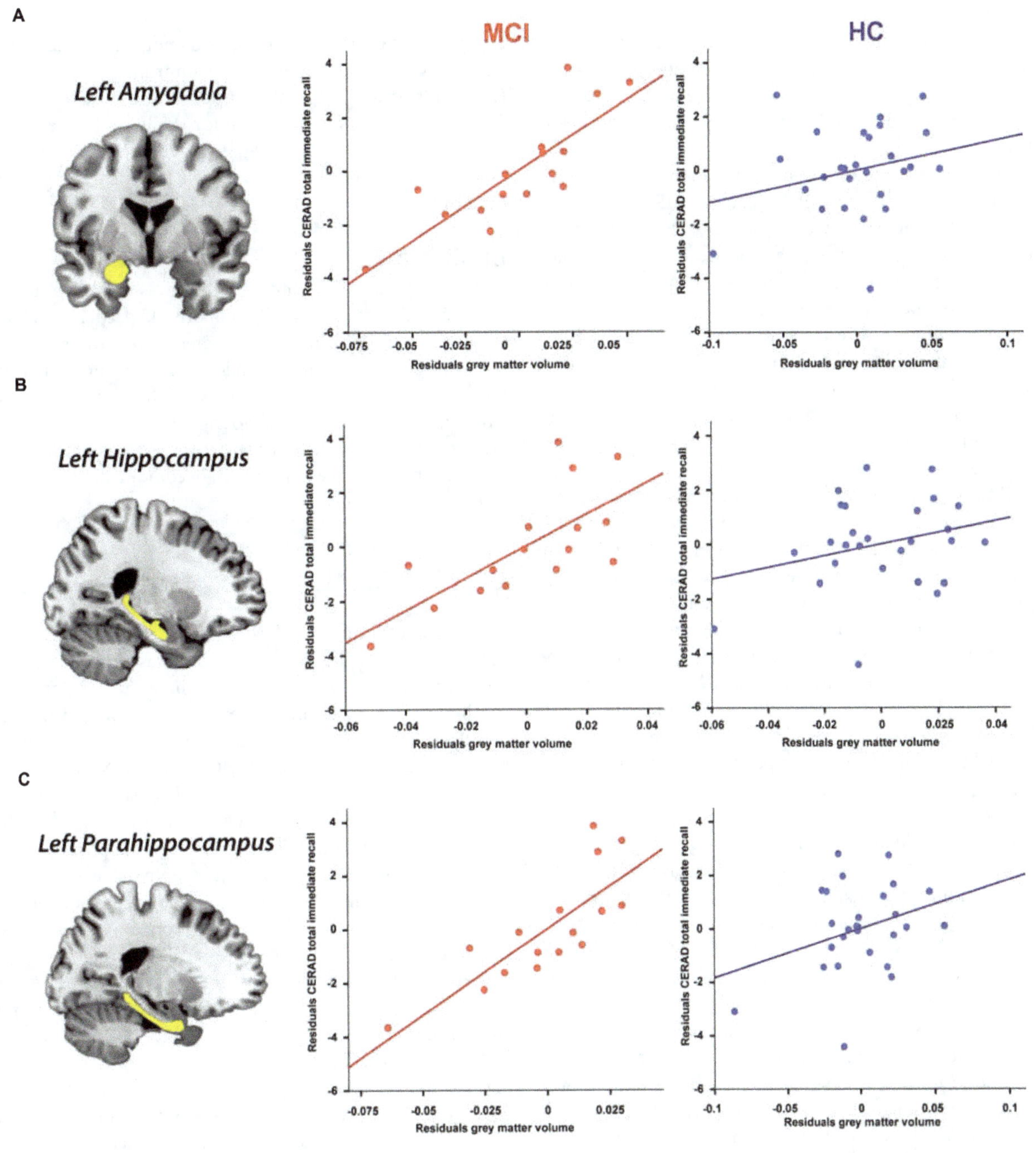

FIGURE 3 | Partial correlations controlling for age, gender, education, and TIV between CERAD total immediate recall performance and ROI GM volume in the MCI and HC group across 3 years (Holm–Bonferroni corrected $p < 0.006$). (A) Left amygdala, **(B)** Left hippocampus, **(C)** Left parahippocampus.

with verbal memory impairment. This finding complements previous observations that cerebral atrophy correlates with measures of general cognition in MCI (Jack et al., 2010). Atrophy rates did not significantly differ between MCI participants and controls, although this might be expected with progressing MCI (e.g., Trivedi et al., 2006; for a review, see Chetelat and Baron, 2003). However, this absence of differences in atrophy rates may be explained by the restricted time frame of the present study, comprising 3 years, which was probably not long enough to capture significant differences in atrophy rates. Moreover, none of the study participants converted to dementia during the course of the investigation, indicating that indeed early-stage MCI was captured here, thus further explaining the absence of group differences in GM atrophy rates. This could also explain why no GM atrophy in the precuneus was identified here, suggesting that atrophy in this region may occur at later stages of MCI. Note that MCI participants exhibited lower GM volumes compared to controls already at the first time point. This suggests that GM atrophy in the MCI group had already begun prior to enrolment in the study, warranting the inclusion of younger participants (<50 years) in future studies to be able to identify the point of divergence in medial temporal GM atrophy between MCI and normal aging.

According to the model of dynamic biomarkers of AD proposed by Jack et al. (2010), structural MRI is the last biomarker in the staging of the disease to become abnormal, preceded by Aβ-plaque biomarkers that are dynamic in early stages before the appearance of clinical symptoms, and by biomarkers of neurodegeneration that occur at later stages and correlate with symptom severity. MRI, FDG-PET, and CSF tau biomarkers are already abnormal in the MCI phase preceding AD. Findings of specific relationships between GM atrophy and neuropsychological impairment as observed in this study may be used in the future to increase prediction accuracy for conversion from MCI to AD.

The MMSE, a general cognitive screening test that has been commonly used to assess MCI in previous research did not show any correlations with GM volumes in the present MCI group and could not distinguish between the MCI and HC group: Both groups had an average score of 29 on the MMSE and MMSE scores remained intact over the course of the 3 years, with none of the participants having less than 27 points on the MMSE at any time point. Thus, the present MCI sample would not have been identified as such based on the results of this general screening test, despite evident cognitive impairment as demonstrated by significantly worse performance on the VLMT and CERAD (and tendencies toward impairment in the Benton and WMS-R). This is in line with previous findings showing that despite good sensitivity and specificity for diagnosing dementia, the commonly used cutoff scores of the MMSE do not show good accuracy for discrimination of MCI, misidentifying most of these subjects as having normal cognitive function (Kaufer et al., 2008). Since the MMSE is widely used in the MCI literature – and considering that individuals are classified as MCI with scores ranging from 23.1 to 28.7 (Nickl-Jockschat et al., 2012) – this not only entails the risk to include already more severely impaired individuals in MCI studies, but also causes problems for the comparison and evaluation of the results due to high variability in MCI diagnosis. Future studies should thus avoid relying on the MMSE alone and instead use a broader, more sensitive neuropsychological test battery to diagnose MCI and assess its severity. According to the present results, the total immediate and delayed recall scales of the VLMT and the CERAD seem especially sensitive to identifying early stage MCI in the absence of subjective awareness of cognitive decline. In contrast to the MMSE, the TFDD, a screening test aiming to detect early signs of dementia while differentiating cognitive problems due to depression, could distinguish between the MCI and the HC group in this study, although no between group differences on depression were detected. Thus, it may be worthwhile using the TFDD as an additional screening tool in future studies.

Importantly, SCCs are currently a diagnostic criterion for MCI. None of the individuals classified as MCI in this study were aware of any cognitive impairment (i.e., had no subjective complaints). Yet, the MCI group showed significantly worse performance on more than one test of the neuropsychological test battery. Confirming previous findings (Edmonds et al., 2014), this supports the idea to not include SCC as a diagnostic criterion for MCI in future studies in order to identify GM atrophy underlying early-stage MCI even without subjective awareness of beginning cognitive impairment.

Limitations

The sample size of the present study was small due to a drop-out rate of almost 50%, resulting in only 43 participants (16 MCI) who completed all three measurement time points. High drop-out rates are an inherent risk in longitudinal studies, particularly those including elderly individuals. Future studies should thus aim to include more as well as younger (<50 years) participants in order to pinpoint at what age structural brain changes in relation to beginning cognitive impairment become evident and divergent from normal aging.

CONCLUSION

The present findings indicate that GM atrophy in the left MTL underlying MCI is specifically associated with verbal memory impairment. This underlines the importance of combining neuroanatomical markers of MCI with specific neuropsychological tests as it implies that age-related GM atrophy is only predictive of MCI if accompanied by specific cognitive deficits. Moreover, our findings show that reductions in GM volume are evident even if individuals are not yet aware of cognitive impairment, demonstrating that individuals with neuroanatomical evidence of atrophy in regions associated with verbal memory impairments do not necessarily need to experience subjective cognitive concerns before meeting neuropsychological criteria for MCI. Further, general cognitive screening test such as the MMSE may not be sensitive enough to identify early-stage MCI. These findings have important clinical implications as they highlight the need to discard SCCs from MCI diagnosis. Moreover, it would be useful to apply comprehensive neuropsychological batteries, possibly by means of computerized cognitive assessments rather than relying on a single cognitive screening test to identify MCI. Lastly, establishing regular neuropsychological testing for MCI already in individuals below the age of 50 years will help identify MCI at early stages, enabling early intervention and a timely start of treatment.

AUTHOR CONTRIBUTIONS

Conception: UH. Organization: UH, KG, and MV. Execution: KG, MV, ED, and SE. Statistical Analysis: KG, MV, and GC. Manuscript: Writing of the first draft: KG and MV. Review and Critique: KG, MV, ED, SE, GC, and UH. All authors approved the final version of the manuscript.

ACKNOWLEDGMENT

This work was supported by the Helmholtz Alliance "Mental Health in an Ageing Society," funded by the Initiative and Networking Fund of the Helmholtz Association, and by the Brain Imaging Facility, a core facility of the Interdisciplinary Center for Clinical Research (IZKF) Aachen within the Faculty of Medicine at RWTH Aachen University.

REFERENCES

Adaszewski, S., Dukart, J., Kherif, F., Frackowiak, R., and Draganski, B. (2013). How early can we predict Alzheimer's disease using computational anatomy? *Neurobiol. Aging* 34, 2815–2826. doi: 10.1016/j.neurobiolaging.2013.06.015

Ashburner, J., and Friston, K. J. (2000). Voxel-based morphometry—the methods. *Neuroimage* 11, 805–821. doi: 10.1006/nimg.2000.0582

Ashburner, J., and Ridgway, G. R. (2013). Symmetric diffeomorphic modeling of longitudinal structural MRI. *Front. Neurosci.* 6:197. doi: 10.3389/fnins.2012.00197

Besson, G., Ceccaldi, M., Tramoni, E., Felician, O., Didic, M., and Barbeau, E. J. (2015). Fast, but not slow, familiarity is preserved in patients with amnestic mild cognitive impairment. *Cortex* 65, 36–49. doi: 10.1016/j.cortex.2014.10.020

Bondi, M. W., Edmonds, E. C., Jak, A. J., Clark, L. R., Delano-Wood, L., Mcdonald, C. R., et al. (2014). Neuropsychological criteria for mild cognitive impairment improves diagnostic precision, biomarker associations, and progression rates. *J. Alzheimers Dis.* 42, 275–289. doi: 10.3233/JAD-140276

Callahan, B. L., Ramirez, J., Berezuk, C., Duchesne, S., Black, S. E., and Initiative, A. S. D. N. (2015). Predicting Alzheimer's disease development: a comparison of cognitive criteria and associated neuroimaging biomarkers. *Alzheimers Res. Ther.* 7, 1–10. doi: 10.1186/s13195-015-0152-z

Chapman, K. R., Bing-Canar, H., Alosco, M. L., Steinberg, E. G., Martin, B., Chaisson, C., et al. (2016). Mini mental state examination and logical memory scores for entry into Alzheimer's disease trials. *Alzheimers Res. Ther.* 8, 9. doi: 10.1186/s13195-016-0176-z

Chechko, N., Drexler, E., Voss, B., Kellermann, T., Finkelmeyer, A., Schneider, F., et al. (2014). Neural correlates of unsuccessful memory performance in MCI. *Front. Aging Neurosci.* 6:201. doi: 10.3389/fnagi.2014.00201

Chetelat, G., and Baron, J.-C. (2003). Early diagnosis of Alzheimer's disease: contribution of structural neuroimaging. *Neuroimage* 18, 525–541. doi: 10.1016/S1053-8119(02)00026-5

Clark, L. R., Koscik, R. L., Nicholas, C. R., Okonkwo, O. C., Engelman, C. D., Bratzke, L. C., et al. (2016). Mild cognitive impairment in late middle age in the wisconsin registry for Alzheimer's prevention study: prevalence and characteristics using robust and standard neuropsychological normative data. *Arch. Clin. Neuropsychol.* doi: 10.1093/arclin/acw024 [Epub ahead of print].

Csukly, G., Sirály, E., Fodor, Z., Horváth, A., Salacz, P., Hidasi, Z., et al. (2016). The differentiation of amnestic type MCI from the non-amnestic types by structural MRI. *Front. Aging Neurosci.* 8:52. doi: 10.3389/fnagi.2016.00052

DeCarli, C. (2003). Mild cognitive impairment: prevalence, prognosis, aetiology, and treatment. *Lancet Neurol.* 2, 15–21. doi: 10.1016/S1474-4422(03)00262-X

Drexler, E., Voss, B., Amunts, K., Schneider, F., and Habel, U. (2013). Mild cognitive impairment: advantages of a comprehensive neuropsychological assessment. *Curr. Alzheimer Res.* 10, 1098–1106. doi: 10.2174/15672050113109990014

Dubois, B., Hampel, H., Feldman, H. H., Scheltens, P., Aisen, P., Andrieu, S., et al. (2016). Preclinical Alzheimer's disease: definition, natural history, and diagnostic criteria. *Alzheimers Dement.* 12, 292–323. doi: 10.1016/j.jalz.2016.02.002

Dugger, B. N., Davis, K., Malek-Ahmadi, M., Hentz, J. G., Sandhu, S., Beach, T. G., et al. (2015). Neuropathological comparisons of amnestic and nonamnestic mild cognitive impairment. *BMC Neurol.* 15, 146. doi: 10.1186/s12883-015-0403-4

Edmonds, E. C., Delano-Wood, L., Galasko, D. R., Salmon, D. P., and Bondi, M. W. (2014). Subjective cognitive complaints contribute to misdiagnosis of mild cognitive impairment. *J. Int. Neuropsychol. Soc.* 20, 836–847. doi: 10.1017/S135561771400068X

Ellendt, S., Voß, B., Kohn, N., Wagels, L., Goerlich, K., Drexler, E., et al. (2016). Predicting stability of mild cognitive impairment (MCI): findings of a community based sample. *Curr. Alzheimer Res.* doi: 10.2174/1567205014666161213120807 [Epub ahead of print].

Ewers, M., Buerger, K., Teipel, S. J., Scheltens, P., Schröder, J., Zinkowski, R. P., et al. (2007). Multicenter assessment of CSF-phosphorylated tau for the prediction of conversion of MCI. *Neurology* 69, 2205–2212. doi: 10.1212/01.wnl.0000286944.22262.ff

Fellhauer, I., Zöllner, F. G., Schröder, J., Degen, C., Kong, L., Essig, M., et al. (2015). Comparison of automated brain segmentation using a brain phantom and patients with early Alzheimer's dementia or mild cognitive impairment. *Psychiatry Res.* 233, 299–305. doi: 10.1016/j.pscychresns.2015.07.011

Ferreira, L. K., Diniz, B. S., Forlenza, O. V., Busatto, G. F., and Zanetti, M. V. (2011). Neurostructural predictors of Alzheimer's disease: a meta-analysis of VBM studies. *Neurobiol. Aging* 32, 1733–1741. doi: 10.1016/j.neurobiolaging.2009.11.008

Forlenza, O. V., Diniz, B. S., Stella, F., Teixeira, A. L., and Gattaz, W. F. (2013). Mild cognitive impairment (part 1): clinical characteristics and predictors of dementia. *Rev. Bras. Psiquiatr.* 35, 178–185. doi: 10.1590/1516-4446-2012-3503

Fragkiadaki, S., Kontaxopoulou, D., Beratis, I. N., Andronas, N., Economou, A., Yannis, G., et al. (2016). Self-awareness of cognitive efficiency: differences between healthy elderly and patients with mild cognitive impairment (MCI). *J. Clin. Exp. Neuropsychol.* 38, 1144–1157. doi: 10.1080/13803395.2016.1198469

Granziera, C., Daducci, A., Donati, A., Bonnier, G., Romascano, D., Roche, A., et al. (2015). A multi-contrast MRI study of microstructural brain damage in patients with mild cognitive impairment. *Neuroimage* 8, 631–639. doi: 10.1016/j.nicl.2015.06.003

Jack, C., Petersen, R., Xu, Y., O'brien, P., Smith, G., Ivnik, R., et al. (2000). Rates of hippocampal atrophy correlate with change in clinical status in aging and AD. *Neurology* 55, 484–490. doi: 10.1212/WNL.55.4.484

Jack, C. R. Jr., Knopman, D. S., Jagust, W. J., Shaw, L. M., Aisen, P. S., Weiner, M. W., et al. (2010). Hypothetical model of dynamic biomarkers of the Alzheimer's pathological cascade. *Lancet Neurol.* 9, 119–128. doi: 10.1016/S1474-4422(09)70299-6

Jak, A. J., Bondi, M. W., Delano-Wood, L., Wierenga, C., Corey-Bloom, J., Salmon, D. P., et al. (2009). Quantification of five neuropsychological approaches to defining mild cognitive impairment. *Am. J. Geriatr. Psychiatry* 17, 368–375. doi: 10.1097/JGP.0b013e31819431d5

Kandel, E. R., Schwartz, J. H., and Jessell, T. M. (2013). *Principles of Neural Science.* New York, NY: McGraw-hill.

Kaufer, D. I., Williams, C. S., Braaten, A. J., Gill, K., Zimmerman, S., and Sloane, P. D. (2008). Cognitive screening for dementia and mild cognitive impairment in assisted living: comparison of 3 tests. *J. Am. Med. Dir. Assoc.* 9, 586–593. doi: 10.1016/j.jamda.2008.05.006

Lenehan, M. E., Klekociuk, S. Z., and Summers, M. J. (2012). Absence of a relationship between subjective memory complaint and objective memory impairment in mild cognitive impairment (MCI): Is it time to abandon subjective memory complaint as an MCI diagnostic criterion? *Int. Psychogeriatr.* 24, 1505–1514. doi: 10.1017/S1041610212000695

Nickl-Jockschat, T., Kleiman, A., Schulz, J. B., Schneider, F., Laird, A. R., Fox, P. T., et al. (2012). Neuroanatomic changes and their association with cognitive decline in mild cognitive impairment: a meta-analysis. *Brain Struct. Funct.* 217, 115–125. doi: 10.1007/s00429-011-0333-x

Petersen, R. C., and Morris, J. C. (2005). Mild cognitive impairment as a clinical entity and treatment target. *Arch. Neurol.* 62, 1160–1163. doi: 10.1001/archneur.62.7.1160

Petersen, R. C., Smith, G. E., Waring, S. C., Ivnik, R. J., Kokmen, E., and Tangelos, E. G. (1997). Aging, memory, and mild cognitive impairment. *Int. Psychogeriatr.* 9, 65–69. doi: 10.1017/S1041610297004717

Petersen, R. C., Smith, G. E., Waring, S. C., Ivnik, R. J., Tangalos, E. G., and Kokmen, E. (1999). Mild cognitive impairment: clinical characterization and outcome. *Arch. Neurol.* 56, 303–308. doi: 10.1001/archneur.56.3.303

Prince, M., Bryce, R., Albanese, E., Wimo, A., Ribeiro, W., and Ferri, C. P. (2013). The global prevalence of dementia: a systematic review and metaanalysis. *Alzheimers Dement.* 9, 63–75.e2. doi: 10.1016/j.jalz.2012.11.007

Purser, J. L., Fillenbaum, G. G., and Wallace, R. B. (2006). Memory complaint is not necessary for diagnosis of mild cognitive impairment and does not predict 10-year trajectories of functional disability, word recall, or short portable mental status questionnaire limitations. *J. Am. Geriatr. Soc.* 54, 335–338. doi: 10.1111/j.1532-5415.2005.00589.x

Reid, L. M., and MacLullich, A. M. (2006). Subjective memory complaints and cognitive impairment in older people. *Dement. Geriatr. Cogn. Disord.* 22, 471–485. doi: 10.1159/000096295

Roberts, J. L., Clare, L., and Woods, R. T. (2009). Subjective memory complaints and awareness of memory functioning in mild cognitive impairment: a systematic review. *Dement. Geriatr. Cogn. Disord.* 28, 95–109. doi: 10.1159/000234911

Ruan, Q., D'onofrio, G., Sancarlo, D., Bao, Z., Greco, A., and Yu, Z. (2016). Potential neuroimaging biomarkers of pathologic brain changes in Mild Cognitive Impairment and Alzheimer's disease: a systematic review. *BMC Geriatr.* 16, 104. doi: 10.1186/s12877-016-0281-7

Shaw, L. M., Vanderstichele, H., Knapik-Czajka, M., Clark, C. M., Aisen, P. S., Petersen, R. C., et al. (2009). Cerebrospinal fluid biomarker signature in Alzheimer's disease neuroimaging initiative subjects. *Ann. Neurol.* 65, 403–413. doi: 10.1002/ana.21610

Sluimer, J. D., Van Der Flier, W. M., Karas, G. B., Fox, N. C., Scheltens, P., Barkhof, F., et al. (2008). Whole-brain atrophy rate and cognitive decline: longitudinal MR study of memory clinic patients 1. *Radiology* 248, 590–598. doi: 10.1148/radiol.2482070938

Trivedi, M. A., Wichmann, A. K., Torgerson, B. M., Ward, M. A., Schmitz, T. W., Ries, M. L., et al. (2006). Structural MRI discriminates individuals with Mild Cognitive Impairment from age-matched controls: a combined neuropsychological and voxel based morphometry study. *Alzheimers Dement.* 2, 296–302. doi: 10.1016/j.jalz.2006.06.001

Tzourio-Mazoyer, N., Landeau, B., Papathanassiou, D., Crivello, F., Etard, O., Delcroix, N., et al. (2002). Automated anatomical labeling of activations in SPM using a macroscopic anatomical parcellation of the MNI MRI single-subject brain. *Neuroimage* 15, 273–289. doi: 10.1006/nimg.2001.0978

Vemuri, P., Wiste, H. J., Weigand, S. D., Shaw, L. M., Trojanowski, J. Q., Weiner, M. W., et al. (2009). MRI and CSF biomarkers in normal, MCI, and AD subjects: predicting future clinical change. *Neurology* 73, 294–301. doi: 10.1212/WNL.0b013e3181af79fb

Weiner, M. W., Veitch, D. P., Aisen, P. S., Beckett, L. A., Cairns, N. J., Green, R. C., et al. (2013). The Alzheimer's disease neuroimaging initiative: a review of papers published since its inception. *Alzheimers Dement.* 9, e111-94. doi: 10.1016/j.jalz.2013.05.1769

Whitwell, J. L., Przybelski, S. A., Weigand, S. D., Knopman, D. S., Boeve, B. F., Petersen, R. C., et al. (2007). 3D maps from multiple MRI illustrate changing atrophy patterns as subjects progress from mild cognitive impairment to Alzheimer's disease. *Brain* 130, 1777–1786. doi: 10.1093/brain/awm112

Winblad, B., Palmer, K., Kivipelto, M., Jelic, V., Fratiglioni, L., Wahlund, L. O., et al. (2004). Mild cognitive impairment–beyond controversies, towards a consensus: report of the international working group on mild cognitive impairment. *J. Intern. Med.* 256, 240–246. doi: 10.1111/j.1365-2796.2004.01380.x

Wittchen, H. U., Wunderlich, U., Gruschwitz, S., and Zaudig, M. (1997). *SCID: Clinical Interview for DSM-IV (German Version).* Göttingen: Verlag für Psychologie.

Yang, J., Pan, P., Song, W., Huang, R., Li, J., Chen, K., et al. (2012). Voxelwise meta-analysis of gray matter anomalies in Alzheimer's disease and mild cognitive impairment using anatomic likelihood estimation. *J. Neurol. Sci.* 316, 21–29. doi: 10.1016/j.jns.2012.02.010

Zetterberg, H., and Mattsson, N. (2014). Understanding the cause of sporadic Alzheimer's disease. *Expert Rev. Neurother.* 14, 621–630. doi: 10.1186/alzrt130

3

Inhibition of PirB Activity by TAT-PEP Improves Mouse Motor Ability and Cognitive Behavior

Ya-Jing Mi [1†], Hai Chen [1,2†], Na Guo [1†], Meng-Yi Sun [3], Zhao-Hua Zhao [1], Xing-Chun Gao [1], Xiao-Long Wang [1], Rui-San Zhang [1], Jiang-Bing Zhou [3] and Xing-Chun Gou [1,3*]*

[1] Institute of Basic and Translational Medicine, and School of Basic Medical Sciences, and Shaanxi Key Laboratory of Brain Disorders, Xi'an Medical University, Xi'an, China, [2] Department of Anesthesiology, Tangdu Hospital, Fourth Military Medical University, Xi'an, China, [3] Department of Neurosurgery, School of Medicine, Yale University, New Haven, CT, United States

***Correspondence:**
Jiang-Bing Zhou
jiangbing.zhou@yale.edu
Xing-Chun Gou
gouxingchun@189.cn

† These authors have contributed equally to this work.

Paired immunoglobulin-like receptor B (PirB), a functional receptor for myelin-associated inhibitory proteins, plays an important role in axon regeneration in injured brains. However, its role in normal brain function with age has not been previously investigated. Therefore in this study, we examined the expression level of PirB in the cerebral cortex, hippocampus and cerebellum of mice at 1 month, 3 months and 18 months of age. The results showed that the expression of PirB increased with age. We further demonstrated that overexpression of PirB inhibited neurite outgrowth in PC12 cells, and this inhibitory activity of PirB could be reversed by TAT-PEP, which is a recombinant soluble PirB ectodomain fused with TAT domain for blood-brain barrier penetration. *In vivo* study, intraperitoneal administration of TAT-PEP was capable of enhancing motor capacity and spatial learning and memory in mice, which appeared to be mediated through regulation of brain-derived neurotrophic factor (BDNF) secretion. Our study suggests that PirB is associated with aging and TAT-PEP may be a promising therapeutic agent for modulation of age-related motor and cognitive dysfunctions.

Keywords: PirB, motor capacity, cognitive behavior, TAT-PEP, BDNF

INTRODUCTION

Paired immunoglobulin-like receptor B (PirB) is a functional receptor for myelin-associated inhibitory proteins, including Nogo, myelin-associated glycoprotein (MAG) and oligodendrocyte-myelin glycoprotein (OMgp), which inhibit axonal regeneration and functional recovery after brain injury (Gou et al., 2014). The expression level of PirB in neurons has been shown to increase after neurological injuries, including spinal cord injuries (Zhou et al., 2010), hypoxic-ischemic brain damage (Adelson et al., 2012; Wang et al., 2012; Guo et al., 2013), encephalitis (Deng et al., 2012), hippocampal aging (VanGuilder Starkey et al., 2012) and retinopathy (Cai et al., 2012). Blocking PirB activity through antibody antagonism or genetic approaches allowed the promotion of axon regeneration and synapse plasticity (Adelson et al., 2012; Wang et al., 2012; Kim et al., 2013; Bochner et al., 2014).

Recent emerging evidence further suggests that PirB may regulate cognitive functions in addition to neurite regeneration. It was found that the expression of PirB in the cortex and hippocampus was significantly upregulated in rats with memory deficits induced by lipopolysaccharide (Deng et al., 2012). The expression of PirB was also found to gradually increase in the CA1 and DG subregions of the hippocampus in aging mice with cognitive behavior deficits (VanGuilder Starkey et al., 2012). Blocking PirB receptor could enhance both the short-term and long-term cognitive functions after bilateral common carotid artery occlusion in mice (Deng et al., 2016; Li et al., 2017). However, neither the association between PirB and cognition in normal brain development nor whether PirB can be used as a pharmacological target for modulating cognitive functions has been previously studied.

In this study, we examined the pattern of PirB expression in the brain of mice at different developmental stages. We found that the expression of PirB in the cerebral cortex, cerebellum and hippocampus increased with age. Then, we explored whether PirB could be targeted to improve age-related cognitive dysfunctions by using TAT-PEP, a recombinant protein consisting of soluble PirB ectodomain fused with TAT. TAT is a cell penetration peptide derived from the TAT-protein in the human immunodeficiency virus and was previously successfully used for facilitating drug delivery to the brain by us and others (Aarts et al., 2002; Wang et al., 2008). We demonstrated that treatment with TAT-PEP significantly increased the length of axons in neurons *in vitro* and improved exhaustive swimming capacity, spatial learning and memory in mice. Our study suggests that PirB plays an important role in aging and is a promising target for pharmacological modulation of cognitive function.

MATERIALS AND METHODS

Animals

All animal procedures were approved by the Animal Care and Ethical Committee at Xi'an Medical University (Permit Number: 2012-8, 7 March 2012). Male C57BL/6 mice of 1 month, 3 months and 18 months were supplied by the Experimental Animal Center of Xi'an Jiao Tong University. Efforts were made to reduce the number of animals used in the study by following the 3Rs (reduction, refinement and replacement). The total number of mice used in our experiments was 180.

Construction, Expression and Purification of TAT-PEP

TAT-PEP (PirB extracellular peptide) construction, expression and purification were carried out as previously reported (Deng et al., 2016). Briefly, cDNA of extracellular domain of PirB was synthesized and cloned into expression vector pTAT-HA-6xHis. For protein expression, pTAT-PEP was transformed into BL21 (DE3). Protein production was induced with 100 mM isopropyl β-D-1-thiogalactopyranoside (TaKaRa, Tokyo, Japan), and purified by Ni-NTA-agarose chromatography (Merck, Darmstadt, Germany). The size and purity were confirmed by sodium dodecyl sulfate-polyacrylamide gel electrophoresis (SDS-PAGE). As a control peptide, the scrambled PEP fusion protein named as TAT-mPEP was expressed and purified according to the same procedure used for TAT-PEP (Deng et al., 2016).

Overexpression PirB in PC12 Cells

PC12 cell lines derived from rat adrenal gland pheochromocytoma were cultured in Dulbecco's Modified Eagle's Medium (DMEM) with 10% horse serum, 5% FBS and 1% penicyline/streptomycine at 37°C and 5% CO_2. Cells with overexpressed PirB were obtained through lentiviral transduction of mouse PirB, which was constructed by HANBIO company (Shanghai, China), and then selected with puromycin (8 μg/ml) according to our recently published procedures (Chen et al., 2015). These cells were named $PC12^{PirB}$ cells.

Determination of the Length of Axons

PC12 cells and $PC12^{PirB}$ cells were plated on glass coverslips, and one half of $PC12^{PirB}$ cells were treated with 150 μg/L TAT-PEP. After 24 h, cells were stained with the anti-β-tubulin antibody (Catalog#: MA5-16308, 1:200, Thermo Scientific) and then the Alexa-594-labeled donkey anti-mouse IgG secondary antibody (1:800, Thermo Scientific). Cells were imaged using a fluorescence microscope (OLYMPUS IX73). The length of an axon was determined as the linear distance from the point of exit to the end of the longest branch of the neurite according to a previous report (Richardson et al., 2007). In every experimental group, 150–200 cells were analyzed.

Design of Animal Studies

A scheme for animal studies was shown in **Figure 4A**. Mice at the selected ages were randomly divided into two groups,

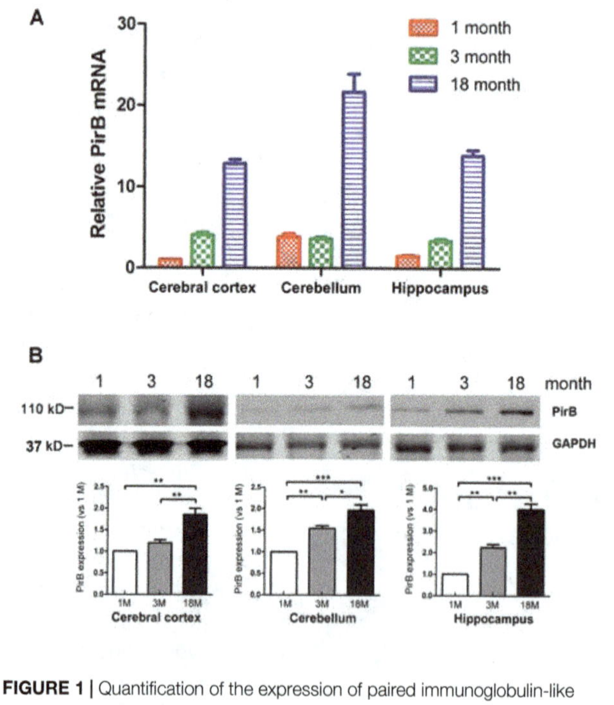

FIGURE 1 | Quantification of the expression of paired immunoglobulin-like receptor B (PirB) in mouse brains ($n = 3$). Expression of PirB at the mRNA level **(A)** and protein level **(B)** in the cerebral cortex, cerebellum and hippocampus of 1 month, 3 months and 18 months mice were quantified using Quantitative Real-time PCR (qPCR) and western blot respectively. $^*p < 0.05$, $^{**}p < 0.01$, $^{***}p < 0.001$.

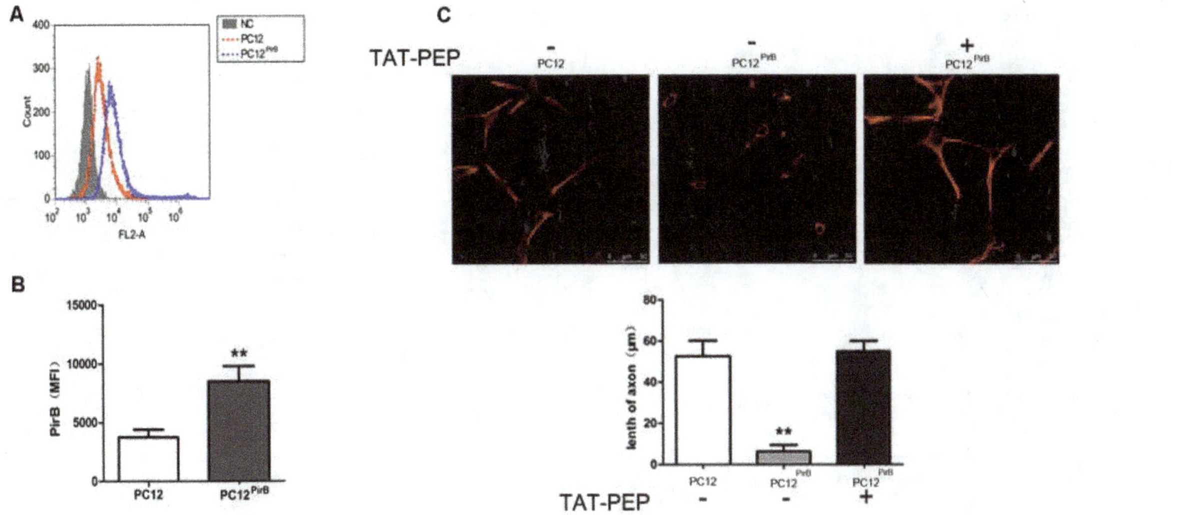

FIGURE 2 | Overexpression of PirB inhibited neurites outgrowth in PC12 cells, which was reversed by TAT-PEP treatment ($n = 4$). Flow cytometry diagram **(A)** and quantification **(B)** of PirB expression in $PC12^{PirB}$ cells (NC means normal PC12 cells without any treatment). **(C)** Representative images of PC12 cells, $PC12^{PirB}$ cells with and without treatment of TAT-PEP. Cells were stained with anti-β-tubulin antibody. The length of axons was measured using fluorescence microscope. $^{**}p < 0.01$.

with 12 mice in each group. One group received treatment of TAT-PEP in saline, another group received TAT-mPEP in saline as control. Treatments were carried out through intraperitoneal administration of TAT-PEP or TAT-mPEP at 8 mg/kg/injection, twice a day, for 30 or 60 days, as indicated in **Figure 4A**. Behavior training and evaluation were performed according to the time points indicated in **Figure 4A**.

Morris Water Maze

Water maze tests were performed as previously described (Torres et al., 2015). The diameter and the depth of the circular pool were 90 cm and 50 cm, respectively. The inner wall was carefully cleaned to eliminate any local cues. The temperature of the room and water was kept at 23 ± 1°C, and the pool was filled with water to a depth of 40 cm and rendered opaque by the addition of milk to hide the escape platform. The plexiglas platform of 9 cm in diameter was placed in the pool 1 cm below the water surface. The recording camera was connected to a digital tracking device, and the water-maze software was used to process the tracking information. The platform position remained constant throughout the training period.

In the training period, each animal performed four trials per session, one session per day, for 4 days. The intertrial interval (ITI) was 1 min. During each session, the mouse started from a random position in the pool, and the maximum time allowed for swimming and searching was 60 s. Mice were allowed to remain on the platform for 10 s after they had found it. The subjects that failed to find the platform were gently guided to it and placed on the platform for 10 s. The average distance traveled to the platform per day was recorded. On the fifth day, probe test was performed with the platform removed from the pool. Mice were allowed to swim for 60 s. The distance traveled and the time spent in target quadrant were recorded, and the percentages were calculated from the recorded data.

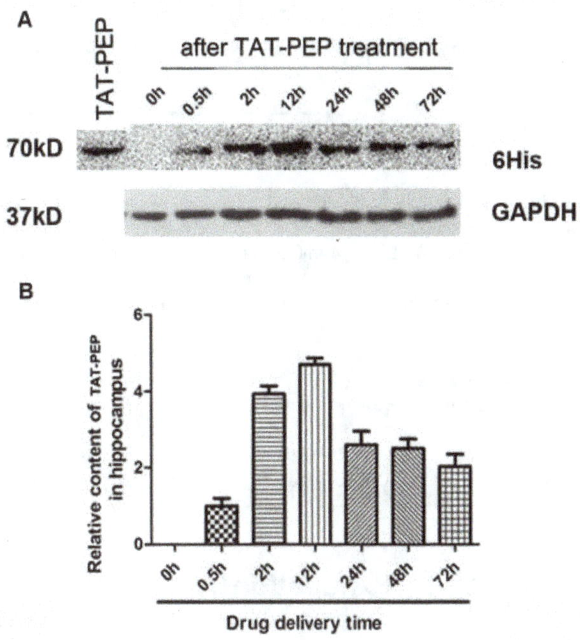

FIGURE 3 | TAT-PEP penetrated the brain after intraperitoneal injection ($n = 4$). Blot **(A)** and quantification **(B)** of TAT-PEP in the hippocampus at the indicated time points after intraperitoneal injection. The first lane was the sample of TAT-PEP protein provided as the positive control.

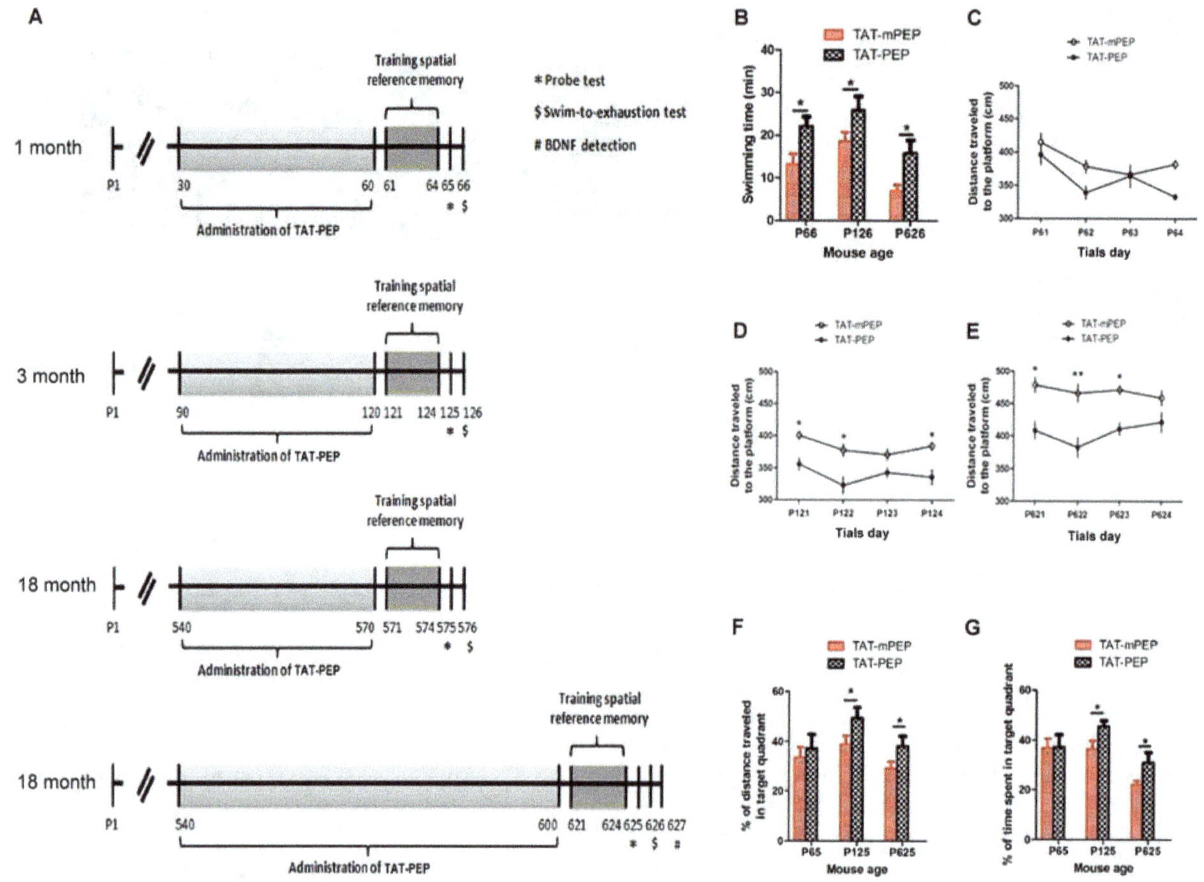

FIGURE 4 | Intraperitoneal administration of TAT-PEP enhanced mouse motor capacity, spatial learning and memory (*n* = 12). **(A)** Schemes of experimental design for mice of different ages. Mice in 1 month, 3 months and the first 18 months groups received injection of TAT-PEP or TAT-mPEP for 30 days. In the second 18 months group, TAT-PEP or TAT-mPEP was given for 60 days. Spatial reference memory training in Morris water maze was performed at P61-P64 (1 month), P121-P124 (3 months), P571-P574 (the first 18 months group) and P621-P624 (the second 18 months group). Probe tests (*) were performed on the next day after the training. Swiming-to-exhaustion test ($) was performed at P66 for 1 month mice, P126 for 3 months mice, P576 for the first 18 months group mice and P626 for the second 18 months group mice. Mice in the second 18 months group were sacrificed at P627 for ELISA analysis of brain-derived neurotrophic factor (BDNF). **(B)** Evaluation of exhaustive swimming capacity was performed in the next day of Probe test. Mice were forced to swim until they were exhausted. The length of swimming time was recorded. **(C–E)** The distance traveled to the platform of different age mouse was recorded in the training of the spatial reference memory task in the Morris water maze. **(F,G)** The spatial learning and memory were measured by Probe test using water maze. Percentage of distance in the target quadrant is relative to the total distance in the water maze **(F)** in indicated groups, and percentage of time in the target quadrant is relative to the total time in the water maze **(G)**. During the above experiments **(B–G)**, there was no significant difference between the 18 months group received TAT-PEP and TAT-mPEP for 30 days. Data was not shown. $^*p < 0.05$, $^{**}p < 0.01$ for mice with TAT-PEP treatment compared with TAT-mPEP treatment.

Swimming-to-Exhaustion Test

On the next day after the probe test, a weight (5% body weight) was attached to the tail of each mouse for the swim-to-exhaustion test (You et al., 2015). The swimming exercise was carried out in a tank filled with water in 38 cm depth and at 34 ± 1°C. Mice were defined to be exhausted when they failed to rise to the surface of the water to breathe within 5–7 s period. Swimming time was recorded for each mouse.

Quantitative Real-Time PCR (qPCR)

Total RNA was isolated using the Trizol reagent (Invitrogen), and treated with RNase-free DNase I (Roche) to remove residual DNA. cDNA was obtained using ReverTra Ace quantitative real-time PCR (qPCR) RT Kit (TOYOBO). qPCR was carried out using ABI Stepone plus and Realtime PCR Master Mix (SYBR Green; TOYOBO). Primers for mouse PirB were: 5′-TACAAGGAAGTACCACGCCC-3′ (forward) and 5′-GGTTCAGCCTTGATGGTTGG-3′ (reverse). GAPDH was used as the endogenous control.

Western Blot

Proteins were prepared using RIPA lysis buffer containing protease and phosphatase inhibitors (Beyotime Biotechnology).

Protein concentrations were determined using BCA protein assay (Thermo Scientific). Proteins were separated using 8% SDS-PAGE and transferred to the polyvinylidene fluoride membranes (Millipore). The membranes were blocked for 1 h, followed by incubation with the primary antibodies overnight, and then incubated with the HRP-conjugated anti-mouse antibody afterwards (1:10,000, Roche). The primary antibodies were anti-6xHis antibody (1:1000, Abcam) and anti-PirB (1:500, Thermo Scientific). GAPDH was used as loading control and determined using the anti-GAPDH antibody (1:2000, Santa Cruz). Blots were detected using BM Chemiluminescence Western Blotting kit (Roche). Densitometry quantification was analyzed using IPP6.0 software.

Flow Cytometry

The cell surface expression level of PirB in transduced cells was determined using flow cytometry. Briefly, the cells were centrifuged and washed with phosphate buffered saline (PBS), followed by incubation with the primary antibody against PirB (1:200, Thermo Scientific) for 1 h on ice. After washing 3 times with PBS, the cells were treated with a 1:50 dilution of FITC-conjugated secondary antibody (1:800, Thermo Scientific). The cells were then washed 3 times with PBS and analyzed using a Accuri C6 flow cytometer (BD Biosciences), and data analysis was performed with Flowjo software.

ELISA Assay

BDNF concentration was determined using the BDNF Emax ImmunoAssay (Promega, Madison, WI, USA) according to the manufacturer's instructions. First, a 96-well microplate was sealed, incubated with anti-BDNF antibody (1:1000) overnight at 4°C, and washed with Tris-buffered saline (TBS). On the next day, the plate was blocked at RT for 1 h and washed. Samples and BDNF standards were added into the plate and incubated at RT for 2 h. After an extensive wash, the anti-BDNF antibody (1:500) was added to each well and the plate was incubated at RT for 2 h. After an additional wash, the HRP-conjugated anti-IgY (1:200) was added. One hour later, the plate was washed and incubated with TMB One solution for 10 min at RT. The reaction was ended by adding 1 M HCl. The absorbance was measured at 450 nm. The same procedures were used to determine the level of nerve growth factor (NGF).

Data Analysis

The data is expressed as the mean ± SD and analyzed with SPSS 13.0 statistical software. The data in **Figures 4C–E** was analyzed using two-way ANOVA with Bonferroni post-test analysis, with the treatments as the between-subject factor and the trial days as the within-subject factors. The data in **Figures 1B, 2C** were analyzed using One-way ANOVA with Dunnett's test. The data in **Figures 2B, 4B,F,G, 5** were analyzed using Student's *t*-test.

RESULTS

Expression of Endogenous PirB

To determine the temporal and spatial expression pattern of endogenous PirB in the brain, we harvested the cerebral cortex, cerebellum and hippocampus from mice at the age of 1 month, 3 months and 18 months. The expression of PirB in different regions was determined by qPCR and western blot. Results in **Figure 1** showed that the expression of PirB increased gradually with age in all compartments at both the mRNA and protein levels, suggesting that PirB is associated with aging.

Over-Expression of PirB Inhibits Axon Outgrowth, Which Can be Reversed by TAT-PEP Treatment

We studied the impact of PirB on axon outgrowth using PirB-overexpressed PC12 cells, $PC12^{PirB}$, which were generated through lentiviral transduction. The results from the flow cytometry showed that the expression level of PirB in $PC12^{PirB}$ cells was 2.4-fold of that in PC12 cells (**Figures 2A,B**). As shown in **Figure 2C**, overexpression of PirB significantly inhibits axon outgrowth. The average length of an axon in $PC12^{PirB}$ cells is 7 μm, compared to 53 μm in control PC12 cells. This result is consistent with previous reports that PirB inhibits axon outgrowth (Gou et al., 2014; Liu et al., 2015).

Next, we investigated whether blocking PirB activity could reverse the axon outgrowth inhibition caused by PirB overexpression. TAT-PEP, a recombinant protein consisting of PirB extracellular motif fused with TAT, which demonstrated the ability to rescue neurite outgrowth inhibition induced by Nogo, MAG and OMgp in stroke (Deng et al., 2016), was used to treat $PC12^{PirB}$. Results in **Figure 2C** showed that treatment with TAT-PEP effectively prolonged the growth of axon.

TAT-PEP Penetrates the Brain

In our previous work, we demonstrated that the TAT peptide mediated efficient delivery of a 40 aa peptide, NEP1-40, to the brain (Han et al., 2016). To evaluate whether the conjugation of TAT enhances brain penetration of PEP, we injected TAT-PEP intraperitoneally into mice. At 0.5 h, 2 h, 12 h, 24 h, 48 h and 72 h after injection, the hippocampus was collected and processed. The presence of TAT-PEP was detected by western blot. Results in **Figure 3** showed that TAT-PEP was detectable at 0.5 h after administration. The concentration of TAT-PEP in the hippocampus peaked at 12 h. The protein sample of the first lane was TAT-PEP synthesized *in vitro*, and here it was used as a positive control.

Intraperitoneal Administration of TAT-PEP Enhances Mouse Motor Capacity, Spatial Learning and Memory

Motor deficit is one of the major results of aging. As the PirB expression is associated with aging, we set to study whether suppression of PirB activity by TAT-PEP could enhance mouse motor capacity. Based on the pharmacokinetic result described in **Figure 3**, TAT-PEP or TAT-mPEP was administered in mice every 12 h. Treatment lasted for 30 days for 1 month, 3 months and 18 months groups. Exhaustive swimming capacities in the three groups of mice were examined (**Figure 4A**). Compared to TAT-mPEP treatment, the time of swimming significantly increased in both 1 month and 3 months groups mice that received the 30-day TAT-PEP treatment (**Figure 4B**). With the same treatment regimen, the difference in the 18 months group between mice with TAT-PEP and TAT-mPEP treatments was insignificant (data not shown). However, the difference reached significance when the 60-day treatment was carried out (**Figure 4B**).

The spatial learning ability and memory in mice was examined using the Morris water maze evaluation method. **Figures 4C–E** showed the performance of both TAT-PEP and TAT-mPEP treated animals on the spatial reference memory tests. The group of 1 month mice injected with TAT-PEP exhibited no significant difference in the acquisition of the spatial reference memory task, as revealed by distance traveled to the platform in **Figure 4C**. For 3 months and 18 months groups, the TAT-PEP treatment notably increased the acquisition of the spatial reference memory task (**Figures 4D,E**). **Figures 4F,G** showed that treatment with TAT-PEP significantly improved the percentage of time and distance traveled in the target quadrant for 3 months and 18 months groups. Similarly, the data for 18 months groups in the Morris water maze evaluation was presented as a 60-day treatment of TAT-PEP, because no significant difference was detected for the 30-day treatment (data not shown).

BDNF Expression but Not NGF Is Upregulated in TAT-PEP Treated Mice

We explored the potential mechanism for TAT-PEP-mediated motor and cognitive behavior enhancement by analyzing the expression of brain-derived neurotrophic factor (BDNF) and NGF in the brain of 18 months mice. Both BDNF and NGF are known to play major roles in promoting neuronal survival, neurite growth and cognitive ability (Lu et al., 2014; Lin et al., 2015). At the end of the behavioral test, the cerebral cortex, cerebellum and hippocampus were harvested and subjected to an ELISA assay. Results in **Figure 5** showed that the 60-day TAT-PEP treatment significantly enhanced the level of BDNF in all three sub-regions. By contrast, no significant difference in NGF expression was seen between mice with TAT-PEP and TAT-mPEP treatment. These results suggest that the motor and cognitive behavior enhancement effect of TAT-PEP is likely mediated by BDNF.

DISCUSSION

As a functional receptor for the myelin inhibitors of axonal regeneration, PirB has been previously characterized in the neurological system with injuries, including spinal cord injuries (Zhou et al., 2010), optic nerve injuries (Cai et al., 2012), hypoxic-ischemic damage (Wang et al., 2012), stroke and lipopolysaccharide-induced chronic neuroinflammation (Deng et al., 2012). Across all these disease conditions, the expression level of PirB was found to be significantly elevated. In this study, we examined both the mRNA and protein levels of PirB in young (1 month), adult (3 months) and aged (18 months) mice, and found that the expression of PirB in the cerebral cortex, cerebellum and hippocampus increased with brain development (**Figure 1**). Our results are consistent with a previous report by VanGuilder Starkey et al. (2012) in which they found that both the mRNA and protein levels of PirB were upregulated in subregions of hippocampus in Fischer 344–Brown Norway rats with advanced aging.

The association of PirB with motor and cognitive functions has been previously reported. In a mouse model of stroke, it was found that knockout of the PirB gene enhanced corticospinal projections and motor recovery (Adelson et al., 2012). However, similar findings were not seen in mouse models of cortical injury (Omoto et al., 2010) nor spinal cord injury (Nakamura et al., 2011). Genetic deletion of PirB leads to activation of alternative

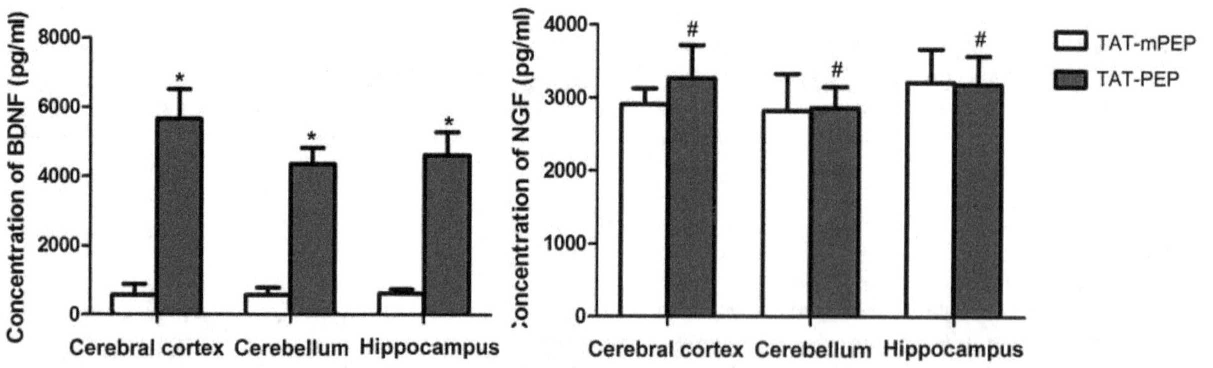

FIGURE 5 | Quantification of BDNF and nerve growth factor (NGF) in 18 months mice with TAT-PEP treatment ($n = 4$). The level of BDNF and the level of NGF in the cerebral cortex, cerebellum and hippocampus of 18 months mice with 60-day TAT-PEP or TAT-mPEP treatment were examined using Emax ImmunoAssay System kits. Data were expressed in pg*ml-1. $^{*}p < 0.05$, $^{\#}p > 0.05$.

axon growth inhibitory receptors, such as NgR, integrin and Ephrin 4A. It is likely that the activated alternative pathways are sufficient to compensate for the loss of PirB in cortical injury or spinal cord injury but not in stroke. In wild type animals, inhibition of PirB prior to the full activation of alternative pathways is likely able to induce significant therapeutic benefits, as seen in an induced stroke model (Li et al., 2017) and in the aging mice described in this study.

The extracellular segment of PirB consists of six extracellular Ig-like domains, D1 to D6 from the N- to the C-terminus (Takai, 2005). Among them, D1-D2 and D3-D6 have high affinities with MHCI and Nogo-66, respectively (Matsushita et al., 2011). It was previously reported that, during the process of age-related hippocampal changes, which were accompanied with cognitive decline, the expression levels of MHCI and PirB were elevated, suggesting that D1-D2 of PirB might promote cognition deficits through interaction with MHCI (VanGuilder Starkey et al., 2012). By contrast, Nogo-66 is correlated with motor behavior, thus we speculate that D3-D6 domain mainly mediates PirB-related motor deficits (Fouad et al., 2001). In this study, TAT-PEP was designed to include all of the six domains. Therefore, the effects of TAT-PEP treatment observed in this study is likely due to the interaction of TAT-PEP with both MHCI and Nogo-66.

We found that the therapeutic benefit of TAT-PEP treatment might be mediated by BDNF. BDNF is known to play an important role in the regulation of learning and memory (Komulainen et al., 2008; Cowansage et al., 2010; Lu et al., 2014; Tong et al., 2015), and can be used as a therapeutic agent to alleviate cognitive impairment (Wu et al., 2015). Recently, Raiker et al. (2010) reported that myelin inhibitors antagonize BDNF-induced signaling cascades through attenuation of Erk1/2 activation. This result suggests that myelin inhibitors and their receptors, such as PirB, may coordinate structural and functional neuronal plasticity in CNS health and disease through regulation of BDNF signaling, and thus, could be targeted for improvement of neurological functions. This hypothesis is well supported by the findings described in this study.

In summary, we found that PirB is correlated with age and might be a promising molecular target for modulation of motor and cognitive dysfunctions. Our results suggest TAT-PEP as a promising therapeutic agent in the future. Of course, TAT-PEP only antagonizes the extracellular segments of PirB and partly inhibits the signaling pathway of axon regeneration. Besides PirB, there are still other receptors such as NgR, integrin and Ephrin 4A that exert similar functions. Therefore, combined antagonists targeting all the receptors will be a more expected treatment strategy.

AUTHOR CONTRIBUTIONS

X-CGou and J-BZ designed the experiments. Y-JM, NG, Z-HZ, X-CGao, R-SZ and M-YS performed the experiments. HC and X-LW did the data analyses. Y-JM, X-CGou and J-BZ wrote the article, with the help of the co-authors.

FUNDING

This work was supported by NSFC grant, 81471415, 31400913, 81402063 and 81271290. Shaanxi Scientific Research Program fund 16JK1655 and 16JK1645, Shaanxi Natural Science Basic Research Plan fund 2016JQ8022, NIH Grants NS095817 and NS095147, and the Leading Disciplines Development Government Foundation of Shaanxi. University's Key Disciplines of Molecular Immunology.

REFERENCES

Aarts, M., Liu, Y., Liu, L., Besshoh, S., Arundine, M., Gurd, J. W., et al. (2002). Treatment of ischemic brain damage by perturbing NMDA receptor-PSD-95 protein interactions. *Science* 298, 846–850. doi: 10.1126/science.1072873

Adelson, J. D., Barreto, G. E., Xu, L., Kim, T., Brott, B. K., Ouyang, Y. B., et al. (2012). Neuroprotection from stroke in the absence of MHCI or PirB. *Neuron* 73, 1100–1107. doi: 10.1016/j.neuron.2012.01.020

Bochner, D. N., Sapp, R. W., Adelson, J. D., Zhang, S., Lee, H., Djurisic, M., et al. (2014). Blocking PirB up-regulates spines and functional synapses to unlock visual cortical plasticity and facilitate recovery from amblyopia. *Sci. Transl. Med.* 6:258ra140. doi: 10.1126/scitranslmed.3010157

Cai, X., Yuan, R., Hu, Z., Chen, C., Yu, J., Zheng, Z., et al. (2012). Expression of PirB protein in intact and injured optic nerve and retina of mice. *Neurochem. Res.* 37, 647–654. doi: 10.1007/s11064-011-0656-2

Chen, Y., Gou, X., Kong, D. K., Wang, X., Wang, J., Chen, Z., et al. (2015). EMMPRIN regulates tumor growth and metastasis by recruiting bone marrow-derived cells through paracrine signaling of SDF-1 and VEGF. *Oncotarget* 6, 32575–32585. doi: 10.18632/oncotarget.5331

Cowansage, K. K., LeDoux, J. E., and Monfils, M. H. (2010). Brain-derived neurotrophic factor: a dynamic gatekeeper of neural plasticity. *Curr. Mol. Pharmacol.* 3, 12–29. doi: 10.2174/1874-470211003010012

Deng, X. H., Ai, W. M., Lei, D. L., Luo, X. G., Yan, X. X., and Li, Z. (2012). Lipopolysaccharide induces paired immunoglobulin-like receptor B (PirB) expression, synaptic alteration, and learning-memory deficit in rats. *Neuroscience* 209, 161–170. doi: 10.1016/j.neuroscience.2012.02.022

Deng, B., Li, L., Gou, X., Xu, H., Zhao, Z., Wang, Q., et al. (2016). TAT-PEP enhanced neurobehavioral functional recovery by facilitating axonal regeneration and corticospinal tract projection after stroke. *Mol. Neurobiol.* doi: 10.1007/s12035-016-0301-9 [Epub ahead of print].

Fouad, K., Dietz, V., and Schwab, M. E. (2001). Improving axonal growth and functional recovery after experimental spinal cord injury by neutralizing myelin associated inhibitors. *Brain Res. Rev.* 36, 204–212. doi: 10.1016/s0165-0173(01)00096-0

Gou, Z., Mi, Y., Jiang, F., Deng, B., Yang, J., and Gou, X. (2014). PirB is a novel potential therapeutic target for enhancing axonal regeneration and synaptic plasticity following CNS injury in mammals. *J. Drug. Target.* 22, 365–371. doi: 10.3109/1061186X.2013.878939

Guo, F., Jin, W. L., Li, L. Y., Song, W. Y., Wang, H. W., Gou, X. C., et al. (2013). M9, a novel region of amino-Nogo-A, attenuates cerebral ischemic injury by inhibiting NADPH oxidase-derived superoxide production in mice. *CNS Neurosci. Ther.* 19, 319–328. doi: 10.1111/cns.12083

Han, L., Cai, Q., Tian, D., Kong, D. K., Gou, X., Chen, Z., et al. (2016). Targeted drug delivery to ischemic stroke via chlorotoxin-anchored, lexiscan-loaded nanoparticles. *Nanomedicine* 12, 1833–1842. doi: 10.1016/j.nano.2016.03.005

Kim, T., Vidal, G. S., Djurisic, M., William, C. M., Birnbaum, M. E., Garcia, K. C., et al. (2013). Human LilrB2 is a β-amyloid receptor and its murine homolog PirB regulates synaptic plasticity in an Alzheimer's model. *Science* 341, 1399–1404. doi: 10.1126/science.1242077

Komulainen, P., Pedersen, M., Hänninen, T., Bruunsgaard, H., Lakka, T. A., Kivipelto, M., et al. (2008). BDNF is a novel marker of cognitive function in ageing women: the DR's EXTRA Study. *Neurobiol. Learn. Mem.* 90, 596–603. doi: 10.1016/j.nlm.2008.07.014

Li, L., Deng, B., Li, S., Liu, Z., Jiang, T., Xiao, Z., et al. (2017). TAT-PEP, a novel blocker of PirB, enhances the recovery of cognitive function in mice after transient global cerebral ischemia. *Behav. Brain Res.* 326, 322–330. doi: 10.1016/j.bbr.2017.03.021

Lin, Y., Wan, J. Q., Gao, G. Y., Pan, Y. H., Ding, S. H., Fan, Y. L., et al. (2015). Direct hippocampal injection of pseudo lentivirus-delivered nerve growth factor gene rescues the damaged cognitive function after traumatic brain injury in the rat. *Biomaterials* 69, 148–157. doi: 10.1016/j.biomaterials.2015.08.010

Liu, J., Wang, Y., and Fu, W. (2015). Axon regeneration impediment: the role of paired immunoglobulin-like receptor B. *Neural Regen. Res.* 10, 1338–1342. doi: 10.4103/1673-5374.162771

Lu, B., Nagappan, G., and Lu, Y. (2014). BDNF and synaptic plasticity, cognitive function, and dysfunction. *Handb. Exp. Pharmacol.* 220, 223–250. doi: 10.1007/978-3-642-45106-5_9

Matsushita, H., Endo, S., Kobayashi, E., Sakamoto, Y., Kobayashi, K., Kitaguchi, K., et al. (2011). Differential but competitive binding of Nogo protein and class i major histocompatibility complex (MHCI) to the PIR-B ectodomain provides an inhibition of cells. *J. Biol. Chem.* 286, 25739–25747. doi: 10.1074/jbc.M110.157859

Nakamura, Y., Fujita, Y., Ueno, M., Takai, T., and Yamashita, T. (2011). Paired immunoglobulin-like receptor B knockout does not enhance axonal regeneration or locomotor recovery after spinal cord injury. *J. Biol. Chem.* 286, 1876–1883. doi: 10.1016/j.bbrc.2017.05.158

Omoto, S., Ueno, M., Mochio, S., Takai, T., and Yamashita, T. (2010). Genetic deletion of paired immunoglobulin-like receptor B does not promote axonal plasticity or functional recovery after traumatic brain injury. *J. Neurosci.* 30, 13045–13052. doi: 10.1523/JNEUROSCI.3228-10.2010

Raiker, S. J., Lee, H., Baldwin, K. T., Duan, Y., Shrager, P., and Giger, R. J. (2010). Oligodendrocyte-myelin glycoprotein and Nogo negatively regulate activity-dependent synaptic plasticity. *J. Neurosci.* 30, 12432–12445. doi: 10.1523/JNEUROSCI.0895-10.2010

Richardson, R. T., Thompson, B., Moulton, S., Newbold, C., Lum, M. G., Cameron, A., et al. (2007). The effect of polypyrrole with incorporated neurotrophin-3 on the promotion of neurite outgrowth from auditory neurons. *Biomaterials* 28, 513–523. doi: 10.1016/j.biomaterials.2006.09.008

Takai, T. (2005). Paired immunoglobulin-like receptors and their MHC class I recognition. *Immunology* 115, 433–440. doi: 10.1111/j.1365-2567.2005.02177.x

Tong, C. W., Wang, Z. L., Li, P., Zhu, H., Chen, C. Y., and Hua, T. M. (2015). Effects of senescence on the expression of BDNF and TrkB receptor in the lateral geniculate nucleus of cats. *Dongwuxue Yanjiu* 36, 48–53. doi: 10.13918/j.issn.2095-8137.2015.1.48

Torres, L. H., Garcia, R. C., Blois, A. M., Dati, L. M., Durão, A. C., Alves, A. S., et al. (2015). Exposure of neonatal mice to tobacco smoke disturbs synaptic proteins and spatial learning and memory from late infancy to early adulthood. *PLoS One* 10:e0136399. doi: 10.1371/journal.pone.0136399

VanGuilder Starkey, H. D., Van Kirk, C. A., Bixler, G. V., Imperio, C. G., Kale, V. P., Serfass, J. M., et al. (2012). Neuroglial expression of the MHCI pathway and PirB receptor is upregulated in the hippocampus with advanced aging. *J. Mol. Neurosci.* 48, 111–126. doi: 10.1007/s12031-012-9783-8

Wang, Q., Gou, X., Xiong, L., Jin, W., Chen, S., Hou, L., et al. (2008). Trans-activator of transcription-mediated delivery of NEP1–40 protein into brain has a neuroprotective effect against focal cerebral ischemic injury via inhibition of neuronal apoptosis. *Anesthesiology* 108, 1071–1080. doi: 10.1097/ALN.0b013e318173f66b

Wang, H., Xiong, Y., and Mu, D. (2012). PirB restricts neuronal regeneration in developing rat brain following hypoxia-ischemia. *Mol. Med. Rep.* 6, 339–344. doi: 10.3892/mmr.2012.907

Wu, Y., Luo, X., Liu, X., Liu, D., Wang, X., Guo, Z., et al. (2015). Intraperitoneal administration of a novel TAT-BDNF peptide ameliorates cognitive impairments via modulating multiple pathways in two Alzheimer's rodent models. *Sci. Rep.* 5:15032. doi: 10.1038/srep15032

You, Y., Kim, K., Yoon, H. G., Choi, K. C., Lee, Y. H., Lee, J., et al. (2015). Sasa borealis extract efficiently enhanced swimming capacity by improving energy metabolism and the antioxidant defense system in mice. *J. Nutr. Sci. Vitaminol. (Tokyo)* 61, 488–496. doi: 10.3177/jnsv.61.488

Zhou, Y., Qian, R., Rao, J., Weng, M., and Yi, X. (2010). Expression of PirB in normal and injured spinal cord of rats. *J. Huazhong Univ. Sci. Technol. Med. Sci.* 30, 482–485. doi: 10.1007/s11596-010-0453-1

4

Acute Stress Affects the Expression of Hippocampal Mu Oscillations in an Age-Dependent Manner

Samir Takillah[1,2,3,4,5*†], *Jérémie Naudé*[1†], *Steve Didienne*[1†], *Claude Sebban*[2,3], *Brigitte Decros*[2,3], *Esther Schenker*[6], *Michael Spedding*[7], *Alexandre Mourot*[1], *Jean Mariani*[2,3‡] *and Philippe Faure*[1*‡]

[1] *Team Neurophysiology and Behavior, Institut de Biologie Paris Seine (IBPS), UMR 8246 Neuroscience Paris Seine (NPS), Sorbonne Universités, Université Pierre et Marie Curie (UPMC), CNRS, INSERM, U1130, Paris, France,* [2] *Team Brain Development, Repair and Ageing, Institut de Biologie Paris Seine (IBPS), UMR 8256 Biological Adaptation and Ageing (B2A), Sorbonne Universités, Université Pierre et Marie Curie (UPMC), CNRS, Paris, France,* [3] *APHP Hôpital Charles Foix, DHU Fast, Institut de la Longévité, Ivry-sur-Seine, France,* [4] *Département Neurosciences et Contraintes Opérationnelles, Institut de Recherche Biomédicale des Armées (IRBA), Unité Fatigue et Vigilance, Brétigny-sur-Orge, France,* [5] *EA7330 VIFASOM, Université Paris Descartes, Paris, France,* [6] *Neuroscience Drug Discovery Unit, Institut de Recherches Servier, Croissy-sur-Seine, France,* [7] *Spedding Research Solutions SARL, Le Vésinet, France*

***Correspondence:**
Samir Takillah
samir.takillah@gmail.com
Philippe Faure
phfaure@gmail.com

† *These authors have contributed equally to this work.*

‡ *These authors have jointly directed this work.*

Anxiolytic drugs are widely used in the elderly, a population particularly sensitive to stress. Stress, aging and anxiolytics all affect low-frequency oscillations in the hippocampus and prefrontal cortex (PFC) independently, but the interactions between these factors remain unclear. Here, we compared the effects of stress (elevated platform, EP) and anxiolytics (diazepam, DZP) on extracellular field potentials (EFP) in the PFC, parietal cortex and hippocampus (dorsal and ventral parts) of adult (8 months) and aged (18 months) Wistar rats. A potential source of confusion in the experimental studies in rodents comes from locomotion-related theta (6–12 Hz) oscillations, which may overshadow the direct effects of anxiety on low-frequency and especially on the high-amplitude oscillations in the Mu range (7–12 Hz), related to arousal. Animals were restrained to avoid any confound and isolate the direct effects of stress from theta oscillations related to stress-induced locomotion. We identified transient, high-amplitude oscillations in the 7–12 Hz range ("Mu-bursts") in the PFC, parietal cortex and only in the dorsal part of hippocampus. At rest, aged rats displayed more Mu-bursts than adults. Stress acted differently on Mu-bursts depending on age: it increases vs. decreases burst, in adult and aged animals, respectively. In contrast DZP (1 mg/kg) acted the same way in stressed adult and age animal: it decreased the occurrence of Mu-bursts, as well as their co-occurrence. This is consistent with DZP acting as a positive allosteric modulator of $GABA_A$ receptors, which globally potentiates inhibition and has anxiolytic effects. Overall, the effect of benzodiazepines on stressed animals was to restore Mu burst activity in adults but to strongly diminish them in aged rats. This work suggests Mu-bursts as a neural marker to study the impact of stress and DZP on age.

Keywords: aging, stress, hippocampus, Mu-rhythm, synchronized oscillation

INTRODUCTION

Stress is a set of physiological responses triggered by an aversive situation (Kim and Diamond, 2002). It is generally associated with anxiety disorder (Pêgo et al., 2008; Bessa et al., 2009), a state characterized by "hypervigilance" (i.e., a high level of arousal) and sustained alertness for potential threats (Sylvers et al., 2011; Adhikari, 2014; Tovote et al., 2015). Stress also promotes avoidance and is often associated with fear generalization (Duvarci et al., 2009; Davis et al., 2010). A key point is that reaction to stress is strongly age-dependent, with elderly people enduring stressful situations more frequently and reacting to pressure more profoundly (Prenderville et al., 2015). In particular, aging may induce sustained stress reactions (Wikinski et al., 2001; Leite-Almeida et al., 2009; Pietrelli et al., 2012). The neurological consequences of stress and age appear furthermore strikingly similar: both are associated with alterations of neuronal plasticity and increased risk of brain disorders (Morrison and Baxter, 2012; Prenderville et al., 2015). These similarities suggest that age itself may act as a stressor factor (Buechel et al., 2014). This link between age and stress is highlighted by an altered brain plasticity in elderly after exposure to new-onset stress (Morrison and Baxter, 2012; Lindenberger, 2014; Prenderville et al., 2015), and that aged individuals often cope with stressful situations (Barrientos et al., 2012; Buechel et al., 2014).

A proper understanding of the interactions between age and stress is crucial when considering the wide use of anxiolytic drugs such as benzodiazepines in the elderly (Gleason et al., 1998; Kirby et al., 1999). Benzodiazepines like diazepam (DZP) have a number of clinically approved uses (reduction of sleep latency, muscle relaxation, anxiolysis...) but also have unwanted side effects, in particular a decreased alertness, anterograde amnesia, dependence and addiction (Tan et al., 2011). Benzodiazepines influence behavioral activity and, accordingly, neural oscillations in cortical circuits. DZP is a positive allosteric modulator of the $GABA_A$ receptor that acts by potentiating the natural ligand GABA (Tan et al., 2011). At the synaptic level, DZP enhances the amplitude and duration of inhibitory postsynaptic events, and thus increases phasic inhibition (Scheffzük et al., 2013). At the network level, this potentiation of inhibition results in characteristic alterations of rhythmic activity patterns (Dimpfel et al., 1988; van Lier et al., 2004; Botta et al., 2015).

The organized activity of neural networks, as reflected in multi-neuronal, extracellular fields potential (EFP) recordings, frequently presents a rhythmic quality. In humans, the central 7–12 Hz rhythm, also called Mu-rhythm in the sensorimotor/parietal area, reflects an idling state (Gastaut et al., 1965). This oscillatory index, characterized by bursts of oscillations of high amplitude, has been mostly observed in somatosensory cortex and is known to be modulated by attention (Wiest and Nicolelis, 2003; Fontanini and Katz, 2005; Tort et al., 2010; Coll et al., 2017). However, other studies found Mu oscillations in many fronto-parietal regions (Sakata et al., 2005; Marini et al., 2008; Tort et al., 2010) and even in the cerebellum (Hartmann and Bower, 1998). In rats, the role of 7–12 Hz cortical rhythm remains a topic of intense debate (Nicolelis et al., 1995; Nicolelis and Fanselow, 2002; Wiest and Nicolelis, 2003; Shaw, 2004, 2007; Fontanini and Katz, 2005). It has been proposed to represent a dynamical filter for detecting weak or novel tactile stimuli (Wiest and Nicolelis, 2003) or a withdrawal state (i.e., with internally-directed attention; Fontanini and Katz, 2005). This rhythm is associated with whisker twitching (WT), during which rats stand still and twitch their whiskers in small-amplitude movements, inducing an increase of sensitivity to weak sensory signals (Nicolelis et al., 1995; Fanselow et al., 2001). However, it remains unknown whether stressful situations can switch the vigilance state towards such quiet alertness, reflected by an increased occurrence of the 7–12 Hz oscillations.

In this study, we recorded EFP in the dorsal and ventral hippocampus (d/v-HPC), prefrontal cortex (PFC) and parietal associative cortex (PAR, formerly called sensorimotor cortex in the somatosensory system) in adult and aged rats, at rest (control) and on an elevated platform (EP; stress condition), with systemic injections of saline or DZP, in order to assess the interactions between stress, age and anxiolytics on alertness-related cortical rhythms. We show that stress increased the 7–12 Hz rhythms of the PFC, PAR and HPC in adult rats but that, inversely, it decreased these rhythms in aged rats. Furthermore, we reveal an interaction between DZP, age and stress that may bear important implications for the anxiolytic effects of DZP in the elderly.

MATERIALS AND METHODS

Animals Care, Housing Conditions and Ethics Statement

All experiments were approved by the Ethic committee CAPSUD/N°26 (Ministère de l'Enseignement Supérieur et de la Recherche, France) and conducted in agreement with institutional guidelines and in compliance with national and European laws and policies (Project no. 01272.01). Experiments were performed on 17 adults (8 months) and 10 aged (strictly speaking, late middle-aged rats, 18 months (Prenderville et al., 2015), but referred to here as "aged") male Wistar rats from Janvier Laboratories. The animals were singly housed, in a 12 h light/dark cycle and temperature-controlled room (22 ± 2°C) with food and water available *ad libitum*.

In Vivo Electrophysiological Recordings

Rats were anesthetized with ketamine and xylazine and placed in a stereotaxic frame. Anesthesia was maintained with inhalation of a mixture of isoflurane 3% and oxygen. Bipolar stainless steel electrodes were chronically implanted bilaterally in each rat into the infralimbic/prelimbic of PFC, the PAR, the CA1 dHPC and the CA1 vHPC. Monopolar ground electrodes were laid over the cortical layer of the cerebellum and the olfactory bulb. Electrodes were connected to an electrode interface board (QuickClip Connect EIB-16-QC-H, Neuralynx) and dental acrylic was used to fix them to the skull during the surgery. Six bipolar electrodes (the distance between the recording tips and the reference tips were 0.7 mm for the PFC or PAR and 0.5 mm for the different part of the HPC) were implanted through burr holes targeting the following coordinates from Bregma: depth over the cortex 3.8 mm, AP +3 mm, ML ± 0.8 mm for the PFC; depth over the cortex 0.7 mm, AP −4 mm, ML ± 4 mm for PAR; depth 2.8 mm, AP −3.6 mm, ML ± 2.2 mm for the dHPC; depth over the cortex 5.3 mm, AP −6.3 mm, ML ± 5.6 mm for the vHPC. The recording tips were located in the deep layers and the local reference tips at the surface of the corresponding cortices.

Finally, to reduce electrical noise, two grounds (monopolar electrodes) were implanted over the cortex at the following coordinates from Bregma, AP +6.7 mm, ML ± 1 mm for the olfactory bulb; AP −11 mm, ML ± 1 mm for the cerebellum (Paxinos and Watson, 2006).

After surgery, an antiseptic (Povidone-iodine solution) and a local anesthetic (lidocaine ointment) were applied in all areas where the scalp had been incised. Animals were permitted to recover until regaining pre-surgery body weight.

Protocol Design

Experimental setting is based on previous studies (Sebban et al., 1999a,b, 2002). EFP obtained from the dHPC generally exhibit prominent theta-frequency oscillations. Two types of hippocampal theta activity were described in the rat. One type was termed atropine-sensitive theta, since it was abolished by the administration of atropine. Atropine-sensitive theta occurred during immobility in rodents in the normal state. The other type of theta was termed atropine-resistant, since it was not sensitive to treatment with atropine but was abolished by locomotors activities or anesthetics. Atropine-sensitive theta became known as type II (immobility-related) theta. Atropine-resistant theta became known as type I theta, since it occurred during Type I (voluntary) motor behaviors, such as walking, rearing and postural adjustments. These oscillations can be modulated by stress, in the case of type II theta, related to cognition (Hsiao et al., 2012) but also by other behavioral variables, in particular by locomotion, in the case of type I theta (Vanderwolf, 1969; Buzsáki, 2002). In the theta frequency range, Mu oscillations are thought to reflect the vigilance state (Kramis et al., 1975; Sakata et al., 2005; Popa et al., 2010) but can be affected by sensory inputs (Fanselow et al., 2001; Tort et al., 2010; Aitake et al., 2011; Fries, 2015). We thus aimed at eliminating potential confounds related to type I theta and sensory influences on Mu oscillations. To minimize the EFP modulations induced by spontaneous locomotor activity (type I theta), rats were restrained in a resting-state environment box and were gradually accustomed to be restricted in their movements, 10 min the first day and with an additional 10 min every day (D1: 10 min, D2: 20 min, D3: 30 min...), until the recording time was reached. This procedure required approximatively 10–14 days for each animal to remain quiet. Furthermore, a cold light source of 100 lux was applied at a distance of 10 cm in front of the rat's nose to keep the animal still, with the head up (the animal voluntarily kept the head up due to the light source) and wide-open eyes (Sebban et al., 1999a,b). During recordings, rats were isolated into a large, electrically and acoustically insulated chamber, in a specific recording room, to eliminate as far as possible to any sensory input that might affect the Mu oscillations.

Recordings were obtained using a Digital Lynx SX (Neuralynx). Sixty minutes baseline EFP recordings were obtained while the animals remained relatively still. The effect of stress was evaluated 1 day later by placing rats on an EP (Xu et al., 1998; Rocher et al., 2004) of small size in the same experimental room and condition. To avoid any bias linked to circadian variation of EFP (Sebban et al., 2002) both recording sessions took place exactly at the same hour of the day. Adult and aged rats were examined simultaneously excepted for five additional adult rats. We checked that the restraining procedure do not produce stress symptoms by itself: no attempts to escape or notable stress reactions were observed (i.e., defecation, urination, freezing) at rest at the end of the habituation procedure, contrarily to the stress condition. Throughout all the recording, rats showed quick reactions when probed by slight sound stimulation, by turning their head toward the sound. We did not observe any difference in the propensity to detect the sound, nor in the reaction times between adult and aged rats, but no quantitative comparison of sensory functions between adult and aged rats were performed.

Neurophysiological Data Analysis

Data were analyzed using Matlab (Matworks®) built-in and custom-written codes. All EFP: (i) were acquired at 1000 Hz and offline band-pass filtered between 0.1 Hz and 100 Hz with a zero-phase shift filter function (zero-phase digital filtering *filtfilt* function); (ii) detrended using local linear regression (*locdetrend* function from the Chronux toolbox; Bokil et al., 2010): window size 1 s, overlap 0.5 s) to remove slow drifts; and (iii) notch-filtered (*iirnotch* function), with the notch located at 50 Hz to remove any possible power line noise. EFP signal was expressed in z-score units. The z-score normalization used the mean and the standard deviation from the baseline (entire rest session) of each electrode. Multitaper *spectrogram* method from the Chronux toolbox (Bokil et al., 2010) with time-bandwidth product of 5 and 10 slepian sequences of orthogonal data tapers was used to calculate power spectral density (PSD) of the EFP data, using a window size of 5 s, with 2 s overlap. PSD was averaged over two similar brain regions (right and left hemisphere) in each animal, for each frequency and time bin. The multitaper *coherogram* method was used to calculate the coherence (normalized spectral covariance) between the EFP from two structures with time-bandwidth product of 30 and 60 slepian sequences of orthogonal data tapers, using a windows size of 30 s without overlap. The signal was bandpass-filtered to extract Mu-oscillations by applying a 7–12 Hz finite impulse response (FIR) bandpass with zero-phase shift filter function (*filtfilt* function).

Instantaneous amplitude and phase from the EFP were obtained using a continuous Morlet wavelet transform, with matcher filter construct parameters: center frequency = 1 and bandwidth = 2, for the 0.1–30 Hz range. Wavelet coherence was computed by smoothing the product of the two relevant wavelet transforms over time (window for time smoothing = 0.6 s) and over scale (pseudo-frequency) steps (window for scale smoothing = 3 Hz).

We measured the phase locking value (as an index for synchrony) between EFP in the PFC and dHPC from the wavelet coherence, using the distribution of the phase differences between EFPs (Lachaux et al., 2002). This measurement is a normalized index of the stability of phase shifts which varies between 0 (random distribution, no phase synchrony) and 1 (perfect phase synchrony locking; Le Van Quyen et al., 2001).

The international classification of the borders between the different frequency bands was arbitrarily drawn (Delta, 0.5–4 Hz; Theta 4–8 Hz; Alpha, 8–12 Hz; Beta, 12–30 Hz; Gamma >30 Hz). In the freely moving rodent, hippocampal theta should be designated theta-alpha, according to the committee's recommendation, since theta varies between 6–7 Hz and 12 Hz (Vanderwolf, 1969; Winson, 1978; Bland, 1986; Buzsáki, 2002; Yamamoto et al., 2014). Hence, we did not separate alpha from theta and considered the whole 7–12 Hz range for statistical testing. A great variety of rhythms in the same 7–12 Hz range have been described in the thalamocortical system, including Mu rhythm (8–12 Hz, sensorimotor system), together with alpha waves (8–12 Hz, visual system), tau rhythms (8–12 Hz, auditory system) or sleep spindles (10–20 Hz). Hence, in rodents, Mu and Theta oscillations share the same frequency component. However, they differ in their voltage intensity i.e., Mu exhibiting higher amplitude of oscillations. These particularly large amplitude oscillations makes sometimes called high-voltage spindle or spike-and-wave discharge (Robinson and Gilmore, 1980; Inoue et al., 1990; Shaw, 2007). We thus separated Mu oscillations from type II Theta rhythm by an amplitude threshold, with the highest voltage events classified as Mu and residual activity considered as theta, with the following procedure. We measured the amplitude in the 7–12 Hz range from the area under the curve (AUC; *trapz* function) of the complex Morlet wavelet transform in this range. Finally, Mu-bursts were extracted by: (i) smoothing the filtered power of 7–12 Hz wavelet transform with a Kalman filter; and (ii) using a double threshold (for the beginning and end of a burst) and a persistence greater than 3 s, i.e., Mu-burst started when the EFP was above the upper thresholds for more than 3 s, and ended after switching below the lowest threshold for a duration greater than 3 s.

Drugs Preparation and Pharmacological Protocol

DZP (Sigma-Aldrich), a standard anxiolytic in humans and rodents (van Lier et al., 2004; Scheffzük et al., 2013), was prepared in a 10% 2-hydroxypropyl-β-cyclodextrin solution and saline. The same solvent was used as vehicle in control experiments. DZP was injected intra-peritoneally at a single dose of 1 mg/kg, which is known to exert an anxiolytic effect. Higher doses were not tested as they may induce sedation (Wikinski et al., 2001; van Lier et al., 2004). Recordings started immediately after DZP administration. Five days before experiments, rats were daily prepared for intra-peritoneal administration by exerting a light pressure on the body with a syringe. The effect of DZP vs. vehicle administration was evaluated in the two conditions, i.e., at rest and under stress (in the EP), for 145 min. Moreover, to avoid the bias linked to circadian variation of EFP, both recording sessions took place exactly at the same hour. The rats were randomly assigned to a given treatment according to a within-subject "Latin square". A free week was imposed between two interventions.

Statistical Analysis

All datasets were tested for normality using Shapiro-Wilk and Lilliefors tests. For statistical comparison, three bands of the PSD were analyzed for each structure: 0.1–4 Hz (Delta), 7–12 Hz (Mu) and 12–30 Hz (Beta). No statistical methods were used to predetermine sample sizes, but our sample sizes are similar to those reported in previous publications.

For single comparisons, paired-sample *T*-tests (normally distributed data) or non-parametric Wilcoxon's signed rank tests (non-Gaussian distribution or for small samples) were used to compare PSD and coherence estimates of the Mu-rhythm from the same animals. Two-sample *T*-tests or nonparametric Wilcoxon's rank-sum tests were used to compare PSD and coherence estimates between adult and aged groups.

For multiple comparisons of normally distributed data, we used one-way ANOVA (e.g., adults/aged rats) or two-way ANOVA (e.g., with frequency bands and stress/rest as factors). For data with non-Gaussian distribution or for small samples, non-parametric tests were used: Kruskal-Wallis test (instead of one-way ANOVA) and Friedman test (instead of two-way ANOVA). *Post hoc* tests were performed to identify which frequency bands differed in the spectral analysis and which groups differed in the wavelet-transform analysis. We did not compare different frequency bands from different conditions (e.g., theta in adults with delta in aged rats). We used respectively the stepwise algorithms Holm-Bonferroni to correct family-wise error rate (i.e., potential interferences during multiple comparisons) by ordering the *p*-values and adjusting the significant level α and Tukey's honest significant difference (HSD) criterion.

Results are expressed as mean ± standard error of the mean (SEM) and were listed in table. SEM intervals were calculated through a jackknife method (Bokil et al., 2010). The level of statistical significance was set at 5% for all tests (two-sided). Significance levels are shown in figures with one to three asterisks ($^{*}p < 0.05$, $^{**}p < 0.005$, $^{***}p < 0.0005$).

RESULTS

Electrophysiological Signatures of Stress

Electrophysiological signatures of stress-induced activities in the PFC and HPC were evaluated by comparing PSD of EFP obtained for adult rats in a state of quiet wakefulness at rest,

TABLE 1 | Interactions of age and stress on prefrontal cortex (PFC) and hippocampus (HPC) oscillations.

Group	Figure	Test	*P* value	*Post hoc*	Correction	*P* value
Adults: Rest/Stress **PFC**: $n = 13$	1C Left	Two-way ANOVA (condition × bands)	$F_{(1,72)} = 119.11$; $P = 0.1719$ (condition)	Not applicable (N/A)	N/A	N/A
Adults: Rest/Stress **dHPC**: $n = 13$	1C Middle	Friedman ANOVA Table (condition × bands)	$\chi^2 = 4.36$; $^*P = 0.0369$ (condition)	Delta: Wilcoxon signed rank test Mu: Wilcoxon signed rank test Beta: Paired sample *t*-test	Holm-Bonferroni: $\alpha < 0.05$ $\alpha/3 < 0.0167$ $\alpha/2 < 0.025$	n/s P_{Delta}: 0.1188 $^{***}P_{Mu}$: 7.3242e-4 $^*P_{Beta}$: 0.0188
Adults: Rest/Stress **vHPC:** $n = 12$	1C Right	Two-way ANOVA (condition × bands)	$F_{(1,66)} = 7.04$; $^*P = 0.01$ (condition)	Delta: Paired sample *t*-test Mu: Wilcoxon signed rank test Beta: Paired sample *t*-test	Holm-Bonferroni: $\alpha/2 < 0.025$ $\alpha/3 < 0.0167$ $\alpha < 0.05$	n/s P_{Delta}: 0.0336 $^{***}P_{Mu}$: 4.8828e-4 n/s P_{Beta}: 0.0345
Adults: Rest/Stress **Coherence$_{PFC\text{-}dHPC}$** $n = 13$	1D Left	Friedman ANOVA Table (condition × bands)	$\chi^2 = 4.61$; $^*P = 0.0318$ (condition)	Delta: Wilcoxon signed rank test Mu: Paired sample *t*-test Beta: Wilcoxon signed rank test	Holm-Bonferroni: $\alpha < 0.05$ $\alpha/3 < 0.0167$ $\alpha/2 < 0.025$	n/s P_{Delta}: 0.2439 $^*P_{Mu}$: 0.0076 $^*P_{Beta}$: 0.0085
Adults: Rest/Stress **Coherence$_{PFC\text{-}vHPC}$** $n = 12$	1D Middle	Two-way ANOVA (condition × bands)	$F_{(1,60)} = 3.98$; $P = 0.0507$ (condition)	N/A	N/A	N/A
Adults: Rest/Stress **Coherence$_{dHPC\text{-}vHPC}$** $n = 12$	1D Right	Two-way ANOVA (condition × bands)	$F_{(1,60)} = 1.31$; $P = 0.2566$ (condition)	N/A	N/A	N/A
Aged: Rest/Stress **PFC**: $n = 10$	5C Left insert	Friedman ANOVA Table (condition × bands)	$\chi^2 = 5.15$, $^*P = 0.0232$ (condition)	Delta: Paired sample *T*-test Mu: Wilcoxon signed rank test Beta: Wilcoxon signed rank test	Holm-Bonferroni: $\alpha/3 < 0.0167$ $\alpha/2 < 0.025$ $\alpha < 0.05$	n/s P_{Delta}: 0.0495 n/s P_{Mu}: 0.3750 n/s P_{Beta}: 0.4316
Aged: Rest/Stress **dHPC**: $n = 10$	5C Middle insert	Friedman ANOVA Table (ages × bands)	$\chi^2 = 15.61$, $^{***}P = 7.781e\text{-}5$ (condition)	Delta: Wilcoxon signed rank test Mu: Paired sample *t*-test Beta: Paired sample *t*-test	Holm-Bonferroni: $\alpha/3 < 0.0167$ $\alpha < 0.05$ $\alpha/2 < 0.025$	$^*P_{Delta}$: 0.0078 $^*P_{Mu}$: 0.0291 $^*P_{Beta}$: 0.0118
Aged: Rest/Stress **vHPC:** $n = 5$	5C Right insert	Friedman ANOVA Table (condition × bands)	$\chi^2 = 5.53$, $^*P = 0.0187$ (condition)	Delta: Paired sample *t*-test Mu: Wilcoxon signed rank test Beta: Paired sample *t*-test	Holm-Bonferroni: $\alpha/2 < 0.025$ $\alpha < 0.05$ $\alpha/3 < 0.0167$	n/s P_{Delta}: 0.1866 n/s P_{Mu}: 0.1875 n/s P_{Beta}: 0.1343
Aged: Rest/Stress **Coherence$_{PFC\text{-}dHPC}$** $n = 10$	5D Left insert	Friedman ANOVA Table (condition × bands)	$\chi^2 = 5.76$, $^*P = 0.0164$ (condition)	Delta: Paired sample *t*-test Mu: Wilcoxon signed rank test Beta: Wilcoxon signed rank test	Holm-Bonferroni: $\alpha < 0.05$ $\alpha/3 < 0.0167$ $\alpha/2 < 0.025$	$^*P_{Delta}$: 0.0166 $^*P_{Mu}$: 0.0098 $^*P_{Beta}$: 0.0137
Aged: Rest/Stress **Coherence$_{PFC\text{-}vHPC}$** $n = 5$	5D Middle insert	Friedman ANOVA Table (condition × bands)	$\chi^2 = 4.98$, $^*P = 0.0257$ (condition)	Delta: Paired sample *t*-test Mu: Wilcoxon signed rank test Beta: Wilcoxon signed rank test	Holm-Bonferroni: $\alpha/3 < 0.0167$ $\alpha < 0.05$ $\alpha/2 < 0.025$	$^*P_{Delta}$: 0.0850 $^*P_{Mu}$: 0.4375 $^*P_{Beta}$: 0.2911
Aged: Rest/Stress **Coherence$_{dHPC\text{-}vHPC}$** $n = 5$	5D Right insert	Two-way ANOVA ANOVA Table (condition × bands)	$F_{(1,24)} = 0.02$, $P = 0.8766$ (condition)	N/A	N/A	N/A

*For multicomparisons tests (Two-way ANOVA or Friedman), significant levels (statistical significance was set at 5%) are presented with one to three asterisks (*P < 0.05, **P < 0.005, ***P < 0.0005) and for post hoc tests (Wilcoxon signed rank test or paired sample t-test) i.e. multicomparisons followed by Holm-Bonferroni corrections, by ordering the p-values p(1) < p(2) < p(3) and adjusting the significant level (1) α/3 < 0.0167, (2) α/2 < 0.025, (3) α < 0.05.*

TABLE 2 | Impact of Mu-bursts on amplitude covariation and phase-locking value.

Group	Figure	Test	*P* value	*Post hoc*/correction	*P* value
Adults rest: Amplitude covariation	3E UP	Kruskal-Wallis ANOVA Table	$\chi^2 = 31.64$; ***$P = 6.238e-7$	Tukey's honest significant Difference criterion	R1-R2: ***$P < 0.0005$ R1-R3: $P = 0.0676$ R1-R4: ***$P < 0.0005$ R2-R3: $P = 0.08$ R2-R4: $P = 0.9715$ R3-R4: $P = 0.1553$
Adults stress: Amplitude covariation	3E UP	Kruskal-Wallis ANOVA Table	$\chi^2 = 31.61$; ***$P = 6.309e-7$	Tukey's honest significant Difference criterion	S1-S2: ***$P < 0.0005$ S1-S3: $P = 0.2571$ S1-S4: ***$P = 0.0003$ S2-S3: **$P = 0.0061$ S2-S4: $P = 0.7691$ S3-S4: $P = 0.0995$
Adults rest: Phase-locking value	3E Down	Kruskal-Wallis ANOVA Table	$\chi^2 = 23.2$; ***$P = 3.661e-5$	Tukey's honest significant Difference criterion	R1-R2: ***$P = 0.0003$ R1-R3: **$P = 0.0013$ R1-R4: $P = 0.0503$ R2-R3: $P = 0.7660$ R2-R4: $P = 0.4318$ R3-R4: $P = 0.8995$
Adults stress: Phase-locking value	3E Down	Kruskal-Wallis ANOVA Table	$\chi^2 = 23.65$; ***$P = 2.960e-5$	Tukey's honest significant Difference criterion	S1-S2: ***$P < 0.0005$ S1-S3: *$P = 0.0119$ S1-S4: *$P = 0.0254$ S2-S3: $P = 0.2533$ S2-S4: $P = 0.3358$ S3-S4: $P = 1$
Aged rest: Amplitude covariation	6E UP	Kruskal-Wallis ANOVA Table	$\chi^2 = 15.16$; **$P = 0.0017$	Tukey's honest significant Difference criterion	R1-R2: **$P = 0.0016$ R1-R3: $P = 0.9065$ R1-R4: $P = 0.1584$ R2-R3: *$P = 0.0209$ R2-R4: $P = 0.5218$ R3-R4: $P = 0.4971$
Aged stress: Amplitude covariation	6E UP	Kruskal-Wallis ANOVA Table	$\chi^2 = 5.41$; $P = 0.1444$	N/A	N/A
Aged rest: Phase-locking value	6E Down	One-way ANOVA	$F_{(3,26)} = 7.66$; **$P = 0.001$	Tukey's honest significant Difference criterion	R1-R2: **$P = 0.0006$ R1-R3: $P = 0.059$ R1-R4: $P = 0.0960$ R2-R3: $P = 0.1663$ R2-R4: $P = 0.1576$ R3-R4: $P = 0.9995$
Aged stress: Phase-locking value	6E Down	One-way ANOVA	$F_{(3,25)} = 9.57$; **$P = 0.0003$	Tukey's honest significant Difference criterion	R1-R2: ***$P = 0.0002$ R1-R3: *$P = 0.0265$ R1-R4: $P = 0.0759$ R2-R3: $P = 0.1745$ R2-R4: $P = 0.0770$ R3-R4: $P = 0.9678$

*Significant levels are presented with one to three asterisks (*P < 0.05, **P < 0.005, ***P < 0.0005).*

TABLE 3 | Baselines for age groups.

Group	Figure	Test	P value	*Post hoc*	Correction	P value
PFC rest Adults/Aged	5C Left	Kruskal-Wallis ANOVA Table	$\chi^2 = 57.19$; ***$P = 3.814e-13$	Delta: Two-sample *t*-test Mu: Wilcoxon rank sum test Beta: Wilcoxon rank sum test	Holm-Bonferroni: $\alpha/2 < 0.025$ $\alpha < 0.05$ $\alpha/3 < 0.0167$	n/s P_{Delta}: 0.3482 n/s P_{Mu}: 0.4025 n/s P_{Beta}: 0.1003
dHPC rest Adults/Aged	5C Middle	One-way ANOVA	$F_{(2,65)} = 132.45$; ***$P = 2.711e-23$	Delta: Two-sample *t*-test Mu: Two-sample *t*-test Beta: Two-sample *t*-test	Holm-Bonferroni: $\alpha < 0.05$ $\alpha/3 < 0.0167$ $\alpha/2 < 0.025$	n/s P_{Delta}: 0.9657 n/s P_{Mu}: 0.1778 n/s P_{Beta}: 0.4458
vHPC rest Adults/Aged	5C Right	Kruskal-Wallis ANOVA Table	$\chi^2 = 41.61$; ***$P = 9.233e-10$	Delta: Two-sample *t*-test Mu: Wilcoxon rank sum test Beta: Two-sample *t*-test	Holm-Bonferroni: $\alpha < 0.05$ $\alpha/2 < 0.025$ $\alpha/3 < 0.0167$	n/s P_{Delta}: 0.4550 n/s P_{Mu}: 0.4421 n/s P_{Beta}: 0.6993
Rest: Adults/Aged **Coherence$_{PFC-dHPC}$**	5D Left	Kruskal-Wallis ANOVA Table	$\chi^2 = 14.81$; ***$P = 0.0006$	Delta: Two-sample *t*-test Mu: Two-sample *t*-test Beta: Wilcoxon rank sum test	Holm-Bonferroni: $\alpha < 0.05$ $\alpha/3 < 0.0167$ $\alpha/2 < 0.025$	n/s P_{Delta}: 0.0675 n/s P_{Mu}: 0.0227 n/s P_{Beta}: 0.0586
Rest: Adults/Aged **Coherence$_{PFC-vHPC}$**	5D Middle	Kruskal-Wallis ANOVA Table	$\chi^2 = 24.26$; ***$P = 5.387e-6$	Delta: Two-sample *t*-test Mu: Wilcoxon rank sum test Beta: Two-sample *t*-test	Holm-Bonferroni: $\alpha/3 < 0.0167$ $\alpha < 0.05$ $\alpha/2 < 0.025$	n/s P_{Delta}: 0.0492 n/s P_{Mu}: 0.8269 n/s P_{Beta}: 0.1883
Rest: Adults/Aged **Coherence$_{dHPC-vHPC}$**	5D Right	One-way ANOVA	$F_{(2,47)} = 1.58$; $P = 0.2165$	N/A	N/A	N/A

For multicomparisons tests (Two-way ANOVA or Friedman), significant levels (statistical significance was set at 5%) are presented with one to three asterisks ($P < 0.05$, **$P < 0.005$, ***$P < 0.0005$) and for post hoc tests (Wilcoxon signed rank test or paired sample t-test) i.e. multicomparisons followed by Holm-Bonferroni corrections, by ordering the p-values $p(1) < p(2) < p(3)$ and adjusting the significant level (1) $\alpha/3 < 0.0167$, (2) $\alpha/2 < 0.025$, (3) $\alpha < 0.05$.*

or in a stressful condition when animals were placed on an EP (**Figures 1A,B**). Restraining rats allowed to avoid theta oscillations related to locomotion (type I theta, prominent in the dHPC, see "Materials and Methods" Section) and thus to correctly evaluate the impact of acute stress on EFP frequency content, and in particular type II theta and Mu oscillations, which are both related to arousal and vigilance (Kramis et al., 1975; Shaw, 2004; Tort et al., 2010; Sobolewski et al., 2011; Wells et al., 2013).

Comparison of EFP content in specific frequency bands (i.e., delta (0.1–4 Hz), Mu (7–12 Hz) and beta (12–30 Hz), see **Table 1**) showed a significant increase in the Mu and Beta ranges of the dHPC EFP (n = 13, χ^2 = 4.36; $^*P$ = 0.0369 Friedman's test followed by Wilcoxon's signed rank-test $^{**}P_{\text{mu}}$ = 7.3242e-4, and paired sample T-test $^*P_{\text{beta}}$ = 0.0188, **Figure 1C**, middle). In contrast, the PSD of vHPC (n = 12) was globally reduced following the stress procedure, in particular in the Mu range ($F_{(1,66)}$ = 7.04; $^*P$ = 0.01 Two-way ANOVA test followed by Wilcoxon's signed-rank test $^{**}P_{\text{mu}}$ = 4.8828e-4, **Figure 1C**, right).

These differences in EFP co-occurred with a modification of the functional connectivity between brain areas. This functional connectivity was evaluated using pairwise coherences (i.e., co-modulation in amplitude and phase-shift stability between two structures) between the PFC, dHPC and vHPC (**Figure 1D**). At rest, coherence in the delta/Mu ranges was relatively higher between the ventral and dorsal HPC than between the PFC and either part of the hippocampus (**Figure 1D**). The stress protocol induced only a clear increase in coherence between the PFC and dHPC in the Mu and beta ranges (**Figure 1D** left (χ^2 = 4.61; $^*P$ = 0.0318 Friedman's test followed by paired T-test: $^*P_{\text{mu}}$ = 0.0076 and Wilcoxon's signed-rank test: $^*P_{\text{beta}}$ = 0.0085). Eliminating potential locomotion-related effects thus revealed that stress increased both the amplitude of the Mu rhythm in the dHPC and its coherence with mPFC in adult rats.

Stress-Induced Modifications of Mu Rhythms Are Composed of Mu-Bursts of Oscillations, Associated with Whisker Twitching and Alertness

We next investigated whether the stress-induced increase in the dHPC Mu rhythm was related to a state of alertness, and thus could reflect an effect of stress on vigilance. Indeed, the time-dependent spectrogram of the dHPC EFP revealed transient bursts of oscillations in the Mu range (**Figure 2A**), thereafter called Mu-bursts, which were observed in every rat. While they rarely occurred in adult rats at rest (**Figure 2A**, left), their occurrence increased under the stress condition (**Figure 2A**, right). Mu-bursts were almost systematically associated with an exploratory behavior of "WT" (**Figure 2B**), i.e., an alert state where rats are still, keep their eyes open, and twitch their whiskers in rhythmic, small-amplitude movements (Fanselow et al., 2001; Sobolewski et al., 2011). This contrasted with the usual behavioral pattern at rest, where rats moved their head left and right, without rhythmic whisker movements. A careful examination of the time-resolved power (of dHPC EFP) obtained from the Morlet wavelet transforms revealed that Mu-bursts were composed of two main frequency contents: one between 7 Hz and 12 Hz, and one at higher frequencies possibly reflecting a "biological harmonic" (**Figure 2C**). PSD obtained from wavelets transforms of the dHPC EFP in the 7–12 Hz range at rest followed a unimodal distribution (**Figure 2D**, black curve), as commonly found throughout cortices (Roberts et al., 2015). This type of distribution indicates that synchronous events, i.e., high-amplitude oscillations, were irregularly interspersed with smaller-sized events. Nevertheless, in the stressful situation, another peak appeared in this distribution for large PSD values, while the rest of the distribution was unchanged (**Figure 2D**, blue). Hence Mu-bursts did not reflect an overall increase in oscillation amplitude, which would have resulted in a rightward shift of the distribution. Rather, they constituted discrete events that were clearly distinct from baseline oscillations and that co-occurred with WT. Furthermore, analysis of the AUC of the wavelet PSD confirmed an increase in the 7–12 Hz oscillations under stress condition ($^{***}p$ = 5e-4, Wilcoxon' sign rank test **Figure 2E**). Overall the increase in the number of Mu-bursts recapitulated the increase in dHPC Mu band induced by stress.

Stress-Induced Mu-Bursts Co-Occur in the dHPC and PFC

We next assessed whether the Mu-bursts observed in the HPC were correlated with similar activity in the PFC. Mu-burst were indeed detected both in the PFC, dHPC (**Figure 3A**, left-middle) and in the parietal cortex (**Figure 4**), but not in the vHPC. Coherence between the dHPC and PFC was maximal during the Mu-bursts (**Figure 3A**, right), which may explain why coherence increases during stress (see **Figure 1D**, left). Individual detection of Mu-bursts (see "Materials and Methods" Section, **Figure 3B**) indicated that they occurred more often in the PFC than in the dHPC, both at rest and under stress (**Figure 3C**, top). At rest, about half (56% ± 16, mean ± SEM) of the dHPC Mu-bursts appeared concomitantly in the PFC, while one fourth (26% ± 10, mean ± SEM) of the PFC Mu-burst were concomitantly detected in the dHPC (**Figure 3C**, top left). Hence, Mu-bursts could occur independently in these two structures. In the stress condition, the total number of Mu-bursts increased (**Figure 3C**, top right) in the dHPC ($^*p$ = 0.0156, Wilcoxon's signed rank test) but not in the PFC (p = 0.8389, Wilcoxon's signed rank test). Moreover, co-occuring Mu-bursts were detected in the PFC first and then in the dHPC, both at rest and under stress ($^{**}p$ = 0.0016 and $^{***}p$ = 8e-15, respectively), with a median delay that was shorter at rest (0.20 s, **Figure 3D**, left) than under stress (0.32 s, **Figure 3D**, right). Hence, stress increased the occurrence of dHPC Mu-bursts, especially after the initiation of a PFC Mu-burst. We also detected Mu-burst in the PAR. These events could also be observed independently from the ones in the two neighboring structures (PAR and dHPC, **Figure 4**).

At a finer timescale (**Figure 3D**, top), phase shifts (derived from wavelet coherence) among simultaneous bursts appeared nearly constant during Mu-bursts (**Figure 3D**, bottom),

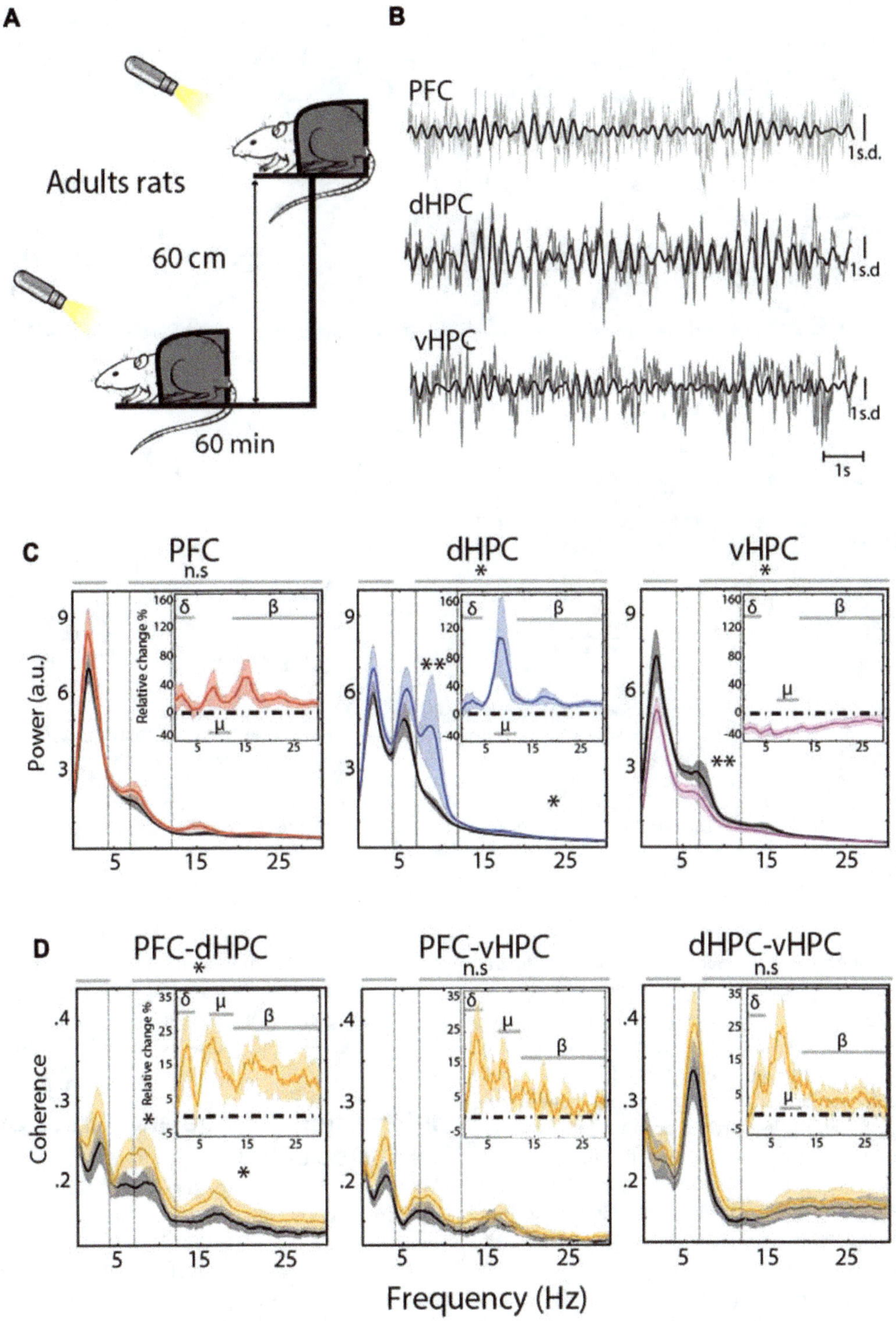

FIGURE 1 | (A) Stress protocol: 60 min at rest, followed 1 day later by 60 min under stress on an elevated platform (EP). A cold light source (100 lux) was applied at a distance of 10 cm in front of the rat's nose to keep the eyes of the animal wide open and its head held up. **(B)** Representative traces of the Z-scored extracellular fields potential (EFP) simultaneously recorded from the same animal in the prefrontal cortex (PFC), dorsal hippocampus (dHPC) and ventral hippocampus (vHPC) at rest. Raw traces are plotted in gray and filtered (7–12 Hz range) traces are overlaid in black. **(C)** Spectral analysis of the EFP recorded at rest for each structure (black) and under acute stress (red: PFC n = 13, blue: dHPC n = 13, purple: vHPC n = 12). The top right insert represents the averaged relative change, expressed in percentage of variation. Horizontal dashed line at zero indicates no change. Data are presented as mean ± standard error of the mean (SEM) and shaded area indicates SEM. **(D)** Coherence for PFC-dHPC, PFC-vHPC and dHPC-vHPC at rest (black) and under stress (orange). In top right insert, averaged relative change expressed in percentage of variation. Horizontal dashed line at zero indicates no change. Data are presented as mean ± SEM and shaded area indicates SEM.

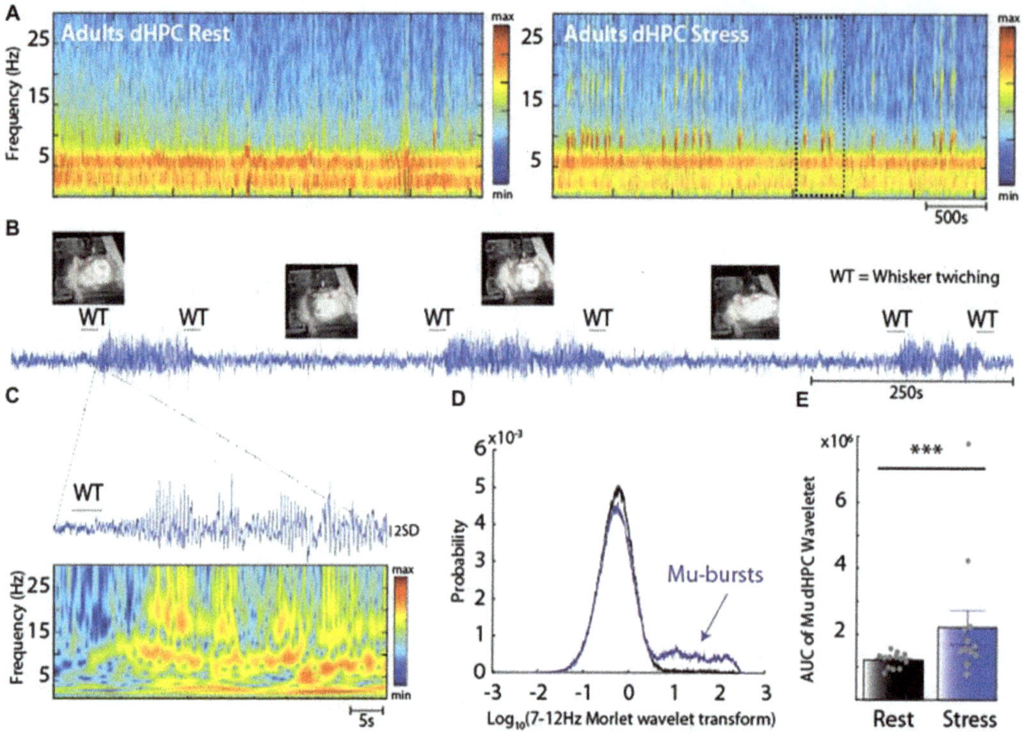

FIGURE 2 | (A) Spectrogram of dHPC at rest (left panel) and under stress (right panel). Note the emergence of intermittent oscillations in the 7–12 Hz range in stress condition. **(B)** Raw trace of the dHPC and its behavioral correlate. Note the prominent increase in the raw signal. Most of the Mu-bursts events were associated with whisker twitching (WT) both at the onset and ending. **(C)** EFP Z-scored trace and time-resolved power spectral density (PSD; using a complex Morlet wavelet transform) during a Mu-burst. Mu-bursts correspond to an oscillation with a dominant frequency peak around 7–12 Hz, together with one to several biological harmonics. **(D)** Distribution of 7–12 Hz power across time at rest (black) and under stress (blue). The bell curve of the distribution after a log transform reveals a unimodal distribution. Note this another peak appearing under stress, with the rest of the distribution unchanged, corresponding to the Mu-bursts associated with WT. **(E)** Area under the curve (AUC) computed from the Morlet wavelet transform (averaged over the 7–12 Hz range) that reflects the overall amplitude of Mu-bursts. The Mu-bursts AUC increased significantly in stress condition (***$p < 0.001$, $n = 13$).

consistent with a value of coherence around one, indicating a strong stability of the phase shift and a high covariation in amplitude. The dHPC PSD amplitude in the Mu-range was low in the absence of Mu-bursts, regardless of the stress or rest condition (**Figure 3E**, top). As expected, amplitude in the 7–12 Hz range increased strikingly during co-occurring Mu-bursts, an effect that was less pronounced when we focused on Mu-bursts occurring in single structures, e.g., only in the PFC or dHPC (Kruskal-Wallis test $\chi^2 = 31.64$; $^{***}P_{\text{rest}} = 6.238\text{e-}7$ and $\chi^2 = 31.61$; $^{***}P_{\text{stress}} = 6.309\text{e-}7$, **Table 2** and **Figure 3E**, top). This profile was similar at rest or in stress condition. More intriguingly, phase-locking was also higher during Mu-bursts in one of the two structure (whatever the context) than in non-bursting episodes, suggesting synchronization processes between the PFC and dHPC even during "subthreshold" oscillations in the Mu range (Kruskal-Wallis test $\chi^2 = 23.2$ $^{***}P_{\text{rest}} = 3.661\text{ e-}5$ and $\chi^2 = 23.65$; $^{***}P_{\text{stress}} = 2.961\text{ e-}5$, **Table 2** and **Figure 3E**, down). These results indicate that Mu-bursts can be generated independently in the PFC and dHPC, while being highly synchronized, and that stress affected the occurrence of Mu-bursts rather than the fine temporal relations between them. Acute stress increased the occurrence of Mu-bursts in both the PFC and dHPC, but impacted the total PSD in the dHPC only. Hence stress can affect the generation of Mu-bursts independently from the basal amplitude and phase of background oscillations in each structure.

Interactions of Age and Stress on PFC and HPC Oscillations

We then characterized the modifications of EFP spectral properties upon aging (late middle aged rats of 18 months, henceforth called "aged rats", $n = 10$ for PFC and dHPC recordings, $n = 5$ for vHPC) and after stress exposure. Strikingly, at rest, aged rats exhibited Mu-bursts in the PFC and in the dHPC (**Figures 5A,B**), reminiscent of the Mu-bursts induced by stress in adults (**Figures 1, 2**), but no Mu-bursts in the vHPC (**Figure 5B**, see below for analysis), as in adults. Moreover, significant differences were observed: (i) between the average spectral properties of adults and aged rats whatever the structure but without specific frequency range (**Figure 5C** and **Table 3**); and (ii) in hippocampal-prefrontal synchrony in the PFC-dHPC and PFC-vHPC. *Post hoc* test showed that this difference did not implicate

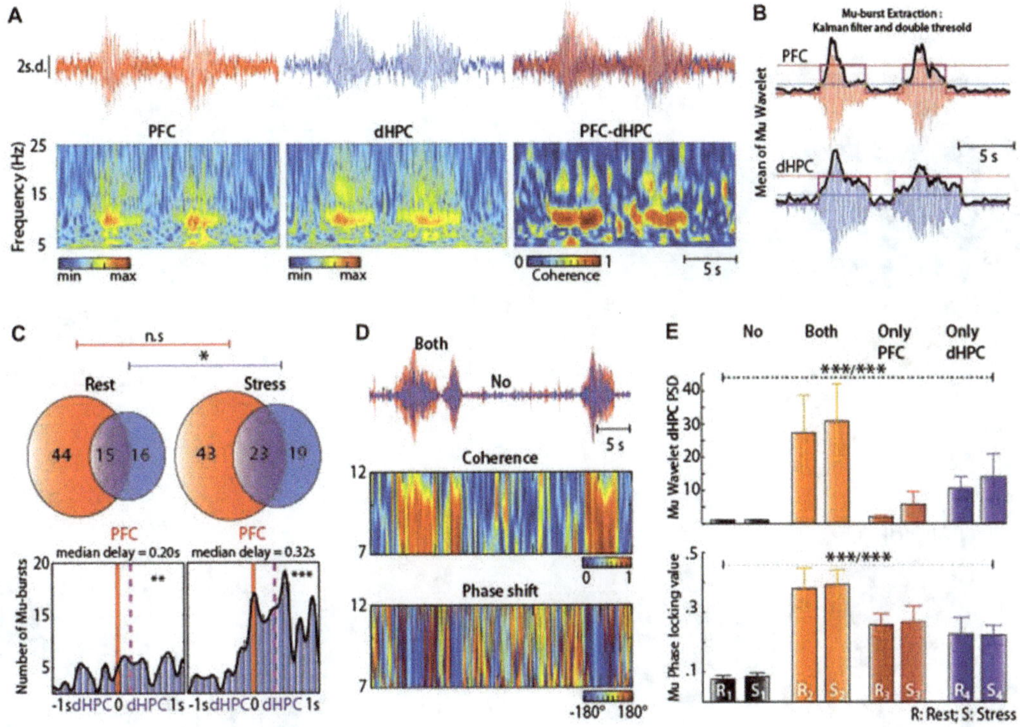

FIGURE 3 | (A) Typical examples of Mu-bursts in Z-scored EFP traces (top) and corresponding time-resolved PSD (bottom) in both the PFC (left) and dHPC (middle), as well as the superposition of these traces (top right) and the time-resolved coherence between the PFC and dHPC (bottom right). These Mu-bursts consisted in oscillations at the same frequencies (7–12 Hz). **(B)** Extraction of discrete Mu-bursts: (i) raw EFP (red: PFC; blue: dHPC) was wavelet-transformed in the 7–12 Hz range, averaged over frequency and smoothed across time (Kalman filter), resulting in the black trace. Mu-bursts starts and stops were determined using a double threshold, one for the onset (blue line) and another for the completion (red line), also constrained by a burst duration greater than 3 s. **(C)** Top: Venn diagram illustrating the average occurrence of Mu-bursts in each structure and their co-occurrence; Bottom: distribution of time lags between Mu-bursts onsets, from dHPC relative to PFC. Red line corresponds to zero-lag and purple line represents the median lag. **(D)** Top: superimposed EFP (red: PFC; blue: dHPC) showing both epochs of Mu-bursts and of baseline oscillations. Middle: time-resolved coherence between the PFC and dHPC. Coherence is maximal during Mu-bursts. Bottom: difference in instantaneous phases from the wavelet transforms (phase-shift) of dHPC and PFC, indicating phase-locking during Mu-bursts. **(E)** Top: square of the absolute value of the wavelet transform when no Mu-bursts occur ("No"), Mu-bursts occur in both the PFC and dHPC ("both") and only in one of the two structures ("Only PFC", "Only dHPC") in two condition (R: rest; S: stress), ($^{***}P_{rest}/^{***}P_{stress}$) Tukey's honest significant difference (HSD) test indicated statistical difference between the following pairs: (Rest: R_1-{R_2, R_4}; R_2-{R_1}; R_3-{naught}; R_4-{R_1}; Stress: S_1-{S_2, S_4}; S_2-{S_1, S_3}; S_3-{S_2}; S_4-{S_1}). Bottom: phase-locking value), ($^{***}P_{rest}/^{***}P_{stress}$). See **Table 2** which indicated statistical difference between pairs.

any specific band after statistical correction (**Figure 5C**, bottom).

Stress in aged animal decreased the PSD amplitude in all brain structures (**Table 1** and **Figure 5C**, insert), contrasting with adult rats where only the vHPC was affected (**Figure 1C**). This decrease was prominent in the dHPC whatever the band ($^*P_{delta} = 0.0078$ Wilcoxon's signed rank test; $^*P_{mu} = 0.0291$ Paired sample t-test; $^*P_{beta} = 0.0118$ Paired sample t-test). This might reflect a different reactivity of the vigilance state to stress in aged rats compared to adults. Furthermore, stress decreased dramatically the coherence between the PFC and dHPC in aged rats, for all frequency ranges taken separately (**Figure 5D**, insert right). This clearly contrasted with the stress-induced increase in coherence observed in adults (**Figure 1D**), and provides evidence for stress impacting cortical activity of aged and adult rats in an opposite fashion. Finally, significant difference was also found in PFC-vHPC coherence without incrimination of a specific frequency band, while coherence between the two parts of the hippocampus was not affected by stress.

We thus characterized the Mu-burst activity to assess the effect of stress in aged rats. Both at rest and under stress (**Figure 6A**), the vast majority of Mu-bursts co-occurred in the two structures PFC and dHPC (**Figure 6B**, top). Under stress, the total number of Mu-bursts decreased in the dHPC ($^*p = 0.0313$ Wilcoxon signed rank test) and in the PFC ($^*p = 0.0298$, paired sample T-test). However, at rest there was no significant delay between the PFC and dHPC bursts on average (**Figure 6B**, bottom left), while under stress, bursts were detected in the dHPC first (**Figure 6B**, bottom right). Hence temporal relations between Mu-bursts in the dHPC and PFC were inverted in adult and aged rats under stress. Finally, at rest, time-dependent spectrogram analysis suggested a high occurrence of Mu-bursts in aged rats in dHPC, similar to adult rats under stress (**Figure 2A**, right). The AUC from wavelet analysis confirmed a reduction under stress of dHPC

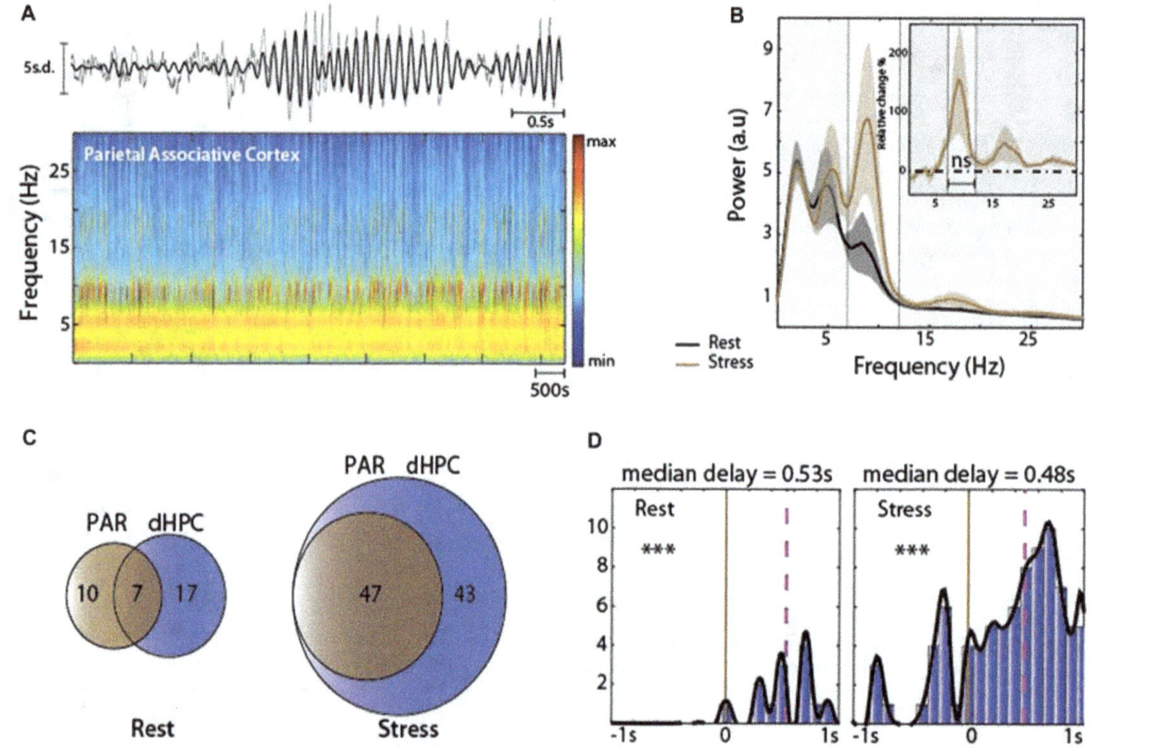

FIGURE 4 | (A) Top: representative traces of the Z-scored EFP in the parietal associative cortex (PAR). Raw traces are plotted in gray and filtered (7–12 Hz range) traces are overlaid in black; Bottom: spectrogram of PAR under stress. **(B)** Spectral analysis of the EFP recorded at rest structure (black) and under acute stress (brown) $N = 5$. **(C)** Venn diagram illustrating the average occurrence of Mu-bursts in dHPC and PAR and their co-occurrence. Note at rest, Mu-burst are observed independently in the two neighboring structures. Under stress condition the total number increased in both structure. Note that all Mu-bursts detected in PAR co-occurred in the dHPC. **(D)** Distribution of time lags between Mu-bursts onsets, from dHPC relative to PAR. Brown line corresponds to zero-lag and purple line represents the median lag. Note that all Mu-bursts detected in PAR co-occurred in the dHPC. Note that the Mu-burst are observed independently in the two neighboring structures. Rest: 0.53 s median delay, paired sample T-test $^{***}P < 0.001$ stress: 0.48 s median delay, Wilcoxon signed rank test $^{***}P < 0.001$.

Mu-bursts in aged rats (**Figure 6C**, $^{**}P_{aged} = 0.0057$ Paired-sample T-test). A similar decrease was observed in dHPC-PFC coherence (**Figure 6D**, $^{**}P_{aged} = 0.0075$ paired sample T-test). Overall, both the occurrence of Mu-bursts in the PFC and dHPC, and the synchrony between these structures, were higher at rest in aged rats when compared to adults, and were differentially affected by stress (i.e., increased in adult vs. decreased in aged rats).

Paradoxically, compared to the adult group, dHPC PSD remained low only in the stress condition, during occurring (in a single structure) and co-occurring (PFC and dHPC) Mu-bursts (Kruskal-Wallis test $\chi^2 = 15.16$, $^{**}P_{rest} = 0.0017$ and $\chi^2 = 5.41$, $P_{stress} = 0.1444$, **Table 2** and **Figure 6E**, top). Interestingly at rest, phase-locking remained significantly higher exclusively when Mu-bursts appeared at the same time in both structures. Lastly, phase locking appeared to be significantly higher when these events were detected together, or only in the PFC, under stress (One-way ANOVA $F_{(3,23)} = 7.66$, $^{**}P_{rest} = 0.001$ and $F_{(3,22)} = 9.57$, $^{***}P_{stress} = 0.0003$, **Table 2** and **Figure 6E**, bottom).

These results appear fully consistent with the notions that aging is itself a stress factor (Morrison and Baxter, 2012; Lindenberger, 2014; Prenderville et al., 2015), and that aged individuals differently cope with stressful situations (Barrientos et al., 2012; Buechel et al., 2014).

Effect of the Anxiolytic Diazepam on PFC and HPC Oscillations

Finally, we assessed how DZP, a widely-used anxiolytic, affects stress- and age-related changes on the dHPC-PFC coherence (145 min, $n = 5$ for each group; **Figures 7A,B**). In the stress condition, for each group, DZP decreased the coherence between the PFC and dHPC in the Mu-range, compared to saline (**Figure 7B**: left, Adults $^{*}P_{mu} = 0.0204$, right, Aged $^{***}P_{mu} = 0.0009$). Time-dependent spectrograms of dHPC suggested that DZP abolished the increase in stress-related Mu-bursts (**Figure 7C**). In the adults group, DZP partially abolished the effects of stress on the coherence of hippocampal and prefrontal field potentials (**Figure 7D**, left). Contrarily, in aged rats, Mu-rhythms were reduced in the stress-DZP condition compared to the stress-vehicle (SV) condition and rest-vehicle (RV) condition (**Figure 7**). Furthermore, the effect of DZP on the Mu-rhythms seemed to be specific to stress: there was no changes in control non-stressed rats treated with DZP (**Figure 8**). Overall, these results suggest an efficient effect of DZP on adults (DZP abolishes stress effects), and an additive effect of

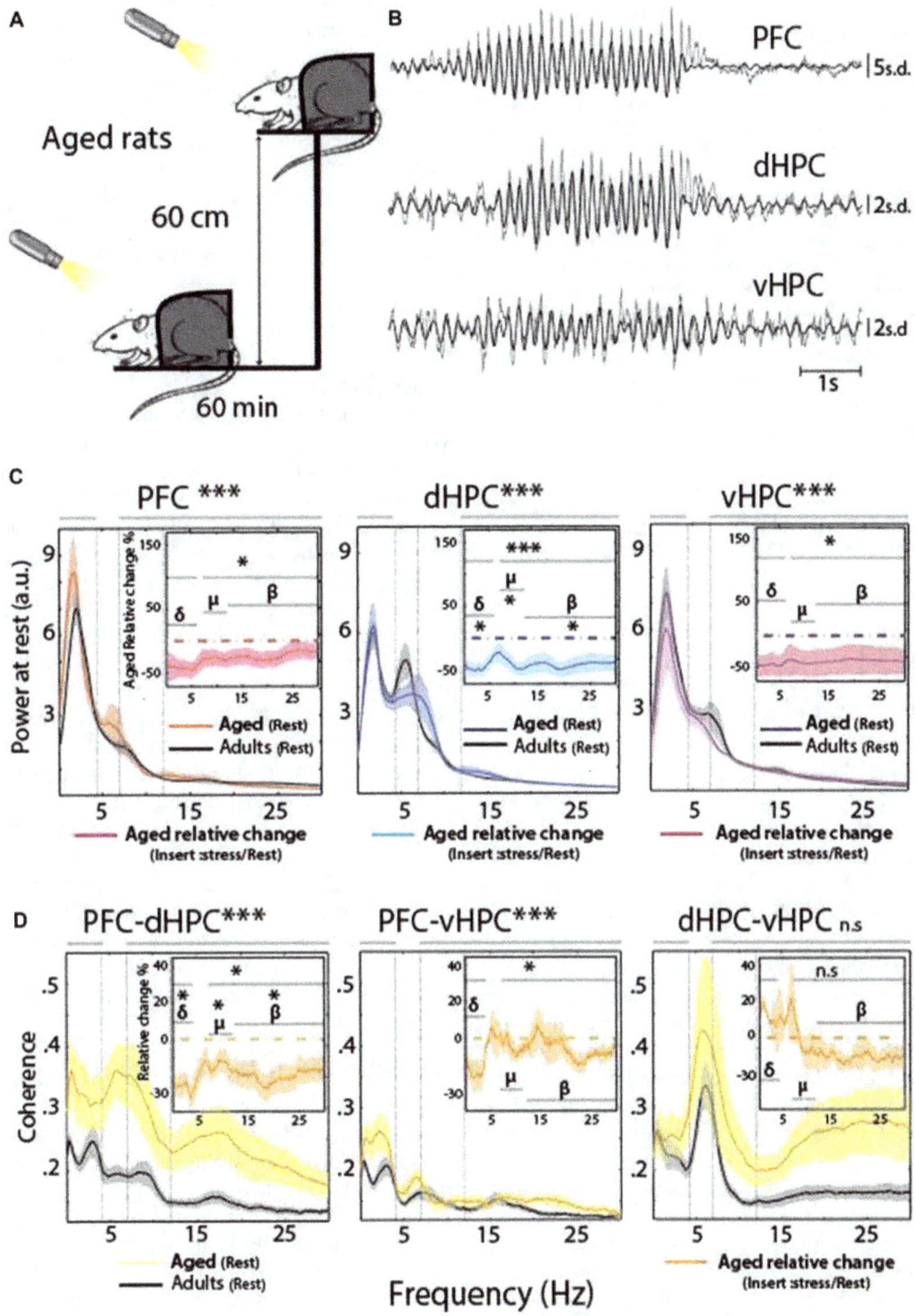

FIGURE 5 | (A) Stress protocol (same as **Figure 1**) in aged rats. **(B)** Representative traces of the Z-scored EFP simultaneously recorded from the same animal in the PFC, dHPC and vHPC at rest. Raw traces are plotted in gray and filtered (Mu range) traces are overlaid in black. **(C)** Spectral analysis of the EFP recorded at rest for each structure and each group. Adults (black) Aged (color); red: PFC $n = 10$, blue: dHPC $n = 9$, purple: vHPC $n = 5$). Differences were observed between the average spectral properties of adults and aged rats at rest, whatever the structure (PFC: $\chi^2 = 57.19$; $^{***}P < 0.001$ Kruskal-Wallis test; dHPC: $F_{(2,63)} = 132.45$; $^{***}P < 0.001$ One-way ANOVA test; vHPC Kruskal-Wallis test $\chi^2 = 41.61$ $^{***}P \leq 0.001$) and without specific frequency range. Inserts corresponded at the average relative changes under stress, expressed in percentage of variation. Stress in aged animal decreased the PSD amplitude in all brain structures (Friedman's test:

(Continued)

FIGURE 5 | Continued
$\chi^2 = 5.15$, $*P < 0.05$ for the PFC; $\chi^2 = 15.61$, $***P \leq 0.001$ for the dHPC; $\chi^2 = 5.53$, $*P < 0.05$ for the vHPC) whatever the band after correction (see text) **(D)** Coherence for PFC-dHPC, PFC-vHPC and dHPC-vHPC at rest for each group (black: Adults; gold: Aged; PFC-dHPC $n = 10$, PFC-vHPC $n = 5$, dHPC-vHPC $n = 5$). Hippocampal-prefrontal synchrony at rest was significantly different between aged and adults rats, in the PFC-dHPC and PFC-vHPC (Kruskal-Wallis test: $\chi^2 = 14.81$ $***PCOH_{PFC\text{-}dHPC} < 0.001$; $\chi^2 = 24.26$, $***PCOH_{PFC\text{-}vHPC} < 0.001$). *Post hoc* (Holm's Bonferroni) test showed that this difference did not implicate any specific band. Top-right insert: relative change after stress, expressed in percentage of variation. Horizontal dashed line at zero indicates no change. Shaded area indicated SEM. Stress decreased dramatically the coherence between PFC and dHPC in aged rats, for all frequency ranges taken separately ($\chi^2 = 5.76$, $*P < 0.05$ Friedman's test followed by *post hoc* tests (Holm's Bonferroni), $*P_{delta} = 0.0166$ paired-sample *t*-test; $*P_{mu} = 0.0098$ Wilcoxon's signed rank test; $*Pbeta = 0.0137$ Wilcoxon's signed rank test). Significant difference was also found in PFC-vHPC coherence without incrimination of a specific frequency band ($\chi^2 = 4.98$, $*P < 0.05$ Friedman's test), but not in dHPC-vHPC ($F_{(1,24)} = 0.02$, $P = 0.8766$ Two-way ANOVA; ns $p > 0.05$; $*p < 0.05$; $**p < 0.01$, $***p < 0.001$).

DZP and stress in aged rats. These results are summarized in the average coherograms from the pharmacological protocol (**Figure 9**).

DISCUSSION

Electrophysiological Markers of Stress in Immobile Rats

There is an ongoing debate on the implication of the different parts of the hippocampus in response to stress (Fanselow and Dong, 2010; Bannerman et al., 2014). While the vHPC is known to be directly implicated in anxiety-related processes through direct connections with the amygdala and bed nucleus of stria terminalis (Adhikari, 2014; Adhikari et al., 2015; Padilla-Coreano et al., 2016), the dHPC is believed to exert a role in contextual fear learning only (Bannerman et al., 2004; Fanselow and Dong, 2010). In most studies in rodents, analysis of hippocampal EFP focused on theta (4–12 Hz) oscillations, which in the dorsal part reveal prominent movement-dependent theta-rhythms (Buzsáki, 2002). Theta rhythms in the dHPC are generally of two types: type I theta, which is related to movement and is generated by the entorhinal cortex; and type II theta, which relates to alert immobility, arousal and anxiety and is generated by the medial septum and diagonal band of Broca (Vanderwolf, 1969; Kramis et al., 1975; Wells et al., 2013). Here we used a setup where rats could not move, enabling us to record type II theta and Mu rhythm, while avoiding contamination by type I theta, and we showed that dHPC rhythms were in fact modified by acute stress.

This is to our best knowledge the first report providing evidence that the dHPC PSD in adult rats significantly increased in the 7–12 Hz band under stress. Interestingly, these changes were exclusively caused by Mu-bursts rather than due to type II theta oscillation. These results were not observed in other studies, most probably because animals were free to move, e.g., in an elevated plus maze or an open field (Adhikari et al., 2010; Jacinto et al., 2013). In our experimental paradigm, changes in dHPC rhythms may be explained by animals being immobile (no theta I) or displaying a form of resignation to the long restraining time, with no escape possible (Balleine and Curthoys, 1991). Whatever the reason, these PSD increases in the 7–12 Hz range can be explained by fear experienced by rats when subjected to the EP, or by memorization of the stress context (but see "Interpretation of Mu Burst Events" Section for alternative interpretations).

Studies suggest that anxiety-like behaviors decrease, together with the activity of the vHPC circuit, when the environment becomes familiar. Likewise, we observed that vHPC PSD was globally desynchronized, probably due to a long exposure of the same environment, which is consistent with previous studies (Jacinto et al., 2013). Indeed, the environment in which the experiments took place was familiar (following habituation) to all groups of rats.

We found that, at rest, coherence in the 7–12 Hz range was very high between the two parts of the hippocampus (vHPC and dHPC). Coherence was also high between the PFC and the hippocampus but, unexpectedly, significantly higher with the dorsal than with the ventral part. Synchronizations were significantly increased by stress, yet only between the PFC and dHPC. These results are somewhat surprising considering the monosynaptic connections between the PFC and vHPC and the role of these structures in in anxiety (Verwer et al., 1997; Parent et al., 2010). Nevertheless, a strong coherence between the PFC and the dHPC is consistent with their anatomical relationship, which includes not only polysynaptic connections but also monosynaptic drive from the dorsal anterior cingulate cortex to the CA1/CA3 subfield (Rajasethupathy et al., 2015). Coherence analysis reflect functional cell assemblies, e.g., related groups of cells in distant brain structures with synchronized discharge to encode and store information (Battaglia et al., 2011). Hence, our results can be explained by a propagation of activity in the 7–12 Hz range from dHPC neurons, a crucial structure for the fast encoding of initial fear information, to the PFC, a structure with larger storage capacity, but slower learning, resulting into the consolidation of the fear memory.

Modulation of Mu-Bursts by Age, Stress and Benzodiazepine

We detected in the PFC and dHPC (but not the vHPC) transient bursts of activity consisting in large amplitude oscillations in the 7–12 Hz frequency range, which we called Mu-bursts, and that seem associated with WT. These events were modulated in the dHPC by multiple factors, including age, stress and benzodiazepines. At rest, we observed a striking effect of the animal's age, with more Mu-bursts in aged rats compared to adults, which is in agreement with previous studies (Aporti et al., 1986; Buzsáki et al., 1988; Ambrosini et al., 1997). This increased occurrence of Mu-bursts with age suggests these one may arise from the pathway specifically alters with aging. An important finding is that the 7–12 Hz rhythm of the dHPC was the frequency range the most impacted by stress, which suggests these events may be used as a biomarker for stress. Yet, stress acted on Mu-bursts in

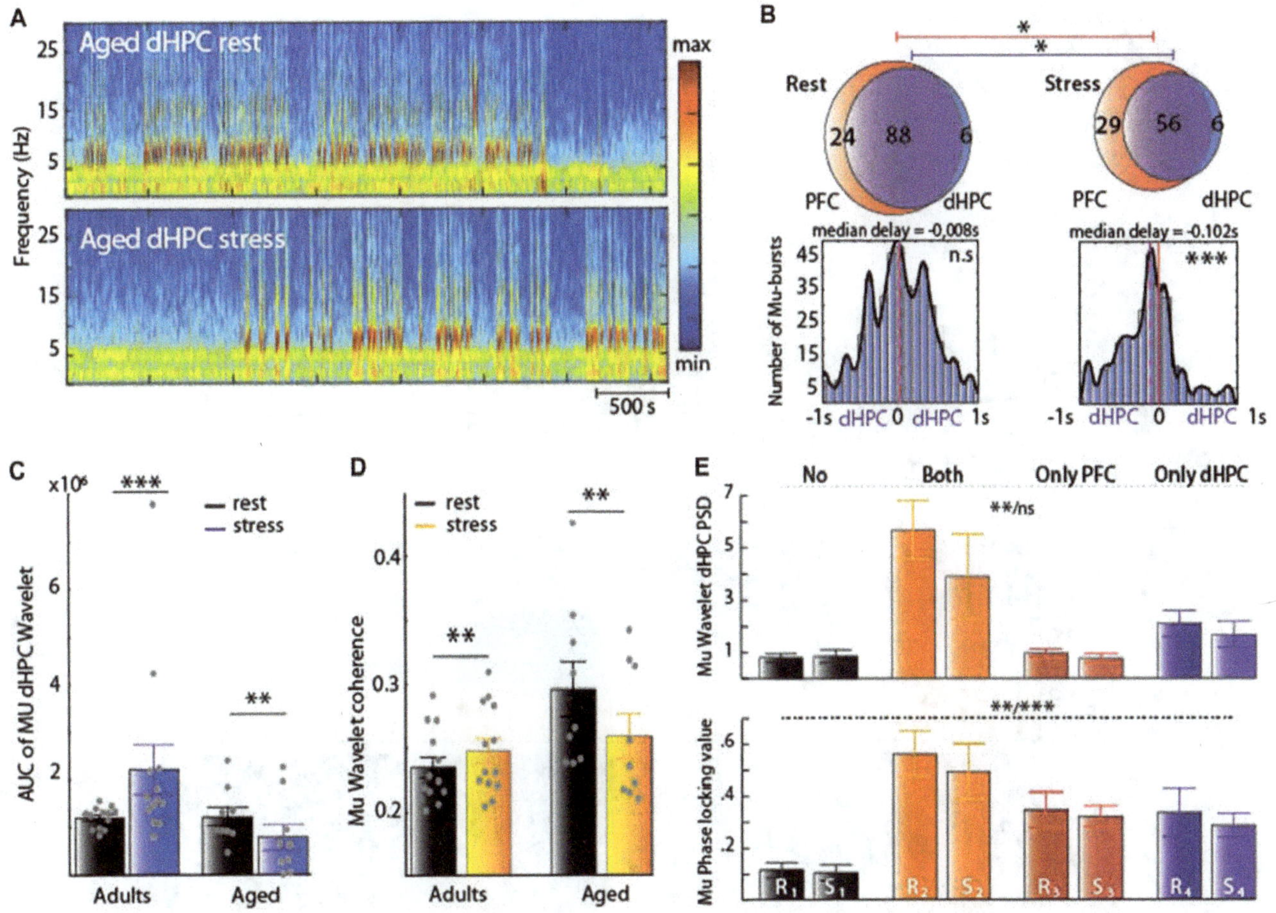

FIGURE 6 | (A) Spectrogram of dHPC at rest (top) and under stress (bottom). Note the decrease of Mu-bursts under stress condition. **(B)** Top: Venn diagram illustrating the average occurrence of Mu-bursts in each structure and their co-occurrence and distribution of time lags between Mu-bursts onsets, from dHPC relative to PFC. Red line corresponds to the zero-lag and the purple line represents the median lag. Under stress condition, the total number of Mu-bursts decreased in the dHPC (*$p < 0.05$, Wilcoxon signed rank test) and in the PFC (*$p < 0.05$, paired sample T-test). At rest, there was on average no significant delay (median delay = −0.004 s) between PFC and dHPC bursts, while under stress, bursts were detected first in the dHPC (median delay = −0.0781 s, Wilcoxon signed rank test, ***$p < 0.001$). **(C,D)** AUC computed from the wavelet transform (left) and the wavelet coherence (right) from the 7–12 Hz range. In aged group, both decreased significantly under stress (black: rest; color: stress). Significant differences were found for AUC (Wilcoxson signed rank test $n = 13$ ***$P_{adults} < 0.001$ and paired sample T-test $n = 9$ **$P_{aged} < 0.001$) and for coherence (paired sample T-test **$P_{adults} < 0.01$ and **$P_{aged} < 0.01$). **(E)** Top: square of the absolute value of the wavelet transform when no Mu-bursts occur ("No"), when Mu-bursts occur in both the PFC and dHPC ("both") or only in one of the two structures ("only PFC" and "only dHPC) in two condition (R: rest; S: stress). dHPC PSD remained low in the absence of Mu-burst and during of occurring and co-occurring Mu-bursts only in the rest condition (Kruskal-Wallis test $\chi^2 = 15.12$, **$P_{rest} < 0.05$ and $\chi^2 = 5.41$, $P_{stress} = 0.1444$) Bottom: phase-locking value still remained significantly higher during co-occurring of the Mu-bursts at rest, and during PFC-occurring only (One-way ANOVA $F_{(3,23)} = 7.66$, **$P_{rest} < 0.01$ and $F_{(3,22)} = 9.57$ ***$P_{stress} < 0.001$). See table which indicated statistical difference between pairs.

opposite fashion, i.e., increase vs. decrease, in adult and aged animals, respectively. Aged rats mays exhibit a hypersecreting HPA axis with increased corticotropin release, and such glucocorticoid signaling might result in an exaggerated stress response (Buechel et al., 2014; Barrientos et al., 2015). This paradoxical result may alternatively be explained by the fact that, at rest, animals already exhibited different levels of Mu-burst activity.

In addition, we show that DZP decreased the occurrence of Mu-bursts, together with their co-occurrence, across all age in the stress condition. This is consistent with DZP acting as a positive allosteric modulator of $GABA_A$ receptors, hence globally potentiating inhibition and inducing anxiolytic effects. However, because stress differently affect adult vs. aged animal, DZP overall reverted Mu-bursts occurrence and coherence in adult animals but almost abolished them in aged rats. Aging is associated with an altered composition in α1 and especially α5 subunits of $GABA_A$ receptors (Yu et al., 2006; Schmidt et al., 2010). The GABAergic inhibition is less active in enhancing benzodiazepine binding in older animals, potentially due to the loss of functional $GABA_A$ subunits (Calderini et al., 1981; Hoekzema et al., 2012). However, an increase in benzodiazepine binding sites was observed in aged rats, mainly in the hippocampus, striatum and cerebellum (Calderini et al., 1981). Hence, starting from

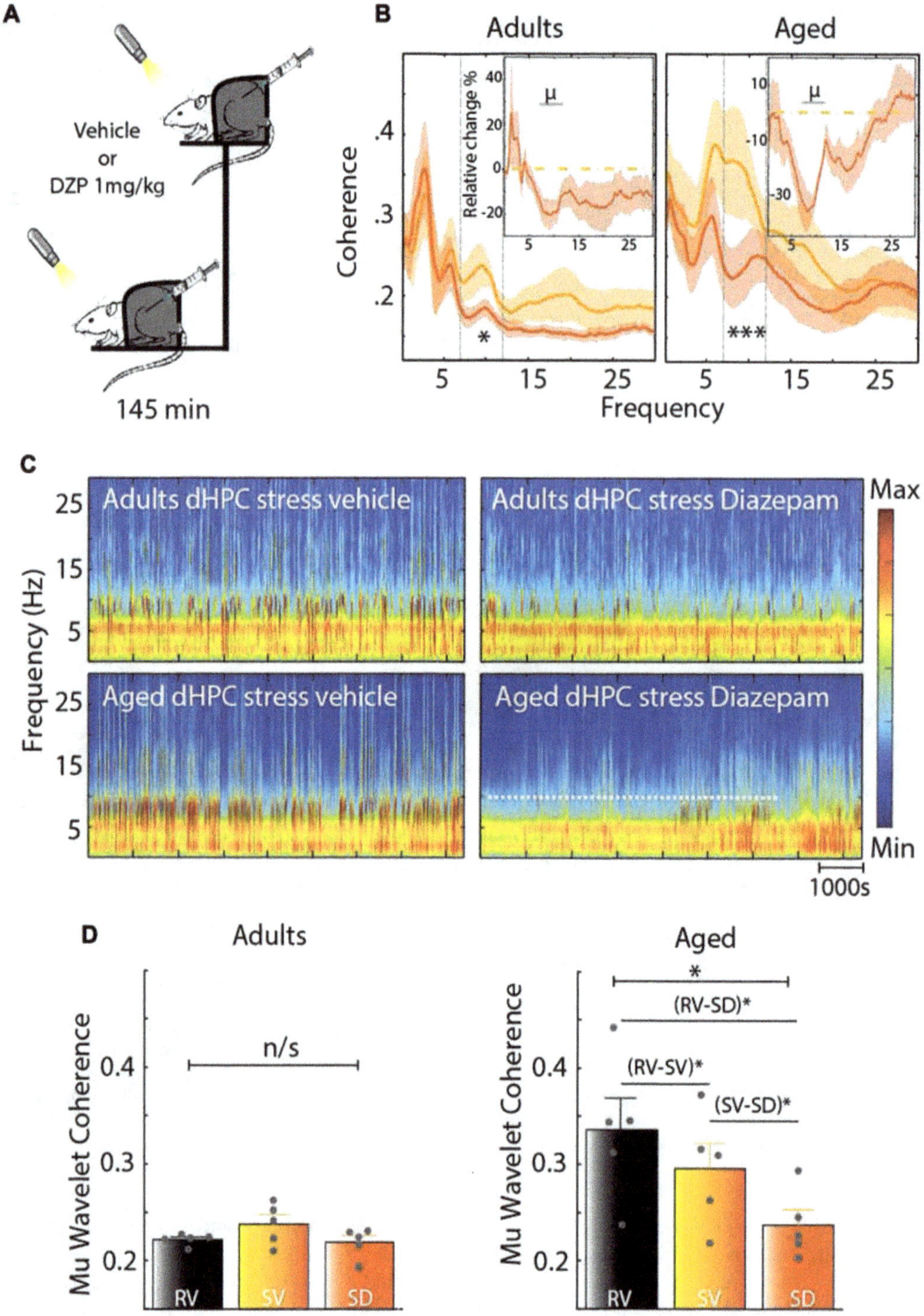

FIGURE 7 | (A) Stress protocol (same as **Figure 1**) with an acute i.p injection of Diazepam (DZP; 1 mg/kg) vs. vehicle, in adult rats (*n* = 5) and aged rats (*n* = 5). **(B)** Coherence for PFC-dHPC in stress condition, under vehicle (orange) and under DZP (orange red). Top right insert: averaged relative change in coherence, expressed in percentage of variation. Horizontal dashed line at zero indicates no change. Shaded area indicates SEM. A significant decrease was found in the Mu band both for adult (left panel) and aged rats (right panel; $*P_{adults} < 0.01$; $***P_{aged} < 0.001$, paired sample *T*-test). **(C)** Spectrogram of dHPC under stress for each group after a vehicle or DZP injection. Note the decrease of Mu-bursts under stress condition after an i.p injection of DZP. **(D)** PFC-dHPC coherence computed from the wavelet transform in the Mu range in three conditions (RV, rest vehicle; SV, stress vehicle; SD, Stress DZP (1 mg/kg)). Adults: $COH_{PFC\text{-}dHPC}$: Kruskal-Wallis test $\chi^2 = 1.63$, $P = 0.4431$ for the PFC-dHPC coherence. Aged: Kruskal-Wallis test: $\chi^2 = 6.02$, $*P < 0.05$, followed by paired-sample *t*-test and Holm-Bonferroni correction $*P_{RV\text{-}SD} = 0.0071$, $*P_{RV\text{-}SV} = 0.0102$, $*P_{SV\text{-}SD} = 0.0146$ for the PFC-dHPC coherence.

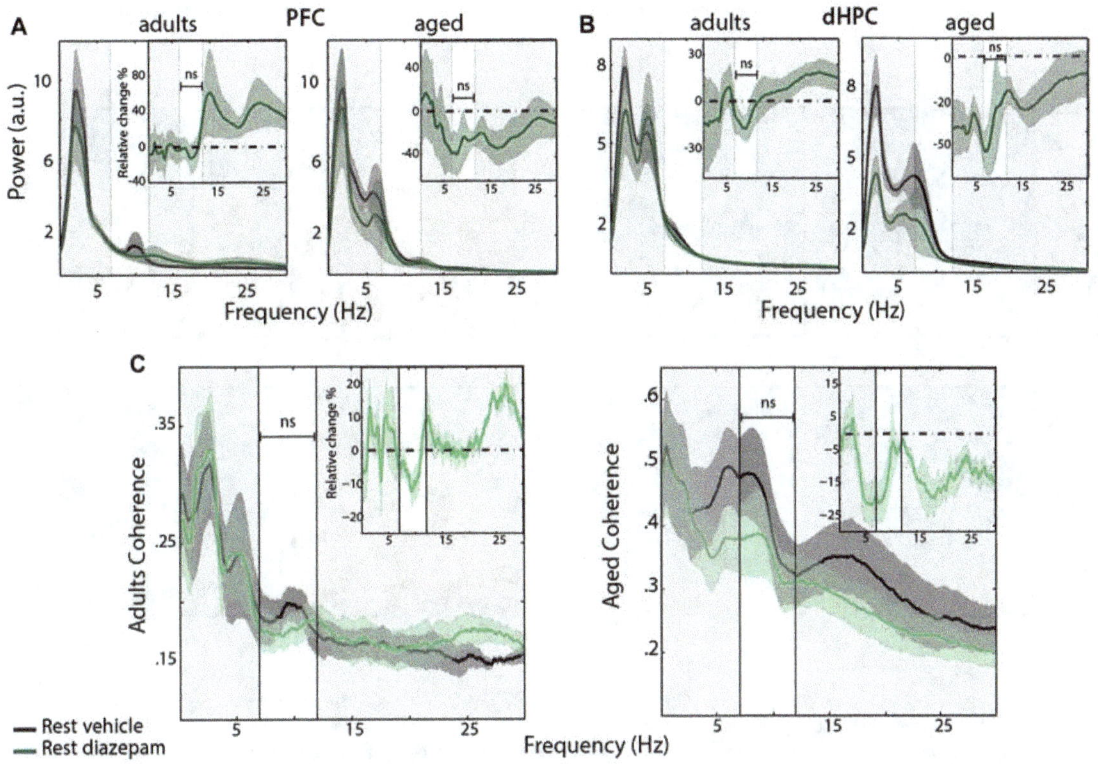

FIGURE 8 | (A,B) Power spectrum density of PFC (left) and dHPC (right) EFP recorded at rest with an acute i.p injection of vehicle (black) vs. DZP 1 mg/kg (green), and the averaged relative change due to DZP (insert). Horizontal dashed line at zero indicates no change. Data are presented as mean ± SEM and shaded area indicates SEM. No significant change was observed in this condition, in both age groups. PFC: $P_{adults} = 0.8491$; $P_{aged} = 0.2694$, paired sample T-test; dHPC: $P_{adults} = 0.4360$; $P_{aged} = 0.1473$, paired sample T-test. **(C)** Coherence for PFC-dHPC (adults (left) and aged (right) rats) in rest condition, under vehicle (black) and DZP (green). Top right insert: averaged relative change in coherence, expressed in percentage of variation. Horizontal dashed line at zero indicates no change. Shaded area indicates SEM. No significant differences were found in Mu band in both group ($P_{adults} = 0.2410$; $P_{aged} = 0.1159$, paired sample T-test).

a reduced inhibitory drive, acute administration of DZP may be more efficient in enhancing $GABA_A$ function in old rats (Reeves and Schweizer, 1983). Our results suggest a definite effect of age on stress response and DZP administration. How this relates to alterations in oscillatory activity will be the focus of further work.

Interpretation of the Mu-Burst Events

Mu-bursts, like spindles, have been traditionally observed in the cortex. Mu-bursts are associated with bursting in thalamic neurons and are believed to support distal communication between cortical areas and with the hippocampus (Fanselow et al., 2001). Although EFP reflect the activity of large groups of synapses, allowing identification of synchronous oscillatory activity within and across the brain areas, the exact anatomical origins of EFP must be tempered as voltage fluctuations can originate from volume conduction of distal signals. Our findings suggest that this was not the case here. First, we used a local reference (bipolar electrode) that minimizes electrical transfer (because common distal signals are subtracted), and provides the "intrinsic" EFP of the structure. Second, these bursts were found in adult rats in different combinations: only in the PFC, only in the dHPC, or in both structures. It is thus unlikely that dHPC bursts originate from the neocortex. Third, we also recorded from the parietal cortex, in the adult group and found that Mu-bursts could also be observed independently in two close neighboring structures (parietal and dHPC **Figure 4**). Therefore, our work, together with a previous study in the cerebellum (Hartmann and Bower, 1998), suggest that a much larger network of somatosensory structures (i.e., rather than the sole somatosensory cortex) may be flexibly involved in Mu-burst generation. The functional role of Mu-bursts is still a subject of debate in the literature: it has been hypothesized to reflect either a pathological (i.e., absence epilepsy, Inoue et al., 1990; Shaw, 2004, 2007) or physiological state (e.g., alertness or idling; Fanselow and Nicolelis, 1999; Fontanini and Katz, 2005). Even though we cannot definitely discard the hypothesis of an epileptic phenomenon, we believe that the effects of stress, age and anxiolytic we have observed on the 7–12 Hz bursts are of physiological background. First, similar "Mu rhythms" occur in 10%–30% of normal human subjects at rest (Nicolelis et al., 1995; Fontanini and Katz, 2005; Sakata et al., 2005; Tort et al., 2010) and have also been observed in cats (Guido and Weyand, 1995; Reinagel et al., 1999), guinea pigs (Edeline et al., 2000), rabbits (Swadlow and Gusev, 2002) and monkeys during periods of sensory processing (Ramcharan et al., 2000).

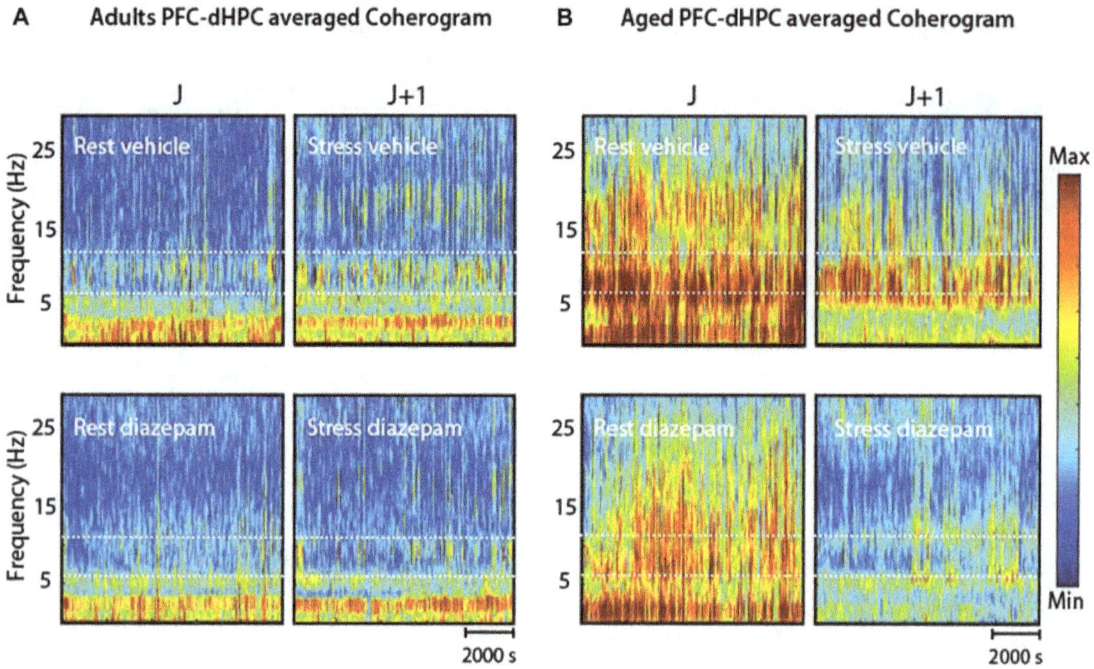

FIGURE 9 | (A) Coherogram (PFC-dHPC coherence over time) in four conditions (RV; SV; rest-DZP; stress-DZP) for adult rats. Stress enhanced synchronization between PFC-dHPC in 7–12 Hz in the adult group compared to rest. Acute DZP injection reduced this synchrony at rest and under stress. **(B)** In aged rats, a global decrease (all frequency ranges) was observed under acute stress, but was less pronounced in the 7–12 Hz range. Conversely, DZP alleviated the coherence mainly in the 7–12 Hz. The combination of DZP and stress nearly abolished PFC-dHPC coherence for all frequency ranges.

These data suggest a functionally important and conserved physiological phenomenon. Second, we and others have observed that rats respond rapidly to stimuli during periods where Mu-bursts are detected (Vergnes et al., 1982; Fanselow et al., 2001) and these prominent oscillatory activities are invariably suppressed by movement, but not affected by eye opening (Buzsaki et al., 1988). This suggests that Mu-bursts do not reflect an epileptic state, which would be associated with an impaired sensory detection, but rather a "hyper alert" state of vigilance (Fanselow et al., 2001; Sobolewski et al., 2011) or, alternatively, an idling state during quiet immobility (Fontanini and Katz, 2005). Finally, Mu bursts have been associated with sensory-motor processing, which may provide an alternative interpretation of the Mu-burst modifications with age we observed. Animals were indeed isolated from any sensory inputs that might affect Mu oscillations, by placing them in an acoustically insolated chamber. Yet we cannot totally exclude the possibility that Mu oscillations reflected the sensory-motor processing of WT, rather than the level of alertness associated with WT. Along the same line, alterations of Mu oscillations in aged rats may have been caused by sensory impairment associated with aging. We did not quantify sensory function *per se*, even if aged rats were able to quickly detect sound.

Given that a high occurrence of Mu rhythms has been observed in humans during mind wandering (Braboszcz and Delorme, 2011; Kerr et al., 2013), we propose Mu-bursts in rats could correspond to a similar state of internal attention (Corballis, 2013a,b). Mind-wandering consists in disengaging from goal-oriented interactions with the external environment, with attention being directed inwardly to self-generated, stimulus-independent and task-unrelated thoughts. It is plausible that stress and age favor this mind state together with a disengagement from the environment (Killingsworth and Gilbert, 2010; Forster et al., 2015). Nonetheless, our study puts forward that stress-induced theta in the HPC and PFC is composed of Mu-bursts related to arousal. This provides an interesting electrophysiological framework to study the neurobiology of anxiety and anxiolytics, especially in the elderly.

AUTHOR CONTRIBUTIONS

CS, ES, MS, PF and JM designed the study. ST and BD performed the manufacture of bipolar electrodes and surgery. ST, BD and SD realized the experiment. ST, SD, JN and PF analyzed the data. JM provided the animal facility, the experimental sites and the electrophysiological equipment. ST, JN, AM and PF wrote the manuscript with inputs from SD and JM.

FUNDING

This work was supported by the Ministère de l'Education nationale de l'Enseignement supérieur et de la Recherche, the region of Ile de France, Centre National de la Recherche

Scientifique (CNRS), the University Pierre et Marie Curie, the Agence Nationale pour la Recherche (ANR Programme Blanc 2012 for PF), the foundation for Medical Research (FRM, Equipe FRM DEQ2013326488 to PF), the Fédération pour la Recherche sur le Cerveau (FRC et les rotariens de France, "espoir en tête" 2012 to PF) and the IMI Newmeds grant (to ST). The laboratories of PF and JM are part of the École des Neurosciences de Paris Ile-de-France RTRA network. PF and JM are members of the Laboratory of Excellence, LabEx Bio-Psy, and of respectively the DHU Pepsy and the DHU Fast.

ACKNOWLEDGMENTS

We thank Marie-Louise Dongelmans and Sebastien Valverde for their critical reading of the article, Amélie Cougny and Vincent Grosjean for help with experiments during their internship, Thomas Watson and Lu Zhang for their critical interpretations of the Mu-bursts and the discussion of wavelet coherence analysis, Soizic Jezequel, Laura Legouestre, Grégoire Mauny and Laurent Poitier, for animal care and the animal facility of Université Pierre et Marie Curie based in the Hôpital Charles Foix.

REFERENCES

Adhikari, A. (2014). Distributed circuits underlying anxiety. *Front. Behav. Neurosci.* 8:112. doi: 10.3389/fnbeh.2014.00112

Adhikari, A., Lerner, T. N., Finkelstein, J., Pak, S., Jennings, J. H., Davidson, T. J., et al. (2015). Basomedial amygdala mediates top-down control of anxiety and fear. *Nature* 527, 179–185. doi: 10.1038/nature15698

Adhikari, A., Topiwala, M. A., and Gordon, J. A. (2010). Synchronized activity between the ventral hippocampus and the medial prefrontal cortex during anxiety. *Neuron* 65, 257–269. doi: 10.1016/j.neuron.2009.12.002

Aitake, M., Hori, E., Matsumoto, J., Umeno, K., Fukuda, M., Ono, T., et al. (2011). Sensory mismatch induces autonomic responses associated with hippocampal theta waves in rats. *Behav. Brain Res.* 220, 244–253. doi: 10.1016/j.bbr.2011.02.011

Ambrosini, M. V., Bruschelli, G., Mariucci, G., Mandile, P., and Giuditta, A. (1997). Post-trial sleep in old rats trained for a two-way active avoidance task. *Physiol. Behav.* 62, 773–778. doi: 10.1016/s0031-9384(97)00196-0

Aporti, F., Borsato, R., Calderini, G., Rubini, R., Toffano, G., Zanotti, A., et al. (1986). Age-Dependent spontaneous EEG bursts in rats: effects of brain phosphatidylserine. *Neurobiol. Aging* 7, 115–120. doi: 10.1016/0197-4580(86)90149-1

Balleine, B. W., and Curthoys, I. S. (1991). Differential effects of escapable and inescapable footshock on hippocampal theta activity. *Behav. Neurosci.* 105, 202–209. doi: 10.1037//0735-7044.105.1.202

Bannerman, D. M., Rawlins, J. N. P., McHugh, S. B., Deacon, R. M. J., Yee, B. K., Bast, T., et al. (2004). Regional dissociations within the hippocampus—memory and anxiety. *Neurosci. Biobehav. Rev.* 28, 273–283. doi: 10.1016/j.neubiorev.2004.03.004

Bannerman, D. M., Sprengel, R., Sanderson, D. J., McHugh, S. B., Rawlins, J. N. P., Monyer, H., et al. (2014). Hippocampal synaptic plasticity, spatial memory and anxiety. *Nat. Rev. Neurosci.* 15, 181–192. doi: 10.1038/nrn3677

Barrientos, R. M., Frank, M. G., Watkins, L. R., and Maier, S. F. (2012). Aging-related changes in neuroimmune-endocrine function: implications for hippocampal-dependent cognition. *Horm. Behav.* 62, 219–227. doi: 10.1016/j.yhbeh.2012.02.010

Barrientos, R. M., Thompson, V. M., Kitt, M. M., Amat, J., Hale, M. W., Frank, M. G., et al. (2015). Greater glucocorticoid receptor activation in hippocampus of aged rats sensitizes microglia. *Neurobiol. Aging* 36, 1483–1495. doi: 10.1016/j.neurobiolaging.2014.12.003

Battaglia, F. P., Benchenane, K., Sirota, A., Pennartz, C. M. A., and Wiener, S. I. (2011). The hippocampus: hub of brain network communication for memory. *Trends Cogn. Sci.* 15, 310–318. doi: 10.1016/j.tics.2011.05.008

Bessa, J. M., Mesquita, A. R., Oliveira, M., Pêgo, J. M., Cerqueira, J. J., Palha, J. A., et al. (2009). A trans-dimensional approach to the behavioral aspects of depression. *Front. Behav. Neurosci.* 3:1. doi: 10.3389/neuro.08.001.2009

Bland, B. H. (1986). The physiology and pharmacology of hippocampal formation theta rhythms. *Prog. Neurobiol.* 26, 1–54. doi: 10.1016/0301-0082(86)90019-5

Bokil, H., Andrews, P., Kulkarni, J. E., Mehta, S., and Mitra, P. P. (2010). Chronux: a platform for analyzing neural signals. *J. Neurosci. Methods* 192, 146–151. doi: 10.1016/j.jneumeth.2010.06.020

Botta, P., Demmou, L., Kasugai, Y., Markovic, M., Xu, C., Fadok, J. P., et al. (2015). Regulating anxiety with extrasynaptic inhibition. *Nat. Neurosci.* 18, 1493–1500. doi: 10.1038/nn1215-1862a

Braboszcz, C., and Delorme, A. (2011). Lost in thoughts: neural markers of low alertness during mind wandering. *Neuroimage* 54, 3040–3047. doi: 10.1016/j.neuroimage.2010.10.008

Buechel, H. M., Popovic, J., Staggs, K., Anderson, K. L., Thibault, O., and Blalock, E. M. (2014). Aged rats are hypo-responsive to acute restraint: implications for psychosocial stress in aging. *Front. Aging Neurosci.* 6:13. doi: 10.3389/fnagi.2014.00013

Buzsáki, G. (2002). Theta oscillations in the hippocampus. *Neuron* 33, 325–340. doi: 10.1016/S0896-6273(02)00586-X

Buzsáki, G., Bickford, R. G., Armstrong, D. M., Ponomareff, G., Chen, K. S., Ruiz, R., et al. (1988). Electric activity in the neocortex of freely moving young and aged rats. *Neuroscience* 26, 735–744. doi: 10.1016/0306-4522(88)90095-4

Buzsaki, G., Bickford, R. G., Ponomareff, G., Thal, L. J., Mandel, R., and Gage, F. H. (1988). Nucleus basalis and thalamic control of neocortical activity in the freely moving rat. *J. Neurosci.* 8, 4007–4026.

Calderini, G., Bonetti, A. C., Aldinio, A., Savoini, G., Di Perri, B., Biggio, G., et al. (1981). Functional interaction between benzodiazepine and GABA recognition sites in aged rats. *Neurobiol. Aging* 2, 309–313. doi: 10.1016/0197-4580(81)90040-3

Coll, M.-P., Press, C., Hobson, H., Catmur, C., and Bird, G. (2017). Crossmodal classification of mu rhythm activity during action observation and execution suggests specificity to somatosensory features of actions. *J. Neurosci.* 37, 5936–5947. doi: 10.1523/jneurosci.3393-16.2017

Corballis, M. C. (2013a). The wandering rat: response to Suddendorf. *Trends Cogn. Sci.* 17:152. doi: 10.1016/j.tics.2013.01.012

Corballis, M. C. (2013b). Wandering tales: Evolutionary origins of mental time travel and language. *Front. Psychol.* 4:485. doi: 10.3389/fpsyg.2013.00485

Davis, M., Walker, D. L., Miles, L., and Grillon, C. (2010). Phasic vs. sustained fear in rats and humans: role of the extended amygdala in fear vs. anxiety. *Neuropsychopharmacology* 35, 105–135. doi: 10.1038/npp.2009.109

Dimpfel, W., Spüler, M., and Borbe, H. O. (1988). Monitoring of the effects of antidepressant drugs in the freely moving rat by radioelectroencephalography (tele-stereo-EEG). *Neuropsychobiology* 19, 116–120. doi: 10.1159/000118445

Duvarci, S., Bauer, E. P., and Paré, D. (2009). The bed nucleus of the stria terminalis mediates inter-individual variations in anxiety and fear. *J. Neurosci.* 29, 10357–10361. doi: 10.1523/JNEUROSCI.2119-09.2009

Edeline, J. M., Manunta, Y., and Hennevin, E. (2000). Auditory thalamus neurons during sleep: changes in frequency selectivity, threshold, and receptive field size. *J. Neurophysiol.* 84, 934–952.

Fanselow, M. S., and Dong, H.-W. (2010). Are the dorsal and ventral hippocampus functionally distinct structures? *Neuron* 65, 7–19. doi: 10.1016/j.neuron.2009.11.031

Fanselow, E. E., and Nicolelis, M. A. (1999). Behavioral modulation of tactile responses in the rat somatosensory system. *J. Neurosci.* 19, 7603–7616.

Fanselow, E. E., Sameshima, K., Baccala, L. A., and Nicolelis, M. A. L. (2001). Thalamic bursting in rats during different awake behavioral states. *Proc. Natl. Acad. Sci. U S A* 98, 15330–15335. doi: 10.1073/pnas.261273898

Fontanini, A., and Katz, D. B. (2005). 7 to 12 Hz activity in rat gustatory cortex reflects disengagement from a fluid self-administration task. *J. Neurophysiol.* 93, 2832–2840. doi: 10.1152/jn.01035.2004

Forster, S., Nunez Elizalde, A. O., Castle, E., and Bishop, S. J. (2015). Unraveling the anxious mind: anxiety, worry, and frontal engagement in sustained attention versus off-task processing. *Cereb. Cortex* 25, 609–618. doi: 10.1093/cercor/bht248

Fries, P. (2015). Rhythms for cognition: communication through coherence. *Neuron* 88, 220–235. doi: 10.1016/j.neuron.2015.09.034

Gastaut, H., Naquet, R., and Gastaut, Y. (1965). A study of the mu rhythm in subjects lacking one or more limbs. *Electroenceph. Clin. Neurophysiol.* 18, 720–721.

Gleason, P. P., Schulz, R., Smith, N. L., Newsom, J. T., Kroboth, P. D., Kroboth, F. J., et al. (1998). Correlates and prevalence of benzodiazepine use in community-dwelling elderly. *J. Gen. Intern. Med.* 13, 243–250.

Guido, W., and Weyand, T. (1995). Burst responses in thalamic relay cells of the awake behaving cat. *J. Neurophysiol.* 74, 1782–1786.

Hartmann, M. J., and Bower, J. M. (1998). Oscillatory activity in the cerebellar hemispheres of unrestrained rats. *J. Neurophysiol.* 80, 1598–1604.

Hoekzema, E., Rojas, S., Herance, R., Pareto, D., Abad, S., Jiménez, X., et al. (2012). *In vivo* molecular imaging of the GABA/benzodiazepine receptor complex in the aged rat brain. *Neurobiol. Aging* 33, 1457–1465. doi: 10.1016/j.neurobiolaging.2010.12.006

Hsiao, Y.-T., Jou, S.-B., Yi, P.-L., and Chang, F.-C. (2012). Activation of GABAergic pathway by hypocretin in the median raphe nucleus (MRN) mediates stress-induced theta rhythm in rats. *Behav. Brain Res.* 233, 224–231. doi: 10.1016/j.bbr.2012.05.002

Inoue, M., Peeters, B. W., van Luijtelaar, E. L., Vossen, J. M., and Coenen, A. M. (1990). Spontaneous occurrence of spike-wave discharges in five inbred strains of rats. *Physiol. Behav.* 48, 199–201. doi: 10.1016/0031-9384(90)90285-c

Jacinto, L. R., Reis, J. S., Dias, N. S., Cerqueira, J. J., Correia, J. H., and Sousa, N. (2013). Stress affects theta activity in limbic networks and impairs novelty-induced exploration and familiarization. *Front. Behav. Neurosci.* 7:127. doi: 10.3389/fnbeh.2013.00127

Kerr, C. E., Sacchet, M. D., Lazar, S. W., Moore, C. I., and Jones, S. R. (2013). Mindfulness starts with the body: somatosensory attention and top-down modulation of cortical α rhythms in mindfulness meditation. *Front. Hum. Neurosci.* 7:12. doi: 10.3389/fnhum.2013.00012

Killingsworth, M. A., and Gilbert, D. T. (2010). A wandering mind is an unhappy mind. *Science* 330:932. doi: 10.1126/science.1192439

Kim, J. J., and Diamond, D. M. (2002). The stressed hippocampus, synaptic plasticity and lost memories. *Nat. Rev. Neurosci.* 3, 453–462. doi: 10.1038/nrn849

Kirby, M., Denihan, A., Bruce, I., Radic, A., Coakley, D., and Lawlor, B. A. (1999). Benzodiazepine use among the elderly in the community. *Int. J. Geriatr. Psychiatry* 14, 280–284. doi: 10.1002/(sici)1099-1166(199904)14:4<280::aid-gps898>3.3.co;2-f

Kramis, R., Vanderwolf, C. H., and Bland, B. H. (1975). Two types of hippocampal rhythmical slow activity in both the rabbit and the rat: relations to behavior and effects of atropine, diethyl ether, urethane, and pentobarbital. *Exp. Neurol.* 49, 58–85. doi: 10.1016/0014-4886(75)90195-8

Lachaux, J. P., Lutz, A., Rudrauf, D., Cosmelli, D., Le Van Quyen, M., Martinerie, J., et al. (2002). Estimating the time-course of coherence between single-trial brain signals: an introduction to wavelet coherence. *Neurophysiol. Clin.* 32, 157–174. doi: 10.1016/s0987-7053(02)00301-5

Leite-Almeida, H., Almeida-Torres, L., Mesquita, A. R., Pertovaara, A., Sousa, N., Cerqueira, J. J., et al. (2009). The impact of age on emotional and cognitive behaviours triggered by experimental neuropathy in rats. *Pain* 144, 57–65. doi: 10.1016/j.pain.2009.02.024

Le Van Quyen, M., Foucher, J., Lachaux, J., Rodriguez, E., Lutz, A., Martinerie, J., et al. (2001). Comparison of Hilbert transform and wavelet methods for the analysis of neuronal synchrony. *J. Neurosci. Methods* 111, 83–98. doi: 10.1016/s0165-0270(01)00372-7

Lindenberger, U. (2014). Human cognitive aging: corriger la fortune? *Science* 346, 572–578. doi: 10.1126/science.1254403

Marini, G., Ceccarelli, P., and Mancia, M. (2008). Characterization of the 7-12 Hz EEG oscillations during immobile waking and REM sleep in behaving rats. *Clin. Neurophysiol.* 119, 315–320. doi: 10.1016/j.clinph.2007.09.142

Morrison, J. H., and Baxter, M. G. (2012). The ageing cortical synapse: hallmarks and implications for cognitive decline. *Nat. Rev. Neurosci.* 13, 240–250. doi: 10.1038/nrn3200

Nicolelis, M., Baccala, L., Lin, R. C., and Chapin, J. K. (1995). Sensorimotor encoding by synchronous neural ensemble activity at multiple levels of the somatosensory system. *Science* 268, 1353–1358. doi: 10.1126/science.7761855

Nicolelis, M. A. L., and Fanselow, E. E. (2002). Thalamocortical [correction of Thalamcortical] optimization of tactile processing according to behavioral state. *Nat. Neurosci.* 5, 517–523. doi: 10.1038/nn0602-517

Padilla-Coreano, N., Bolkan, S. S., Pierce, G. M., Blackman, D. R., Hardin, W. D., Garcia-Garcia, A. L., et al. (2016). Direct ventral hippocampal-prefrontal input is required for anxiety-related neural activity and behavior. *Neuron* 89, 857–866. doi: 10.1016/j.neuron.2016.01.011

Parent, M. A., Wang, L., Su, J., Netoff, T., and Yuan, L. L. (2010). Identification of the hippocampal input to medial prefrontal cortex *in vitro*. *Cereb. Cortex* 20, 393–403. doi: 10.1093/cercor/bhp108

Paxinos, G., and Watson, C. (2006). *The Rat Brain in Stereotaxic Coordinates*. 6th Edn., Cambridge, MA: Academic Press.

Pêgo, J. M., Morgado, P., Pinto, L. G., Cerqueira, J. J., Almeida, O. F. X., and Sousa, N. (2008). Dissociation of the morphological correlates of stress-induced anxiety and fear. *Eur. J. Neurosci.* 27, 1503–1516. doi: 10.1111/j.1460-9568.2008.06112.x

Pietrelli, A., Lopez-Costa, J., Goñi, R., Brusco, A., and Basso, N. (2012). Aerobic exercise prevents age-dependent cognitive decline and reduces anxiety-related behaviors in middle-aged and old rats. *Neuroscience* 202, 252–266. doi: 10.1016/j.neuroscience.2011.11.054

Popa, D., Duvarci, S., Popescu, A. T., Léna, C., and Paré, D. (2010). Coherent amygdalocortical theta promotes fear memory consolidation during paradoxical sleep. *Proc. Natl. Acad. Sci. U S A* 107, 6516–6519. doi: 10.1073/pnas.0913016107

Prenderville, J. A., Kennedy, P. J., Dinan, T. G., and Cryan, J. F. (2015). Adding fuel to the fire: the impact of stress on the ageing brain. *Trends Neurosci.* 38, 13–25. doi: 10.1016/j.tins.2014.11.001

Rajasethupathy, P., Sankaran, S., Marshel, J. H., Kim, C. K., Ferenczi, E., Lee, S. Y., et al. (2015). Projections from neocortex mediate top-down control of memory retrieval. *Nature* 526, 653–659. doi: 10.1038/nature15389

Ramcharan, E. J., Cox, C. L., Zhan, X. J., Sherman, S. M., and Gnadt, J. W. (2000). Cellular mechanisms underlying activity patterns in the monkey thalamus during visual behavior. *J. Neurophysiol.* 84, 1982–1987.

Reeves, P. M., and Schweizer, M. P. (1983). Aging, diazepam exposure and benzodiazepine receptors in rat cortex. *Brain Res.* 270, 376–379. doi: 10.1016/0006-8993(83)90618-2

Reinagel, P., Godwin, D., Sherman, S. M., and Koch, C. (1999). Encoding of visual information by LGN bursts. *J. Neurophysiol.* 81, 2558–2569.

Roberts, J. A., Boonstra, T. W., and Breakspear, M. (2015). The heavy tail of the human brain. *Curr. Opin. Neurobiol.* 31, 164–172. doi: 10.1016/j.conb.2014.10.014

Robinson, P. F., and Gilmore, S. A. (1980). Spontaneous generalized spike-wave discharges in the electrocorticograms of albino rats. *Brain Res.* 201, 452–458. doi: 10.1016/0006-8993(80)91052-5

Rocher, C., Spedding, M., Munoz, C., and Jay, T. M. (2004). Acute stress-induced changes in hippocampal/prefrontal circuits in rats: effects of antidepressants. *Cereb. Cortex* 14, 224–229. doi: 10.1093/cercor/bhg122

Sakata, S., Yamamori, T., and Sakurai, Y. (2005). 7–12 Hz cortical oscillations: behavioral context and dynamics of prefrontal neuronal ensembles. *Neuroscience* 134, 1099–1111. doi: 10.1016/j.neuroscience.2005.05.018

Scheffzük, C., Kukushka, V. I., Vyssotski, A. L., Draguhn, A., Tort, A. B. L., and Brankačk, J. (2013). Global slowing of network oscillations in mouse neocortex by diazepam. *Neuropharmacology* 65, 123–133. doi: 10.1016/j.neuropharm.2012.09.014

Schmidt, S., Redecker, C., Bruehl, C., and Witte, O. W. (2010). Age-related decline of functional inhibition in rat cortex. *Neurobiol. Aging* 31, 504–511. doi: 10.1016/j.neurobiolaging.2008.04.006

Sebban, C., Tesolin-Decros, B., Ciprian-Ollivier, J., Perret, L., and Spedding, M. (2002). Effects of phencyclidine (PCP) and MK 801 on the EEGq in the prefrontal cortex of conscious rats; antagonism by clozapine, and antagonists of AMPA-, α_1- and 5-HT$_{2A}$-receptors. *Br. J. Pharmacol.* 135, 65–78. doi: 10.1038/sj.bjp.0704451

Sebban, C., Tesolin-Decros, B., Millan, M. J., and Spedding, M. (1999a). Contrasting EEG profiles elicited by antipsychotic agents in the prefrontal cortex of the conscious rat: antagonism of the effects of clozapine by modafinil. *Br. J. Pharmacol.* 128, 1055–1063. doi: 10.1038/sj.bjp.0702893

Sebban, C., Zhang, X. Q., Tesolin-Decros, B., Millan, M. J., and Spedding, M. (1999b). Changes in EEG spectral power in the prefrontal cortex of conscious rats elicited by drugs interacting with dopaminergic and noradrenergic transmission. *Br. J. Pharmacol.* 128, 1045–1054. doi: 10.1038/sj.bjp.0702894

Shaw, F.-Z. (2004). Is spontaneous high-voltage rhythmic spike discharge in Long Evans rats an absence-like seizure activity? *J. Neurophysiol.* 91, 63–77. doi: 10.1152/jn.00487.2003

Shaw, F.-Z. (2007). 7–12 Hz high-voltage rhythmic spike discharges in rats evaluated by antiepileptic drugs and flicker stimulation. *J. Neurophysiol.* 97, 238–247. doi: 10.1152/jn.00340.2006

Sobolewski, A., Swiejkowski, D. A., Wróbel, A., and Kublik, E. (2011). The 5–12Hz oscillations in the barrel cortex of awake rats—sustained attention during behavioral idling? *Clin. Neurophysiol.* 122, 483–489. doi: 10.1016/j.clinph.2010.08.006

Swadlow, H. A., and Gusev, A. G. (2002). Receptive-field construction in cortical inhibitory interneurons. *Nat. Neurosci.* 5, 403–404. doi: 10.1038/nn847

Sylvers, P., Lilienfeld, S. O., and LaPrairie, J. L. (2011). Differences between trait fear and trait anxiety: implications for psychopathology. *Clin. Psychol. Rev.* 31, 122–137. doi: 10.1016/j.cpr.2010.08.004

Tan, K. R., Rudolph, U., and Lüscher, C. (2011). Hooked on benzodiazepines: GABA$_A$ receptor subtypes and addiction. *Trends Neurosci.* 34, 188–197. doi: 10.1016/j.tins.2011.01.004

Tort, A. B. L., Fontanini, A., Kramer, M. A., Jones-Lush, L. M., Kopell, N. J., and Katz, D. B. (2010). Cortical networks produce three distinct 7–12 Hz rhythms during single sensory responses in the awake rat. *J. Neurosci.* 30, 4315–4324. doi: 10.1523/JNEUROSCI.6051-09.2010

Tovote, P., Fadok, J. P., and Lüthi, A. (2015). Neuronal circuits for fear and anxiety. *Nat. Rev. Neurosci.* 16, 317–331. doi: 10.1038/nrn3945

van Lier, H., Drinkenburg, W. H. I. M., van Eeten, Y. J. W., and Coenen, A. M. L. (2004). Effects of diazepam and zolpidem on EEG β frequencies are behavior-specific in rats. *Neuropharmacology* 47, 163–174. doi: 10.1016/j.neuropharm.2004.03.017

Vanderwolf, C. H. (1969). Hippocampal electrical activity and voluntary movement in the rat. *Electroencephalogr. Clin. Neurophysiol.* 26, 407–418. doi: 10.1016/0013-4694(69)90092-3

Vergnes, M., Marescaux, C., Micheletti, G., Reis, J., Depaulis, A., Rumbach, L., et al. (1982). Spontaneous paroxysmal electroclinical patterns in rat: a model of generalized non-convulsive epilepsy. *Neurosci. Lett.* 33, 97–101. doi: 10.1016/0304-3940(82)90136-7

Verwer, R. W., Meijer, R. J., Van Uum, H. F., and Witter, M. P. (1997). Collateral projections from the rat hippocampal formation to the lateral and medial prefrontal cortex. *Hippocampus* 7, 397–402. doi: 10.1002/(sici)1098-1063(1997)7:4<397::aid-hipo5>3.3.co;2-a

Wells, C. E., Amos, D. P., Jeewajee, A., Douchamps, V., Rodgers, J., O'Keefe, J., et al. (2013). Novelty and anxiolytic drugs dissociate two components of hippocampal theta in behaving rats. *J. Neurosci.* 33, 8650–8667. doi: 10.1523/JNEUROSCI.5040-12.2013

Wiest, M. C., and Nicolelis, M. A. L. (2003). Behavioral detection of tactile stimuli during 7–12 Hz cortical oscillations in awake rats. *Nat. Neurosci.* 6, 913–914. doi: 10.1038/nn1107

Wikinski, S. I., Acosta, G. B., Gravielle, M. C., Bonavita, C. D., Bisagno, V., Fiszer de Plazas, S., et al. (2001). Diazepam fails to potentiate GABA-induced chloride uptake and to produce anxiolytic-like action in aged rats. *Pharmacol. Biochem. Behav.* 68, 721–727. doi: 10.1016/s0091-3057(01)00480-4

Winson, J. (1978). Loss of hippocampal theta rhythm results in spatial memory deficit in the rat. *Science* 201, 160–163. doi: 10.1126/science.663646

Xu, L., Holscher, C., Anwyl, R., and Rowan, M. J. (1998). Glucocorticoid receptor and protein/RNA synthesis-dependent mechanisms underlie the control of synaptic plasticity by stress. *Proc. Natl. Acad. Sci. U S A* 95, 3204–3208. doi: 10.1073/pnas.95.6.3204

Yamamoto, J., Suh, J., Takeuchi, D., and Tonegawa, S. (2014). Successful execution of working memory linked to synchronized high-frequency γ oscillations. *Cell* 157, 845–857. doi: 10.1016/j.cell.2014.04.009

Yu, Z. Y., Wang, W., Fritschy, J. M., Witte, O. W., and Redecker, C. (2006). Changes in neocortical and hippocampal GABA$_A$ receptor subunit distribution during brain maturation and aging. *Brain Res.* 1099, 73–81. doi: 10.1016/j.brainres.2006.04.118

5

Brain Network Modularity Predicts Exercise-Related Executive Function Gains in Older Adults

Pauline L. Baniqued [1,2*], *Courtney L. Gallen* [1], *Michelle W. Voss* [3], *Agnieszka Z. Burzynska* [4], *Chelsea N. Wong* [2], *Gillian E. Cooke* [2,5], *Kristin Duffy* [2], *Jason Fanning* [6,7], *Diane K. Ehlers* [6], *Elizabeth A. Salerno* [6], *Susan Aguiñaga* [6], *Edward McAuley* [2,6], *Arthur F. Kramer* [2,8] and *Mark D'Esposito* [1]

[1] Helen Wills Neuroscience Institute, University of California, Berkeley, Berkeley, CA, United States, [2] Beckman Institute for Advanced Science and Technology, University of Illinois at Urbana-Champaign, Urbana, IL, United States, [3] Department of Psychological and Brain Sciences, University of Iowa, Iowa City, IA, United States, [4] Department of Human Development and Family Studies, Colorado State University, Fort Collins, CO, United States, [5] Interdisciplinary Health Sciences Institute, University of Illinois at Urbana-Champaign, Urbana, IL, United States, [6] Department of Kinesiology and Community Health, University of Illinois at Urbana-Champaign, Urbana, IL, United States, [7] Department of Internal Medicine-Gerontology, Wake Forest School of Medicine, Winston-Salem, NC, United States, [8] Psychology Department and Mechanical and Industrial Engineering Department, Northeastern University, Boston, MA, United States

***Correspondence:**
Pauline L. Baniqued
paulineb@berkeley.edu

Recent work suggests that the brain can be conceptualized as a network comprised of groups of sub-networks or modules. The extent of segregation between modules can be quantified with a modularity metric, where networks with high modularity have dense connections within modules and sparser connections between modules. Previous work has shown that higher modularity predicts greater improvements after cognitive training in patients with traumatic brain injury and in healthy older and young adults. It is not known, however, whether modularity can also predict cognitive gains after a physical exercise intervention. Here, we quantified modularity in older adults (N = 128, mean age = 64.74) who underwent one of the following interventions for 6 months (NCT01472744 on ClinicalTrials.gov): (1) aerobic exercise in the form of brisk walking (Walk), (2) aerobic exercise in the form of brisk walking plus nutritional supplement (Walk+), (3) stretching, strengthening and stability (SSS), or (4) dance instruction. After the intervention, the Walk, Walk+ and SSS groups showed gains in cardiorespiratory fitness (CRF), with larger effects in both walking groups compared to the SSS and Dance groups. The Walk, Walk+ and SSS groups also improved in executive function (EF) as measured by reasoning, working memory, and task-switching tests. In the Walk, Walk+, and SSS groups that improved in EF, higher baseline modularity was positively related to EF gains, even after controlling for age, in-scanner motion and baseline EF. No relationship between modularity and EF gains was observed in the Dance group, which did not show training-related gains in CRF or EF control. These results are consistent with previous studies demonstrating that individuals with a more modular brain network organization are more responsive to cognitive training. These findings suggest that the predictive power of modularity may be generalizable across interventions aimed to enhance aspects of cognition and that, especially in low-performing individuals, global network properties can capture individual differences in neuroplasticity.

Keywords: executive function, cognitive control, functional connectivity, exercise, brain network modularity

INTRODUCTION

Aging is accompanied by changes in cognition and brain function, yet there is individual variability in the extent to which older adults experience such effects (Wilson et al., 2002; Raz et al., 2005; Fabiani, 2012; Burzynska et al., 2015; Salthouse, 2016). Individual differences in age-related cognitive decline, particularly in executive function processes, are related to changes in structural and functional connectivity between brain regions (Andrews-Hanna et al., 2007; Damoiseaux et al., 2008; Kennedy and Raz, 2009; Madden et al., 2009, 2012). One method to quantify these complex interactions is to conceptualize the brain as a network comprised of sub-networks, or modules (Newman and Girvan, 2004; Newman, 2006b; Chen et al., 2008; Bullmore and Sporns, 2009; Meunier et al., 2010; Betzel et al., 2014; Bertolero et al., 2015). The extent of a module's segregation from the rest of the network can be quantified with a modularity metric (Newman and Girvan, 2004), where networks with high modularity have many connections within modules and fewer connections between modules. Computational models suggest that a modular network organization allows for a system that is more adaptable to new environments (Kashtan and Alon, 2005; Clune et al., 2013; Tosh and McNally, 2015), suggesting a role for network modularity in supporting complex behaviors like executive function. Compared to young adults, older adults have less modular brain networks (Chen et al., 2011; Onoda and Yamaguchi, 2013; Betzel et al., 2014; Geerligs et al., 2015) with pronounced age-related differences in sub-networks that support "associative" processes, such as executive function (Chan et al., 2014). Taken together, these findings suggest that more modular brain networks enable complex cognitive processes and neuroplasticity and, further, may provide insight into the mechanisms underlying the effectiveness of interventions geared toward ameliorating age-related cognitive decline.

Recent work has demonstrated that individual differences in brain network modularity can predict the extent to which individuals improve after cognitive interventions aimed to improve executive function. Specifically, higher baseline modularity (i.e., measured prior to the intervention) quantified during a task-free "resting state" predicted greater improvements after cognitive training in patients with traumatic brain injury (Arnemann et al., 2015) and more recently, in healthy older (Gallen et al., 2016) and young adults (Baniqued et al., 2015). Importantly, modularity predicted training gains even after controlling for baseline cognitive performance. These findings suggest that the informative nature of such individual differences in brain network organization can be used to maximize intervention effectiveness, such as by modifying training intensity or duration, especially in populations where behavioral measures may be difficult to collect (Gabrieli et al., 2015). Previous studies have examined other neural metrics in relation to learning and training responses (Erickson et al., 2010; Basak et al., 2011; Vo et al., 2011; Mathewson et al., 2012), but have often focused on specific brain regions related to specific types of interventions. As modularity has been shown to be reliable in individuals across sessions (Stevens et al., 2012; Cao et al., 2014) and predictive of cognitive gains across a variety of populations and training protocols, modularity may be a unifying biomarker that indexes an individual's potential for adaptive reorganization with intervention.

In addition to cognitive training interventions, cost-effective and easily accessible physical activity interventions involving brisk walking have been shown to have rehabilitative and protective effects on brain function in older adults (Kramer et al., 2006; Voss et al., 2013c). Further, there are significant individual differences in responsiveness to exercise training, with factors such as initial levels of heart rate and blood pressure determining gains in cardiorespiratory fitness (Bouchard and Rankinen, 2001). Although we have previously found that individual differences in brain network modularity can predict training-related gains after cognitive training (Arnemann et al., 2015; Baniqued et al., 2015; Gallen et al., 2016), it is not yet known whether the relationship between modularity and training gains is generalizable to interventions aimed to enhance executive function in older adults. Although there are several graph theoretical metrics, we were specifically interested if this relationship between pre-intervention brain modularity and training gains can also be found in a different, non-cognitive training intervention, such as a physical exercise intervention.

Specifically, we hypothesize that modularity reflects an individual's readiness to engage in and benefit from training. A recent study demonstrated that individuals with higher general intelligence show smaller connectivity changes between a resting state and task states, suggesting the existence of a more "optimal" network organization that provides more efficient reconfiguration during performance of various tasks (Schultz and Cole, 2016). Similar to this idea, we hypothesize that a more optimal—more modular network configuration is better able to transition to task states demanded by the interventions; it is more adaptable. In the context of the current study, a more modular brain network may potentiate the rehabilitative and protective effects of physical exercise on the aging brain, leading to greater improvements in executive function.

Here, we examined brain network modularity in older adults who underwent a 6-month exercise training intervention. Specifically, we tested the hypothesis that higher baseline modularity predicts larger exercise-related gains in cognition. The current study employed a broad battery of cognitive tests to assess intervention-related gains in executive function, episodic memory, vocabulary and perceptual speed. Here, we focused on the relationship between baseline modularity and improvements in executive function, as these processes show pronounced age-related decline and exercise-related changes (Hillman et al., 2008; Voss et al., 2013c; Kawagoe et al., 2017).

MATERIALS AND METHODS

Participants

Healthy, low active, older adults (N = 247) aged 60–80 from the Urbana-Champaign community participated in a randomized controlled exercise trial (https://clinicaltrials.gov/ct2/show/NCT01472744; see Voss et al., 2016; Burzynska et al., 2017; Ehlers et al., 2017a,b; Fanning et al., 2017, for data published from this same cohort). All participants provided informed consent and the University of Illinois Institutional Review Board approved all procedures used in the study. Selection criteria consisted of the following, (1) >75% right-handed on the Edinburgh Handedness Questionnaire; (2) normal or corrected-to-normal vision of at least 20/40; (3) no color-blindness; (4) no history of stroke, transient ischemic attack, or head trauma; (5) >23 score on Mini-Mental State Examination (MMSE); (6) >21 score on Telephone Interview of Cognitive Status (TICS); (7) <10 score on Geriatric Depression Scale (GDS); (8) reported that they engaged in moderate intensity exercise for 30+ min no more than twice a week in the last 6 months and 9) screened for safe participation in an MRI environment (e.g., no claustrophobia or metallic implants). In all analyses presented here, we further excluded participants with MMSE scores less than 27 ($N = 26$), as a more stringent criterion is recommended in highly educated samples such as in the current study (O'Bryant et al., 2008). Summary demographics for included participants are provided in **Table 1**. Additional data were excluded on a case-by-case basis during data quality procedures applied to each behavioral measure. Specifically, cognitive measures greater than 3 SD from the mean were excluded. After this step, to reduce the influence of remaining extreme values, scores greater than 3 SD from the recomputed mean were winsorized (Tukey, 1962; Wilcox, 2005) to the appropriate cut-off value (3 SD below or above the mean). Analyses involving only fitness or behavioral scores were performed on the larger sample ($N = 188$), prior to exclusion due to MRI data quality, but effects were similar in the MRI sample ($N = 128$).

For the MRI data, we excluded one participant with incomplete resting state data, one participant with structural abnormalities (see section MRI Acquisition and Processing for more details), and 39 participants who reported taking medications known to influence the central nervous system. Thirty-five participants whose resting state scans contained more than 10% of volumes with movement greater than 0.50 framewise displacement (FD) or any volume with a maximum absolute displacement of 4.0 mm were excluded. MRI data were not collected for five subjects. Demographics for this reduced sample are provided in **Table 1**.

Protocol Summary

All participants underwent MRI, behavioral, and fitness testing sessions before and after a 6-month long physical exercise intervention. Participants were paid for the pre- and post-testing sessions at a rate of $10/h. Participants were randomly assigned to one of four intervention groups, which met for an hour three times a week. All group sessions were led by trained exercise specialists. In the walking group (Walk), participants were instructed to walk within their target heart rate (50–60% of their maximal heart rate for first 6 weeks, 60–75% for last 18 weeks). A second group was also instructed to walk within the same target heart rate and was provided with a daily milk-based supplement formula provided by Abbott Nutrition that contained beta-alanine (Walk+). A third group was instructed in exercises focusing on stretching, strengthening and stability (SSS). A fourth group (Dance) was instructed in social dance sequences (i.e., Contra and English country dancing) by experienced dance instructors. Since the focus of this study is on the utility of brain modularity in predicting intervention-related gains, we limit our discussion of the intervention approach and choice of training regimen (for detailed information, see Ehlers et al., 2016; Burzynska et al., 2017).

Cardiorespiratory Fitness Testing

Participants underwent cardiorespiratory fitness (CRF) testing before and after the intervention. CRF reflects the integrated ability of the cardiovascular and respiratory systems to deliver oxygen during sustained physical effort (Ross et al., 2016), and regular physical exercise increases the efficiency of these systems (Wenger and Bell, 1986). CRF testing involves gradually increasing exercise intensity to tax the aerobic system and measuring the corresponding increase in oxygen consumption. Physician's approval was solicited prior to testing. CRF, operationally defined as peak oxygen consumption (VO_2peak in mL/kg/min, relative rate in milliliters of oxygen per kilogram of body mass per minute), was measured with indirect calorimetry during a modified Balke graded maximal exercise test on a motor-driven treadmill (Balke and Ware, 1959; Froelicher et al., 1975). Participants walked on a treadmill at a constant pace while the incline was increased 2–3% every 2 min. Expired air was sampled at 30-s intervals until maximal VO_2 was reached or the test was terminated due to volitional exhaustion and/or symptom limitation. Maximal VO_2 was determined after two of three criteria were met: (1) a plateau in VO_2 after increase in workload; (2) a respiratory exchange ratio (ratio of CO_2 production and O_2 consumption, reflecting limits of cardiovascular system) >1.10, and (3) a maximal heart rate within 10 bpm of their age-predicted maximum. VO_2peak was the highest VO_2 recorded during the test. For the correlation analyses, we calculated a standardized CRF gain score for each individual by taking the difference between post-and pre-scores and dividing this by the standard deviation of pre-test scores (SD collapsed across groups).

Behavioral Testing

Participants underwent cognitive testing before and after the interventions. With the exception of the Switching Task and the Spatial Working Memory Task, all tests were taken from the Virginia Cognitive Aging Project (VCAP) (Salthouse and Ferrer-Caja, 2003; Salthouse, 2004, 2005, 2010). The VCAP tests were categorized into four categories: vocabulary, perceptual speed, episodic memory, and fluid reasoning. In the analyses, we grouped the Switching Task and Spatial Working Memory Task together with the fluid reasoning tasks to create an "executive function" component score, given previously demonstrated relationships between cognitive control and fluid reasoning abilities (Kane et al., 2005; Salthouse, 2005). We also performed a principal components analysis (PCA) on all the pre-test measures to confirm the VCAP construct groupings and to confirm that the Switching and Spatial Working Memory Tasks were related to performance on the fluid reasoning tests (**Table 2**, Supplementary Table 1). For each pre-test and post-test measure, we calculated standardized scores (z-scores) and averaged these z-scores according to the task groupings specified above, resulting in

TABLE 1 | Demographics.

	Walk	Walk+	Dance	SSS	Group effect
FULL SAMPLE*					
Age	64.82 (4.55), 60–77	64.51 (4.47), 60–78	65.58 (4.57), 60–78	65.52 (4.43), 60–78	$F_{(3, 217)} = 0.75, p = 0.53$
Education	16.13 (3.31), 12–26	15.60 (2.26), 12–20	15.54 (3.17), 12–25	16.44 (3.14), 12–26	$F_{(3, 217)} = 1.19, p = 0.31$
MMSE	28.86 (1.02), 27–30	28.80 (0.94), 27–30	28.90 (0.94), 27–30	28.94 (1.08), 27–30	$F_{(3, 217)} = 0.20, p = 0.90$
VO_2peak	19.97 (5.11), 12–34	19.78 (4.15), 9–28	19.98 (4.69), 10–33	19.22 (4.73), 6–30	$F_{(3, 215)} = 0.35, p = 0.79$
Female	34	33	42	40	$\chi^2_{(3)} = 0.18, p = 0.98$
N	49	49	59	64	221
BEH + CRF					
Age	64.64 (4.06), 60–75	64.80 (4.49), 60–77	65.50 (4.50), 60–78	65.81 (4.43), 60–78	$F_{(3, 184)} = 0.78, p = 0.51$
Education	16.43 (3.30), 12–26	15.74 (2.21), 12–20	15.52 (3.12), 12–25	16.70 (3.22), 12–26	$F_{(3, 184)} = 1.70, p = 0.17$
MMSE	28.93 (1.02), 27–30	28.82 (0.95), 27–30	28.92 (0.94), 27–30	28.89 (1.11), 27–30	$F_{(3, 184)} = 0.11, p = 0.96$
VO_2peak	20.21 (5.04), 12–34	19.76 (4.06), 9–28	19.99 (4.07), 13–29	19.53 (4.69), 7–30	$F_{(3, 182)} = 0.20, p = 0.90$
Female	28	29	34	36	$\chi^2_{(3)} = 0.32, p = 0.96$
N	42	44	48	54	188
MRI SAMPLE					
Age	63.83 (3.96), 60–75	64.59 (4.27), 60–77	65.06 (4.00), 60–73	65.29 (4.18), 60–75	$F_{(3, 124)} = 0.78, p = 0.51$
Education	16.59 (2.80), 12–24	15.66 (2.31), 12–20	15.78 (3.16), 12–26	17.22 (3.40), 12–26	$F_{(3, 124)} = 2.06, p = 0.11$
MMSE	29.07 (0.92), 27–30	28.86 (0.92), 27–30	28.94 (0.98), 27–30	29.08 (1.08), 27–30	$F_{(3, 124)} = 0.36, p = 0.78$
VO_2peak	21.60 (5.39), 12–34	20.12 (4.14), 11–28	20.11 (4.00), 13–27	19.70 (4.60), 7–30	$F_{(3, 122)} = 1.02, p = 0.39$
Female	18	19	23	27	$\chi^2_{(3)} = 0.93, p = 0.82$
N	29	29	32	38	128

*Mean (SD) and range for age, education, MMSE and VO_2peak. *Full sample excludes participants with MMSE scores lower than 27. Two participants are missing VO_2peak data.*

four component scores representing baseline cognitive abilities in vocabulary, perceptual speed, episodic memory and executive function (fluid reasoning plus switching and working memory). For each test, we also calculated standardized gain scores by subtracting pre-test performance from post-test performance, and dividing this value by the standard deviation of raw pre-test scores (collapsed across groups). We averaged the standardized gain scores accordingly to create composite gain scores in vocabulary, perceptual speed, episodic memory, and executive function. The following sections have brief descriptions of each test and the specific measure used for analyses.

TABLE 2 | PCA standardized loadings (pattern matrix) based upon correlation matrix of baseline scores.

	PC1	PC2	PC4	PC3
Digit symbol	0.19	*0.85*	0.07	0.17
Pattern comparison	0.19	*0.79*	0.07	0.05
Letter comparison	0.01	*0.83*	0.18	0.02
Word recall	−0.01	0.23	0.34	*0.75*
Logical memory	0.23	0.16	0.34	*0.69*
Paired associates	0.18	0.04	0.12	*0.83*
Shipley abstraction	*0.56*	0.30	0.46	0.27
Form boards	*0.69*	0.28	0.21	0.00
Letter sets	*0.50*	0.40	0.38	0.25
Matrix reasoning	*0.65*	0.26	0.28	0.29
Paper folding	*0.77*	0.05	0.13	0.18
Spatial relations	*0.85*	0.20	0.15	0.04
Word vocabulary	0.13	0.13	*0.85*	0.25
Picture vocabulary	0.39	0.02	*0.74*	0.11
Synonym-antonym	0.22	0.04	*0.82*	0.24
Spatial working memory	*0.29*	0.53	0.03	0.12
Task switching bin score	*−0.23*	−0.44	0.12	−0.33

Performed varimax rotation and extraction of 4 components, which accounted for 67% of total variance. Italics denote component groupings.

Task-Switching (Kramer et al., 1999; Voss et al., 2010a,b, 2013b; Leckie et al., 2014)

On each trial, participants were shown a number between 1 and 9 (except 5) against a colored background: (1) on a pink background, participants were instructed to determine whether the number was odd or even, (2) on a blue background, they were to determine if the number was higher or lower than 5. Participants completed a high/low practice block (40 trials) an odd/even practice block (40 trials), a single high/low task block (40 trials), a single odd/even task block (40 trials), a mixed practice block (64 trials) and a mixed task block (160 trials). We analyzed performance on the mixed task block and extracted (1) local switch cost (mixed switch reaction time; RT—mixed non-switch RT) and (2) task switching bin score (combination of accuracy and RT measures) (Draheim et al., 2016). The task switching bin score was used in the principal components and correlation analyses to better examine the relationship between task switching performance and performance on other tests (Draheim et al., 2016). Local RT switch cost was used in the analyses of intervention effects, consistent with previous studies (Voss et al., 2010a, 2013b). The two measures were correlated (Supplementary Table 1; baseline measures: $r_{(211)} = 0.322, p < 0.001$, two-tailed; standardized gain scores: $r_{(159)} = 0.267, p < 0.001$, two-tailed), and the intervention effects were similar when using bin score instead of local RT switch cost.

Spatial Working Memory (Erickson et al., 2011)

On each trial, an arrangement of two, three, or four black dots was briefly presented on the screen. After a delay, a red dot appeared and participants were instructed to determine if the red dot matched the position of one of the black dots presented earlier in that trial (match or non-match). Participants performed a practice block of 12 trials, and a task block of 120 trials (40 trials per condition). We analyzed mean accuracy during the task block for the more difficult three-dot and four-dot trial conditions.

Shipley Abstraction (Zachary, 1986)

Participants were given a list of word, letter, or number sequences on a piece of paper and were instructed to write the missing item/s (word, letter or number) in each sequence. Participants were given 5 min to answer 20 items. We analyzed the total number of correctly answered items.

Matrix Reasoning (Ravens, 1962)

On each trial, participants were shown a 3 × 3 grid, with each cell except for one containing an abstract pattern. Participants were instructed to select which among eight options best completes the matrix along both the rows and columns. Participants performed two practice trials and were then given 10 min to complete a maximum of 18 items. We analyzed the total number of correctly answered items.

Paper Folding (Ekstrom et al., 1976)

On each trial, participants were presented with images that show a sheet of paper folded in a certain sequence and a hole punched through the folded sheet. Participants were asked to select which among five options matched the pattern of holes that would result when the paper was unfolded. They were given 10 min to complete a maximum of 12 trials. We analyzed the total number of correctly answered items.

Spatial Relations (Bennett et al., 1997)

On each trial, participants were presented with a 2-dimensional object pattern and instructed to identify which among four three-dimensional figures would match the 2-dimensional pattern when folded. Participants were given 10 min to complete a maximum of 20 trials. We analyzed the total number of correctly answered items.

Form Boards (Ekstrom et al., 1976)

On each trial, participants were presented with a specific shape and instructed to choose which pieces (five total options) will exactly fill the space inside the shape. They were given 8 min to complete a maximum of 24 trials. We analyzed the total number of correctly answered items.

Letter Sets (Ekstrom et al., 1976)

On each trial, participants were presented with five sets of four-letter strings and asked to determine which set was different from the other four. Participants were given 10 min to complete a maximum of 15 trials. We analyzed the total number of correctly answered items.

Digit-Symbol Coding (Wechsler, 1997a)

Participants were presented with a sheet of paper containing a series of numbers between 1 and 9, were asked to fill in the corresponding symbol based on a digit-symbol key provided. Participants completed 7 practice items and were given 2 min to complete a maximum of 133 items. We analyzed the number of correctly answered items.

Pattern Comparison (Salthouse and Babcock, 1991)

Participants were given a sheet of paper with a set of line patterns and were tasked to determine whether a pair of line patterns was the same or different. Participants completed three practice items, followed by two task sets, each set with a maximum number of 30 items to be completed within 30 s. We analyzed the number of correctly answered items, averaged across two sets of problems.

Letter Comparison (Salthouse and Babcock, 1991)

Participants were given a sheet of paper with a set of non-word letter strings and were tasked to determine whether a pair of letter strings was the same or different. Participants completed three practice items, followed by two task sets, each set with a maximum number of 30 items to be completed within 30 s. We analyzed the number of correctly answered items, averaged across two sets of problems.

Logical Memory (Wechsler, 1997b)

Participants listened to stories narrated by an experimenter and after each reading, were asked to recall each story in detail. We analyzed the number of correctly recalled story details, summed across three story-tellings (first story, second story, re-reading of second story).

Paired Associates (Salthouse et al., 1996)

Participants listened to a list of six word pairs read aloud by an experimenter. The experimenter then read the first word of each pair and asked participants to recall the paired second word. We analyzed the number of correctly recalled items, averaged across two sets of six pairs each.

Word Recall (Wechsler, 1997b)

Participants listened to a list of words and were given 90 s to recall the words in any order. Participants listed to the same list three more times and were asked to recall as many words as possible after each reading. Participants were then read a new list of words, asked to recall as many words as possible from the new list, and then asked to recall words from the old list. We analyzed the total number of correctly recalled items.

Word Vocabulary (Wechsler, 1997a)

Experimenters read aloud a list of 33 words and asked participants to verbally give the meaning of each word. Responses are scored 0–2 points according to the quality of the definition (based on provided word and phrase guidelines). The test is discontinued after six consecutive scores of 0. We analyzed the total number of points.

Picture Vocabulary (Woodcock and Johnson, 1989)

Experimenters present a maximum of 30 images and participants are tasked to name the objects presented. The test is discontinued after a participant fails to name six consecutive items. We analyzed the total number of correctly named items.

Synonym-Antonym (Salthouse, 1993)

On each trial, participants are presented a target word and are tasked to select which among five word options is most similar (synonym) or opposite (antonym) in meaning to the target word. Participants completed a synonym block followed by an antonym block, each with a maximum of 10 items to be completed within 5 min. We analyzed the total number of correctly identified words across the synonym and antonym blocks.

MRI Acquisition and Processing

Participants underwent MRI scanning on a 3 Tesla Siemens Trio Tim System with a 12-channel head coil before and after the intervention; however, only the pre-intervention scans were analyzed in this study given our hypotheses regarding correlations between baseline brain modularity and cognitive gains. The anatomical scan consisted of T1-weighted MPRAGE images acquired with the following parameters: GRAPPA acceleration factor 2, voxel size $= 0.9 \times 0.9 \times 0.9$ mm, $TR = 1{,}900$ ms, $TI = 900$ ms, $TE = 2.32$ ms, flip angle $= 9°$, FoV $= 230$ mm. To analyze network properties during a task-free "resting state," a 6-min functional scan was obtained using a T2*-weighted echoplanar imaging (EPI) pulse sequence with the following parameters: GRAPPA acceleration factor 2, 180 volumes, in-plane resolution $= 3.4$ mm^2, $TR = 2{,}000$ ms, $TE = 25$ ms, flip angle $= 80°$, 35 4 mm ascending slices, no slice gap. Participants were instructed to lie still with their eyes closed.

Brain extraction from anatomical scans was performed with Advanced Normalization Tools (ANTs; Avants et al., 2010, 2011) using the Kirby/MMRR template (Landman et al., 2011). When this skull-stripping procedure failed, brain extraction was instead performed using the IXI template (Heckemann et al., 2003; Ericsson et al., 2008). The skull-stripped anatomical images and raw functional images were preprocessed through the Configurable Pipeline for Connectomes (CPAC; Giavasis et al., 2015). Anatomical images were registered to the MNI152 template (Fonov et al., 2009) using ANTs and segmented into gray matter (probability threshold $= 0.7$), white matter (probability threshold $= 0.98$) and cerebrospinal fluid (CSF; probability threshold $= 0.98$) using FSL/FAST (Zhang et al., 2001). Functional images were slice-time corrected, motion-corrected (Friston et al., 1996) and co-registered to the anatomical images. Nuisance signal removal was performed by regressing out the aforementioned motion parameters, signals from the first five components from white matter and CSF voxels (Compcor; Behzadi et al., 2007; Muschelli et al., 2014), and linear and quadratic trends. Signals were bandpass filtered at 0.009–0.08 Hz. Participants whose resting state scan contained (1) more than 10% of volumes with framewise displacement (FD) greater than 0.5 mm ($N = 23$) or (2) maximum absolute displacement greater than 4.0 mm were excluded from subsequent analyses (additional $N = 12$). One participant was excluded because structural abnormalities caused anatomical-to-MNI registration to fail (spatial warping) during preprocessing, such that we could not reliably extract ROIs.

Functional Connectivity and Modularity Analyses

Functional scans were warped to the MNI template and parcellated into 264 regions of interest (Power et al., 2011). Due to uneven partial coverage of the cerebellum across subjects in the functional data, we excluded the four cerebellum module ROIs prior to analysis. Eight additional ROIs were excluded due to lack of functional coverage in at least one participant, leaving a total of 252 ROIs. For each individual, time series from all voxels within each ROI were averaged together. Average ROI time series were correlated between each pair of ROIs (Pearson's coefficient), and the resulting ROI-to-ROI correlation matrices were Fisher z-transformed. Matrices were binarized over a range of connection density thresholds (costs): 2–10% of all possible connections, in 2% increments, following (Power et al., 2011; Power and Petersen, 2013). These thresholded matrices were used to create unweighted, undirected whole-brain graphs for each participant, from which network metrics were derived using the BrainX (https://github.com/nipy/brainx) and NetworkX Python package (Hagberg et al., 2008). Network modularity was quantified separately for each connection threshold to examine the consistency of results across thresholds. We use the middle 6% threshold for all our primary analyses, but verified effects at the other thresholds (Supplementary Material).

For our primary analysis, we quantified modularity, a network measure that compares the number of connections within modules to the number of connections across modules (Newman and Girvan, 2004). Modularity is defined as $\sum_{i=1}^{m} (e_{ii} - a_i^2)$, where e_{ii} is the fraction of connections that connect two nodes within module i, a_i is the fraction of connections connecting a node in module i to any other node, and m is the total number of modules in the network (Newman and Girvan, 2004). There are multiple methods for identifying network modules. Here, we used a spectral algorithm (Newman, 2006a) to identify the partition that maximizes modularity for each participant at each threshold.

Further, to confirm that our effects were not driven by a specific partitioning algorithm, we also computed modularity using partitions identified in Power et al. (2011) using the Infomap algorithm (Rosvall and Bergstrom, 2008; Fortunato, 2010). Here, every node was assigned to one of thirteen modules (as identified in Power et al., 2011): default mode (DMN), fronto-parietal (FP), cingulo-opercular (CO), salience (Sal), dorsal attention (DAN), ventral attention (VAN), auditory (Aud), visual (Vis), memory (Mem), sensory/somatomotor hand (SM-hand), sensory/somatomotor mouth (SM-mouth), subcortical (Subcort) and a module containing unassigned nodes. The modularity values derived from the Power partition were highly correlated with the modularity values obtained using the spectral clustering partition (all $r > 0.761$, all $p > 0.001$, two-tailed for all five cost thresholds).

Potential Confounds

Before examining the relationship between brain modularity and intervention-related gains, we examined relationships between potential confounding variables and our measures of interest (i.e., baseline modularity and intervention-related gains), including age, in-scanner motion (i.e., frame-wise displacement or FD; Power et al., 2012; Satterthwaite et al., 2012; Siegel et al., 2016), and baseline cognitive performance. All the analyses include only subjects with usable baseline MRI scans, baseline EF scores, and EF gain scores ($N = 128$). If a significant relationship between potential confounding variables and our dependent measures was found, we then used these variables as covariates in our primary analyses examining correlations between modularity and intervention-related gains. For all analyses, we also controlled for age and in-scanner motion (i.e., FD). For all correlation analyses, we computed bias-corrected and accelerated (BCa) confidence intervals (CI) using 5,000 bootstrapped samples.

There is considerable variability in brain volume in older adults (Salat et al., 2004; Raz et al., 2005; Raz and Rodrigue, 2006). Thus, for participants with structural volume data, we also tested whether the pattern of brain-behavior relationships from the network analyses could have been confounded by gross individual differences in brain structure. We extracted measures of brain volume using Freesurfer v5.3 (Dale et al., 1999); http://surfer.nmr.mgh.harvard.edu), which performs segmentation of cortical and subcortical matter using automated and probabilistic algorithms (Fischl et al., 2002, 2004a,b; Desikan et al., 2006). AZB inspected the segmentation output and performed appropriate corrections. Using the anatomical scans obtained at baseline, we obtained measures of total intracranial volume, white matter, and total gray matter volume, described in more detail on the Freesurfer website (https://surfer.nmr.mgh.harvard.edu/fswiki/MorphometryStats). We included estimated intracranial volume as a covariate in volumetric analyses to control for differences in overall brain volume (Jack et al., 1989; Buckner et al., 2004). Since not all participants had high-quality structural scans for volumetric analysis ($N = 15$), we conducted this analysis as a follow-up to the primary analyses of modularity vs. intervention-related gains.

RESULTS

Exercise-Related Changes in Cardiorespiratory Fitness (CRF)

We first verified that the groups demonstrated the expected patterns of fitness improvements. At baseline, the groups did not differ in CRF $F_{(3, 182)} = 0.199$, $p = 0.897$, $\eta_p^2 = 0.003$. A mixed ANOVA with VO_2peak scores over time (pre- and post-testing) as a within-subjects factor and group as a between-subjects factor revealed a main effect of time $F_{(1, 182)} = 21.737$, $p < 0.001$,

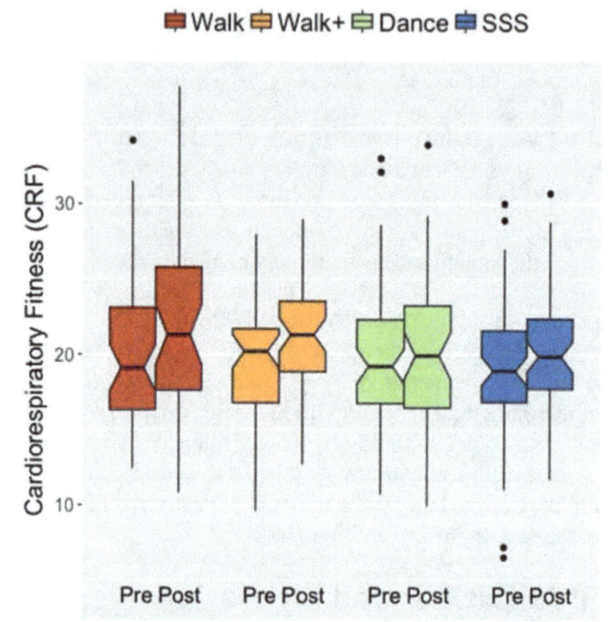

FIGURE 1 | Notched box plots show the distribution of CRF values before and after the intervention. The horizontal line marks the median. The notches extend to ±1.58 IQR/sqrt(n). The upper and lower hinges correspond to the first and third quartiles. The whiskers extend from the hinge to ±1.5*IQR of the hinge. IQR, inter-quartile range.

$\eta_p^2 = 0.107$, and an interaction of group and time $F_{(3, 182)} = 2.792$, $p = 0.042$, $\eta_p^2 = 0.044$. Follow-up analyses showed that the Walk and Walk+ groups showed greater improvements in CRF compared to the SSS and Dance groups (**Figure 1**). Separate comparisons of pre- and post-test scores within each group showed significant gains in the Walk and Walk+ groups (both $p = 0.001$, both $d \geq 0.539$) and marginal gains in the SSS group ($p = 0.059$, $d = 0.225$). There were no significant gains in the Dance group ($p = 0.345$, $d = 0.062$).

Exercise-Related Changes in Cognitive Function

To determine the effects of the exercise intervention on cognitive function and to minimize measurement error and multiple comparison issues in analyzing each test separately, we analyzed cognitive effects at the construct level using composite scores. The creation of composite scores was guided by previous literature (Kane et al., 2005; Salthouse, 2005), correlations (Supplementary Table 1), and a PCA on the baseline test scores (**Table 2**), which confirmed the grouping of the cognitive tests into categories of vocabulary, episodic memory, perceptual speed, and executive function.

At baseline, the groups did not differ in EF, $F_{(3, 187)} = 1.191$, $p = 0.315$, $\eta_p^2 = 0.019$, perceptual speed $F_{(3, 185)} = 0.525$, $p = 0.665$, $\eta_p^2 = 0.008$, episodic memory, $F_{(3, 187)} = 0.098$, $p = 0.961$, $\eta_p^2 = 0.002$, and vocabulary, $F_{(3, 184)} = 0.619$, $p = 0.604$, $\eta_p^2 = 0.010$. With the exception of a correlation between vocabulary gain and perceptual speed gain

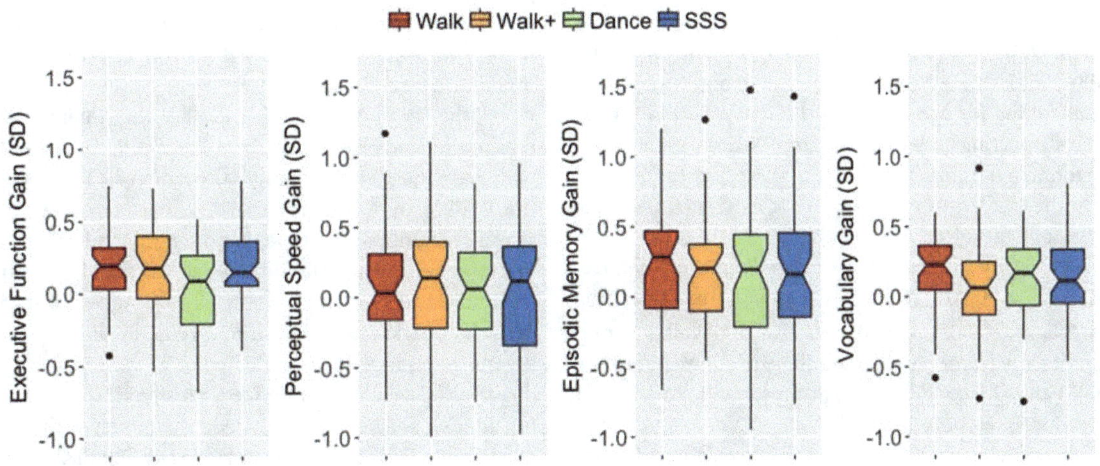

FIGURE 2 | Notched box plots show the distribution of composite gain scores before and after the intervention. The horizontal line marks the median. The notches extend to ±1.58 IQR/sqrt(n). The upper and lower hinges correspond to the first and third quartiles. The whiskers extend from the hinge to ±1.5*IQR of the hinge. IQR, inter-quartile range.

[$r_{(186)} = 0.152$, 95% *CI* [−0.002, 0.304], $p = 0.039$, two-tailed], and between vocabulary gain and EF gain [$r_{(188)} = 0.147$, 95% *CI* [0.011, 0.275], $p = 0.043$, two-tailed], the composite scores of cognitive change scores (i.e., gains) were not significantly correlated with each other (all others $p > 0.05$, two-tailed). Therefore, we conducted separate ANOVAs on the composite gain scores to examine the differential effects of the intervention on cognitive function (Huberty and Morris, 1989).

An ANOVA on the EF gain score with intervention group as a between-subjects factor yielded a significant group effect $F_{(3,187)} = 3.899$, $p = 0.010$, $\eta_p^2 = 0.059$. The Walk, Walk+ and SSS groups showed greater EF gains compared to the Dance group (all $p < 0.05$ for each group vs. Dance, Dance vs. Walk+ is $p < 0.10$ with Bonferroni correction; **Figure 2**). Tests for significance of gain scores (i.e., test against a comparison value of zero) separately in each group showed significant EF gains in the Walk, Walk+ and SSS groups (all $p < 0.001$), but not in the Dance group ($p = 0.703$). Since baseline EF was moderately correlated with EF gain, $r_{(189)} = -0.140$, 95% *CI* [−0.255, −0.026] $p = 0.053$, two-tailed, we verified that the group effect in EF gain remained significant after controlling for baseline EF, $F_{(3, 186)} = 3.498$, $p = 0.017$, $\eta_p^2 = 0.053$. No group effects were observed for gains in perceptual speed, $F_{(3, 185)} = 0.129$, $p = 0.943$, $\eta_p^2 = 0.002$, episodic memory, $F_{(3, 187)} = 0.086$, $p = 0.968$, $\eta_p^2 = 0.001$, and vocabulary, $F_{(3, 184)} = 1.376$, $p = 0.251$, $\eta_p^2 = 0.022$ (**Figure 2**).

Relationship between Fitness and Cognitive Effects

Given that the groups that improved in EF were also those that showed larger CRF gains (i.e., Walk, Walk+, SSS groups), we tested whether the degree of CRF improvement was related to EF improvement. Across the whole sample with CRF data and behavioral data, there was no significant relationship between CRF gain and EF gain, $r_{(184)} = 0.104$, 95% CI [−0.045, 0.251], $p = 0.157$, two-tailed, even when excluding the Dance group which did not show CRF and EF gains, $r_{(138)} = 0.080$, 95% CI [−0.045, 0.251], $p = 0.352$, two-tailed. The correlations were also not significant within each group (all $|r|$ <0.25, all $p > 0.05$, two-tailed).

Examination of Potential Confounds

Across the whole sample with quality MRI data, we first examined relationships between group assignment (i.e., to confirm that groups did not differ in baseline characteristics), potential confounding variables (i.e., age, years of education, mean FD) and our measures of interest (i.e., baseline modularity and EF gain). In the case of a non-significant relationship between variables when analyzing the whole MRI sample, we also verified that the relationship was not significant when analyzing each group separately, as the primary analyses of baseline modularity and EF gain were conducted within group.

Age did not differ across groups (**Table 1**), but was significantly correlated with baseline modularity, $r_{(126)} = 0.239$, 95% CI [0.102, 0.370], $p = 0.007$, two-tailed, and was not correlated with EF gain, $r_{(126)} = -0.008$, 95% CI [−0.211, 0.197], $p = 0.932$, two-tailed. We verified that there was no significant relationship between age and EF gain within each group (all $|r|$ <0.314, all $p > 0.097$, two-tailed).

Years of education did not significantly differ across groups (**Table 1**), even after accounting for age $F_{(3,123)} = 2.117$, $p = 0.101$, $\eta_p^2 = 0.049$. Education was not significantly correlated with baseline modularity, $r_{(126)} = -0.031$, 95% CI [−0.183, 0.124], $p = 0.730$, or EF gain, $r_{(126)} = -0.041$, 95% CI [−0.216, 0.137], $p = 0.649$, even after accounting for age, and when examining within each group separately (all $|r| < 0.295$, all $p > 0.101$, two-tailed).

Mean FD did not differ across groups, $F_{(3, 124)} = 0.938$, $p = 0.425$, $\eta_p^2 = 0.022$, even after controlling for age,

$F_{(3, 123)} = 0.935$, $p = 0.426$, $\eta_p^2 = 0.022$. Mean FD was not correlated with baseline modularity, $r_{(126)} = -0.087$, 95% CI [−0.272, 0.092], $p = 0.328$, two-tailed or with EF gain, $r_{(126)} = 0.039$, 95% CI [−0.138, 0.197], $p = 0.666$, two-tailed, even after controlling for age (all $|r| < 0.122$, all $p > 0.173$, two-tailed). When inspecting these relationships within each group however, we found a trending relationship between mean FD and modularity in the Walk group, $r_{(27)} = -0.359$, 95% CI [−0.666, 0.005], $p = 0.056$, two-tailed.

Baseline modularity differed across groups, $F_{(3, 124)} = 4.628$, $p = 0.004$, $\eta_p^2 = 0.101$, even after accounting for age, $F_{(3, 123)} = 4.495$, $p = 0.005$, $\eta_p^2 = 0.099$, with the Walk+ group showing significantly lower baseline modularity compared to the SSS ($p = 0.005$) and Dance ($p = 0.011$) groups, but not compared to the Walk group ($p = 0.116$).

Lastly, given previously documented relationships between modularity and cognitive function (Kitzbichler et al., 2011; Stevens et al., 2012; Stanley et al., 2014; Sadaghiani et al., 2015), we examined whether baseline modularity was related to baseline EF. Across the whole MRI sample, there was no significant relationship between baseline modularity and baseline EF, $r_{(126)} = 0.023$, 95% CI [−0.167, 0.207], $p = 0.798$, two-tailed, even after accounting for age and/or mean FD and examining each group separately (all $|r| < 0.319$, all $p > 0.098$, two-tailed). Thus, potential relationships between modularity and EF gains cannot be attributed to correlations between modularity and EF performance at baseline.

The above results were similar when using modularity values derived from other thresholds and when using modularity values derived from the Power partition (see Supplementary Material). Thus, given these findings that age and mean FD showed some relationship with modularity, and given that baseline EF was moderately related to EF gain, we used age, mean FD and baseline EF as covariates in the primary analyses of modularity and exercise-related gains.

Relationship between Baseline Modularity and Exercise-Related Gains

We next examined the relationship between baseline modularity and intervention-related effects on EF, having confirmed EF and CRF improvements in the Walk, Walk+ and SSS groups (**Figure 3**). For each group, we first performed linear regression analyses with EF gain as the dependent variable, age, mean FD and baseline EF as covariates, and independent variables of baseline EF, baseline modularity, and an interaction term of baseline EF and baseline modularity. Importantly, the interaction term was included to test whether the relationship between baseline modularity and EF gain was moderated by baseline EF (i.e., whether the modularity-gain relationship was stronger in high or low performing individuals at baseline).

The model (**Table 3**) with all three terms and covariates was significant in the Walk [$R^2 = 0.450$, Adjusted $R^2 = 0.330$, $F_{(5, 23)} = 3.756$, $p = 0.012$] and Walk+ groups [$R^2 = 0.375$, Adjusted $R^2 = 0.239$, $F_{(5, 23)} = 2.762$, $p = 0.043$].

In the Walk group, age, mean FD, modularity, and the interaction term of modularity and baseline EF were significant predictors of EF gain (**Table 3**). Critically, modularity positively predicted EF gain, while the interaction showed that individuals with lower baseline EF showed a stronger relationship between modularity and EF gain.

In the Walk+ group, age and the interaction term of modularity and baseline EF were significant predictors of EF gain, with baseline EF as a marginal predictor (**Table 3**). Similar to the Walk group, individuals with lower baseline EF showed a stronger relationship between modularity and EF gain.

In the SSS group, the full model was not significant [**Table 3**; $R^2 = 0.094$, Adjusted $R^2 = -0.048$, $F_{(5, 32)} = 0.661$, $p = 0.656$]. Modularity was not a significant predictor, although it explained the most variance and was related to EF gain in a similar positive direction. Given that there were no significant predictors in the full model, we performed a reduced model with only baseline modularity. This model was marginally significant [$R^2 = 0.083$, Adjusted $R^2 = 0.057$, $F_{(1, 36)} = 3.246$, $p = 0.080$], with modularity marginally related to EF gain ($B = 1.218$, $p = 0.080$, BCa 95% CI [−0.439, 2.276]).

As expected, in the Dance group, the full model [**Table 3**; $R^2 = 0.217$, Adjusted $R^2 = 0.066$, $F_{(5, 26)} = 1.437$, $p = 0.244$], and a reduced model with only baseline modularity [$R^2 = 0.002$, Adjusted $R^2 = -0.032$, $F_{(1, 30)} = 0.045$, $p = 0.833$] were not significant, with no factor emerging as a significant predictor.

In summary, we find that baseline modularity was related to EF gains in groups that showed training-related gains. For illustrative purposes, **Figure 3** shows the relationship between baseline modularity and EF gain with and without controlling for age, mean FD and baseline EF.

Controlling for Individual Differences in Brain Volume

Age-related differences in white and gray matter volume loss may influence brain function (Persson et al., 2006; Chadick et al., 2014; Pudas et al., 2017), functional connectivity patterns (Meunier et al., 2014), and in turn, the pattern of brain-behavioral results we find here. On the sample of participants with high-quality anatomical data, we ran partial correlation analyses of baseline modularity and EF gain within each of the four groups (one-tailed tests to confirm initial results), controlling for estimated intra-cranial volume, gray matter volume, and white matter volume in addition to age, mean FD and baseline EF. Critically, the pattern of relationships remained the same, Walk: $rp_{(16)} = 0.369$, 95% CI [−0.339, 0.884], $p = 0.066$; Walk+: $rp_{(20)} = 0.098$, 95% CI [−0.519, 0.628], $p = 0.331$; SSS: $rp_{(25)} = 0.408$, 95% CI [−0.024, 0.709], $p = 0.017$, Dance: $rp_{(20)} = -0.017$, 95% CI [−0.496, 0.635], $p = 0.469$, suggesting that individual differences in brain volume did not contribute to the relationship between baseline modularity and EF gain.

Exploratory Analyses: Sub-network Contribution to Relationship between Baseline Modularity and Training-Related Gains

Brain modules show distinct age-related connectivity changes (Chan et al., 2014), and modularity in the association systems

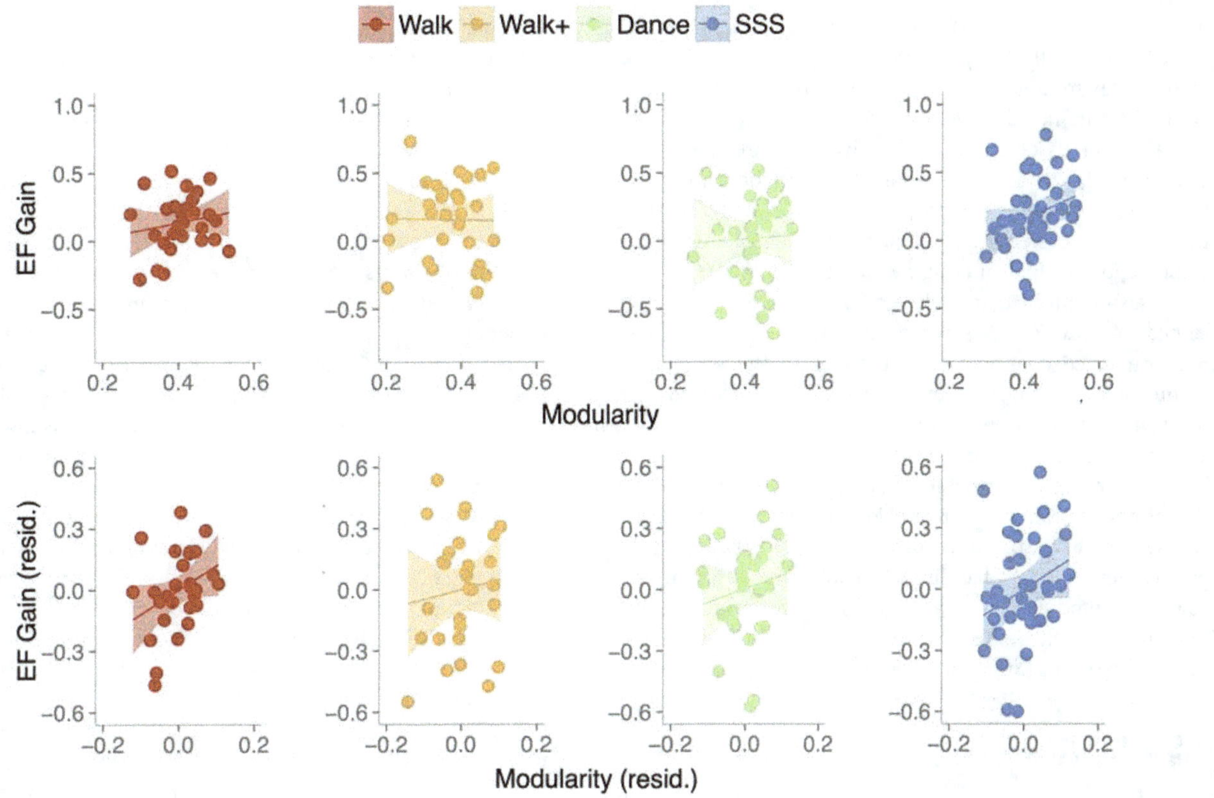

FIGURE 3 | Scatterplots show the relationship between baseline modularity (6% threshold) and executive function gain in each group, without controlling for any other factors **(top)** and after controlling for age, mean FD and baseline EF **(bottom)**. Shaded areas represent 95% confidence region of the regression line.

TABLE 3 | Multiple linear regression models.

	Walk		Walk+		Dance		SSS	
	***B* 95% CI**	***p***	***B* 95% CI**	***p***	***B* 95% CI**	***p***	***B* 95% CI**	***p***
Intercept	0.156 [0.090, 0.221]	<0.001***	0.173 [0.067, 0.263]	0.001**	0.030 [−0.069, 0.143]	0.594	0.190 [0.103, 0.286]	<0.001***
Age	−0.021 [−0.032, −0.003]	0.022*	−0.041 [−0.073, −0.004]	0.022*	−0.009 [−0.051, 0.033]	0.582	0.004 [−0.022, 0.023]	0.710
Mean FD	1.036 [−0.248, 2.226]	0.037*	−0.560 [−1.686, 0.488]	0.277	0.778 [−0.403, 2.242]	0.196	0.166 [−1.015, 1.352]	0.747
Baseline EF	−0.011 [−0.124, 0.082]	0.812	−0.190 [−0.434, −0.025]	0.067~	−0.155 [−0.289, 0.101]	0.113	0.007 [−0.113, 0.146]	0.929
Modularity	1.823 [0.343, 3.309]	0.006**	0.445 [−1.127, 1.909]	0.553	−0.064 [−2.496, 1.454]	0.951	1.182 [−0.518, 2.624]	0.114
Baseline EF × Modularity	−2.365 [−4.038, 0.197]	0.005**	−5.007 [−8.738, −1.301]	0.003**	1.406 [−1.730, 5.369]	0.267	−0.261 [−2.612, 1.584]	0.802

****p* < 0.001, ***p* < 0.01, **p* < 0.05, ~*p* < 0.10.*

(DMN, FP, CO, Sal, DAN, VAN) has been found to drive the correlation between global modularity and training-related gains (Gallen et al., 2016). Given this, we examined whether specific networks contribute to the modularity vs. gain relationship. Similar to previous findings, sensory-motor modularity was higher than association cortex modularity both when analyzing the whole sample, $t_{(127)} = 24.954$, $p < 0.001$, and each group separately (all $p < 0.001$). We then examined the contribution of each sub-network to the modularity vs. EF gain relationship. For these analyses, we performed partial correlation analyses with age, mean FD and baseline EF as covariates. To reduce the number of analyses, we combined the three groups (Walk, Walk+ and SSS) given the similarity in their intervention-related effects.

Across the three groups, EF gain was marginally correlated with baseline association sub-network modularity $r_{(91)} = 0.159$, 95% CI [−0.053, 0.346], $p = 0.064$, one-tailed, but not sensory-motor cortex modularity $r_{(91)} = 0.003$, 95% CI [−0.188, 0.209], $p = 0.488$, one-tailed. Given the trending relationship between EF gain and association modularity and previous findings (Gallen et al., 2016), we examined the relationship between EF gain and each association sub-network. After Bonferroni correction however, none of the six modules showed a significant relationship with EF Gain (Supplementary Material).

We also quantified module segregation (Chan et al., 2014), defined as $(Z_w\text{-}Z_b)/Z_w$, where Z_w is the average Fisher-transformed correlation between nodes in the same module (within-module connectivity) and Z_b is the average Fisher-transformed correlation between nodes in a module to nodes in any other module (between-module connectivity). Importantly, this metric retains the weights of all connections (lower than 2–10% of connections). Given previous findings, we focused our analyses on the association cortex modules. When controlling for age, mean FD, and baseline EF, whole-brain segregation and association module segregation were not significantly related to EF gain, although the results were in the same direction as the modularity results (Supplementary Material).

DISCUSSION

We examined whether baseline brain network modularity predicts cognitive improvements in older adults after an exercise intervention. We found that in the groups that showed gains in fitness and cognitive function (Walk, Walk+, and SSS), higher baseline brain modularity predicted greater gains in executive function, even after accounting for individual differences in baseline performance, age, in-scanner motion, and individual differences in brain volume. These results parallel findings in TBI patients (Arnemann et al., 2015), older adults (Gallen et al., 2016), and young adults who underwent cognitive training (Baniqued et al., 2015). Given that we find a similar relationship between modularity and cognitive gains after an exercise intervention in older adults suggests that the predictive power of brain modularity may be generalizable across populations and interventions aimed to enhance executive function. Moreover, these findings point to the potential of global network properties to capture individual differences in neuroplasticity.

Modularity and Exercise-Related Gains in Executive Function

Our findings demonstrating a relationship between baseline brain network modularity and EF improvements with exercise training add to a series of studies that find a similar relationship with cognitive gains from cognitive training interventions (Arnemann et al., 2015; Baniqued et al., 2015; Gallen et al., 2016). Importantly, the current study shows that the pattern of results holds after controlling for factors such as baseline cognitive performance, age, and individual differences in brain volume—the latter of which can present a confound, especially when analyzing measures of brain function in older adults, who show considerable variability in age-related atrophy and lesions (Hedden et al., 2012; Grady, 2013). In the current study, the modularity-gain correlations were found in two (Walk, SSS) out of the three groups that showed some improvement in CRF and EF. In the Walk and Walk+ groups, the modularity-gain relationship was moderated by baseline EF, which together with previous findings in older adults (Arnemann et al., 2015; Gallen et al., 2016) underscores the utility of the network modularity measure in lower-performing individuals. These results suggest that the two measures of baseline performance and modularity together may be a better predictor of training-related gains than either alone.

The relevance of the modularity metric in neuroplasticity, specifically, in predicting response to an intervention, can be linked back to computational models showing that modular networks more rapidly reconfigure in response to new environments (Kashtan and Alon, 2005; Clune et al., 2013; Tosh and McNally, 2015), such that reorganization is more efficiently achieved by slight modifications within and between relatively specialized modules than by a large-scale overhaul of a highly interdependent network. Moreover, individuals with disrupted modular brain organization (Fornito et al., 2015), such as those with focal lesions to brain regions important for between-module connectivity (Nomura et al., 2010; Gratton et al., 2012; Warren et al., 2014) show widespread cognitive dysfunction and thus underscore the role of a modular structure in enabling brain processes that support a wide range of behaviors. In a recent study, individuals who scored higher on general intelligence tests tended to show smaller functional connectivity changes between a "resting state" and task performance states (Schultz and Cole, 2016), suggesting that they adapt more efficiently to task demands. In this sense, the architecture of brain networks at rest guides the connectivity patterns that emerge during the performance of various tasks. Indeed, modularity measured during "resting states" has been found to predict working memory performance (Stevens et al., 2012), and stimulus detection in a perceptual task (Sadaghiani et al., 2015). Taken together, these findings suggest that an "optimally" organized network requires less reorganization to be receptive to new input encountered during learning or training, or to capitalize from intervention-related changes in brain function. In the context of the current study, a more modular brain network may potentiate the rehabilitative and protective effects of physical exercise on the aging brain. In fitness interventions, for example, exercise-associated up-regulation in neurotrophic factors has been related to greater exercise-related changes in brain connectivity (Voss et al., 2013a). Given previous findings and the results of the current study, an optimal network for intervention-related cognitive gains is modularly organized at rest, with a balance of within-module connections that support local processing and across-module connections that support global processing (Meunier et al., 2009, 2010). Indeed, recent studies have shown that increased brain modularity post-therapy correlated with greater speech improvement in aphasic patients (Duncan and Small, 2016), and that greater structural modularity prior to carotid artery intervention predicted reduced risk of cognitive decline after carotid intervention (Soman et al., 2016).

Additionally, connectivity measures obtained during preclinical stages, when combined with biomarkers such as amyloid-beta, have been shown to predict later cognitive decline (Buckley et al., 2017), suggesting that these metrics have the potential to provide actionable information when clinical symptoms have yet to manifest.

We found that modularity predicted training gains, beyond the baseline behavioral EF measure. This is a promising finding given that behavioral or cognitive measures may be confounded in certain populations (Gabrieli et al., 2015), such as in older adults, where factors such as mobility or visual acuity interact with task performance. While typical behavioral measures may not reliably distinguish between individual differences in cognitive ability, brain network measures provide a way to gauge training responsiveness. Although this study involved a fairly large sample, functional connectivity was assessed during a relatively short resting-state scan. More reliable measures and more information regarding network structure, particularly in higher performing individuals, may be gleaned from a longer scan period (Birn et al., 2013; Laumann et al., 2015; Gordon et al., 2017). Nonetheless, the pattern of higher baseline modularity predicting intervention-related cognitive gains is now consistent across four studies (Arnemann et al., 2015; Baniqued et al., 2015; Gallen et al., 2016). Using brain network measures in combination with behavioral, demographic, lifestyle, and other brain measures could also help customize intervention protocols to maximize effectiveness, especially in the context of dose-response relationships, for example by increasing the intensity, frequency, or duration of exercises, or including pre-intervention lifestyle or behavioral protocols geared to promote or maintain optimal levels of brain modularity. Nonetheless, future work may identify behavioral measures that are sensitive to the information captured by network measures; the relationship between baseline modularity and future behavior (i.e., training gains) suggests that modularity may be reflected in baseline behavior to some extent, a brain characteristic that the current study's behavioral measures are not designed to capture. In addition, more work is needed to examine the mechanisms in which a modular architecture interacts with changes in neural and vascular function to enable benefits from cognitive and fitness interventions, and whether such interventions lead to changes in brain modularity. In the current study, we found a marginal correlation between EF gain and baseline association cortex modularity, which suggests that association sub-networks drive the relationship between baseline modularity and EF gain, similar to our previous study (Gallen et al., 2016). Relatedly, association sub-networks have also been shown to increase in functional connectivity after a physical exercise intervention (Voss et al., 2010b), concomitant with improvements in EF.

In our dataset, we found a positive correlation between age and baseline modularity, unlike previous studies that found lower modularity in older adults compared to young adults (Meunier et al., 2009; Betzel et al., 2014; Song et al., 2014; Geerligs et al., 2015). Importantly, our study only included older adults, whereas reductions in modularity are typically found when comparing older and young populations. In addition, some studies show no correlation between modularity and age within older adults (Geerligs et al., 2015; Gallen et al., 2016), no difference in modularity *per se* when comparing young and old adults (Meunier et al., 2009) and observations that modularity variability was higher in older adults (Song et al., 2014). Moreover, our older adult sample may not be representative of the general population, as participants were relatively healthy and free of major health incidents despite being generally inactive or sedentary prior to participating in the study. Notably however, the relationship between baseline modularity and training gain in the current study remained even after accounting for age.

Neurovascular coupling is an important issue to consider when conducting fMRI studies in older adults, where age-related vascular changes may lead to age-related BOLD differences in the absence of "true" neural differences (D'Esposito et al., 2003; Samanez-Larkin and D'Esposito, 2008). The current study however, does not compare heterogeneous groups (e.g., young vs. old, low-fit vs. high-fit)—all participants were low-fit but relatively healthy older adults, and all analyses controlled for age. Moreover, across the whole sample, baseline VO_2 and baseline modularity were not significantly correlated (all $|r| < 0.067$, all $p > 0.457$, two-tailed), even after controlling for mean FD. In addition, controlling for baseline VO_2 in the modularity vs. training gain analyses does not change the results. Future studies can include taking into account indicators of cerebrovascular health such as cerebral blood flow (Brown et al., 2010; Zimmerman et al., 2014) to determine whether and/or to what extent it relates to connectivity measures. In the current study, we controlled for measures such as age, medication, and structural brain measures to examine the potential effects of confounds common to studying an older population. Nonetheless, methodological considerations such as the use of population-specific brain templates may help increase the reliability of brain measures (Buckner et al., 2004).

Fitness and Cognitive Gains after Exercise Intervention

The cognitive improvements in the current study are similar to previous studies that find the largest gains in executive function after aerobic exercise training (Colcombe and Kramer, 2003; Guiney and Machado, 2013; Voss et al., 2013c; Kelly et al., 2014). Here, we used a composite score to analyze training effects instead of assessing group by time interactions in each cognitive task, which can be problematic given the multitude of tasks which requires multiple statistical comparisons. Nonetheless, it is possible that the cognitive effects of the current intervention are driven by specific tasks. For example, the task-switching and spatial working memory tasks in the current study are similar to previous tasks that are sensitive to fitness-related improvements (Hawkins et al., 1992; Kramer et al., 2001; Colcombe and Kramer, 2003; Erickson et al., 2011). On the other hand, improvements in reasoning tasks have been less studied in fitness interventions, although aerobic-related gains in visuo-spatial processes have been documented in younger populations (Stroth et al., 2009; Monti et al., 2012), and improvement in reasoning skills have been found after cognitive training interventions in older adults (Ball et al., 2002; Willis et al., 2006; Lustig et al., 2009). Moreover, compared to previous studies (Colcombe and Kramer, 2003; Voss et al., 2010b; Erickson et al., 2011), the current intervention lasted only 6 months, and it is likely that larger cognitive effects would result from a longer intervention (Colcombe and Kramer, 2003; Kelly et al., 2014). In addition, aerobic exercise has been shown to improve hippocampal function in animal and human studies (Berchtold et al., 2010; Voss et al., 2013c), increase hippocampal volume in humans (Erickson et al., 2011) and to relate to hippocampal-dependent functions such as spatial memory (Erickson et al., 2011) and relational memory (Chaddock et al., 2010). Given these previous findings, we would have expected exercise-related effects not only in the spatial working memory task, but also in the episodic memory tasks. The null findings of the current study may in part reflect a lack of sensitivity in these relatively brief memory tasks in measuring intervention-related change, but may also stem from comparable effects across the four groups, with similar improvements from the different interventions.

In the current study, the SSS group performed exercises that involved some form of resistance training, which has also shown to be beneficial for executive functioning in older adults when performed at a higher intensity (Liu-Ambrose et al., 2010, 2012). Although the strength portion of the SSS exercises in the current study is not comparable to the intensive strength training regimens of other studies, the similarity in exercise style may present an issue for analyzing the effects of interventions such as these, since strength training exercise and aerobic-walking exercise may benefit cognitive function in both differential and overlapping ways. Thus, "null effects" in terms of a lack of differential improvement (i.e., group by time interaction) in other cognitive domains may instead partly reflect comparable gains from the different types of interventions (in addition to gains attributable to test-retest effects) and contamination effects from self-initiated exercise (Ehlers et al., 2016). The Dance group, despite the cognitive demands thought to be involved in the learning and execution of dance steps, showed the smallest effects post-intervention; the group as a whole did not improve in CRF and showed the smallest changes in cognitive function. These findings may in part stem from the heterogeneity and lack of intensity in the Dance sessions, which varied in form (i.e., type of dance) across sessions, and may have thus failed to consistently and intensively train specific physical and cognitive skills. Indeed, Dance participants perceived their in-class sessions as less intensive (Ehlers et al., 2016). Nonetheless, the Dance intervention in the current study has been shown to improve white matter microstructure in the fornix, with baseline fornix fractional anisotropy correlating with baseline processing speed (Burzynska et al., 2017). This paper focuses on EF and connectivity in gray matter, and it is likely that different brain measures reflect distinct aspects of cognitive function. Moreover, the sixth month duration before pre- and post-testing may not adequately reflect longer-term neural and behavioral effects of each intervention.

EF improvements were not directly related to CRF improvements. Combining the test scores into a composite score may have diluted any relationship between CRF gain and gains in a specific test, but no robust correlations were found when examining the relationship between CRF gain and gain on each test measure. In addition, it is possible that intervention-related gains in CRF *per se* does not lead to cognitive improvements, and that indirect effects of exercise on stress, sleep and overall health lead to positive cognitive outcomes (King et al., 1997; Etnier et al., 2006; Cotman et al., 2007; Bherer et al., 2013; Awick et al., 2015). Furthermore, CRF as measured using VO_2 peak in the current study, indexes an array of bodily functions (Dustman et al., 1984; Etnier et al., 2006; Jain et al., 2010) and may not adequately capture cerebrovascular changes.

AUTHOR CONTRIBUTIONS

Conceptualization and study design: PB, CG, MV, EM, AK, and MD. Data collection: PB, MV, AB, CW, GC, KD, JF, DE, ES, and SA. Data analysis: PB and CG. Writing—original draft: PB and CG. Writing—review and editing: PB, CG, MV, AB, JF, DE, ES, EM, AK, and MD.

ACKNOWLEDGMENTS

This work was supported by the National Science Foundation (IGERT Grant 0903622 to PB), Beckman Institute for Advanced Science and Technology (Graduate Fellowship to PB), Department of Defense (NDSEG to CG), National Institutes of Health (Grant R37 AG025667 to AK and EM, Grant NS079698 to MD), Center for Nutrition Learning and Memory, UIUC (Grant 2012-04673 to AK and EM), and the American Cancer Society (Postdoctoral Fellowship Grant PF-16-021-01-CPPB to DE). We thank Anya Knecht and Susan Houseworth for coordinating the intervention, Nancy Dodge and Holly Tracy for assistance in MRI data collection, Kathleen Kramer and Kishan Patel for assistance with Freesurfer processing, and members of the Lifelong Brain and Cognition Laboratory and Exercise Psychology Laboratory for assistance in data collection.

REFERENCES

Andrews-Hanna, J. R., Snyder, A. Z., Vincent, J. L., Lustig, C., Head, D., Raichle, M. E., et al. (2007). Disruption of large-scale brain systems in advanced aging. *Neuron* 56, 924–935. doi: 10.1016/j.neuron.2007.10.038

Arnemann, K. L., Chen, A. J. W., Novakovic-Agopian, T., Gratton, C., Nomura, E. M., and D'Esposito, M. (2015). Functional brain network modularity predicts response to cognitive training after brain injury. *Neurology* 84, 1568–1574. doi: 10.1212/WNL.0000000000001476

Avants, B. B., Tustison, N. J., Song, G., Cook, P. A., Klein, A., and Gee, J. C. (2011). A reproducible evaluation of ANTs similarity metric performance in brain image registration. *Neuroimage* 54, 2033–2044. doi: 10.1016/j.neuroimage.2010.09.025

Avants, B. B., Yushkevich, P., Pluta, J., Minkoff, D., Korczykowski, M., Detre, J., et al. (2010). The optimal template effect in hippocampus studies of diseased populations. *Neuroimage* 49, 2457–2466. doi: 10.1016/j.neuroimage.2009.09.062

Awick, E. A., Wójcicki, T. R., Olson, E. A., Fanning, J., Chung, H. D., Zuniga, K., et al. (2015). Differential exercise effects on quality of life and health-related quality of life in older adults: a randomized controlled trial. *Qual. Life Res.* 24, 455–462. doi: 10.1007/s11136-014-0762-0

Balke, B., and Ware, R. W. (1959). *The Present Status of Physical Fitness in the Air Force.* Fort Belvoir, VA: Defense Technical Information Center.

Ball, K., Berch, D. B., Helmers, K. F., Jobe, J. B., Leveck, M. D., Marsiske, M., et al. (2002). Effects of cognitive training interventions with older adults: a randomized controlled trial. *JAMA* 288, 2271–2281. doi: 10.1001/jama.288.18.2271

Baniqued, P. L., Gallen, C. L., Kranz, M. B., Kramer, A. F., and D'Esposito, M. (2015). "Brain network predictors of cognitive training-related gains in young adults," in *Society for Neuroscience Annual Meeting* (Chicago, IL).

Basak, C., Voss, M. W., Erickson, K. I., Boot, W. R., and Kramer, A. F. (2011). Regional differences in brain volume predict the acquisition of skill in a complex real-time strategy videogame. *Brain Cogn.* 76, 407–414. doi: 10.1016/j.bandc.2011.03.017

Behzadi, Y., Restom, K., Liau, J., and Liu, T. T. (2007). A component based noise correction method (CompCor) for BOLD and perfusion based fMRI. *Neuroimage* 37, 90–101. doi: 10.1016/j.neuroimage.2007.04.042

Bennett, G. K., Seashore, H. G., and Wesman, A. G. (1997). *Differential Aptitude Test.* San Antonio, TX: Psychological Corporation.

Berchtold, N. C., Castello, N., and Cotman, C. W. (2010). Exercise and time-dependent benefits to learning and memory. *Neuroscience* 167, 588–597. doi: 10.1016/j.neuroscience.2010.02.050

Bertolero, M. A., Yeo, B. T., and D'Esposito, M. (2015). The modular and integrative functional architecture of the human brain. *Proc. Natl. Acad. Sci. U.S.A.* 112, E6798–E6807. doi: 10.1073/pnas.1510619112

Betzel, R. F., Byrge, L., He, Y., Goñi, J., Zuo, X.-N., and Sporns, O. (2014). Changes in structural and functional connectivity among resting-state networks across the human lifespan. *Neuroimage* 102, 345–357. doi: 10.1016/j.neuroimage.2014.07.067

Bherer, L., Erickson, K. I., and Liu-Ambrose, T. (2013). A review of the effects of physical activity and exercise on cognitive and brain functions in older adults. *J. Aging Res.* 2013, 1–8. doi: 10.1155/2013/657508

Birn, R. M., Molloy, E. K., Patriat, R., Parker, T., Meier, T. B., Kirk, G. R., et al. (2013). The effect of scan length on the reliability of resting-state fMRI connectivity estimates. *Neuroimage* 83, 550–558. doi: 10.1016/j.neuroimage.2013.05.099

Bouchard, C., and Rankinen, T. (2001). Individual differences in response to regular physical activity. *Med. Sci. Sports Exerc.* 33, S446–S451. discussion: S452–S453. doi: 10.1097/00005768-200106001-00013

Brown, A. D., McMorris, C. A., Longman, R. S., Leigh, R., Hill, M. D., Friedenreich, C. M., et al. (2010). Effects of cardiorespiratory fitness and cerebral blood flow on cognitive outcomes in older women. *Neurobiol. Aging* 31, 2047–2057. doi: 10.1016/j.neurobiolaging.2008.11.002

Buckley, R. F., Schultz, A. P., Hedden, T., Papp, K. V., Hanseeuw, B. J., Marshall, G., et al. (2017). Functional network integrity presages cognitive decline in preclinical Alzheimer disease. *Neurology* 89, 29–37. doi: 10.1212/WNL.0000000000004059

Buckner, R. L., Head, D., Parker, J., Fotenos, A. F., Marcus, D., Morris, J. C., et al. (2004). A unified approach for morphometric and functional data analysis in young, old, and demented adults using automated atlas-based head size normalization: reliability and validation against manual measurement of total intracranial volume. *Neuroimage* 23, 724–738. doi: 10.1016/j.neuroimage.2004.06.018

Bullmore, E., and Sporns, O. (2009). Complex brain networks: graph theoretical analysis of structural and functional systems. *Nat. Rev. Neurosci.* 10, 186–198. doi: 10.1038/nrn2575

Burzynska, A. Z., Jiao, Y., Knecht, A. M., Fanning, J., Awick, E. A., Chen, T., et al. (2017). White matter integrity declined over 6-months, but dance intervention improved integrity of the fornix of older adults. *Front. Aging Neurosci.* 9:59. doi: 10.3389/fnagi.2017.00059

Burzynska, A. Z., Wong, C. N., Voss, M. W., Cooke, G. E., McAuley, E., and Kramer, A. F. (2015). White matter integrity supports BOLD signal variability and cognitive performance in the aging human brain. *PLoS ONE* 10:e0120315. doi: 10.1371/journal.pone.0120315

Cao, H., Plichta, M. M., Schäfer, A., Haddad, L., Grimm, O., Schneider, M., et al. (2014). Test–retest reliability of fMRI-based graph theoretical properties during working memory, emotion processing, and resting state. *Neuroimage* 84, 888–900. doi: 10.1016/j.neuroimage.2013.09.013

Chaddock, L., Erickson, K. I., Prakash, R. S., Kim, J. S., Voss, M. W., VanPatter, M., et al. (2010). A neuroimaging investigation of the association between aerobic fitness, hippocampal volume, and memory performance in preadolescent children. *Brain Res.* 1358, 172–183. doi: 10.1016/j.brainres.2010.08.049

Chadick, J. Z., Zanto, T. P., and Gazzaley, A. (2014). Structural and functional differences in medial prefrontal cortex underlie distractibility and suppression deficits in ageing. *Nat. Commun.* 5:4223. doi: 10.1038/ncomms5223

Chan, M. Y., Park, D. C., Savalia, N. K., Petersen, S. E., and Wig, G. S. (2014). Decreased segregation of brain systems across the healthy adult lifespan. *Proc. Natl. Acad. Sci. U.S.A.* 111, E4997–E5006. doi: 10.1073/pnas.1415122111

Chen, Z. J., He, Y., Rosa-Neto, P., Germann, J., and Evans, A. C. (2008). Revealing modular architecture of human brain structural networks by using cortical thickness from MRI. *Cereb. Cortex* 18, 2374–2381. doi: 10.1093/cercor/bhn003

Chen, Z. J., He, Y., Rosa-Neto, P., Gong, G., and Evans, A. C. (2011). Age-related alterations in the modular organization of structural cortical network by using cortical thickness from MRI. *Neuroimage* 56, 235–245. doi: 10.1016/j.neuroimage.2011.01.010

Clune, J., Mouret, J.-B., and Lipson, H. (2013). The evolutionary origins of modularity. *Proc. R. Soc. B* 280:20122863. doi: 10.1098/rspb.2012.2863

Colcombe, S., and Kramer, A. F. (2003). Fitness effects on the cognitive function of older adults: a meta-analytic study. *Psychol. Sci.* 14, 125–130. doi: 10.1111/1467-9280.t01-1-01430

Cotman, C. W., Berchtold, N. C., and Christie, L.-A. (2007). Exercise builds brain health: key roles of growth factor cascades and inflammation. *Trends Neurosci.* 30, 464–472. doi: 10.1016/j.tins.2007.06.011

Dale, A. M., Fischl, B., and Sereno, M. I. (1999). Cortical surface-based analysis. *Neuroimage* 9, 179–194. doi: 10.1006/nimg.1998.0395

Damoiseaux, J. S., Beckmann, C. F., Arigita, E. J., Barkhof, F., Scheltens, P., Stam, C. J., et al. (2008). Reduced resting-state brain activity in the "default network" in normal aging. *Cereb. Cortex* 18, 1856–1864. doi: 10.1093/cercor/bhm207

Desikan, R. S., Ségonne, F., Fischl, B., Quinn, B. T., Dickerson, B. C., Blacker, D., et al. (2006). An automated labeling system for subdividing the human cerebral cortex on MRI scans into gyral based regions of interest. *Neuroimage* 31, 968–980. doi: 10.1016/j.neuroimage.2006.01.021

D'Esposito, M., Deouell, L. Y., and Gazzaley, A. (2003). Alterations in the BOLD fMRI signal with ageing and disease: a challenge for neuroimaging. *Nat. Rev. Neurosci.* 4, 863–872. doi: 10.1038/nrn1246

Draheim, C., Hicks, K. L., and Engle, R. W. (2016). Combining reaction time and accuracy. *Perspect. Psychol. Sci.* 11, 133–155. doi: 10.1177/1745691615596990

Duncan, E. S., and Small, S. L. (2016). Increased modularity of resting state networks supports improved narrative production in aphasia recovery. *Brain Connect.* 6, 524–529. doi: 10.1089/brain.2016.0437

Dustman, R. E., Ruhling, R. O., Russell, E. M., Shearer, D. E., Bonekat, H. W., Shigeoka, J. W., et al. (1984). Aerobic exercise training and improved neuropsychological function of older individuals. *Neurobiol. Aging* 5, 35–42. doi: 10.1016/0197-4580(84)90083-6

Ehlers, D. K., Banducci, S. E., Daugherty, A. M., Fanning, J., Awick, E. A., Porter, G. C., et al. (2017a). Effects of gait self-efficacy and lower-extremity physical function on dual-task performance in older adults. *Biomed Res. Int.* 2017:8570960. doi: 10.1155/2017/8570960

Ehlers, D. K., Daugherty, A. M., Burzynska, A. Z., Fanning, J., Awick, E. A., Chaddock-Heyman, L., et al. (2017b). Regional brain volumes moderate, but do not mediate, the effects of group-based exercise training on reductions in loneliness in older adults. *Front. Aging Neurosci.* 9:110. doi: 10.3389/fnagi.2017.00110

Ehlers, D. K., Fanning, J., Awick, E. A., Kramer, A. F., and McAuley, E. (2016). Contamination by an active control condition in a randomized exercise trial. *PLoS ONE* 11:e0164246. doi: 10.1371/journal.pone.0164246

Ekstrom, R. B., French, J. W., Harman, H. H., and Dermen, D. (1976). *Manual for Kit of Factor-Referenced Cognitive Tests.* Princeton, NJ: Educational Testing Service.

Ericsson, A., Aljabar, P., and Rueckert, D. (2008). "Construction of a patient-specific atlas of the brain: application to normal aging," in *5th IEEE International Symposium on Biomedical Imaging: From Nano to Macro, 2008. ISBI 2008* (Paris: IEEE), 480–483.

Erickson, K. I., Boot, W. R., Basak, C., Neider, M. B., Prakash, R. S., Voss, M. W., et al. (2010). Striatal volume predicts level of video game skill acquisition. *Cereb. Cortex* 20, 2522–2530. doi: 10.1093/cercor/bhp293

Erickson, K. I., Voss, M. W., Prakash, R. S., Basak, C., Szabo, A., Chaddock, L., et al. (2011). Exercise training increases size of hippocampus and improves memory. *Proc. Natl. Acad. Sci. U.S.A.* 108, 3017–3022. doi: 10.1073/pnas.1015950108

Etnier, J. L., Nowell, P. M., Landers, D. M., and Sibley, B. A. (2006). A meta-regression to examine the relationship between aerobic fitness and cognitive performance. *Brain Res. Rev.* 52, 119–130. doi: 10.1016/j.brainresrev.2006.01.002

Fabiani, M. (2012). It was the best of times, it was the worst of times: a psychophysiologist's view of cognitive aging. *Psychophysiology* 49, 283–304. doi: 10.1111/j.1469-8986.2011.01331.x

Fanning, J., Porter, G., Awick, E. A., Ehlers, D. K., Roberts, S. A., Cooke, G., et al. (2017). Replacing sedentary time with sleep, light, or moderate-to-vigorous physical activity: effects on self-regulation and executive functioning. *J. Behav. Med.* 40, 332–342. doi: 10.1007/s10865-016-9788-9

Fischl, B., Salat, D. H., Busa, E., Albert, M., Dieterich, M., Haselgrove, C., et al. (2002). Whole brain segmentation: automated labeling of neuroanatomical structures in the human brain. *Neuron* 33, 341–355. doi: 10.1016/S0896-6273(02)00569-X

Fischl, B., Salat, D. H., van der Kouwe, A. J. W., Makris, N., Ségonne, F., Quinn, B. T., et al. (2004a). Sequence-independent segmentation of magnetic resonance images. *Neuroimage* 23, S69–S84. doi: 10.1016/j.neuroimage.2004.07.016

Fischl, B., van der Kouwe, A., Destrieux, C., Halgren, E., Ségonne, F., Salat, D. H., et al. (2004b). Automatically parcellating the human cerebral cortex. *Cereb. Cortex* 14, 11–22. doi: 10.1093/cercor/bhg087

Fonov, V. S., Evans, A. C., McKinstry, R. C., Almli, C. R., and Collins, D. L. (2009). Unbiased nonlinear average age-appropriate brain templates from birth to adulthood. *Neuroimage* 47:S102. doi: 10.1016/S1053-8119(09)70884-5

Fornito, A., Zalesky, A., and Breakspear, M. (2015). The connectomics of brain disorders. *Nat. Rev. Neurosci.* 16, 159–172. doi: 10.1038/nrn3901

Fortunato, S. (2010). Community detection in graphs. *Phys. Rep.* 486, 75–174. doi: 10.1016/j.physrep.2009.11.002

Friston, K. J., Williams, S., Howard, R., Frackowiak, R. S., and Turner, R. (1996). Movement-related effects in fMRI time-series. *Magn. Reson. Med.* 35, 346–355. doi: 10.1002/mrm.1910350312

Froelicher, V. F. Jr., Thompson, A. J. Jr., Noguera, I., Davis, G., Stewart, A. J., and Triebwasser, J. H. (1975). Prediction of maximal oxygen consumption. *Chest* 68, 331–336. doi: 10.1378/chest.68.3.331

Gabrieli, J. D., Ghosh, S. S., and Whitfield-Gabrieli, S. (2015). Prediction as a humanitarian and pragmatic contribution from human cognitive neuroscience. *Neuron* 85, 11–26. doi: 10.1016/j.neuron.2014.10.047

Gallen, C. L., Baniqued, P. L., Chapman, S. B., Aslan, S., Keebler, M., Didehbani, N., et al. (2016). Modular brain network organization predicts response to cognitive training in older adults. *PLoS ONE* 11:e0169015. doi: 10.1371/journal.pone.0169015

Geerligs, L., Renken, R. J., Saliasi, E., Maurits, N. M., and Lorist, M. M. (2015). A Brain-wide study of age-related changes in functional connectivity. *Cereb. Cortex* 25, 1987–1999. doi: 10.1093/cercor/bhu012

Giavasis, S., Khanuja, R., Sikka, S., Shehzad, Z., Clark, D., Cheung, B., et al. (2015). *C-PAC: CPAC Version 0.3.9 Alpha.*

Gordon, E. M., Laumann, T. O., Gilmore, A. W., Newbold, D. J., Greene, D. J., Berg, J. J., et al. (2017). Precision functional mapping of individual human Brains. *Neuron* 95, 791–807.e7. doi: 10.1016/j.neuron.2017.07.011

Grady, C. (2013). Trends in neurocognitive aging. *Nat. Rev. Neurosci.* 13, 491–505. doi: 10.1038/nrn3256

Gratton, C., Nomura, E. M., Pérez, F., and D'Esposito, M. (2012). Focal brain lesions to critical locations cause widespread disruption of the modular organization of the brain. *J Cogn. Neurosci.* 24, 1275–1285. doi: 10.1162/jocn_a_00222

Guiney, H., and Machado, L. (2013). Benefits of regular aerobic exercise for executive functioning in healthy populations. *Psychon. Bull. Rev.* 20, 73–86. doi: 10.3758/s13423-012-0345-4

Hagberg, A. A., Schult, D. A., and Swart, P. J. (2008). "Exploring network structure, dynamics, and function using NetworkX," in *Proceedings of the 7th Python in Science Conference (SciPy2008)*, eds G. Varoquaux, T. Vaught, and J. Millman (Pasadena, CA: Los Alamos National Laboratory (LANL)), 11–15.

Hawkins, H. L., Kramer, A. F., and Capaldi, D. (1992). Aging, exercise, and attention. *Psychol. Aging* 7, 643–653. doi: 10.1037/0882-7974.7.4.643

Heckemann, R. A., Hartkens, T., Leung, K. K., Zheng, Y., Hill, D. L., Hajnal, J. V., et al. (2003). "Information extraction from medical images: developing an e-Science application based on the Globus toolkit," in *Proceedings of the 2nd UK e-Science All Hands Meeting* (Nottingham).

Hedden, T., Mormino, E. C., Amariglio, R. E., Younger, A. P., Schultz, A. P., Becker, J. A., et al. (2012). Cognitive profile of amyloid burden and white matter hyperintensities in cognitively normal older adults. *J. Neurosci.* 32, 16233–16242. doi: 10.1523/JNEUROSCI.2462-12.2012

Hillman, C. H., Erickson, K. I., and Kramer, A. F. (2008). Be smart, exercise your heart: exercise effects on brain and cognition. *Nat. Rev. Neurosci.* 9, 58–65. doi: 10.1038/nrn2298

Huberty, C. J., and Morris, J. D. (1989). Multivariate analysis versus multiple univariate analyses. *Psychol. Bull.* 105, 302–308. doi: 10.1037/0033-2909.105.2.302

Jack, C. R. Jr., Twomey, C. K., Zinsmeister, A. R., Sharbrough, F. W., Petersen, R. C., and Cascino, G. D. (1989). Anterior temporal lobes and hippocampal formations: normative volumetric measurements from MR images in young adults. *Radiology* 172, 549–554. doi: 10.1148/radiology.172.2.2748838

Jain, V., Langham, M. C., and Wehrli, F. W. (2010). MRI estimation of global brain oxygen consumption rate. *J. Cereb. Blood Flow Metab.* 30, 1598–1607. doi: 10.1038/jcbfm.2010.49

Kane, M. J., Hambrick, D. Z., and Conway, A. R. A. (2005). Working memory capacity and fluid intelligence are strongly related constructs: comment on ackerman, beier, and boyle (2005). *Psychol. Bull.* 131, 66–71. doi: 10.1037/0033-2909.131.1.66

Kashtan, N., and Alon, U. (2005). Spontaneous evolution of modularity and network motifs. *Proc. Natl. Acad. Sci. U.S.A.* 102, 13773–13778. doi: 10.1073/pnas.0503610102

Kawagoe, T., Onoda, K., and Yamaguchi, S. (2017). Associations among executive function, cardiorespiratory fitness, and brain network properties in older adults. *Sci. Rep.* 7:40107. doi: 10.1038/srep40107

Kelly, M. E., Loughrey, D., Lawlor, B. A., Robertson, I. H., Walsh, C., and Brennan, S. (2014). The impact of exercise on the cognitive functioning of healthy older adults: a systematic review and meta-analysis. *Ageing Res. Rev.* 16, 12–31. doi: 10.1016/j.arr.2014.05.002

Kennedy, K. M., and Raz, N. (2009). Aging white matter and cognition: differential effects of regional variations in diffusion properties on memory, executive functions, and speed. *Neuropsychologia* 47, 916–927. doi: 10.1016/j.neuropsychologia.2009.01.001

King, A. C., Oman, R. F., Brassington, G. S., Bliwise, D. L., and Haskell, W. L. (1997). Moderate-intensity exercise and self-rated quality of sleep in older adults: a randomized controlled trial. *JAMA* 277, 32–37. doi: 10.1001/jama.1997.03540250040029

Kitzbichler, M. G., Henson, R. N., Smith, M. L., Nathan, P. J., and Bullmore, E. T. (2011). Cognitive effort drives workspace configuration of human brain functional networks. *J. Neurosci.* 31, 8259–8270. doi: 10.1523/JNEUROSCI.0440-11.2011

Kramer, A. F., Erickson, K. I., and Colcombe, S. J. (2006). Exercise, cognition, and the aging brain. *J. Appl. Physiol.* 101, 1237–1242. doi: 10.1152/japplphysiol.00500.2006

Kramer, A. F., Hahn, S., and Gopher, D. (1999). Task coordination and aging: explorations of executive control processes in the task switching paradigm. *Acta Psychol.* 101, 339–378. doi: 10.1016/S0001-6918(99)00011-6

Kramer, A. F., Hahn, S., McAuley, E., Cohen, N. J., Banich, M. T., Harrison, C., et al. (2001). "Exercise, aging and cognition: healthy body, healthy mind?," in *Human Factors Interventions for the Health Care of Older Adults*, eds A. D. Fisk and W. Rogers (Hillsdale, NJ: Erlbaum), 91–120.

Landman, B. A., Huang, A. J., Gifford, A., Vikram, D. S., Lim, I. A., Farrell, J. A., et al. (2011). Multi-parametric neuroimaging reproducibility: a 3-T resource study. *Neuroimage* 54, 2854–2866. doi: 10.1016/j.neuroimage.2010.11.047

Laumann, T. O., Gordon, E. M., Adeyemo, B., Snyder, A. Z., Joo, S. J., Chen, M.-Y., et al. (2015). Functional system and areal organization of a highly sampled individual human brain. *Neuron* 87, 657–670. doi: 10.1016/j.neuron.2015.06.037

Leckie, R. L., Oberlin, L. E., Voss, M. W., Prakash, R. S., Szabo-Reed, A., Chaddock-Heyman, L., et al. (2014). BDNF mediates improvements in executive function following a 1-year exercise intervention. *Front. Hum. Neurosci.* 8:985. doi: 10.3389/fnhum.2014.00985

Liu-Ambrose, T., Nagamatsu, L. S., Graf, P., Beattie, B. L., Ashe, M. C., and Handy, T. C. (2010). Resistance training and executive functions: a 12-month randomized controlled trial. *Arch. Intern. Med.* 170, 170–178. doi: 10.1001/archinternmed.2009.494

Liu-Ambrose, T., Nagamatsu, L. S., Voss, M. W., Khan, K. M., and Handy, T. C. (2012). Resistance training and functional plasticity of the aging brain: a 12-month randomized controlled trial. *Neurobiol. Aging* 33, 1690–1698. doi: 10.1016/j.neurobiolaging.2011.05.010

Lustig, C., Shah, P., Seidler, R., and Reuter-Lorenz, P. A. (2009). Aging, training, and the brain: a review and future directions. *Neuropsychol. Rev.* 19, 504–522. doi: 10.1007/s11065-009-9119-9

Madden, D. J., Bennett, I. J., Burzynska, A., Potter, G. G., Chen, N.-K., and Song, A. W. (2012). Diffusion tensor imaging of cerebral white matter integrity in cognitive aging. *Biochim. Biophys. Acta* 1822, 386–400. doi: 10.1016/j.bbadis.2011.08.003

Madden, D. J., Bennett, I. J., and Song, A. W. (2009). Cerebral white matter integrity and cognitive aging: contributions from diffusion tensor imaging. *Neuropsychol. Rev.* 19, 415–435. doi: 10.1007/s11065-009-9113-2

Mathewson, K. E., Basak, C., Maclin, E. L., Low, K. A., Boot, W. R., Kramer, A. F., et al. (2012). Different slopes for different folks: alpha and delta EEG power predict subsequent video game learning rate and improvements in cognitive control tasks. *Psychophysiology* 49, 1558–1570. doi: 10.1111/j.1469-8986.2012.01474.x

Meunier, D., Achard, S., Morcom, A., and Bullmore, E. (2009). Age-related changes in modular organization of human brain functional networks. *Neuroimage* 44, 715–723. doi: 10.1016/j.neuroimage.2008.09.062

Meunier, D., Lambiotte, R., and Bullmore, E. T. (2010). Modular and hierarchically modular organization of brain networks. *Front. Neurosci.* 4:200. doi: 10.3389/fnins.2010.00200

Meunier, D., Stamatakis, E. A., and Tyler, L. K. (2014). Age-related functional reorganization, structural changes, and preserved cognition. *Neurobiol. Aging* 35, 42–54. doi: 10.1016/j.neurobiolaging.2013.07.003

Monti, J. M., Hillman, C. H., and Cohen, N. J. (2012). Aerobic fitness enhances relational memory in preadolescent children: the FITKids randomized control trial. *Hippocampus* 22, 1876–1882. doi: 10.1002/hipo.22023

Muschelli, J., Nebel, M. B., Caffo, B. S., Barber, A. D., Pekar, J. J., and Mostofsky, S. H. (2014). Reduction of motion-related artifacts in resting state fMRI using aCompCor. *Neuroimage* 96, 22–35. doi: 10.1016/j.neuroimage.2014.03.028

Newman, M. E. (2006a). Finding community structure in networks using the eigenvectors of matrices. *Phys. Rev. E* 74:036104. doi: 10.1103/PhysRevE.74.036104

Newman, M. E. (2006b). Modularity and community structure in networks. *Proc. Natl. Acad. Sci. U.S.A.* 103, 8577–8582. doi: 10.1073/pnas.0601602103

Newman, M. E., and Girvan, M. (2004). Finding and evaluating community structure in networks. *Phys. Rev. E* 69:026113. doi: 10.1103/PhysRevE.69.026113

Nomura, E. M., Gratton, C., Visser, R. M., Kayser, A., Perez, F., and D'Esposito, M. (2010). Double dissociation of two cognitive control networks in patients with focal brain lesions. *Proc. Natl. Acad. Sci. U.S.A.* 107, 12017–12022. doi: 10.1073/pnas.1002431107

O'Bryant, S. E., Humphreys, J. D., Smith, G. E., Ivnik, R. J., Graff-Radford, N. R., Petersen, R. C., et al. (2008). Detecting dementia with the mini-mental state examination in highly educated individuals. *Arch. Neurol.* 65, 963–967. doi: 10.1001/archneur.65.7.963

Onoda, K., and Yamaguchi, S. (2013). Small-worldness and modularity of the resting-state functional brain network decrease with aging. *Neurosci. Lett.* 556, 104–108. doi: 10.1016/j.neulet.2013.10.023

Persson, J., Nyberg, L., Lind, J., Larsson, A., Nilsson, L.-G., Ingvar, M., et al. (2006). Structure-function correlates of cognitive decline in aging. *Cereb. Cortex* 16, 907–915. doi: 10.1093/cercor/bhj036

Power, J. D., Barnes, K. A., Snyder, A. Z., Schlaggar, B. L., and Petersen, S. E. (2012). Spurious but systematic correlations in functional connectivity MRI networks arise from subject motion. *Neuroimage* 59, 2142–2154. doi: 10.1016/j.neuroimage.2011.10.018

Power, J. D., Cohen, A. L., Nelson, S. M., Wig, G. S., Barnes, K. A., Church, J. A., et al. (2011). Functional network organization of the human brain. *Neuron* 72, 665–678. doi: 10.1016/j.neuron.2011.09.006

Power, J. D., and Petersen, S. E. (2013). Control-related systems in the human brain. *Curr. Opin. Neurobiol.* 23, 223–228. doi: 10.1016/j.conb.2012.12.009

Pudas, S., Josefsson, M., Rieckmann, A., and Nyberg, L. (2017). Longitudinal evidence for increased functional response in frontal cortex for older adults with hippocampal atrophy and memory decline. *Cereb. Cortex.* doi: 10.1093/cercor/bhw418. [Epub ahead of print].

Ravens, J. C. (1962). *Advanced Progressive Matrices.* London: HK Lewis.

Raz, N., Lindenberger, U., Rodrigue, K. M., Kennedy, K. M., Head, D., Williamson, A., et al. (2005). Regional brain changes in aging healthy adults: general trends, individual differences and modifiers. *Cereb. Cortex* 15, 1676–1689. doi: 10.1093/cercor/bhi044

Raz, N., and Rodrigue, K. M. (2006). Differential aging of the brain: patterns, cognitive correlates and modifiers. *Neurosci. Biobehav. Rev.* 30, 730–748. doi: 10.1016/j.neubiorev.2006.07.001

Ross, R., Blair, S. N., Arena, R., Church, T. S., Després, J.-P., Franklin, B. A., et al. (2016). Importance of assessing cardiorespiratory fitness in clinical practice: a case for fitness as a clinical vital sign: a scientific statement from the american heart association. *Circulation* 134, e653–e699. doi: 10.1161/CIR.0000000000000461

Rosvall, M., and Bergstrom, C. T. (2008). Maps of random walks on complex networks reveal community structure. *Proc. Natl. Acad. Sci. U.S.A.* 105, 1118–1123. doi: 10.1073/pnas.0706851105

Sadaghiani, S., Poline, J.-B., Kleinschmidt, A., and D'Esposito, M. (2015). Ongoing dynamics in large-scale functional connectivity predict perception. *Proc. Natl. Acad. Sci. U.S.A.* 112, 8463–8468. doi: 10.1073/pnas.1420687112

Salat, D. H., Buckner, R. L., Snyder, A. Z., Greve, D. N., Desikan, R. S. R., Busa, E., et al. (2004). Thinning of the cerebral cortex in aging. *Cereb. Cortex* 14, 721–730. doi: 10.1093/cercor/bhh032

Salthouse, T. A. (2004). Localizing age-related individual differences in a hierarchical structure. *Intelligence* 32, 541–561. doi: 10.1016/j.intell.2004.07.003

Salthouse, T. A. (1993). Speed and knowledge as determinants of adult age differences in verbal tasks. *J. Gerontol.* 48, P29–P36. doi: 10.1093/geronj/48.1.P29

Salthouse, T. A. (2005). Relations between cognitive abilities and measures of executive functioning. *Neuropsychology* 19, 532–545. doi: 10.1037/0894-4105.19.4.532

Salthouse, T. A. (2010). Influence of age on practice effects in longitudinal neurocognitive change. *Neuropsychology* 24, 563–572. doi: 10.1037/a0019026

Salthouse, T. A. (2016). Contributions of the individual differences approach to cognitive aging. *J. Gerontol. B Psychol. Sci. Soc. Sci.* 72, 7–15. doi: 10.1093/geronb/gbw069

Salthouse, T. A., and Babcock, R. L. (1991). Decomposing adult age differences in working memory. *Dev. Psychol.* 27, 763–776. doi: 10.1037/0012-1649.27.5.763

Salthouse, T. A., and Ferrer-Caja, E. (2003). What needs to be explained to account for age-related effects on multiple cognitive variables? *Psychol. Aging* 18, 91–110. doi: 10.1037/0882-7974.18.1.91

Salthouse, T. A., Fristoe, N., and Rhee, S. H. (1996). How localized are age-related effects on neuropsychological measures? *Neuropsychology* 10:272. doi: 10.1037/0894-4105.10.2.272

Samanez-Larkin, G. R., and D'Esposito, M. (2008). Group comparisons: imaging the aging brain. *Soc. Cogn. Affect. Neurosci.* 3, 290–297. doi: 10.1093/scan/nsn029

Satterthwaite, T. D., Wolf, D. H., Loughead, J., Ruparel, K., Elliott, M. A., Hakonarson, H., et al. (2012). Impact of in-scanner head motion on multiple measures of functional connectivity: relevance for studies of neurodevelopment in youth. *Neuroimage* 60, 623–632. doi: 10.1016/j.neuroimage.2011.12.063

Schultz, D. H., and Cole, M. W. (2016). Higher intelligence is associated with less task-related brain network reconfiguration. *J. Neurosci.* 36, 8551–8561. doi: 10.1523/JNEUROSCI.0358-16.2016

Siegel, J. S., Mitra, A., Laumann, T. O., Seitzman, B. A., Raichle, M., Corbetta, M., et al. (2016). Data quality influences observed links between functional connectivity and behavior. *Cereb.Cortex.* 27, 4492–4502. doi: 10.1093/cercor/bhw253

Soman, S., Prasad, G., Hitchner, E., Massaband, P., Moseley, M. E., Zhou, W., et al. (2016). Brain structural connectivity distinguishes patients at risk for cognitive decline after carotid interventions. *Hum. Brain Mapp.* 37, 2185–2194. doi: 10.1002/hbm.23166

Song, J., Birn, R. M., Boly, M., Meier, T. B., Nair, V. A., Meyerand, M. E., et al. (2014). Age-related reorganizational changes in modularity and functional connectivity of human brain networks. *Brain Connect.* 4, 662–676. doi: 10.1089/brain.2014.0286

Stanley, M. L., Dagenbach, D., Lyday, R. G., Burdette, J. H., and Laurienti, P. J. (2014). Changes in global and regional modularity associated with increasing working memory load. *Front. Hum. Neurosci.* 8:954. doi: 10.3389/fnhum.2014.00954

Stevens, A. A., Tappon, S. C., Garg, A., and Fair, D. A. (2012). Functional brain network modularity captures inter- and intra-individual variation in working memory capacity. *PLoS ONE* 7:e30468. doi: 10.1371/journal.pone.0030468

Stroth, S., Hille, K., Spitzer, M., and Reinhardt, R. (2009). Aerobic endurance exercise benefits memory and affect in young adults. *Neuropsychol. Rehabil.* 19, 223–243. doi: 10.1080/09602010802091183

Tosh, C. R., and McNally, L. (2015). The relative efficiency of modular and non-modular networks of different size. *Proc. R. Soc. B* 282:20142568. doi: 10.1098/rspb.2014.2568

Tukey, J. W. (1962). The future of data analysis. *Ann. Math. Stat.* 33, 1–67. doi: 10.1214/aoms/1177704711

Vo, L. T., Walther, D. B., Kramer, A. F., Erickson, K. I., Boot, W. R., Voss, M. W., et al. (2011). Predicting individuals' learning success from patterns of pre-learning MRI activity. *PLoS ONE* 6:e16093. doi: 10.1371/journal.pone.0016093

Voss, M. W., Erickson, K. I., Prakash, R. S., Chaddock, L., Kim, J. S., Alves, H., et al. (2013a). Neurobiological markers of exercise-related brain plasticity in older adults. *Brain Behav. Immun.* 28, 90–99. doi: 10.1016/j.bbi.2012.10.021

Voss, M. W., Erickson, K. I., Prakash, R. S., Malkowski, E., Kim, J. S., Morris, K. S., et al. (2010a). Functional connectivity: a source of variance in the association between cardiorespiratory fitness and cognition? *Neuropsychologia* 48, 1394–1406. doi: 10.1016/j.neuropsychologia.2010.01.005

Voss, M. W., Heo, S., Prakash, R. S., Erickson, K. I., Alves, H., Chaddock, L., et al. (2013b). The influence of aerobic fitness on cerebral white matter integrity and cognitive function in older adults: results of a one-year exercise intervention. *Hum. Brain Mapp.* 34, 2972–2985. doi: 10.1002/hbm.22119

Voss, M. W., Prakash, R. S., Erickson, K. I., Basak, C., Chaddock, L., Kim, J. S., et al. (2010b). Plasticity of brain networks in a randomized intervention trial of exercise training in older adults. *Front. Aging Neurosci.* 2:32. doi: 10.3389/fnagi.2010.00032

Voss, M. W., Vivar, C., Kramer, A. F., and van Praag, H. (2013c). Bridging animal and human models of exercise-induced brain plasticity. *Trends Cogn. Sci.* 17, 525–544. doi: 10.1016/j.tics.2013.08.001

Voss, M. W., Weng, T. B., Burzynska, A. Z., Wong, C. N., Cooke, G. E., Clark, R., et al. (2016). Fitness, but not physical activity, is related to functional integrity of brain networks associated with aging. *Neuroimage* 131, 113–125. doi: 10.1016/j.neuroimage.2015.10.044

Warren, D. E., Power, J. D., Bruss, J., Denburg, N. L., Waldron, E. J., Sun, H., et al. (2014). Network measures predict neuropsychological outcome after brain injury. *Proc. Natl. Acad. Sci. U.S.A.* 111, 14247–14252. doi: 10.1073/pnas.1322173111

Wechsler, D. (1997a). *WAIS-III: Administration and Scoring Manual: Wechsler Adult Intelligence Scale.* San Antonix, TX: The Psychological Corporation.

Wechsler, D. (1997b). *Wechsler Memory Scale (WMS-III).* San Antonio, TX: The Psychological Corporation.

Wenger, H. A., and Bell, G. J. (1986). The interactions of intensity, frequency and duration of exercise training in altering cardiorespiratory fitness. *Sports Med.* 3, 346–356. doi: 10.2165/00007256-198603050-00004

Wilcox, R. R. (2005). *Outlier Detection, 3rd Edn.* Chichester: John Wiley & Sons, Ltd.

Willis, S. L., Tennstedt, S. L., Marsiske, M., Ball, K., Elias, J., Koepke, K. M., et al. (2006). Long-term effects of cognitive training on everyday functional outcomes in older adults. *JAMA* 296, 2805–2814. doi: 10.1001/jama.296.23.2805

Wilson, R. S., Beckett, L. A., Barnes, L. L., Schneider, J. A., Bach, J., Evans, D. A., et al. (2002). Individual differences in rates of change in cognitive abilities of older persons. *Psychol. Aging* 17, 179–193. doi: 10.1037/0882-7974.17.2.179

Woodcock, R. W., and Johnson, M. B. (1989). *Woodcock-Johnson PsychoEducational Battery—Revised.* Allen, TX: DLM.

Zachary, R. (1986). *Shipley Institue of Living Scale-Revised.* Los Angeles, CA: Western Psychological Services.

Zhang, Y., Brady, M., and Smith, S. (2001). Segmentation of brain MR images through a hidden Markov random field model and the expectation-maximization algorithm. *IEEE Trans. Med. Imaging* 20, 45–57. doi: 10.1109/42.906424

Zimmerman, B., Sutton, B. P., Low, K. A., Fletcher, M. A., Tan, C. H., Schneider-Garces, N., et al. (2014). Cardiorespiratory fitness mediates the effects of aging on cerebral blood flow. *Front. Aging Neurosci.* 6:59. doi: 10.3389/fnagi.2014.00059

6

Racial Differences in Insular Connectivity and Thickness and Related Cognitive Impairment in Hypertension

Ganesh B. Chand[1], Junjie Wu[2], Deqiang Qiu[2,3†] and Ihab Hajjar[1,4†]*

[1] *Division of General Internal Medicine and Geriatrics, Department of Medicine, Emory University School of Medicine, Atlanta, GA, United States,* [2] *Department of Radiology and Imaging Sciences, Emory University School of Medicine, Atlanta, GA, United States,* [3] *Department of Biomedical Engineering, Georgia Institute of Technology, Emory University, Atlanta, GA, United States,* [4] *Department of Neurology, Emory Alzheimer's Disease Research Center, Emory University School of Medicine, Atlanta, GA, United States*

Correspondence:
Ganesh B. Chand
ganesh.chand@emory.edu
ganeshchand64@gmail.com

† These authors have contributed equally to this work.

Hypertensive African–Americans have a greater risk of cognitive impairment than hypertensive Caucasian–Americans. The neural basis of this increased risk is yet unknown. Neuroimaging investigations suggest that the normal neural activity comprises complex interactions between brain networks. Recent studies consistently demonstrate that the insula, part of the salience network, provides modulation effects (information flow) over the default-mode and central-executive networks in cognitively normal subjects, and argue that the modulation effect is declined in cognitive impairment. The purpose of this study is to examine the information flow at the nodes of three networks using resting state functional magnetic resonance imaging (MRI) data in cognitively impaired hypertensive individuals with the African–Americans and the Caucasian–Americans races, and to compare the thickness of impaired node between two racial groups. Granger causality methodology was used to calculate information flow between networks using resting state functional MRI data, and FreeSurfer was used to measure cortical thickness from T1-weighted structural images. We found that negative information flow of the insula in both African–Americans and Caucasian–Americans, which was in contrast with previously reported positive information flow in this region of normal individuals. Also, significantly greater negative information flow in insula was found in African–Americans than Caucasian–Americans (Wilcoxon rank sum; $Z = 2.06$; $p < 0.05$). Significantly, lower insula thickness was found in African–Americans compared with Caucasian–Americans (median = 2.797 mm vs. 2.897 mm) (Wilcoxon rank sum; $Z = 2.09$; $p < 0.05$). Finally, the insula thickness correlated with the global cognitive testing measured by Montreal cognitive assessment (Spearman's correlation; $r = 0.30$; $p < 0.05$). These findings suggest that the insula is a potential biomarker for the racial disparity in cognitive impairment of hypertensive individuals.

Keywords: cognitive impairment, cognitive racial disparity, salience network, default-mode network, central-executive network, Granger causality, cortical thickness, functional magnetic resonance imaging (fMRI)

INTRODUCTION

It is estimated that above 30% of population and 65% of older population have hypertension worldwide (Novak and Hajjar, 2010). Previous studies suggest that hypertensive individuals have a greater chance of occurring the dementia and physical disability than normotensive individuals (Johnson et al., 2008; Elias et al., 2012; Faraco and Iadecola, 2013). Cognitive functions, especially the executive functions (Chand and Dhamala, 2016b), are widely reported of being impaired in hypertensive individuals (Vicario et al., 2005; Gorelick and Nyenhuis, 2012; Hajjar et al., 2016). Individuals with hypertension have higher chances of occurring executive dysfunction earlier than individuals with normotension, which indicates a potential vascular-cognitive association (Oveisgharna and Hachinski, 2010). However, there are very limited neuroimaging studies that investigated the neural bases of hypertension in cognitive decline (Li et al., 2015). Former non-neuroimaging case studies further report that the African-Americans bear the greater burden of hypertension in the United States and have earlier onset of hypertension and larger hypertension-associated cognitive symptomatology and mortality than the other racial groups, including the Caucasian-Americans (Redmond et al., 2011; Hajjar et al., 2016). The neural mechanisms underlying this racial disparity is largely under-investigated so far. A triple brain network model—a model consisting of the brain's default-mode, salience, and central-executive networks and their interactions—has been recently employed in the neuroimaging field to elucidate the differences in the connectivity patterns associated with the different levels of cognitive impairments such as higher versus lower impairment (Menon, 2011; Uddin, 2015). We therefore use this model to investigate whether there is a difference in the impairment at the nodes of triple network between the African-Americans and the Caucasian-Americans hypertensive cognitively impaired individuals.

Resting state functional MRI (rsfMRI) has been used to investigate the functional brain areas or neurocognitive networks (Biswal et al., 1995; Raichle, 2015). Recent neuroimaging investigations suggest that the neural basis of cognitive activity is related to a dynamically modulating interaction between multiple networks, including the salience, default-mode, and central-executive networks (Bressler and Menon, 2010; Menon, 2015; Uddin, 2015; Chand and Dhamala, 2016a). The key nodes of the default-mode network include the posterior cingulate and the ventromedial prefrontal cortices, the salience network encompasses the insula and the dorsal anterior cingulate cortices, and the central-executive network comprises the posterior parietal and the dorsolateral prefrontal cortices (Chen et al., 2013). It has been demonstrated that the insula and dorsal anterior cingulate of salience network are anatomically connected (Bonnelle et al., 2012; Jilka et al., 2014) and consist of a special type of neurons named von Economo neurons that relay information processed within these regions to other brain regions, including the nodes of default-mode and central-executive networks (Allman et al., 2005, 2010; Watson et al., 2006; Sridharan et al., 2008). This control signal by the insula and the dorsal anterior cingulate cortex has been suggested to be crucial for cognitive maintenance, including a rest, in cognitively normal individuals (Sridharan et al., 2008; Goulden et al., 2014; Chand and Dhamala, 2016a). Alternation in insula connectivity has been consistently implicated in diseases, including autism, frontotemporal dementia, and schizophrenia (Menon, 2011; Uddin, 2015), but it has not been elucidated in cognitively impaired hypertensive patients. Literature suggests that the insula and anterior cingulate cortex—the key regions of salience network—respond as the racially biased brain regions (Cao et al., 2015), such as the greater activity of insula to faces of foreign races than faces of the same race of the subject (Lieberman et al., 2005; Liu et al., 2015). However, the difference in information flow—a measure from information theory that can be quantified using Granger Causality analysis (Dhamala et al., 2008b; Chand and Dhamala, 2017)—in these regions between the African-Americans and the Caucasian-Americans themselves has not been previously investigated. Previous investigations consistently report that the functional changes of brain regions (or networks) are associated with the underlying structural changes of those regions (or networks) with the progression of diseases (Xie et al., 2012; Menon, 2015). Specifically, recent studies suggest that the insula thickness decreases with the progression of cognitive decline in mild cognitive impairment (MCI) patients (Hartikainen et al., 2012; Moretti, 2015). However, whether there is a difference in insula thickness of the cognitively impaired hypertensive patients between the African-Americans and the Caucasian-Americans races has not been reported.

Here, we seek to examine the difference in information flow using Granger causality (Dhamala et al., 2008b; Chand and Dhamala, 2017) at the default-mode, salience and central-executive nodes between the African-Americans and the Caucasian-Americans hypertensive cognitive impaired individuals. As the African-Americans have higher hypertension-associated cognitive symptomatology and mortality than the other racial groups (Redmond et al., 2011; Hajjar et al., 2016), we *hypothesized* that (1) the control signal of the insula of salience network over the default-mode and central-executive nodes is more impaired (more negative value) in the African-Americans than in the Caucasian-Americans. We further seek to examine the structural difference that could substrate this racial disparity by comparing the insula thickness between the two racial groups. To test this, we further *hypothesized* that (2) the insula thickness is lower in the African-Americans than in the Caucasian-Americans, and finally (3) lower insula thickness is associated with poorer cognitive performance.

MATERIALS AND METHODS

Participants

This study was carried out in accordance with the recommendations of "Institutional Review Board (IRB) of Emory University" with written informed consent from all subjects. All subjects gave written informed consent in accordance with the Declaration of Helsinki. The study and the protocol were reviewed and approved by Institutional Review Board of Emory University. The informed written consent was provided by the participants before data collection. We recorded magnetic resonance imaging (MRI) data from 78 individuals who had hypertension and MCI. The inclusion criteria were: (a) age $\geq$ 55 years, (b) hypertension defined by systolic blood pressure $\geq$ 140 mm Hg or diastolic blood pressure $\geq$ 90 mm Hg and (c) MCI was assessed based on previously defined Diagnostic and Statistical Manual of Mental Disorders (DSM) criteria (Chao et al., 2009; Pa et al., 2009): Montreal cognitive assessment (MoCA) $\leq$ 26, clinical dementia rating score of 0.5, minimal functional limitation as reflected by the functional assessment questionnaire $\leq$ 7, and cognitive performance at the 10th percentile or below till the 2nd percentile on at least one of four screening tests—trail marking test B (Reitan, 1958; Tombaugh, 2004), Stroop interference (Stroop, 1935; Kimble et al., 2009), digit span forward and digit span backward (Humstone, 1919; Pa et al., 2009), verbal fluency and abstraction (Henley, 1969; Troyer et al., 1997). Trail marking test B screens the participant's executive ability to draw a line from a 'number' to a 'letter' in ascending order such as '1' to 'A', 'A' to '2', '2' to 'B', and so on. Strop interference effect measures the interference of predominant response in the reaction time of a task such as when the name of a word (say 'red') is printed in a different color (say 'blue'), it takes longer time to name the color of that word compared to when the word ('red') matches the name of color ('red'). Digit span forward and digit span backward test consists of two parts: first, the participant listens to and repeats a sequence of numbers, and second, the participant listens to a sequence of numbers and repeats those numbers in reverse order. The former part screens the short-term auditory memory while the latter part screens the participant's ability to manipulate the verbal information based on the auditory information. The verbal fluency screens the participant's fluency such as the participant is asked to tell as many words as the participant can that begin with certain letter (say 'A') in a limited time and the abstraction test screens the participant's ability to deal with ideas such as how an orange and a banana are alike. These tests have been commonly used to screen the MCI patients (Chao et al., 2009; Pa et al., 2009). The participants exclusion criteria were: (a) systolic blood pressure > 200 mm Hg or diastolic blood pressure > 110 mm Hg, (b) renal disease or hyperkalemia, (c) active medical or psychiatric problems, (d) uncontrolled congestive heart failure (shortness of breath at rest or evidence of pulmonary edema on exam), (e) history of stroke in the past 3 years, (f) ineligibility for MRI (metal implants or cardiac pacemaker), (g) inability to complete cognitive test and MRI scan, (h) women of childbearing potential and (i) diagnosis of dementia (self-reported or care-giver reported). In total sample, the mean age was 66.9 years (*SD*: 9.7), 55.1% were women, mean education was 14.9 years (*SD*: 2.6), mean systolic blood pressure 144.4 mm of Hg (*SD*: 22.6), mean diastolic blood pressure 86.4 mm of Hg (*SD*: 12.8), and MoCA ranged from 11 (minimum value) to 26 (maximum value) with mean score of 21.9 (*SD*: 3.1). Out of 78 participants, there were 50 African-Americans and 28 Caucasian-Americans. In the African-Americans, the mean age was 66.3 years (*SD*: 8.9), 60% were women, mean education was 14.9 years (*SD*: 2.5), mean systolic blood pressure 141.8 mm of Hg (*SD*: 21.3), mean diastolic blood pressure 85.4 mm of Hg (*SD*: 12.0), and mean MoCA score was 21.2 (*SD*: 3.2). In the Caucasian-Americans, the mean age was 68.5 years (*SD*: 10.7), 46.4% were women, mean education was 15.0 years (*SD*: 2.9), mean systolic blood pressure 147.6 mm of Hg (*SD*: 24.0), mean diastolic blood pressure 87.0 mm of Hg (*SD*: 12.7), and mean MoCA score was 23.4 (*SD*: 2.4). The age, sex, education year, systolic blood pressure, and diastolic blood pressure were not statistically significant different between the African-Americans and the Caucasian-Americans, but the MoCA score was significantly lower in the African-Americans compared to the Caucasian-Americans ($p < 0.003$) as shown in **Table 1**.

MRI Acquisition

Magnetic resonance imaging data were acquired on a SIEMENS Trio 3-Tesla scanner available at Center for Systems Imaging of Emory University, Atlanta, GA, United States. Foam padding and ear forms were used to limit head motion and reduce scanner noise to the participants. High-resolution 3D anatomical images were acquired using sagittal T1-weighted magnetization-prepared rapid gradient echo with repetition time = 2300 ms, echo time = 2.89 ms, inversion time = 800 ms, flip angle = 8°, resolution = 256 × 256 matrix, slices = 176, thickness = 1 mm. The rsfMRI were collected axially for 170 volumes during 7.14 min by using an echo-planar imaging (EPI) sequence with repetition time = 2500 ms, echo time = 27 ms, flip

TABLE 1 | Mean scores (standard deviations) and statistical comparison between the African-Americans (AA) and the Caucasian-Americans (CA) regarding their age, sex, education, blood pressure (BP), and Montreal cognitive assessment (MoCA) score.

Characteristic *N*	Total sample 78	AA 50	CA 28	*p*-Value
Age, year	66.9 (9.7)	66.3 (8.9)	68.5 (10.7)	0.44
Sex, women	43 (55.1%)	30 (60%)	13 (46.4%)	0.25
Education, year	14.9 (2.6)	14.9 (2.5)	15.0 (2.9)	0.54
Systolic BP, mm Hg	144.4 (22.6)	141.8 (21.3)	147.6 (24.0)	0.14
Diastolic BP, mm Hg	86.4 (12.8)	85.4 (12.0)	87.0 (12.7)	0.71
MoCA score	21.9 (3.1)	21.2 (3.2)	23.4 (2.4)	0.003

p-Value indicates the level of statistical significance of the comparisons between the African-Americans and the Caucasian-Americans using non-parametric Wilcoxon rank sum for age, education, blood pressure and MoCA, and chi-square test for sex.

angle = 90°, field of view = 22 cm, resolution = 74 × 74 matrix, slices = 48, thickness = 3 mm and bandwidth = 2598 Hz/pixel. We requested the participants to hold still, keep their eyes open and think nothing during the rsfMRI scan.

Image Preprocessing and Time Series Extraction

Images were preprocessed for slice-timing correction, motion correction, co-registration to individual anatomical image, normalization to the Montreal Neurological Institute (MNI) template, and spatial smoothing of the normalized images with a 6 mm isotropic Gaussian kernel. The SPM12 (Wellcome Trust Centre for Neuroimaging, London, United Kingdom[1]) was used to perform those steps. We defined spherical regions of interest with 6 mm radius based on MNI coordinates centered at the posterior cingulate cortex (7, −43, 33) and ventromedial prefrontal cortex (2, 36, −10) of default-mode network, the insula (37, 25, −4) and dorsal anterior cingulate cortex (4, 30, 30) of salience network, and the posterior parietal cortex (54, −50, 50) and dorsolateral prefrontal cortex (45, 16, 45) of central-executive networks (see **Figure 1**) similar to the previous studies (Sridharan et al., 2008; Chand and Dhamala, 2016a). We selected the nodes only in the right hemisphere based on most prior neuroimaging studies that report the right-lateralized activations (Sridharan et al., 2008; Chen et al., 2013; Chand and Dhamala, 2016a). The MarsBaR software package[2] was used to extract the voxel time courses of those nodes.

Granger Causality Analysis

Multivariate analysis has become a commonplace to investigate the information flow between the brain areas and to study how such coordinated brain activity disrupts in diseases (Dhamala et al., 2008a,b; Chiong et al., 2013; Friston et al., 2013). Here we used Granger causality although other methods such as dynamic causal modeling, directed transfer function, and partial directed coherence provide the similar goals and results (Bajaj et al., 2016; Chand et al., 2016). The main benefits of using Granger causality are that it is a data-driven method and therefore computes the information flow based on the data itself at the nodes and networks level, relies on fewer assumptions about the underlying interactions, and does not need computationally intensive time/efforts as opposed to other methods such as dynamical causal modeling (Stephan et al., 2010; Chand and Dhamala, 2016b, 2017). Recent studies by our group and by other groups have successfully applied Granger causality to resting state and/or task fMRI data in both health and disease and have produced meaningful results in terms of information flow at the brain nodes and networks (Sridharan et al., 2008; Chiong et al., 2013; Liang et al., 2014; Bajaj et al., 2016; Chand and Dhamala, 2016a).

Granger causality can be mathematically expressed by considering simultaneously measured time series. Suppose we have two simultaneously recorded time series represented as, (1) $X_1(1), X_1(2),..., X_1(t),...$ and (2) $X_2(1), X_2(2),..., X_2(t)$. Granger causality analysis in the frequency (f) domain examines the strengths, directions, and frequencies of interactions between dynamic processes. Granger causality from the second time series '2' to the first time series '1' (i.e., from brain region '2' to brain region '1') is computed as (Dhamala et al., 2008a,b; Chand and Dhamala, 2016b),

$$M_{2\to 1}(f) = -\ln\left(1 - \frac{(\Sigma_{22} - \Sigma_{12}^2/\Sigma_{11})|H_{12}(f)|^2}{S_{11}(f)}\right) \quad (1)$$

where H is a transfer function, f represents a frequency-domain, S is spectral power, and $\sum$ is noise covariance. The value of Granger causality (M) varies between 0 and $+\infty$, representing zero connectivity strength and maximum connectivity strength, respectively. If there are 'N' numbers of brain areas, the information outflow (F) at a node i can be calculated as,

$$F_i = \frac{1}{N-1}\sum_{j}^{N}(M_{i\to j} - M_{j\to i}). \quad (2)$$

In our case, we have six nodes (two key nodes from each network). Therefore, an index j can be 1, 2, 3, 4, 5, and 6 nodes. The Granger causality outflow (also referred as the net information outflow) from the first node is $F_1 = [(M_{1\to 2} - M_{2\to 1}) + (M_{1\to 3} - M_{3\to 1}) + (M_{1\to 4} - M_{4\to 1}) + (M_{\to 5} - M_{5\to 1}) + (M_{1\to 6} - M_{6\to 1})]/5$, where $M_{1\to 2}$ is Granger causality from the first node to the second node, and $M_{2\to 1}$ is Granger causality from the second node to the first node. Similarly, we calculate Granger causality outflows for other nodes. If the net outflow is negative at a node instead of the previously reported positive value in healthy individuals, then that node is said to have impaired directional connections.

Cortical Thickness Calculation

FreeSurfer version 5.3[3] was used to calculate the cortical thickness from T1-structural images. Briefly, this technique included spatial and intensity normalization, skull stripping, and an automated segmentation of cerebral white matter to locate the gray-white boundary (Dale et al., 1999). Cortical thickness

[1] www.fil.ion.ucl.ac.uk/spm/software/spm12

[2] http://marsbar.sourceforge.net

[3] https://surfer.nmr.mgh.harvard.edu/

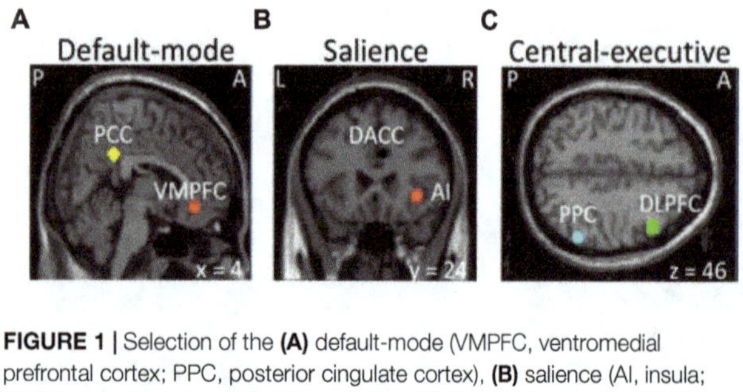

FIGURE 1 | Selection of the **(A)** default-mode (VMPFC, ventromedial prefrontal cortex; PPC, posterior cingulate cortex), **(B)** salience (AI, insula; DACC, dorsal anterior cingulate cortex), and **(C)** central-executive (DLPFC, dorsolateral prefrontal cortex; PPC, posterior parietal cortex) networks (P, posterior; A, anterior; L, left; R, right).

was then computed from the distance between the gray–white boundary and the pial-surface (Fischl and Dale, 2000).

Cognitive Test

We assessed the MoCA (Nasreddine et al., 2005) of each participant. The MoCA is a 30-point scale test administered in 10 min and assesses the global cognitive abilities. It encompasses the following sub-tests. The short-term memory recall (five points) consists of two learning trials of five nouns and delayed recall after 5 min. Visuospatial test includes a clock-drawing (three points) and a three-dimensional cube copy (one point). Executive functions test comprises the trail-making time B (one point), a phonemic fluency (one point), and a two-item verbal abstraction (two points). Attention, concentration, and working memory include a sustained attention (one point), a serial subtraction (three points), and digit forward (one point) and digit backward (one point). Language test consists of naming animals (three points), repetition of two syntactically complex sentences and fluency (two points). Orientation test comprises orientation to time and place (six points). Moreover, if participant's formal education is 12 years or less, one point is added to his/her score. Previous studies (Nasreddine et al., 2005; Hachinski et al., 2006; Dong et al., 2010; Rossetti et al., 2011) suggest that the MoCA is more sensitive screening tool to define the MCI as compared with other existing screening tools such as mini-mental state examination (MMSE).

Statistical Analysis

We first checked whether the data are normally distributed or not using Kolmogorov–Smirnov test. The age, education, MoCA, insular thickness and net flow were negatively skewed and the systolic and diastolic blood pressures were positively skewed (asymptotic p-value in the range 6.17×10^{-71} to 8.42×10^{-14}) at the 0.05 significance level. As data variables did not show normal distributions before and after applying the appropriate transformations (square root, log, and reciprocal), we therefore chose the non-parametric alternative. We compared the sample characteristics between the African–Americans and the Caucasian–Americans using non-parametric Wilcoxon rank sum and/or chi-square test for discrete variables (e.g., sex). Net information outflows between the nodes of three networks were compared using non-parametric Wilcoxon rank sum test. The correlation analysis was performed using Spearman's correlation. A p-value less than 0.05 was considered a statistically significant. MATLAB (Natick, MA, United States[4]) was used for analyzing the data.

RESULTS

Interactions among the Salience, Central-Executive, and Default-Mode Nodes

We computed the Granger causality between all possible pairs of the salience, central-executive, and default-mode nodes and calculated the net information outflow from each node. Our net outflow calculation showed that the nodes of salience network have significantly lower outflow than that of the central-executive and default-mode nodes (**Figure 2**) (Wilcoxon rank sum; $Z = 10.52$; $p < 0.05$). This negative information outflow of salience network nodes compared to previously reported positive flow in healthy individuals implied the impaired salience network nodes in our overall cohort. We compared the net information outflow between African Americans and Caucasian–Americans and found that the insula of salience network has significantly lower (negative value) in the African–Americans than in the Caucasian–Americans (Wilcoxon rank sum; $Z = 2.06$; $p < 0.05$) as shown in **Figure 3**.

Cortical Thickness Comparison and Correlation

To evaluate whether structural alterations explain these connectivity differences, we measured the insular cortical thickness and compared the values between African–Americans and Caucasian–Americans as displayed in **Figure 4**. Cortical thickness in the African–Americans (median = 2.797 mm) and in the Caucasian–Americans (median = 2.897 mm) was significantly different (Wilcoxon rank sum; $Z = 2.09$; $p < 0.05$). To investigate how the thickness of impaired insular cortex relates with the performance on global cognitive testing, we performed a correlation analysis between the thickness and the MoCA scores. We found that a lower thickness was associated with lower performance reflected by MoCA scores ($r = 0.30$; $p < 0.05$). These results are provided in **Figure 5**. Furthermore, we found that the lower cortical thickness was correlated with the lower net information outflow at the insular cortex ($r = 0.31$; $p < 0.05$) as shown in **Figure 6**.

DISCUSSION

Here, we investigated the pattern of connectivity among the key brain areas of the salience, central-executive, and default-mode networks in hypertensive individuals with MCI and we compared African–Americans to Caucasian–Americans within this group. We found larger impairment in the control signal of the insula (of salience network) in the African Americans than in the Caucasian–Americans, as reflected by negative net information outflow metrics measured by Granger causality analysis. Although, there are very limited neuroimaging studies that investigate the neural bases of hypertension in cognitive decline (Li et al., 2015), our findings of greater information flow impairment in the African–Americans were in line with the previous non-neuroimaging reports that the African–Americans bear a greater risk of hypertension-associated cognitive impairment than the Caucasian–Americans (Redmond et al., 2011; Hajjar et al., 2016). We further examined the cortical thickness of impaired insula between the African–Americans and the Caucasian–Americans and found that the insula thickness of the African–Americans is significantly lower than that of the Caucasian–Americans. The insula thickness

[4]https://www.mathworks.com

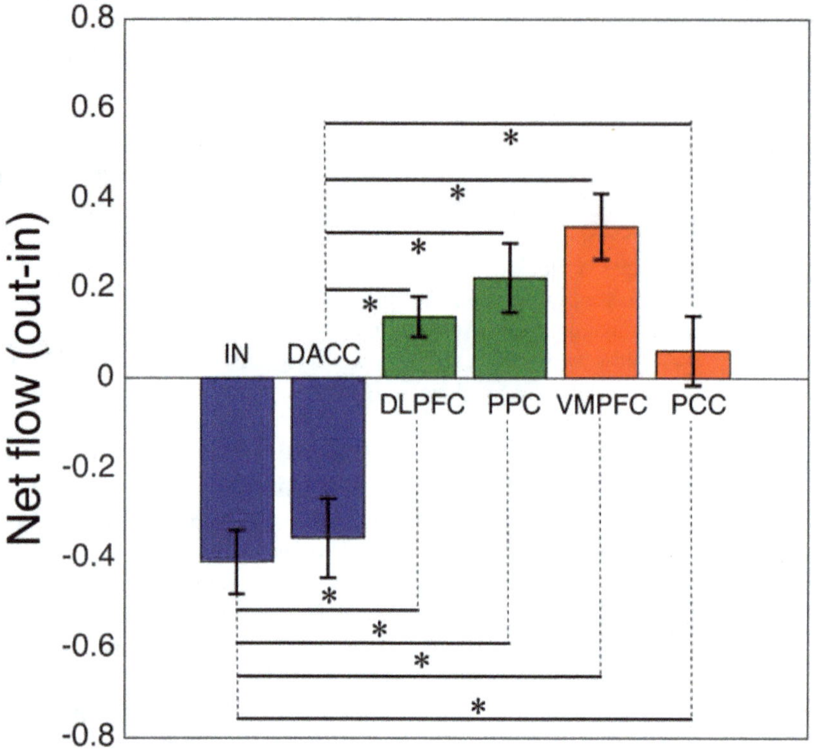

FIGURE 2 | Net flow (information outflow minus information inflow) of the key nodes of the salience (IN, insula; DACC, dorsal anterior cingulate cortex), central-executive (DLPFC, dorsolateral prefrontal cortex; PPC, posterior parietal cortex) and default-mode (VMPFC, ventromedial prefrontal cortex; PPC, posterior cingulate cortex) networks. The AI and DACC of the salience network had a significantly lower net information flow compared with the central-executive and default-mode nodes (*indicates statistical significance).

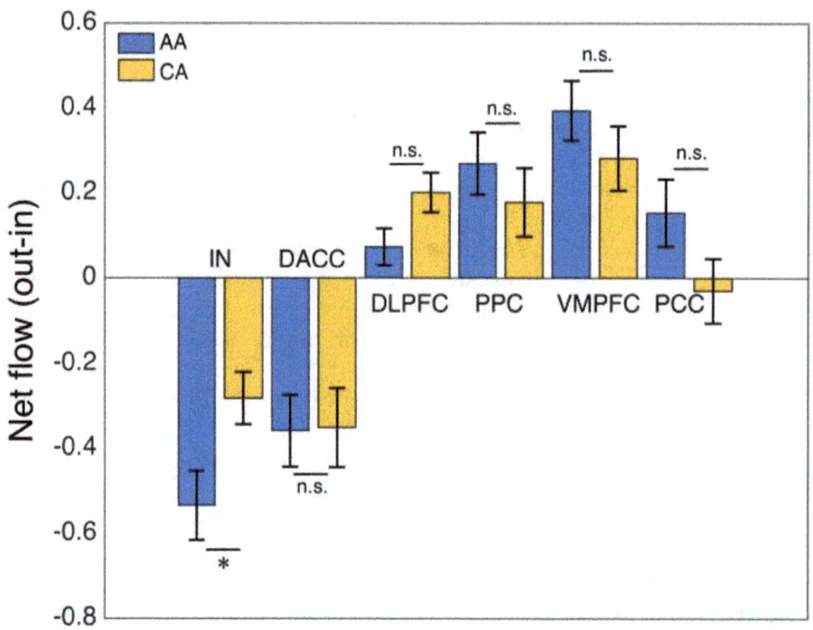

FIGURE 3 | African–Americans (AA) versus Caucasian–Americans (CA) comparison: net flow (out-in) of the key nodes of the salience (IN, insula; DACC, dorsal anterior cingulate cortex), central-executive (DLPFC, dorsolateral prefrontal cortex; PPC, posterior parietal cortex) and default-mode (VMPFC, ventromedial prefrontal cortex; PPC, posterior cingulate cortex) networks. The AI of AA group had a significantly lower net flow (out-in) compared with that of CA group (*indicates statistical significance; ns indicates not significant).

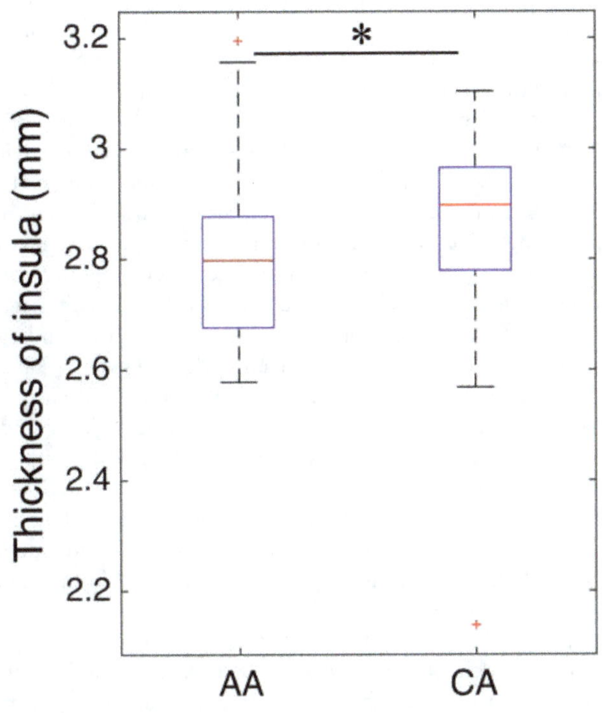

FIGURE 4 | Comparison of insular thickness between African–Americans (AA) and Caucasian–Americans (CA). The thickness had a significantly lower value in AA group than that of CA group (*indicates statistical significance).

was found to be correlated with the behavior performance and with the net information flow at the insula cortex, respectively. Those results about insula thickness were also consistent with the existing literature that insula thickness decreases with cognitive decline (Hartikainen et al., 2012; Moretti, 2015), however the difference in insula thickness between the African–Americans and the Caucasian–Americans has not been previously explored.

Former studies consistently reported that the nodes of salience network render modulation effects over the default-mode and central-executive in healthy individuals (Sridharan et al., 2008; Goulden et al., 2014; Chand and Dhamala, 2016a). The controlling role of salience nodes over the other two networks has been argued to be structurally supported by direct white matter connections between the insula and the dorsal anterior cingulate cortex (Bonnelle et al., 2012; Jilka et al., 2014) and by their unique sharing of cytoarchitecture at neuronal level, i.e., only these regions consist of special type of neurons—von Economo neurons—that relay information processed within those nodes to other nodes, including the default-mode and executive nodes (Allman et al., 2005, 2010; Watson et al., 2006; Sridharan et al., 2008). Literature also shows that the insula of salience network is functionally connected to the central-executive network (Vincent et al., 2008), and has direct white matter connections to the other areas, including the inferior parietal lobe (Uddin et al., 2010), and temporo-parietal junction (Kucyi et al., 2012). These structural and functional settings show the great involvement of insula in many cognitive processes such as in the evaluation of task performance across varying perceptual and response demands (Uddin et al., 2010), the reorientation of attention in conscious error perception (or error awareness) (Ullsperger et al., 2010), and the switching between available cognitive resources to integrate external sensory information with internal states (Uddin and Menon, 2009). The dorsal anterior cingulate cortex of salience network is known for enhanced cognitive control

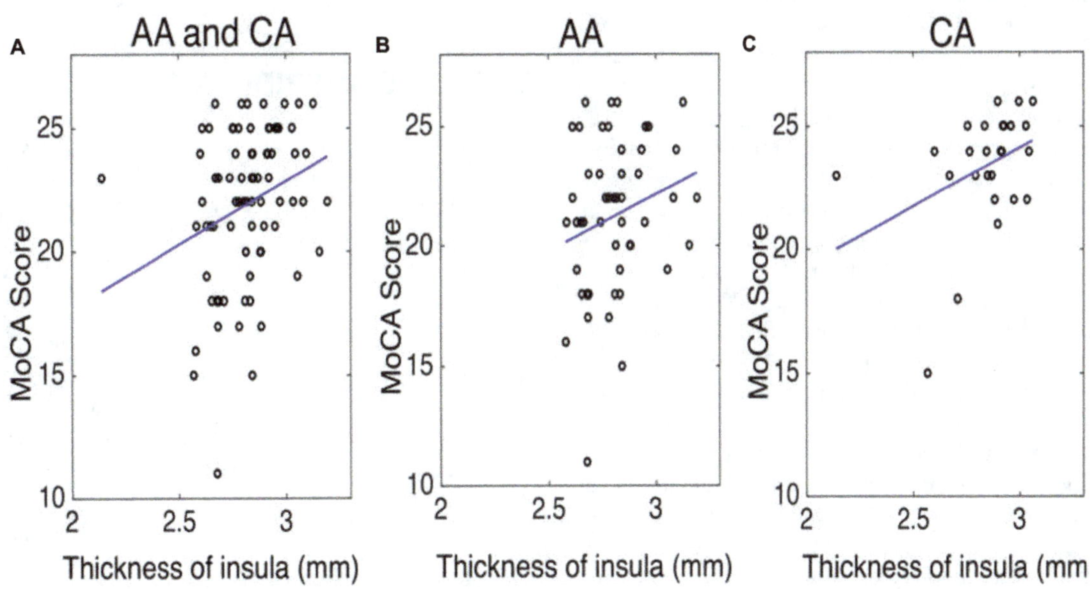

FIGURE 5 | The correlation between the thickness of insula and the Montreal cognitive assessment (MoCA) score in **(A)** both African–Americans (AA) and Caucasian–Americans (CA) (r = 0.30 and p < 0.05), **(B)** AA (r = 0.19 and p = 0.18), and **(C)** CA (r = 0.40 and p < 0.05).

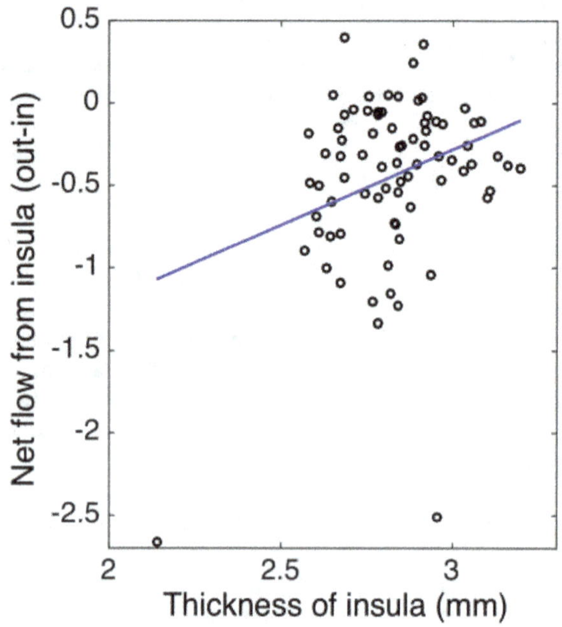

FIGURE 6 | The correlation between the thickness and the net flow (out-in) of insula in both African–Americans (AA) and Caucasian–Americans (CA) (r = 0.31 and p < 0.05).

(Egner, 2009) such as in switching activity in association with the insula during behaviorally harder tasks (Chand and Dhamala, 2016a). The above mentioned neural basis of control signal of the insula and the dorsal anterior cingulate cortex network (salience nodes) has been suggested to be crucial for cognitive maintenance in both task and resting states in cognitively healthy individuals, whereas impairment to such control activity might be caused by the underlying neuroanatomical changes, including the injuries to the highly sensitive/vulnerable von Economo neurons (Allman et al., 2005, 2010; Watson et al., 2006; Sridharan et al., 2008; Bonnelle et al., 2012).

Emerging evidence suggest atypical engagement of the insula of salience network in disease, including frontotemporal dementia, autism, schizophrenia, and Alzheimer's disease (Menon, 2015; Uddin, 2015). The structural changes of the cortex, including the cortical thinning of insula with disease progression to MCI and/or Alzheimer's disease, is widely reported in elderly people (Singh et al., 2006; Hartikainen et al., 2012; Moretti, 2015). Previous studies also suggested the link between the underlying structural changes and the corresponding functional changes of brain nodes and networks (Xie et al., 2012; Menon, 2015). Our connectivity findings indicated that the control mechanism of the salience network was impaired (negative value) in both the African–Americans and the Caucasian–Americans, and the insula was more impaired in the African–Americans than in the Caucasian–Americans. Although, the cortical thinning of insula has been consistently reported in cognitive impairment (Hartikainen et al., 2012; Moretti, 2015), there are no neuroimaging studies so far to our knowledge that report the racial disparity of insula thickness. Neuroimaging literature suggests that the insula and dorsal anterior cingulate cortex—the key regions of salience network—respond as the racially biased brain regions (Cao et al., 2015), especially the greater activity of insula to out-group race than in-group race (Lieberman et al., 2005; Liu et al., 2015), but there are no previous reports about the difference in connectivity patterns of those regions between the African–Americans and the Caucasian–Americans groups with hypertension and cognitive impairment. Prior non-neuroimaging studies repeatedly report that the African–Americans bear the greater risk of hypertension-associated cognitive impairment than the Caucasian–Americans (Redmond et al., 2011; Hajjar et al., 2016). Thus, our findings and existing neuroimaging/non-neuroimaging evidence taken together suggest that the insula is crucial in racial disparity in cognitively impaired individuals with hypertension. This study can be further extended in the future by including the groups of African–Americans and Caucasian–Americans with MCI but without a history of hypertension and by also including the cognitively healthy hypertensive and normotensive individuals to better dissociate the effect of hypertension alone in the brain nodes and networks.

In summary, we evaluated the patterns of interactions among the salience, default-mode, and central-executive nodes in the African–Americans and the Caucasian–Americans race groups, who had hypertension and cognitive impairment. We found that the insula of the salience network was functionally impaired greater, and had lower thickness in the African–Americans than in the Caucasian–Americans. Existing literature and our findings taken together thus suggest that the insula is potential biomarker in the cognitive disorders, including the racial disparity of cognitively impaired hypertensive population. It is worth nothing that the future research should direct toward dissociating the role of hypertension alone between the race groups in the insula and the other possible regions that are functionally and/or structurally connected to the insula.

AUTHOR CONTRIBUTIONS

Conceived and designed the experiment: IH, DQ. Performed the experiment: GC, JW, DQ, IH. Analyzed the data: GC, DQ, IH. Wrote the paper: GC, DQ, IH. Participated in the discussion and provided the comments: GC, JW, DQ, IH.

FUNDING

This research was conducted with NIA/NIH grants RF1AG051633 and R01AG042127 to IH. DQ is supported by NIH grants AG25688, AG42127, AG49752, AG51633, and has received research support from Medtronic and Siemens Medical Solutions.

ACKNOWLEDGMENT

We would like to thank the members of our team and the participants who volunteered for the study.

REFERENCES

Allman, J. M., Tetreault, N. A., Hakeem, A. Y., Manaye, K. F., Semendeferi, K., Erwin, J. M., et al. (2010). The von Economo neurons in frontoinsular and anterior cingulate cortex in great apes and humans. *Brain Struct. Funct.* 214, 495–517. doi: 10.1007/s00429-010-0254-0

Allman, J. M., Watson, K. K., Tetreault, N. A., and Hakeem, A. Y. (2005). Intuition and autism: a possible role for Von Economo neurons. *Trends Cogn. Sci.* 9, 367–373. doi: 10.1016/j.tics.2005.06.008

Bajaj, S., Adhikari, B. M., Friston, K. J., and Dhamala, M. (2016). Bridging the gap: dynamic causal modeling and Granger causality analysis of resting state fMRI. *Brain Connect.* 6, 652–661. doi: 10.1089/brain.2016.0422

Biswal, B., Haughton, V. M., and Hyde, J. (1995). Functional connectivity in the motor cortex resting human brain using echo-planar MRI. *Magn. Reson. Med.* 34, 537–541. doi: 10.1002/mrm.1910340409

Bonnelle, V., Ham, T. E., Leech, R., Kinnunen, K. M., Mehta, M. A., Greenwood, R. J., et al. (2012). Salience network integrity predicts default mode network function after traumatic brain injury. *Proc. Natl. Acad. Sci. U.S.A.* 109, 4690–4695. doi: 10.1073/pnas.1113455109

Bressler, S. L., and Menon, V. (2010). Large-scale brain networks in cognition: emerging methods and principles. *Trends Cogn. Sci.* 14, 277–290. doi: 10.1016/j.tics.2010.04.004

Cao, Y., Contreras-Huerta, L. S., McFadyen, J., and Cunnington, R. (2015). Racial bias in neural response to others' pain is reduced with other-race contact. *Cortex* 70, 68–78. doi: 10.1016/j.cortex.2015.02.010

Chand, G. B., and Dhamala, M. (2016a). Interactions among the brain default-mode, salience, and central-executive networks during perceptual decision-making of moving dots. *Brain Connect.* 6, 249–254. doi: 10.1089/brain.2015.0379

Chand, G. B., and Dhamala, M. (2016b). The salience network dynamics in perceptual decision-making. *Neuroimage* 134, 85–93. doi: 10.1016/j.neuroimage.2016.04.018

Chand, G. B., and Dhamala, M. (2017). Interactions between the anterior cingulate-insula network and the fronto-parietal network during perceptual decision-making. *Neuroimage* 152, 381–389. doi: 10.1016/j.neuroimage.2017.03.014

Chand, G. B., Lamichhane, B., and Dhamala, M. (2016). Face or house image perception: beta and gamma bands of oscillations in brain networks carry out decision-making. *Brain Connect.* 6, 621–631. doi: 10.1089/brain.2016.0421

Chao, L. L., Pa, J., Duarte, A., Schuff, N., Weiner, M. W., Kramer, J. H., et al. (2009). Patterns of cerebral hypoperfusion in amnestic and dysexecutive MCI. *Alzheimer Dis. Assoc. Disord.* 23, 245–252. doi: 10.1097/WAD.0b013e318199ff46

Chen, A. C., Oathes, D. J., Chang, C., Bradley, T., Zhou, Z. W., Williams, L. M., et al. (2013). Causal interactions between fronto-parietal central executive and default-mode networks in humans. *Proc. Natl. Acad. Sci. U.S.A.* 110, 19944–19949. doi: 10.1073/pnas.1311772110

Chiong, W., Wilson, S. M., D'Esposito, M., Kayser, A. S., Grossman, S. N., Poorzand, P., et al. (2013). The salience network causally influences default mode network activity during moral reasoning. *Brain* 136(Pt 6), 1929–1941. doi: 10.1093/brain/awt066

Dale, A., Fischl, B., and Sereno, M. (1999). Cortical surface-based analysis. *Neuroimage* 9, 179–194. doi: 10.1006/nimg.1998.0395

Dhamala, M., Rangarajan, G., and Ding, M. (2008a). Analyzing information flow in brain networks with nonparametric Granger causality. *Neuroimage* 41, 354–362. doi: 10.1016/j.neuroimage.2008.02.020

Dhamala, M., Rangarajan, G., and Ding, M. (2008b). Estimating granger causality from Fourier and wavelet transforms of time series data. *Phys. Rev. Lett.* 100:018701. doi: 10.1103/PhysRevLett.100.018701

Dong, Y., Sharma, V. K., Chan, B. P., Venketasubramanian, N., Teoh, H. L., Seet, R. C., et al. (2010). The Montreal Cognitive Assessment (MoCA) is superior to the mini-mental state examination (MMSE) for the detection of vascular cognitive impairment after acute stroke. *J. Neurol. Sci.* 299, 15–18. doi: 10.1016/j.jns.2010.08.051

Egner, T. (2009). Prefrontal cortex and cognitive control: motivating functional hierarchies. *Nat. Neurosci.* 12, 821–822. doi: 10.1038/nn0709-821

Elias, M. F., Goodell, A. L., and Dore, G. A. (2012). Hypertension and cognitive functioning: a perspective in historical context. *Hypertension* 60, 260–268. doi: 10.1161/HYPERTENSIONAHA.111.186429

Faraco, G., and Iadecola, C. (2013). Hypertension: a harbinger of stroke and dementia. *Hypertension* 62, 810–817. doi: 10.1161/HYPERTENSIONAHA.113.01063

Fischl, B., and Dale, A. (2000). Measuring the thickness of the human cerebral cortex from magnetic resonance images. *Proc. Natl. Acad. Sci. U.S.A.* 97, 11050–11055. doi: 10.1073/pnas.200033797

Friston, K., Moran, R., and Seth, A. K. (2013). Analysing connectivity with Granger causality and dynamic causal modelling. *Curr. Opin. Neurobiol.* 23, 172–178. doi: 10.1016/j.conb.2012.11.010

Gorelick, P. B., and Nyenhuis, D. (2012). Blood pressure and treatment of persons with hypertension as it relates to cognitive outcomes including executive function. *J. Am. Hypertens.* 6, 309–315. doi: 10.1016/j.jash.2012.08.004

Goulden, N., Khusnulina, A., Davis, N. J., Bracewell, R. M., Bokde, A. L., McNulty, J. P., et al. (2014). The salience network is responsible for switching between the default mode network and the central executive network: replication from DCM. *Neuroimage* 99, 180–190. doi: 10.1016/j.neuroimage.2014.05.052

Hachinski, V., Iadecola, C., Petersen, R. C., Breteler, M. M., Nyenhuis, D. L., Black, S. E., et al. (2006). National Institute of Neurological Disorders and Stroke-Canadian Stroke Network vascular cognitive impairment harmonization standards. *Stroke* 37, 2220–2241. doi: 10.1161/01.STR.0000237236.88823.47

Hajjar, I., Wharton, W., Mack, W. J., Levey, A. I., and Goldstein, F. C. (2016). Racial disparity in cognitive and functional disability in hypertension and all-cause mortality. *Am. J. Hypertens.* 29, 185–193. doi: 10.1093/ajh/hpv084

Hartikainen, P., Rasanen, J., Julkunen, V., Niskanen, E., Hallikainen, M., Kivipelto, M., et al. (2012). Cortical thickness in frontotemporal dementia, mild cognitive impairment, and Alzheimer's disease. *J. Alzheimers Dis.* 30, 857–874. doi: 10.3233/JAD-2012-112060

Henley, N. M. (1969). A psychological study of the semantics of animal terms. *J. Verbal Learn. Verbal Behav.* 8, 176–184. doi: 10.1016/S0022-5371(69)80058-7

Humstone, H. J. (1919). Memory span tests. *Psychol. Clin.* 12, 196–200.

Jilka, S. R., Scott, G., Ham, T., Pickering, A., Bonnelle, V., Braga, R. M., et al. (2014). Damage to the Salience Network and interactions with the Default Mode Network. *J. Neurosci.* 34, 10798–10807. doi: 10.1523/JNEUROSCI.0518-14.2014

Johnson, K. C., Margolis, K. L., Espeland, M. A., Colenda, C. C., Fillit, H., Manson, J. E., et al. (2008). A prospective study of the effect of hypertension and baseline blood pressure on cognitive decline and dementia in postmenopausal women: the Women's Health Initiative Memory Study. *J. Am. Geriatr. Soc.* 56, 1449–1458. doi: 10.1111/j.1532-5415.2008.01806.x

Kimble, M. O., Frueh, B. C., and Marks, L. (2009). Does the modified Stroop effect exist in PTSD? Evidence from dissertation abstracts and the peer reviewed literature. *J. Anxiety Disord.* 23, 650–655. doi: 10.1016/j.janxdis.2009.02.002

Kucyi, A., Moayedi, M., Weissman-Fogel, I., Hodaie, M., and Davis, K. D. (2012). Hemispheric asymmetry in white matter connectivity of the temporoparietal junction with the insula and prefrontal cortex. *PLoS ONE* 7:e35589. doi: 10.1371/journal.pone.0035589

Li, X., Liang, Y., Chen, Y., Zhang, J., Wei, D., Chen, K., et al. (2015). Disrupted frontoparietal network mediates white matter structure dysfunction associated with cognitive decline in hypertension patients. *J. Neurosci.* 35, 10015–10024. doi: 10.1523/JNEUROSCI.5113-14.2015

Liang, P., Li, Z., Deshpande, G., Wang, Z., Hu, X., and Li, K. (2014). Altered causal connectivity of resting state brain networks in amnesic MCI. *PLoS ONE* 9:e88476. doi: 10.1371/journal.pone.0088476

Lieberman, M. D., Hariri, A., Jarcho, J. M., Eisenberger, N. I., and Bookheimer, S. Y. (2005). An fMRI investigation of race-related amygdala activity in African-American and Caucasian-American individuals. *Nat. Neurosci.* 8, 720–722. doi: 10.1038/nn1465

Liu, Y., Lin, W., Xu, P., Zhang, D., and Luo, Y. (2015). Neural basis of disgust perception in racial prejudice. *Hum. Brain Mapp.* 36, 5275–5286. doi: 10.1002/hbm.23010

Menon, V. (2011). Large-scale brain networks and psychopathology: a unifying triple network model. *Trends Cogn. Sci.* 15, 483–506. doi: 10.1016/j.tics.2011.08.003

Menon, V. (2015). Salience Network. *Brain Mapp.* 2, 597–611. doi: 10.1016/b978-0-12-397025-1.00052-x

Moretti, D. V. (2015). Conversion of mild cognitive impairment patients in Alzheimer's disease: prognostic value of Alpha3/ Alpha 2 electroencephalographic rhythms power ratio. *Alzheimers Res. Ther.* 7:80. doi: 10.1186/s13195-015-0162-x

Nasreddine, Z. S., Phillips, N. A., Bedirian, V., Charbonneanu, S., Whitehead, V., Collin, I., et al. (2005). The montreal cognitive assessment, MoCA: a brief screening tool for mild cognitive impairment. *J. Am. Geriatr. Soc.* 53, 695–699. doi: 10.1111/j.1532-5415.2005.53221.x

Novak, V., and Hajjar, I. (2010). The relationship between blood pressure and cognitive function. *Nat. Rev. Cardiol.* 7, 686–698. doi: 10.1038/nrcardio.2010.161

Oveisgharna, S., and Hachinski, V. (2010). Hypertension, executive dysfunction, and progression to dementia. *Arch. Neurol.* 67, 187–192. doi: 10.1001/archneurol.2009.312

Pa, J., Boxer, A., Chao, L. L., Gazzaley, A., Freeman, K., Kramer, J., et al. (2009). Clinical-neuroimaging characteristics of dysexecutive mild cognitive impairment. *Ann. Neurol.* 65, 414–423. doi: 10.1002/ana.21591

Raichle, M. E. (2015). The restless brain: how intrinsic activity organizes brain function. *Philos. Trans. R. Soc. Lond. B Biol. Sci.* 370, 20140172. doi: 10.1098/rstb.2014.0172

Redmond, N., Baer, H. J., and Hicks, L. S. (2011). Health behaviors and racial disparity in blood pressure control in the national health and nutrition examination survey. *Hypertension* 57, 383–389. doi: 10.1161/HYPERTENSIONAHA.110.161950

Reitan, R. M. (1958). Validity of the trail marking test as an indicator of organic brain damage. *Percept. Mot. Skills* 8, 271–276. doi: 10.2466/pms.1958.8.3.271

Rossetti, H. C., Lacritz, L. H., Cullum, C. M., and Weiner, M. F. (2011). Normative data for the Montreal Cognitive Assessment (MoCA) in a population-based sample. *Neurology* 77, 1272–1275. doi: 10.1212/WNL.0b013e318230208a

Singh, V., Chertkow, H., Lerch, J. P., Evans, A. C., Dorr, A. E., and Kabani, N. J. (2006). Spatial patterns of cortical thinning in mild cognitive impairment and Alzheimer's disease. *Brain* 129(Pt 11), 2885–2893. doi: 10.1093/brain/awl256

Sridharan, D., Levitin, D. J., and Menon, V. (2008). A critical role for the right fronto-insular cortex in switching between central-executive and default-mode networks. *Proc. Natl. Acad. Sci. U.S.A.* 105, 12569–12574. doi: 10.1073/pnas.0800005105

Stephan, K. E., Penny, W. D., Moran, R. J., den Ouden, H. E., Daunizeau, J., and Friston, K. J. (2010). Ten simple rules for dynamic causal modeling. *Neuroimage* 49, 3099–3109. doi: 10.1016/j.neuroimage.2009.11.015

Stroop, J. R. (1935). Studies of interference in serial verbal reactions. *J. Exp. Psychol.* 18, 643–662. doi: 10.1037/h0054651

Tombaugh, T. N. (2004). Trail making test A and B: normative data stratified by age and education. *Arch. Clin. Neuropsychol.* 19, 203–214. doi: 10.1016/s08876177(03)00039-8

Troyer, A. K., Moscovitch, M., and Winocur, G. (1997). Clustering and switching as two components of verbal fluency: evidence from younger and older healthy adults. *Neuropshychology* 11, 138–146. doi: 10.1037/0894-4105.11.1.138

Uddin, L. Q. (2015). Salience processing and insular cortical function and dysfunction. *Nat. Rev. Neurosci.* 16, 55–61. doi: 10.1038/nrn3857

Uddin, L. Q., and Menon, V. (2009). The anterior insula in autism: under-connected and under-examined. *Neurosci. Biobehav. Rev.* 33, 1198–1203. doi: 10.1016/j.neubiorev.2009.06.002

Uddin, L. Q., Supekar, K., Amin, H., Rykhlevskaia, E., Nguyen, D. A., Greicius, M. D., et al. (2010). Dissociable connectivity within human angular gyrus and intraparietal sulcus: evidence from functional and structural connectivity. *Cereb. Cortex* 20, 2636–2646. doi: 10.1093/cercor/bhq011

Ullsperger, M., Harsay, H. A., Wessel, J. R., and Ridderinkhof, K. R. (2010). Conscious perception of errors and its relation to the anterior insula. *Brain Struct. Funct.* 214, 629–643. doi: 10.1007/s00429-010-0261-1

Vicario, A., Martinez, C. D., Baretto, D., Casale, A. D., and Nicolosi, L. (2005). Hypertension and cognitive decline: impact on executive function. *J. Clin. Hypertens.* 7, 598–604. doi: 10.1111/j.1524-6175.2005.04498.x

Vincent, J. L., Kahn, I., Snyder, A. Z., Raichle, M. E., and Buckner, R. L. (2008). Evidence for a frontoparietal control system revealed by intrinsic functional connectivity. *J. Neurophysiol.* 100, 3328–3342. doi: 10.1152/jn.90355.2008

Watson, K. K., Jones, T. K., and Allman, J. M. (2006). Dendritic architecture of the von Economo neurons. *Neuroscience* 141, 1107–1112. doi: 10.1016/j.neuroscience.2006.04.084

Xie, C., Bai, F., Yu, H., Shi, Y., Yuan, Y., Chen, G., et al. (2012). Abnormal insula functional network is associated with episodic memory decline in amnestic mild cognitive impairment. *Neuroimage* 63, 320–327. doi: 10.1016/j.neuroimage.2012.06.062

7

Functional Re-Organization of Cortical Networks of Senior Citizens after a 24-Week Traditional Dance Program

Vasiliki I. Zilidou[1,2], *Christos A. Frantzidis*[1*], *Evangelia D. Romanopoulou*[1], *Evangelos Paraskevopoulos*[1], *Styliani Douka*[2] *and Panagiotis D. Bamidis*[1]

[1]*Laboratory of Medical Physics, Medical School, Aristotle University of Thessaloniki, Thessaloniki, Greece,* [2]*Department of Physical Activity and Recreation, School of Physical Education and Sport Science, Aristotle University of Thessaloniki, Thessaloniki, Greece*

Correspondence:
Christos A. Frantzidis
christos.frantzidis@gmail.com

Neuroscience is developing rapidly by providing a variety of modern tools for analyzing the functional interactions of the brain and detection of pathological deviations due to neurodegeneration. The present study argues that the induction of neuroplasticity of the mature human brain leads to the prevention of dementia. Promising solution seems to be the dance programs because they combine cognitive and physical activity in a pleasant way. So, we investigated whether the traditional Greek dances can improve the cognitive, physical and functional status of the elderly always aiming at promoting active and healthy aging. Forty-four participants were randomly assigned equally to the training group and an active control group. The duration of the program was 6 months. Also, the participants were evaluated for their physical status and through an electroencephalographic (EEG) examination at rest (eyes-closed condition). The EEG testing was performed 1–14 days before (pre) and after (post) the training. Cortical network analysis was applied by modeling the cortex through a generic anatomical model of 20,000 fixed dipoles. These were grouped into 512 cortical regions of interest (ROIs). High quality, artifact-free data resulting from an elaborate pre-processing pipeline were segmented into multiple, 30 s of continuous epochs. Then, functional connectivity among those ROIs was performed for each epoch through the relative wavelet entropy (RWE). Synchronization matrices were computed and then thresholded in order to provide binary, directed cortical networks of various density ranges. The results showed that the dance training improved optimal network performance as estimated by the small-world property. Further analysis demonstrated that there were also local network changes resulting in better information flow and functional re-organization of the network nodes. These results indicate the application of the dance training as a possible non-pharmacological intervention for promoting mental and physical well-being of senior citizens. Our results were also compared with a combination of computerized cognitive and physical training, which has already been demonstrated to induce neuroplasticity (LLM Care).

Keywords: dancing, electroencephalography, neuroplasticity, dementia, active aging, functional connectivity, neurodegeneration, brain networks

INTRODUCTION

As the number of elderly people worldwide is constantly increasing, important changes regarding the mental, physical and emotional condition occurred. These changes refer to the brain structure, as well as to various functions related to aging. The alterations of the structure and function of the brain associated closely with changes in cognitive function. The most important cognitive functions affected by aging are considered to be memory, attention and movement that may lead to dementia or even Alzheimer's disease.

Different parts of the brain, frontal cortex and hippocampus, were mostly affected by aging leading to the reduction of blood flow in the vessels by causing changes in amyloid plaques. High level of education, healthy lifestyle and regular exercise seem to be essential factors contributing on keeping older adults healthy, preventing diseases and reducing associated complications (Erickson et al., 2011). In recent decades, studies show that regular physical activity and exercise could mediate the negative effects of aging on both body and mind (Billis et al., 2010). The growing proportion of elderly people demonstrates the need of maintaining the independent living, the social integration and the active life for a longer period.

Neuroscience research has provided insights into the brain functions and behaviors with the main focus on the Mild Cognitive Impairment (MCI) transition by contributing to the development of neurodegenerative diseases. Therefore, a plethora of non-pharmacological interventions have been developed. During the last decades there is a steady interest on the investigation of the aging negative effects that can be eliminated through the physical and/or cognitive training. These training procedures aim to induce the neuroplasticity of the mature human brain (Bamidis et al., 2014). The brain is adapted to the new environment (brain and cognitive alterations) by enhancing existing or creating new connections. It is reported that aerobic exercise induces neurogenesis of hippocampus (Erickson et al., 2011) and physical activity is associated with the reduction of risk factors that may accelerate neurodegeneration (Cotman et al., 2007). Research findings show that physical activity is a promising non-pharmaceutical intervention to prevent cognitive impairment associated with age and neurodegenerative diseases (Bherer et al., 2013). In another study, the computerized physical training presented positive effects in the physical and cognitive capacity as well as the participants' quality of life (Zilidou et al., 2016).

Long lasting memories (LLM) is developed as an integrated platform of existing technological achievements in the field of computer-aided physical/cognitive training and ambient assisted living (AAL) solutions for elderly people and vulnerable groups (Romanopoulou et al., 2015). LLM offers an opportunity to improve cognitive and physical condition, being able to continue feeling an active part of society. The core of the LLM service is an integrated ICT platform which combines state-of-the-art cognitive exercises with physical activity in the framework of an advanced AAL environment (Konstantinidis et al., 2010). LLM proved the capacities for improving the mental and physical condition of the elderly that adhered to it. The results from 322 individuals participated in the project shown an improvement in the working and episodic memory, as well as in the executive functions (Bamidis et al., 2015). Moreover, 70 elderlies with MCI were subjected to electroencephalographic (EEG) recording in a resting state to investigate whether or not the combination of cognitive and physical activity, induces changes in brain cortical activity. The results revealed a significant reduction in the delta, theta and beta brain rhythms, and a decrease in the activity of certain brain regions (PCU/PCC) associated with functional plasticity. They also discovered that the greater the decrease in the delta and the theta rate, the higher the neuropsychological assessment through Mini Mental State Examination (MMSE; Styliadis et al., 2015). Moreover, graph analysis in brain networks demonstrated the ability of the brain to be "educated" in order to reorganize the functional connectivity to prevent the effects of neurodegenerative phenomena and normal aging (Klados et al., 2016). An additional study was conducted to investigate whether the combination of physical and mental exercise may lead to the enhancement of the brain functional reorganization in the beta band which is considered to be particularly important for mental functioning. Also, an increase in the functional connection of two brain hemispheres of occipital, temporal, parietal and pre-frontal lobe has been occurred (Frantzidis et al., 2014a).

The aforementioned approach is based on a combination of computerized cognitive and physical training, which is performed intensively (more than four times) for a period of approximately 2 months. Both cognitive and physical training are widely used to induce neuroplasticity on the mature human brain and to delay or even prevent neurodegeneration (Heyn et al., 2004; Voss et al., 2010; Frantzidis et al., 2014b; Bamidis et al., 2015). However, there is an active debate on the optimal intervention design and its effect size and sustainability of the positive effects observed. It seems that improvement is greater when the intervention is performed in day care centers under supervision and not at home installations (Lampit et al., 2014). Similarly, multi-domain physical intervention demonstrated improvement or at least preservation of an adequate cognitive functioning in senior citizens (Ngandu et al., 2015). Combination of cognitive and physical training was proven to induce a more pronounced neuroplasticity effect (Frantzidis et al., 2014b; Bamidis et al., 2015). Although, the aforementioned studies demonstrated the applicability of cognitive and physical interventions as well as the robustness of their combination, the research community recently investigates new training approaches which would be more ecologically valid and applicable on non-clinical settings in order to further enhance the adherence rate and to improve drop-outs. Given also the fact that beneficial effects of the training are evident for a given time period after the intervention's cessation, novel approaches should be adopted as a life-style habit and be performed on a regular basis.

An ideal, non-pharmacological intervention that fulfils the aforementioned criteria is dance. A previous study showed 7% lower risk for developing dementia for elderly people who involved in dancing, playing a musical instrument, reading and playing board games once a week (Verghese et al., 2003). Previous research studies have investigated the potential benefits of dancing interventions to senior citizens. Dance is a less-threatening exercise for many elderlies, since they had many positive and enjoyable experiences in their youth. Also, dancing is an important factor for health and well-being aging. Dance offers the opportunity to maintain a connection with everyday life as it encourages fun and enjoyment, social interaction, team spirit, health, physical activity and mobility. Dance, is considered to be a form of physical exercise that may be adopted as part of many interventions for the elderly instead of other (Wikström, 2004; Lima and Vieira, 2007). Dance improves energy, increases mood and reduces stress or anxiety in ways similar to aerobic exercise (Kim and Kim, 2007). Also, studies have reported that the traditional dances as a physical activity prevent cognitive decline and improve the coordination and control of body movements (Balkus, 1989).

Dance training has been associated with positive behavioral effects in various populations. However, only few studies have evaluated the functional brain correlations in dance interventions as they have not investigated the structural correlations of brain changes due to the dance exercise. It is necessary to perform additional research on brain related networks and correlative behaviors of dance interventions, so as to better understand and validate the dance-related neuroplasticity mechanisms. Thus, there is a huge need to further study the neuroscience of dance in order to provide an increasing multidisciplinary area that may offer information on the interactions between the brain and arts (Karpati et al., 2015).

Thus, traditional dancing may induce many feelings as it is achieved in groups of 15–20 participants who simultaneously perform dancing movements which require balance, flexibility, rhythm, orientation and cognitive functions. More even it does not require any special equipment and can be applied easily by Day Centers with low cost.

Despite the promising results, the majority of studies that are employed dancing training have not been evaluated under medical and neuroscientific criteria. Therefore, we studied an experimental group who performed traditional dancing for 6 months. This group was compared with a control group which performed a cognitive stimulation program. Both groups were assessed in terms of a detailed neurophysiological assessments and neurophysiological (EEG) examination which aimed to assess the brain functioning of the participants before and after the training. This examination evaluates the brain functions in terms of each functional organization through a system level approach employed analysis of brain networks based on graph theory.

This piece of work aims to investigate whether traditional dancing could improve cognitive and brain functioning of elderly compared with a cognitive stimulation program (Active Control Group). We also attempt to answer the following research questions:

- Is traditional dancing intervention an effective approach for promoting active and healthy aging?
- Which are the brain alterations induced by dancing?
- Which is the type of such alterations?

According to previous studies we hypothesize that traditional dancing may be more effective than active stimulation. It would also induce functional re-organization of the brain networks that would shift brain function to a more optimal mood. The latter is hypothesized to be achieved by more efficiency and faster communication among distant brain regions.

MATERIALS AND METHODS

Participants

The study initially employed 54, non-demented, senior citizens, who were randomly assigned either to an active control (mean age 66 ± 5.51 years) or to a traditional dance training group (mean age 68.73 ± 4.73 years). However, five participants from the training-group refused to repeat the neurophysiological intervention at the post level and they excluded from the study. There were also five participants who did not complete the active control program and also excluded. So, the study resulted in 44 senior citizens. Both groups consisted of equal number of participants. Neuropsychological, physical status evaluation and neurophysiological by an electroencephalogram (EEG) were performed. The evaluation took place 1–14 days before/after the training initiation/finalization respectively. Prior to their enrolment in the study activities all participants were informed about the study hypotheses and aims as well as the underlying activities. Inclusion criteria were the following: (1) age to be greater than 60 years; (2) participants should be sedentary or mild sedentary with an upper threshold of 150 min of moderate to vigorous exercise per week; (3) lack of participation in any other physical training intervention within the last year; and (4) performance of medical examination assessing their safe participation in the study. People with heart failure, hypertension and respiratory insufficiency and patients suffering from dementia were excluded from the program as they who participated in other Greek Traditional Dances programs. Also, participants who did not complete at least 80% of the total of hours of program were excluded from further analysis. They had the opportunity to discuss any issues raised and then they signed a written informed consent form. The study was based on specific guidelines and regulations, which were approved by the ethics committee of the Aristotle University of Thessaloniki (AUTH) according to international principles. Group demographics and information about the participants' age, education, body mass index (BMI) and cognitive status, is depicted in **Table 1**. The groups did not significantly differ in baseline cognitive level, mean age, education and gender (all $ps > 0.05$).

Intervention

The active group participated in cognitive intervention with the use of Video GRade software that was developed by the Lab of Medical Physics at the AUTH. Video GRade is an inspired environment for cognitive training[1], which consists of a set of

[1] www.llmcare.gr

TABLE 1 | Number of participants per intervention group, age, education, Body Mass Index (BMI) and cognitive status as measured by the Mini Mental State Examination (MMSE), Trail B and Geriatric Depression Scale (GDS).

	Active group *n* = 22		Dance group *n* = 22		*p*-value
	Mean	SD	Mean	SD	
Age (years)	66	5.51	68.73	4.73	0.091
Education (years)	8.64	3.79	9.55	4.63	0.481
% Female	77.3		95.5		
BMI	30.14	2.92	29.10	4.90	0.408
MMSE	26.73	2.88	27.05	2.75	0.710
Trail B	146.30	51.99	194.11	82.33	0.036
GDS	2.76	3.0	2.00	2.6	0.427

50-min educational video from YouTube that includes content with history, art, culture, dance and music. At the end of each video, participants were asked to answer eight multiple choice questions. Participants performed 24 sessions during a period of 8–10 weeks.

The intervention group was conducted through traditional dances from all over Greece that were divided into three categories according to the number of steps and complexity, the intensity of the pace (slow-fast), as well as the upper limbs position and movement. A 24-week period program was performed for 60 min two times per week, taking place at Day Care Centers of Municipality of Thessaloniki located in Greece. The intervention duration was much longer than the active (Video Grade) control group, due to the annual organizational structure of the local Day Care Centers. So, the maximum number of available sessions was 48. However, the long duration of the intervention overlapped with Christmas and Easter holidays. During that period, many senior citizens preferred to stay at home and did not attend 1–4 (maximum two successive weeks) sessions per occasion. Considering the abovementioned pragmatic limitations and aiming to have a similar number of sessions between the control and the training group we kept the mean number of 28 sessions within the 24-week period.

Neuropsychological and Physical Assessments

Cognitive functioning was estimated through the MMSE (Folstein et al., 1975), Trail Making B Test (Butler et al., 1991) and the Geriatric Depression Scale (GDS short version; Yesavage et al., 1982–1983).

Their physical status and functional ability was evaluated through the following tests: (i) Fullerton Senior Fitness Test which contains six domains: chair Stand (assessed lower body strength), 8 Foot Up and Go (assessed complex coordination, agility and dynamic balance), Back Scratch (assessed flexibility of upper body), Chair Sit and Reach (assessed flexibility of the lower back and hamstring muscles), Arm Curl (assessed upper body strength) and 2 Min Step (assessed aerobic capacity; Jones and Rikli, 2002); (ii) Berg Balance Scale which assessed balance and risk of falls (Berg et al., 2009); (iii) Tinetti Test which assessed walking and risk of falls (Tinetti, 1986); and (iv) Stork Balance Stand Test which assessed balance when standing on one leg (Johnson and Nelson, 1969). Body composition was also calculated.

EEG Analysis

Data Acquisition

The EEG data acquisition was performed through a Nihon Kohden JE-207A device and 57 active electrodes attached on a cap (EASYCAP) fitted directly to the participant's head. Two more electrodes were placed on positions behind the participant's ears and a third active electrode, placed on a left anterior position, served as ground electrode. The electrode impedances were kept lower than 5 KΩs. The sampling frequency was set at 500 Hz. The participants sat on a comfortable, armed chair, which was located in a quiet room with minimal, ambient light. They were instructed to close their eyes for 5 min and avoid any movement, especially of their upper part. The subsequent processing and analysis steps are visualized in **Figure 1** and are the following: (i) electroencephalographic (EEG) data acquisition; (ii) artifact removal and sensor data epoching; (iii) generic anatomy head and cortex modeling; (iv) estimation of the cortical activity for anatomically relevant regions of interest (ROIs); (v) quantification of the co-operative degree (functional connectivity analysis) among ROIs cortical activity through the notion of Relative Wavelet Entropy (RWE); and (vi) formation of functional brain networks regarding the ROIs as network nodes and their connectivity values as edges. The analysis is performed through contemporary mathematical tools derived from graph theory and involves both global and local network properties.

Pre-processing

The 57 active electrodes recording brain signals were re-referenced through the common average model. Then, digital filtering through 3rd order Butterworth filters was applied as follows: (a) high-pass filter with cut-off frequency at 1 Hz; (b) band-stop (notch) filter with cut-off frequency at the 47–53 range; (c) low-pass filter with cut-off frequency at 100 Hz; (d) band-stop (notch) filter with cut-off frequency at the 97–103 Hz range; and (e) band-stop (notch) filter with cut-off frequency at the 147–153 Hz range. Independent Component Analysis was then applied to identify and reject potentially contaminated source components due to eye blinks, muscle artifacts, bad electrode placement, high frequency noise, ECG modulation, linear trends. Finally, the data were epoched. The epoch duration was 1,024 sample points (2.048 s). Epochs still containing artifacts were visually rejected. The pre-processing was performed through built-in code based on the Matlab Signal Processing Toolbox and EEGLAB software (Delorme and Makeig, 2004).

Cortical Activity Estimation

The Brainstorm software package was used for the computation of the inverse problem, which results in the reconstruction of the cortical activity (Tadel et al., 2011). Default anatomy modeling was employed in terms of magnetic resonance imaging (MRI) volume (Colin 27 stereotaxic T1-weighted MRI volume). The head modeling was computed through the Open

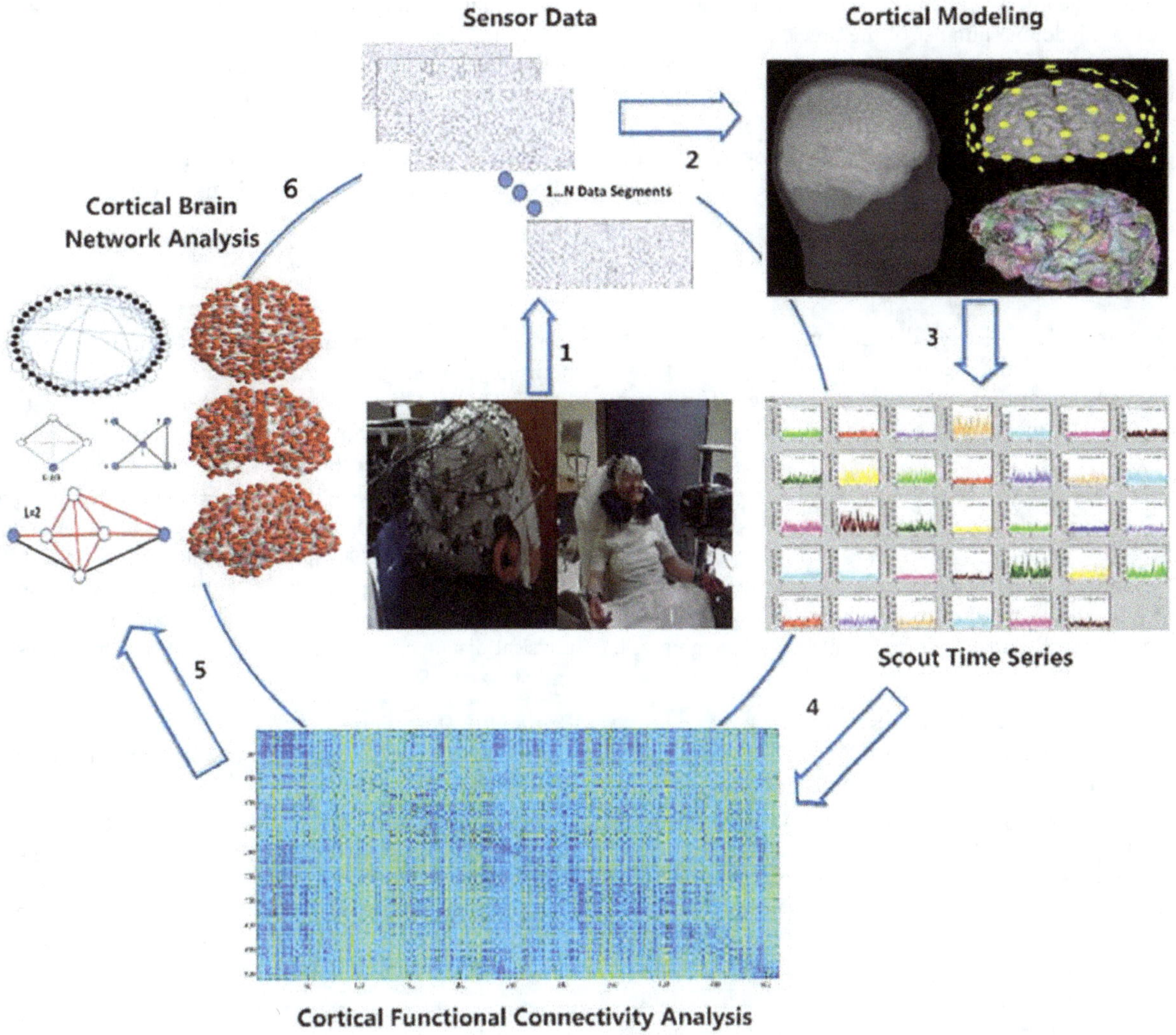

FIGURE 1 | Visualization of the electroencephalographic (EEG) methodology from transforming the raw EEG data (1) to the cortical activity (2), estimation of regions of interest (ROIs) cortical activity (3), quantification of functional connectivity matrix (4) and finally cortical brain network analysis (5) through graph theory (6).

MEEG Boundary Elements Method (BEM head model). The solution space was constrained to the cerebral cortex which was modeled as a 3-dimensional grid of 20,000 fixed dipoles oriented normally to the cortical surface. Then, the inverse solution was estimated by means of the sLORETA methodology (Pascual-Marqui, 2002). The study analysis, employed the entire cortex analysis through the definition of 512 cortical regions of interest (ROIs), which were defined according to the deterministic process implemented by the Brainstorm software. Since, the source analysis requires a symmetric electrode map of 64 electrodes, seven additional electrode activations were inserted through first-neighborhood activity interpolation.

Cortical Synchronization Analysis

The synchronization analysis aims to quantify the co-operative degree among the ROIs by comparing their cortical time series activity. Therefore, it was performed for each participant on the average scout cortical activity. The Orthogonal Discrete Wavelet Transform (ODWT) was applied and the analysis was based on the relative wavelet entropy (RWE) metric. Bi-orthogonal wavelets of 5th order were selected as the family wavelet class (Frantzidis et al., 2010, 2014b; Chriskos et al., 2018). Optimal time-frequency analysis is obtained since the mother wavelet is subjected to scaling and translation. The ODWT analysis framework is based on an iterative decomposition scheme, which employs recursive, low-pass filters for estimating the activity of the five frequency bands (delta, theta, alpha, beta and gamma) through the estimation of the wavelet coefficients. The decomposition scheme involves $j = 1...5$ layers. The amplitude of the wavelet coefficients quantifies the wavelet's correlation with the actual rhythmic activity, while the coefficient's sign is an index of either positive or negative correlation. The ODWT framework involves a periodization mode. So, the final decomposition layer (j = 5) contains one wavelet coefficient and corresponds to the lowest rhythms (delta and theta). Each other step contains the double number of the previous one. So, there are two coefficients for the alpha, four for beta and eight for the gamma rhythm. In this way, non-redundancy and optimal resolution is facilitated through a parameter-free methodology. The energy of each frequency band is estimated by squaring the amplitude of the corresponding wavelet coefficients. Then, the overall energy is estimated as following:

$$E_{tot} = \sum_{j<0} \sum_{k} |C_j(k)|^2 \tag{1}$$

In this way, the relative energy distribution of each frequency band is obtained and the synchronization degree among two ROIs was quantified as the similarity of their energy distribution (p_j and q_j, j = 1. . .5) given by the following formula of the RWE:

$$RWE = \sum_{j=1}^{5} p_j \times \ln\left(\frac{p_j}{q_j}\right) \tag{2}$$

The RWE metric may be then used as a dissimilarity matrix (the larger the value the greater the desynchronization), which may be used as an adjacency matrix for network analysis through graph theory.

Cortical Brain Network Analysis

Functional Connectome Estimation

For each participant and for each time condition (pre/post-intervention) all the available data epochs were used. For each epoch the resulting RWE matrix was used to create a functional brain network, which is defined as a graph G = (V, E). The graph contains a set V of nodes (here V = 512 cortical ROIs) and a number E of edges quantifying the co-operative degree as estimated through the RWE analysis. The RWE matrix is used as it is, but the auto-synchronization information of the main diagonal is discarded from further analysis. Therefore, the resulting adjacency matrix forms a weighted and directed network. Subsequent analysis was performed on binary networks. The thresholding was dynamically configured for each network instance in order to result in fixed density ranges of 10,000, 12,500 and 15,000 edges. The density range was similar as in previous studies (Frantzidis et al., 2014a).

Global Network Characteristics

Global network analysis was applied by computation of both the cluster coefficient for each node and the characteristic path length for each pair of ROIs. Then, their mean values were used for the estimation of the small-world property. While, the interested reader may find detailed information on these fundamental network properties in classical textbooks and studies, in brief the cluster coefficient is an index of local information processing, while the characteristic path length quantifies the integration of information and the network's flow. More specifically, the cluster coefficient (C) for a given node is the number of the existing connections of the node's direct neighborhood to the total number of the possible ones. The set of the node's direct neighborhood contains the ROIs with which the node under consideration is connected. So, C is actually a possibility of the local information capacity for each node. The characteristic path length (L) is applied on node pairs and quantifies the shortest distance among those nodes. The mean values of these two characteristics are computed for both the actual brain network and for a number (N = 100) of random networks with the same characteristics (nodes and density). Then, the small world property (sigma) is computed as follows:

$$sigma = \frac{\frac{L}{L_{\text{rand}}}}{\frac{C}{C_{\text{rand}}}} \tag{3}$$

In the case that the mean cluster coefficient of the actual brain network is much larger than the mean value of the random ones and simultaneously the characteristic path length of the actual and the random networks are quite similar, we have sigma >1. The greater the sigma the more prominent the small-world property is. According to these, small-world is an index of non-random clustering and near-random path length. So, it is a property of the optimal network configuration since it implies strong local information processing which may be transferred from every individual node to every other, regardless of their physical distance, through a small set of intermediaries (Watts and Strogatz, 1998).

Brain Hub Detection

Functional hubs of the cortical connectome were identified based on the betweenness centrality (BC) metric (Bi). It is an index of the information amount transferred through a given node, since it is computed as the number of the network's shortest paths that pass through the specific node (Rubinov and Sporns, 2010). Hub detection was performed based on a criterion of Bi ≥1.5, which was firstly introduced by Seo et al. (2013) and previously applied by Frantzidis et al. (2014b).

Functional Cartography and Node Roles

Aiming to ensure that putative effects were not biased by the particular hub definition, we also followed an alternative approach of applying a previously proposed functional cartography technique (Guimerà and Nunes Amaral, 2005). This framework involves the computation of the community structure (modularity analysis) and then the estimation of the within-module z-score and the participation coefficient (PC). Based on these two metrics a specific role is assigned to each network node. The network's community structure was performed based on the Brain Connectivity Toolbox (BCT; Rubinov and Sporns, 2010). Then, the within-module z-score was used to estimate the connection strength of a given node with the other nodes of its own module. The greater the z-score is, the larger the connection strength. The PC (P) is a probability value, which quantifies the connection distribution of a given node across all the feasible modules of the specific network. The closer the coefficient's value to 1, the more uniform the distribution across modules is. The role assignment to each node is defined based on the node's position to the z-P parameter space. Heuristically, in case a node has within-module z-score greater or equal to 1.5 then it is regarded as a hub and otherwise as non-hub node. Both node categories

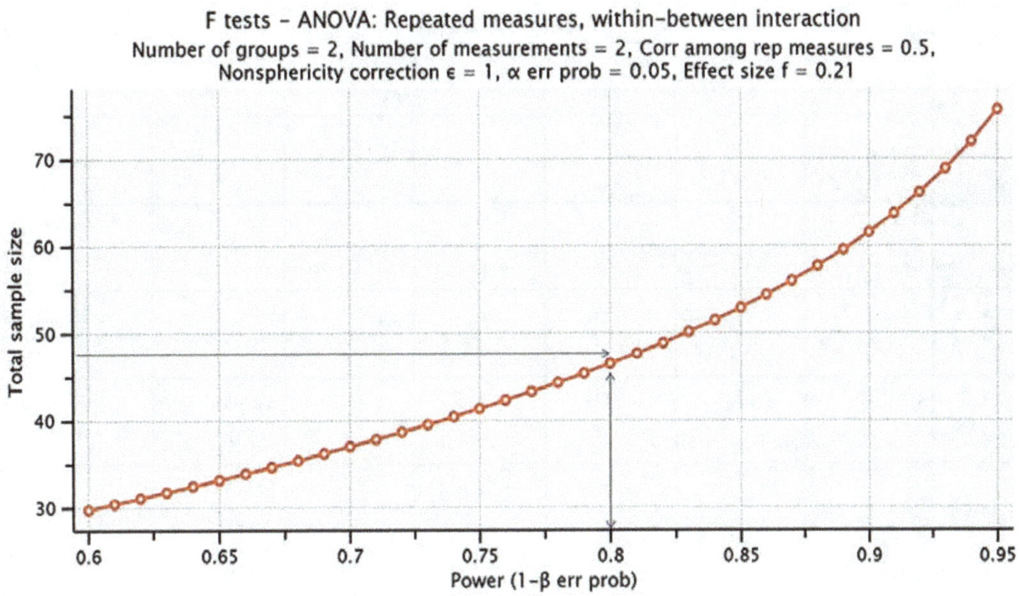

FIGURE 2 | Visualization of the analysis performed for estimating the proper sample size for the proposed statistical analysis. The power analysis indicated that the proper sample size was 48 (24 participants per group), whereas we have included 44 senior citizens (22 participant per group).

are then further characterized according to their PC value. More specifically non-hubs are further characterized as ultra-peripheral ($p \leq 0.05$), peripheral ($0.05 < p \leq 0.45$), connector ($0.45 < p \leq 0.70$) and kinless ($p > 0.70$). Hub nodes are assigned as provincial ($p \leq 0.25$), connector ($0.25 < p \leq 0.50$) and kinless ($p > 0.50$).

RESULTS

Analysis of Global Network Characteristics

The statistical analysis was conducted *via* a 2 × 2 mixed model ANOVA. The groups of intervention (Dance and Active) served as between-subjects factor whereas the time (pre-post) as within-subject factor and the three inter-related dependent variables (small-world value, cluster coefficient and characteristic path value).

Aiming to investigate whether the sample size was adequate for the statistical analysis we performed power analysis. It was conducted in G-Power 3.1 to determine a sufficient sample size using an alpha of 0.05, a power of 0.80, and a medium effect size ($f = 0.21$; Faul et al., 2013). Based on the aforementioned assumptions, a total sample size of 48 people would be sufficient to detect significant interaction effects. Specifically, the appropriate number for each group of intervention (Dance and Active) is 24, in order for group differences to reach statistical significance at the 0.05 level. Our sample size is estimated 44, 22 per group which is adequate for our experimental design and the analysis performed. The results obtained from the statistical analysis are visualized in **Figure 2**.

Results revealed an interaction between time and intervention for the small world property for 10,000 edges, $F_{(1,42)} = 20.56$; $p < 0.05$, as well as the small world property for 12,500 edges $F_{(1,42)} = 19.53$; $p < 0.05$. Furthermore, an interaction between time and intervention was also revealed for the characteristic path for 15,000, $F_{(1,42)} = 5.16$; $p < 0.05$ as you can see in **Table 2**.

TABLE 2 | 2 × 2 mixed model ANOVA statistical analysis.

Variables	Edges	$F_{(1,42)}$	Time/Interv.	Between intervention
Small world value	10,000	20,565	**0.00**	**0.033**
	12,500	19,530	**0.00**	0.19
Characteristic path	15,000	5,163	**0.028**	**0.005**

The groups of intervention (Dance and Active) served as between-subjects factor whereas the time (pre-post) as within-subject factor and the three inter-related dependent variables were the small-world value, cluster coefficient and characteristic path length. The p-values that reached statistical significance (p < 0.05) are displayed in bold.

Correlation With Cognitive and Physical Status

Pearson's correlations were computed, in order to test if there was a linear relationship between cognitive status as measured with the MMSE assessment and physical status as measured with the Fullerton Senior Fitness Test, as well as the Small-World property value. The analysis revealed a significant positive correlation between the Back-Scratch Test score and the Small World property at 12,500 edges, $r = 0.301$, $n = 43$, $p = 0.05$ and between the Chair Sit and Reach Test score and the Small World property at 15,000 edges, $r = 0.385$, $n = 43$, $p = 0.01$. Furthermore, a significant negative correlation was also revealed between the Back-Scratch Test score and the PC of the fronto-parietal network (FPN) score, $r = -0.32$, $n = 43$, $p = 0.039$.

TABLE 3 | Statistically significant changes of each group regarding the Fullerton examination.

TEST	Subdomain	Active group (N = 22)		Dance group (N = 22)	
		$t_{(20)}$	p value	$t_{(21)}$	p-value
Fullerton	Chair stand	−3.700	**0.001**	−3.926	**0.001**
	Arm Curl	−1.407	0.175	−1.588	0.127
	2-min walk in place	0.541	0.595	−0.606	0.551
	Chair sit and reach	−1.494	0.151	−3.023	**0.006**
	Back scratch	−0.583	0.567	−1.648	0.114
	8-Foot-Up-and-Go	1.303	0.207	3.925	**0.001**

Bold values denote statistical significance.

TABLE 4 | Statistically significant changes regarding local network (betweenness centrality, participation coefficient, within-module z-score) at pre-post level for both groups.

Network	Features	$F_{(1,42)}$	Time/Interv.	Between intervention
Executive	Betweenness centrality (BC)	23.246	**0.000**	0.164
	Participation coefficient (PC)	0.219	0.642	0.079
	Within module z-score (ZM)	37.262	**0.000**	0.695
Fronto-parietal	Betweenness centrality (BC)	9.291	**0.004**	0.364
	Participation coefficient (PC)	25.695	**0.000**	0.490
	Within module z-score (ZM)	22.284	**0.000**	0.494
Default mode network (DMN)	Betweenness centrality (BC)	0.860	0.359	0.068
	Participation coefficient (PC)	7.740	**0.008**	**0.002**
	Within module z-score (ZM)	1.450	0.235	0.417
Contribution of all	Betweenness centrality (BC)	1.926	0.172	**0.001**
	Participation coefficient (PC)	11.069	**0.002**	**0.020**
	Within module z-score (ZM)	3.286	0.077	0.180

The p-values that reached statistical significance ($p < 0.05$) are displayed in bold.

Analysis of Physical Status Assessments

A paired-samples t-test was conducted to investigate the effectiveness of Greek traditional dancing on dependent measures of functional connectivity. **Table 3** presents the results (post–pre-intervention differences and p-value) concerning the physical assessment tests. More specifically, the results indicate that the intervention group evoked statistically significant improvement in the Chair Stand, Chair Sit and Reach and 8-Foot-Up-and-Go. Active Control group showed statistically significant improvement in Chair Stand test.

Local Network Analysis

From the 512 ROIs we further analyzed the 22 being part of the default mode network (DMN), FPN, and executive network (EN) according to Voss et al. (2010). For these three networks as well as for their combination we estimated the following local graph properties: PC, BC and within module z-score (ZM). We selected these metrics in order to define node hierarchy according to Guimerà and Nunes Amaral (2005) and Seo et al. (2013). The statistical analysis was conducted *via* a 2 × 2 mixed model ANOVA. The groups of intervention (Dance and Active) served as between-subjects factor whereas the time (pre-post) as within-subject factor and the three inter-related dependent variables (BC, PC and within Module z-score value). **Table 4** presents the results that revealed an interaction between time and intervention for the EN for the BC $F_{(1,42)} = 23.246$ $p < 0.05$ and Within module z-score $F_{(1,42)} = 37.262$ $p < 0.05$. Furthermore, an interaction between time and intervention was also revealed for FPN for BC $F_{(1,42)} = 9.291$ $p < 0.05$, PC $F_{(1,42)} = 25.695$ $p < 0.05$ and Within module z-score $F_{(1,42)} = 22.284$ $p < 0.05$. Finally, PC was also statistically significant feature for DMN $F_{(1,42)} = 7.740$ $p < 0.05$ and contribution of all $F_{(1,42)} = 11.069$; $p < 0.05$.

Hub Identification

As described within the "Methodology" section (Brain Hub Detection), hubs were identified according to their relative BC value (B_i). The B_i value for both groups and both conditions as well as their post-pre/intervention difference are visualized for each cortical node in the **Figure 3**.

Functional Cartography Analysis

The **Figure 4** describes the two-dimensional distribution in terms or PC and within-module z-score for each cortical node, for both groups and conditions.

Pearson analysis revealed statistically significant correlations among the node roles (both positive and negative) as visualized in the following **Figure 5**.

DISCUSSION

This study investigated dancing induced neuroplasticity effects of the mature human brain. We employed an objective evaluation framework based on contemporary mathematical tools such as cortical functional connectivity and graph theory. Network neuroscience has been applied until now to quantify physiological aging mechanisms (Micheloyannis et al., 2009) and neurodegeneration phenomena (Sanz-Arigita et al., 2010; Tijms et al., 2013; Frantzidis et al., 2014a). However, there are only a few preliminary attempts on how cognitive and physical training

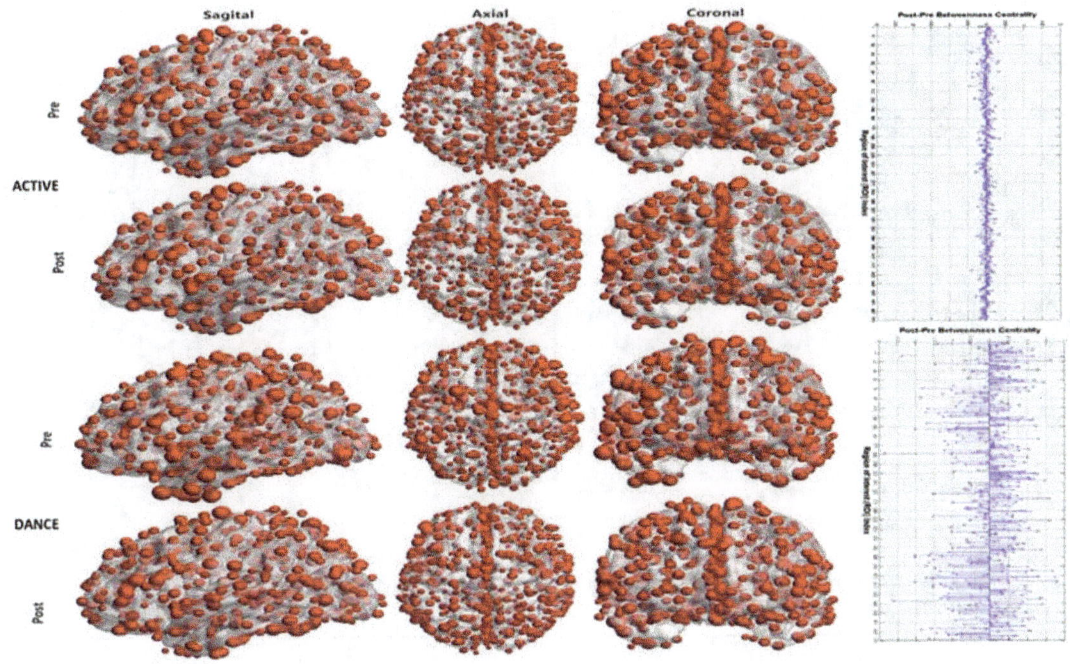

FIGURE 3 | Visualization of the hub significance of each node in terms of betweenness centrality (BC). The first column (from the left) displays a sagittal view of the cortex, the middle one an axial view and the right one a coronal view. Rows 1–2 are for the active control group for pre and post conditions respectively. Rows 3–4 are for the Dance group. The right plot denotes the pre-post differences in the hub strength for the active (upper plot) and for the dance (lower plot).

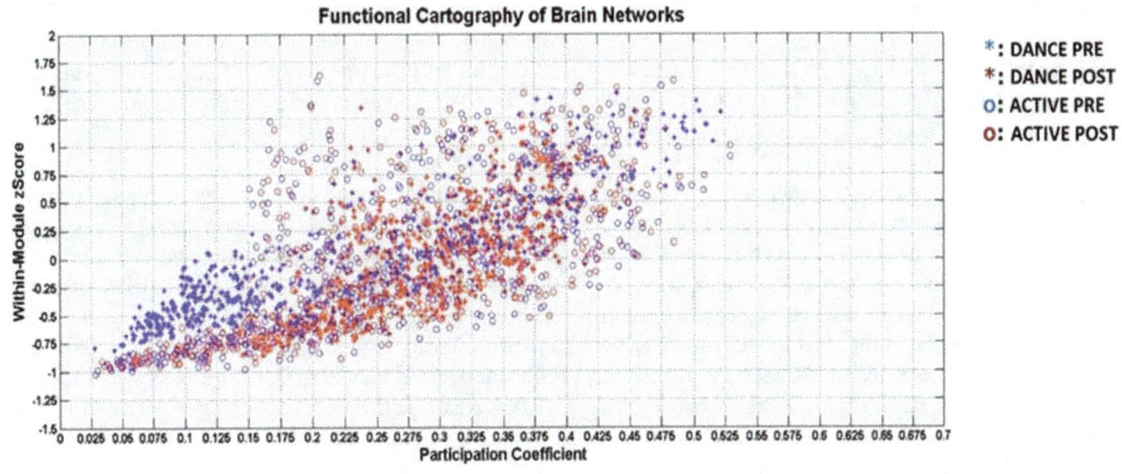

FIGURE 4 | Visualization of the functional cartography in terms of participation coefficient (PC; horizontal axis) and within-module z-score (vertical axis). The DANCE group is denoted with asterisk and the ACTIVE group with circle. The pre-intervention is denoted with blue color and the post condition with red color.

improved brain network functioning (Burdette et al., 2010; Voss et al., 2010; Klados et al., 2016). The pioneering work of Voss et al. (2010) employed functional MRI (fMRI) and showed that aerobic training increases the functional connectivity of the Default Mode and the Fronto-Executive resting state network. The authors found that this type of intervention may increase restoration mechanisms in fronto-temporal, brain networks affected by physiological aging. However, they did not investigate how aerobics improve the functional organization of these networks as an entire system. A similar type of training was also employed by Burdette et al. (2010) and validated that physical exercise increases hippocampal connectivity in comparison to a control group. The authors employed graph theory tools to evaluate these changes and showed that physical training enhanced the hippocampus degree and its connectivity with the anterior cingulate cortex. These two regions were part

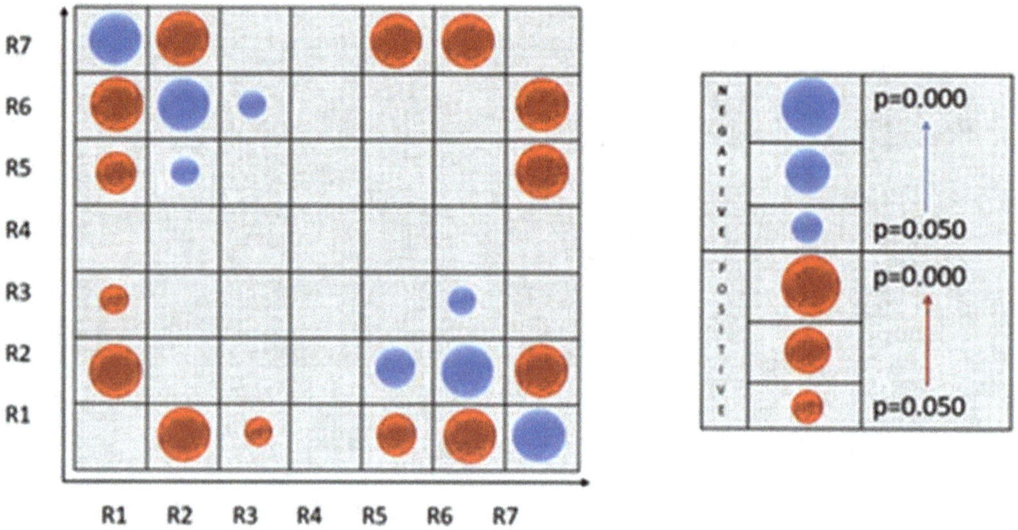

FIGURE 5 | Visualization of the Pearson correlation among nodes' roles. Positive correlations are denoted with blue color and negative correlations with red color. The circle's size is proportional to the strength of the statistical significance.

of the same sub-network (module) for the training group. A more recent work by Klados et al. (2016) examined whether a combination of computerized cognitive and physical training would induce changes in a cortical functional network. They evaluated these changes in terms of alterations in network's density and node's strength. They focused on beta band and on cortical estimations of 305 regions defined by sLORETA software.

Despite the impact of these three studies, they introduced only a partial estimation of the network properties associated with neuroplasticity. Due to methodological limitations attributed either to the low temporal resolution of fMRI (Burdette et al., 2010; Voss et al., 2010) or to the cortical estimation employed by Klados et al. (2016), the previous studies failed to track a global perspective of how training changed the cortical functional organization of the mature human brain. Moreover, the local analysis they performed was minimal since it focused only on modularity analysis of central brain regions (Burdette et al., 2010) or node strength in beta band (Klados et al., 2016). Although these analyses were significant since they shed light at the prominent role of hippocampus and anterior cingulate cortex (Burdette et al., 2010) and the hub strength of cortical regions (Klados et al., 2016) they did not provide answers whether physical intervention increases local information processing or information flow resulting thus in better functional organization as estimated by small-world property (Watts and Strogatz, 1998; Frantzidis et al., 2014a). Moreover, the hub definition through node strength as defined in Klados et al. (2016) is mainly a connectivity-driven metric that may also incorporate compensatory mechanisms and did not regard the node's contribution to the global information flow. Therefore, we employed the BC metric as defined in Seo et al. (2013) and Frantzidis et al. (2014a). Finally, we proposed a more detailed network analysis through the notion of functional cartography as defined in the article of Guimerà and Nunes Amaral (2005). We used that type of analysis to assign to each cortical node a specific role, but we also investigated correlations (either positive or negative) among these nodes and how intervention changes the node distribution to these specific roles. The network analysis was applied to a detailed cortical parcellation (512 nodes) but also in known resting state networks (DMN, FPN and EN) as defined in Voss et al. (2010). So, we believe that the main novelty of our study is the proposal of a holistic intervention evaluation framework based on network neuroscience and covering most of the aspects of graph theory.

Our results regarding global network characteristics demonstrated significant time by intervention interactions for both small-world metric (in density ranges of 10,000 and 12,500 edges) and for characteristic path length regarding 15,000 edges. This was because the participants in dance training showed a significant increase of small-world property at two density ranges mainly attributed to a decrease of characteristic path length which was significant only for 15,000 edges. Although there are not previous global network results regarding intervention evaluation, there is a plethora of studies reporting disrupted functional organization of brain networks due to neurodegeneration. More specifically, the pioneering work of Stam et al. (2008) showed that both cluster coefficient and characteristic path length obtained through Phase Lag Index (PLI)-weighted connected networks were decreased for AD patients. Similarly, sensor-based EEG analysis showed decreased small-world property in the AD group within the beta band (de Haan et al., 2009). The first fMRI-based study performed by Supekar et al. (2008) showed loss of small-world property in AD patients due to decrease in local information processing (cluster coefficient). Another study through fMRI found that AD patients showed increased cluster coefficient and characteristic path length in comparison with a healthy control group (Zhao et al., 2012). Finally, a recent study employing healthy elderly and patients suffering either from amnestic MCI (aMCI) or from mild dementia (MD) reported functional disorganization of small-world brain networks for both pathological groups (Frantzidis et al., 2014a). This decline was mainly attributed to the loss of local information processing capacity (mean cluster coefficient). The aforementioned studies indicate that functional brain networks are vulnerable to neurodegeneration phenomena, which affect brain networks through a multi-level way. The proposed dancing intervention seems to improve functional network performance as estimated through small-world property by reducing the average length of characteristic paths. This implies minimization of functional disconnection patterns and better transmission of the information across network nodes. This finding is of particular importance since Alzheimer's dementia is regarded as a disconnection syndrome resulting thus in longer characteristic path lengths (Stam et al., 2007; Frantzidis et al., 2014a). The specific hypothesis is supported by previous studies which linked longer path lengths and preserved cluster coefficient with a loss of complexity and a less optimal organization (Stam et al., 2007). Among the first findings of the network neuroscience were that increases of characteristic path length induce functional degradation of brain network and reduced interaction among brain nodes (Sporns and Zwi, 2004) which was also correlated with cognitive decline (Stam et al., 2007). So, the present study results regarding global network analysis (increase of small world property due to preservation of cluster coefficient and reduction of characteristic path length) may be attributed to neuroplasticity findings due to the dance intervention which seems robust for promoting active and healthy aging.

We also investigated whether the improvement of physical activity may be correlated with neuroplasticity effects. The study demonstrated positive correlations among the small-world property and the *Back Scratch* ($r = 0.301$, $p = 0.05$) and *Chair Sit and Reach* ($r = 0.385$, $p = 0.01$) domains of the Fullerton Senior Fitness test. These two tests quantified the flexibility of the upper and the lower body respectively. Flexibility is regarded as an index of functional status of the elderly and could be benefited from physical training (Heyn et al., 2004). Dance training induces greater improvement on trunk flexibility and hip-joint mobility (Sofianidis et al., 2009). According to that study, traditional Greek dancing seems to be an ideal candidate for improving flexibility since it involves activities of single-limb standing, while the dancer's body should be flexed/extended, and many steps require forward/backward leaning (Sofianidis et al., 2009). However, previous studies have not investigated how such an intervention affects the functional organization of brain networks. Positive correlations imply that flexibility improvement may be induced by a more efficient function of the mature human brain as quantified by the small-world property. This finding is novel since it identified for first time a positive relationship among flexibility increase and global network performance.

Although, positive correlation of physical activity with global network characteristics is a novel finding which has not been earlier demonstrated to the best of our knowledge, it does not provide information about the mechanism that traditional Greek dance induces neuroplasticity. Aiming to further investigate this issue we performed local network analysis by investigating functional cartography (Guimerà and Nunes Amaral, 2005) and hub identification (Seo et al., 2013; Frantzidis et al., 2014a). This analysis was performed in order to define the functional node hierarchy both on the entire set of nodes and on specific resting-state (Default Mode, Fronto-Parietal and Executive) networks according to (Voss et al., 2010). We computed the BC as a generic hub index, PC as an index of how well a node is connected with nodes belonging to other modules and within-module z-score which quantifies the connection strength of a given node with the other nodes of its own module. The previous finding of positively correlating flexibility improvement with better functional organization (small-world increase) was further validated by the negative correlation observed among the *Back Scratch* and the PC for the nodes of the FPN ($r = -0.32$, $p = 0.039$). FPN seems to be greatly affected by the proposed intervention since there were also statistically significant changes in BC, PC and within module z-score for that network. FPN functioning was linked with goal-directed attention (Uddin, 2015), motor planning and execution (Hsu et al., 2017). It was also shown that fitness gains were associated with greater activation of the FPN and better executive functioning (Colcombe et al., 2004). Combining the previous neuroimaging findings with our results regarding the re-organization of the fronto-parietal and executive resting state network, we may conclude that traditional Greek dance is a potentially robust approach for improving the flexibility of senior citizens. This was achieved by inducing neuroplasticity effects on the modular architecture of resting-state networks known to be affected by increased physical activity (Colcombe et al., 2004; Voss et al., 2010). These networks were also previously demonstrated to govern complex motor planning and executive functioning resulting thus in improved flexibility which is essential during dancing. Neuroplasticity was also evident and for the DMN, as denoted by PC changes, but its effect was more attenuated in comparison to the aforementioned networks.

The aim of the present study was to examine whether a program of traditional Greek dance could induce neuroplasticity effects on the mature human brain. Dancing involves learning of motor skills through physical practice and observation (Kirsch et al., 2018), while it combines cognitive and physical training (Rehfeld et al., 2018). Although it involves a moderate level of physical activity, poses several sensorimotor and cognitive challenges. It also facilitates social interaction enriched with emotional stimulation (Kattenstroth et al., 2013). So, dancing is regarded as a promising intervention for promoting neuroplasticity, healthy and active aging (Merom et al., 2016). The pioneering work of Kattenstroth et al. (2013) demonstrated positive effects on posture, reaction time, cognition, motor performance and quality of life, when compared with a control group. Despite their novelty, the aforementioned studies did not investigated changes in terms of functional or structural neuroimaging, even though dance often involves the activation of premotor, parietal and occipito-temporal cortices (Vogt and Thomaschke, 2007). However, these brain regions are known to be affected by aging mechanisms, resulting thus in poor performance during complex motor sequences like those required for dancing (Kirsch et al., 2018). Our hypothesis was that an intervention based on traditional Greek dance would challenge mental, cognitive and physical abilities of senior citizens. This would be achieved through music stimuli stemming from their youth and requiring execution of complex motor sequences. During the choreography performance, dancers need to co-ordinate their body posture and movement according to the time-varying music characteristics. This would be achieved by improving their balance, flexibility and strength through the functional re-organization of the mature human cortex. Neuroplasticity effects were evident at a global network level denoted by faster information flow among distant brain regions. This may imply the optimized performance of specific neural networks governing elaborate cognitive processing, balance and entire body co-ordination (Voss et al., 2010). Our results validated previous studies that compared a challenging 6-month dance training program with a conventional fitness intervention of equal intensity (Rehfeld et al., 2018). Although both interventions increased physical fitness, dancing was associated with greater brain volume increase and with an increase in plasma BDNF level (Rehfeld et al., 2018). Longer duration of dance intervention was associated with greater activation of the left hippocampal volume and with improved balance performance (Rehfeld et al., 2017). These studies employed advanced neuroimaging techniques for localizing either structural (Rehfeld et al., 2017, 2018) or functional (Kirsch et al., 2018) changes associated with dancing. Our approach aims to provide an evaluation framework, quantifying dynamical interactions among cortical regions based on contemporary mathematical tools derived from graph theory. So, we focused not only on how the dance training changed the macroscopic functional organization of the human brain, but we also investigated local changes on the default-mode, fronto-parietal and executive resting state networks.

Although our results and their interpretations shed light into the neuroplasticity induced by dancing interventions, they should be considered in the context of several limitations. Firstly, the analysis employed an EEG device with 57 active electrodes. Similar EEG recording settings have been used successfully in previous studies (Styliadis et al., 2015; Klados et al., 2016), nonetheless one should take into account in the interpretation of the results the low spatial resolution of such a setting. High density EEG systems with 128 channels may identify with greater accuracy the cortical activations obtained as outcome measures from similar intervention procedures. Moreover, our brain network analysis was based on a generic head anatomy modeling which could not deal with inter-subject variability and therefore may be vulnerable to errors due to atrophy, life style factors, tissue conductivity or injuries. Given that the local network analysis was based on ROIs defined by a previous neuroimaging study (Voss et al., 2010), estimation of cortical activity for these ROIs may be prune to methodological limitations and results should be interpreted with caution. However, our results identifying a major re-organization of fronto-parietal and ENs are in line with a plethora of previous neuroimaging studies (Colcombe et al., 2004; Voss et al., 2010; Hsu et al., 2017; Kirsch et al., 2018). Future studies may also avoid using thresholding of the connectivity values and employ weighted networks. An important aspect of future research will be the validation of our results with resting state data derived from other recording modalities such as magnetoencephalography (MEG) or fMRI. Another possible limitation is the relatively small sample size of participants we employed. Although, power analysis indicated that the proper number of participants is close to the actual one (48 vs. 44), larger cohorts is expected to provide more definitive results regarding the neuroplastic changes due to the dance intervention. We should also mention that the present study enrolled only Greek senior citizens and lacks diversity concerning ethnic background. Our future aim is to investigate the generalizability of the intervention to other sample cohorts across the world and to compare it with other traditional dance types. Finally, future studies should investigate whether the beneficial effects of dancing are dependent from demographic factors (age, gender), education, cognitive reserve, socioeconomic status, etc.

To sum up, the present study investigated whether traditional Greek dance training would induce neuroplasticity effects on senior citizens. It employed network neuroscience in order to investigate the beneficial role of dancing on both global and local cortical level. To the best of our knowledge, it is the first attempt that demonstrated improved functional performance on cortical level through increased small world-property. This finding was mainly attributed to faster information flow and more accurate information integration among distant cortical regions (smaller characteristic path length). Neuroplasticity was more evident on specific modules such as the fronto-parietal and executive resting state networks known for being responsible for attention, motor planning and execution. The present computational approach seems to provide an integrative framework for evaluating the intervention impact on groups of senior citizens and to be robust for quantifying neuroplasticity effects on multi-level aspects of the functional cortical networks.

AUTHOR CONTRIBUTIONS

VZ designed and implemented the dance program, collected the data and prepared the initial draft of the manuscript. CF collected and analyzed the EEG data, guided the analysis, wrote EEG methodological parts, discussed the results and revised the manuscript. ER conceived the analysis of data. EP revised the manuscript. SD guided the study. PB co-guided the study and revised the manuscript.

FUNDING

This work has been partially funded by the European Union's Horizon 2020 research and innovation programme under grant agreement No 643555 Ubiquitous iNteroperable Care for Ageing People (http://www.uncap.eu).

REFERENCES

Balkus, P. L. (1989). "Municipal dance for delayed individuals," in *Proceedings of the 3rd International Congress, Popular Dance and Education* (Athens: D.O.L.T.), 13–17.

Bamidis, P. D., Fissler, P., Papageorgiou, S. G., Zilidou, V., Konstantinidis, E. I., Billis, A. S., et al. (2015). Gains in cognition through combined cognitive and physical training: the role of training dosage and severity of neurocognitive disorder. *Front. Aging Neurosci.* 7:152. doi: 10.3389/fnagi.2015.00152

Bamidis, P. D., Vivas, A. B., Styliadis, C., Frantzidis, C., Klados, M., Schlee, W., et al. (2014). A review of physical and cognitive interventions in aging. *Neurosci. Biobehav. Rev.* 44, 206–220. doi: 10.1016/j.neubiorev.2014.03.019

Berg, K., Wood-Dauphine, S., Williams, J. I., and Gayton, D. (2009). Measuring balance in the elderly: preliminary development of an instrument. *Physiother. Can.* 41, 304–311. doi: 10.3138/ptc.41.6.304

Bherer, L., Erickson, K. I., and Liu-Ambrose, T. (2013). A review of the effects of physical activity and exercise on cognitive and brain functions in older adults. *J. Aging Res.* 2013:657508. doi: 10.1155/2013/657508

Billis, A. S., Konstantinidis, E. I., Mouzakidis, C., Tsolaki, M. N., Pappas, C., and Bamidis, P. D. (2010). "A game-like interface for training seniors' dynamic balance and coordination," in *Proceedings of 12th Mediterranean Conference on Medical and Biological Engineering and Computing 2010 SE—174*, eds P. D. Bamidis and N. Pallikarakis (Heidelberg: IFMBE Proceedings Springer), 691–694.

Burdette, J. H., Laurienti, P. J., Espeland, M. A., Morgan, A., Telesford, Q., Vechlekar, C. D., et al. (2010). Using network science to evaluate exercise-associated brain changes in older adults. *Front. Aging Neurosci.* 2:23. doi: 10.3389/fnagi.2010.00023

Butler, M., Retzlaff, P., and Vanderploeg, R. (1991). Neuropsychological test usage. *Prof. Psychol. Res. Pr.* 22, 510–512. doi: 10.1037/0735-7028.22.6.510

Chriskos, P., Frantzidis, C. A., Gkivogkli, P. T., Bamidis, P. D., and Kourtidou-Papadeli, C. (2018). Achieving accurate automatic sleep staging on manually pre-processed EEG data through synchronization feature extraction and graph metrics. *Front. Hum. Neurosci.* 12:110. doi: 10.3389/fnhum.2018.00110

Colcombe, S. J., Kramer, A. F., Erickson, K. I., Scalf, P., McAuley, E., Cohen, N. J., et al. (2004). Cardiovascular fitness, cortical plasticity, and aging. *Proc. Natl. Acad. Sci. U S A* 101, 3316–3321. doi: 10.1073/pnas.0400266101

Cotman, C. W., Berchtold, N. C., and Christie, L. A. (2007). Exercise builds brain health: key roles of growth factor cascades and inflammation. *Trends Neurosci.* 30, 464–472. doi: 10.1016/j.tins.2007.06.011

de Haan, W., Pijnenburg, Y. A., Strijers, R. L., van der Made, Y., van der Flier, W. M., Scheltens, P., et al. (2009). Functional neural network analysis in frontotemporal dementia and Alzheimer's disease using EEG and graph theory. *BMC Neurosci.* 10:101. doi: 10.1186/1471-2202-10-101

Delorme, A., and Makeig, S. (2004). EEGLAB: an open source toolbox for analysis of single-trial eeg dynamics including independent component analysis. *J. Neurosci. Methods* 134, 9–21. doi: 10.1016/j.jneumeth.2003.10.009

Erickson, K. I., Voss, M. W., Prakash, R. S., Basak, C., Szabo, A., Chaddock, L., et al. (2011). Exercise training increases size of hippocampus and improves memory. *Proc. Natl. Acad. Sci. U S A* 108, 3017–3022. doi: 10.1073/pnas.1015950108

Faul, F., Erdfelder, E., Buchner, A., and Lang, A.-G. (2013). *G*Power Version 3.1.7 [Computer Software].* Germany: Uiversität Kiel. Available online at: http://www.psycho.uni-duesseldorf.de/abteilungen/aap/gpower3/download-and-register

Folstein, M. F., Folstein, S. E., and McHugh, P. R. (1975). "Mini-mental state". A practical method for grading the cognitive state of patients for the clinician. *J. Psychiatr. Res.* 12, 189–198. doi: 10.1016/0022-3956(75)90026-6

Frantzidis, C. A., Bratsas, C., Papadelis, C. L., Konstantinidis, E., Pappas, C., and Bamidis, P. D. (2010). Toward emotion aware computing: an integrated approach using multichannel neurophysiological recordings and affective visual stimuli. *IEEE Trans. Inf. Technol. Biomed.* 14, 589–597. doi: 10.1109/titb.2010.2041553

Frantzidis, C. A., Ladas, A. K., Vivas, A. B., Tsolaki, M., and Bamidis, P. D. (2014a). Cognitive and physical training for the elderly: evaluating outcome efficacy by means of neurophysiological synchronization. *Int. J. Psychophysiol.* 93, 1–11. doi: 10.1016/j.ijpsycho.2014.01.007

Frantzidis, C. A., Vivas, A. B., Tsolaki, A., Klados, M. A., Tsolaki, M., and Bamidis, P. D. (2014b). Functional disorganization of small-world brain networks in mild Alzheimer's disease and amnestic mild cognitive impairment: an eeg study using relative wavelet entropy (RWE). *Front. Aging Neurosci.* 6:224. doi: 10.3389/fnagi.2014.00224

Guimerà, R., and Nunes Amaral, L. A. (2005). Functional cartography of complex metabolic networks. *Nature* 433, 895–900. doi: 10.1038/nature03288

Heyn, P., Abreu, B. C., and Ottenbacher, K. J. (2004). The effects of exercise training on elderly persons with cognitive impairment and dementia: a meta-analysis. *Arch. Phys. Med. Rehab.* 85, 1694–1704. doi: 10.1016/j.apmr.2004.03.019

Hsu, C. L., Best, J. R., Wang, S., Voss, M. W., Hsiung, R. G., Munkacsy, M., et al. (2017). The impact of aerobic exercise on Fronto-parietal network connectivity and its relation to mobility: an exploratory analysis of a 6-month randomized controlled trial. *Front. Hum. Neurosci.* 11:344. doi: 10.3389/fnhum.2017.00344

Johnson, B. L., and Nelson, J. K. (1969). *Practical Measurements for Evaluation in Physical Education.* Minnesota, MN: Burgess.

Jones, C. J., and Rikli, R. E. (2002). Measuring functional fitness of older adults. *Int. J. Act. Aging* 1, 25–30.

Karpati, F. J., Giacosa, C., Foster, N. E. V., Penhune, V. B., and Hyde, K. L. (2015). Dance and the brain: a review. *Ann. N Y Acad. Sci.* 1337, 140–146. doi: 10.1111/nyas.12632

Kattenstroth, J. C., Kalisch, T., Holt, S., Tegenthoff, M., and Dinse, H. R. (2013). Six months of dance intervention enhances postural, sensorimotor, and cognitive performance in elderly without affecting cardio-respiratory functions. *Front. Aging Neurosci.* 5:5. doi: 10.3389/fnagi.2013.00005

Kim, S., and Kim, J. (2007). Mood after various brief exercise and sport modes: aerobics, hip-hop dancing, ICE skating, and body conditioning. *Percept. Mot. Skills* 104, 1265–1270. doi: 10.2466/pms.104.4.1265-1270

Kirsch, L. P., Diersch, N., Sumanapala, D. K., and Cross, E. S. (2018). Dance training shapes action perception and its neural implementation within the young and older adult brain. *Neural Plast.* 2018:5459106. doi: 10.1155/2018/5459106

Klados, M. A., Styliadis, C., Frantzidis, C. A., Paraskevopoulos, E., and Bamidis, P. D. (2016). β-band functional connectivity is reorganized in mild cognitive impairment after combined computerized physical and cognitive training. *Front. Neurosci.* 10:55. doi: 10.3389/fnins.2016.00055

Konstantinidis, E., Billis, A., Hlauschek, W., Panek, P., and Bamidis, P. (2010). Integration of cognitive and physical training in a smart home environment for the elderly people. *Stud. Health Technol. Inform.* 160, 58–62.

Lampit, A., Hallock, H., and Valenzuela, M. (2014). Computerized cognitive training in cognitively healthy older adults: a systematic review and meta-analysis of effect modifiers. *PLoS Med.* 11:e1001756. doi: 10.1371/journal.pmed.1001756

Lima, M. M., and Vieira, A. P. (2007). Ballroom dance as therapy for the elderly in Brazil. *Am. J. Dance Ther.* 29, 129–142. doi: 10.1007/s10465-007-9040-9

Merom, D., Grunseit, A., Eramudugolla, R., Jefferis, B., Mcneill, J., and Anstey, K. J. (2016). Cognitive benefits of social dancing and walking in old age: the Dancing Mind randomized controlled trial. *Front. Aging Neurosci.* 8:26. doi: 10.3389/fnagi.2016.00026

Micheloyannis, S., Vourkas, M., Tsirka, V., Karakonstantaki, E., Kanatsouli, K., and Stam, C. J. (2009). The influence of ageing on complex brain networks: a graph theoretical analysis. *Hum. Brain Mapp.* 30, 200–208. doi: 10.1002/hbm.20492

Ngandu, T., Lehtisalo, J., Solomon, A., Levälahti, E., Ahtiluoto, S., Antikainen, R., et al. (2015). A 2 year multidomain intervention of diet, exercise, cognitive training, and vascular risk monitoring versus control to prevent cognitive decline in at-risk elderly people (FINGER): a randomised controlled trial. *Lancet* 385, 2255–2263. doi: 10.1016/S0140-6736(15)60461-5

Pascual-Marqui, R. D. (2002). Standardized low-resolution brain electromagnetic tomography (sLORETA): technical details. *Methods Find. Exp. Clin. Pharmacol.* 24, 5–12.

Rehfeld, K., Lüders, A., Hökelmann, A., Lessmann, V., Kaufmann, J., Brigadski, T., et al. (2018). Dance training is superior to repetitive physical exercise in inducing brain plasticity in the elderly. *PLoS One* 13:e0196636. doi: 10.1371/journal.pone.0196636

Rehfeld, K., Müller, P., Aye, N., Schmicker, M., Dordevic, M., Kaufmann, J., et al. (2017). Dancing or fitness sport? The effects of two training programs on hippocampal plasticity and balance abilities in healthy seniors. *Front. Hum. Neurosci.* 11:305. doi: 10.3389/fnhum.2017.00305

Romanopoulou, E., Zilidou, V., and Antoniou, P. (2015). "Spinning off gerotechnology business activities: the LLM care best practice paradigm," in *Handbook of Research on Innovations in the Diagnosis and Treatment of Dementia*, eds P. Bamidis, I. Tarnanas, L. Hadjileontiadis and M. Tsolaki (Hershey, PA: IGI Global), 426–436.

Rubinov, M., and Sporns, O. (2010). Complex network measures of brain connectivity: uses and interpretations. *Neuroimage* 52, 1059–1069. doi: 10.1016/j.neuroimage.2009.10.003

Sanz-Arigita, E. J., Schoonheim, M. M., Damoiseaux, J. S., Rombouts, S. A., Maris, E., Barkhof, F., et al. (2010). Loss of 'small-world' networks in Alzheimer's disease: graph analysis of FMRI resting-state functional connectivity. *PLoS One* 5:e13788. doi: 10.1371/journal.pone.0013788

Seo, E. H., Lee, D. Y., Lee, J. M., Park, J. S., Sohn, B. K., Lee, D. S., et al. (2013). Whole-brain functional networks in cognitively normal, mild cognitive impairment, and Alzheimer's disease. *PLoS One* 8:e53922. doi: 10.1371/journal.pone.0053922

Sofianidis, G., Hatzitaki, V., Douka, S., and Grouios, G. (2009). Effect of a 10-week traditional dance program on static and dynamic balance control in elderly adults. *J. Aging Phys. Act.* 17, 167–180. doi: 10.1123/japa.17.2.167

Stam, C. J., de Haan, W., Daffertshofer, A., Jones, B. F., Manshanden, I., van Cappellen van Walsum, A. M., et al. (2008). Graph theoretical analysis of magnetoencephalographic functional connectivity in Alzheimer's disease. *Brain* 132, 213–224. doi: 10.1093/brain/awn262

Stam, C. J., Jones, B. F., Nolte, G., Breakspear, M., and Scheltens, P. (2007). Small-world networks and functional connectivity in Alzheimer's disease. *Cereb. Cortex* 17, 92–99. doi: 10.1093/cercor/bhj127

Styliadis, C., Kartsidis, P., Paraskevopoulos, E., Ioannides, A. A., and Bamidis, P. (2015). Neuroplastic effects of combined computerized physical and cognitive training in elderly individuals at risk for dementia: an eLORETA controlled study on resting states. *Neural Plast.* 2015:172192. doi: 10.1155/2015/172192

Supekar, K., Menon, V., Rubin, D., Musen, M., and Greicius, M. D. (2008). Network analysis of intrinsic functional brain connectivity in Alzheimer's disease. *PLoS Comput. Biol.* 4:e1000100. doi: 10.1371/journal.pcbi.1000100

Tadel, F., Baillet, S., Mosher, J. C., Pantazis, D., and Leahy, R. M. (2011). Brainstorm: a user-friendly application for MEG/EEG analysis. *Comput. Intell. Neurosci.* 2011:879716. doi: 10.1155/2011/879716

Tinetti, M. E. (1986). Performance-oriented assessment of mobility problems in elderly patients. *J. Am. Geriatr. Soc.* 34, 119–126. doi: 10.1111/j.1532-5415.1986.tb05480.x

Tijms, B. M., Wink, A. M., de Haan, W., van der Flier, W. M., Stam, C. J., Scheltens, P., et al. (2013). Alzheimer's disease: connecting findings from graph theoretical studies of brain networks. *Neurobiol. Aging* 34, 2023–2036. doi: 10.1016/j.neurobiolaging.2013.02.020

Uddin, L. Q. (2015). Salience processing and insular cortical function and dysfunction. *Nat. Rev. Neurosci.* 16, 55–61. doi: 10.1038/nrn3857

Verghese, J., Lipton, R. B., Katz, M. J., Hall, C. B., Derby, C. A., Kuslanisky, G., et al. (2003). Leisure activities and the risk of dementia in the elderly. *N. Engl. J. Med.* 348, 2508–2516. doi: 10.1056/NEJMoa022252

Vogt, S., and Thomaschke, R. (2007). From visuo-motor interactions to imitation learning: behavioural and brain imaging studies. *J. Sports Sci.* 25, 497–517. doi: 10.1080/02640410600946779

Voss, M. W., Prakash, R. S., Erickson, K. I., Basak, C., Chaddock, L., Kim, J. S., et al. (2010). Plasticity of brain networks in a randomized intervention trial of exercise training in older adults. *Front. Aging Neurosci.* 2:32. doi: 10.3389/fnagi.2010.00032

Watts, D. J., and Strogatz, S. H. (1998). Collective dynamics of 'small-world's networks. *Nature* 393, 440–442. doi: 10.1038/30918

Wikström, B. M. (2004). Older adults and the arts: the importance of aesthetic forms of expression in later life. *J. Gerontol. Nurs.* 30, 30–36. doi: 10.3928/0098-9134-20040901-07

Yesavage, J. A., Brink, T. L., Rose, T. L., Lum, O., Huang, V., Adey, M., et al. (1982–1983). Development and validation of a geriatric depression screening scale: a preliminary report. *J. Psychiatr. Res.* 17, 37–49. doi: 10.1016/0022-3956(82)90033-4

Zhao, X., Liu, Y., Wang, X., Liu, B., Xi, Q., Guo, Q., et al. (2012). Disrupted small-world brain networks in moderate Alzheimer's disease: a resting-state FMRI study. *PLoS One* 7:e33540. doi: 10.1371/journal.pone.0033540

Zilidou, V. I., Konstantinidis, E. I., Romanopoulou, E. D., Karagianni, M., Kartsidis, P., and Bamidis, P. D. (2016). "Investigating the effectiveness of physical training through exergames: focus on balance and aerobic protocols (2016)," in *Proceedings of the 1st International Conference on Technology and Innovation in Sports* (Vila Real: Health and Wellbeing (TISHW)), 1–6.

8

Disconnectivity between Dorsal Raphe Nucleus and Posterior Cingulate Cortex in Later Life Depression

Toshikazu Ikuta [1], Koji Matsuo [2], Kenichiro Harada [2], Mami Nakashima [2,3], Teruyuki Hobara [2,4], Naoko Higuchi [2], Fumihiro Higuchi [2], Koji Otsuki [2], Tomohiko Shibata [2,5], Toshio Watanuki [2], Toshio Matsubara [2,6], Hirotaka Yamagata [2] and Yoshifumi Watanabe [2]*

[1]Department of Communication Sciences and Disorders, School of Applied Sciences, University of Mississippi, University, MS, United States, [2]Division of Neuropsychiatry, Department of Neuroscience, Graduate School of Medicine, Yamaguchi University, Ube, Japan, [3]Nagato-Ichinomiya Hospital, Shimonoseki, Japan, [4]Department of Psychiatry, Yamaguchi Grand Medical Center, Hofu, Japan, [5]Shinwaen Hospital, Onoda, Japan, [6]Health Administration Center, Yamaguchi University Organization for University Education, Yamaguchi City, Japan

***Correspondence:**
Toshikazu Ikuta
tikuta@olemiss.edu

The dorsal raphe nucleus (DRN) has been repeatedly implicated as having a significant relationship with depression, along with its serotoninergic innervation. However, functional connectivity of the DRN in depression is not well understood. The current study aimed to isolate functional connectivity of the DRN distinct in later life depression (LLD) compared to a healthy age-matched population. Resting state functional magnetic resonance imaging (rsfMRI) data from 95 participants (33 LLD and 62 healthy) were collected to examine functional connectivity from the DRN to the whole brain in voxel-wise fashion. The posterior cingulate cortex (PCC) bilaterally showed significantly smaller connectivity in the LLD group than the control group. The DRN to PCC connectivity did not show any association with the depressive status. The findings implicate that the LLD involves disruption of serotoninergic input to the PCC, which has been suggested to be a part of the reduced default mode network in depression.

Keywords: depression, neuroimaging, geriatric psychiatry, magnetic resonance imaging, dorsal raphe nucleus

INTRODUCTION

Disruption of the dorsal raphe nucleus (DRN) is implicated in depression, given that the DRN serves as the major source of 5-HT release in the brain. In neuroanatomical studies, the area of the DRN is reduced in major depression (Matthews and Harrison, 2012). The number and density of neurons in this region is higher in suicide victims (Underwood et al., 1999). Physiologically, serotonin transporter dysfunction has been found in the DRN of patients with major depression (Hahn et al., 2014), and binding potentials for the 5-HT1A receptor have been found to be reduced in depression (Drevets et al., 1999). Polymorphisms in 5-HT1A gene have been found to be associated with antidepressants (Kato et al., 2009). Genetic variations of tryptophan hydroxylase 2 (*TPH2*) are also associated with major depression (Zill et al., 2004), and are further found to be associated with *TPH2* mRNA expression in the pons including the DRN (Lim et al., 2006). Single nucleotide polymorphisms of the 5-HT1A receptor and *TPH2* have been suggested to interact with the severity of depression and respond to SSRIs (Serretti et al., 2011; Jacobsen et al., 2012). Meanwhile, the DRN is understood to be critical for the actions of antidepressants including

SSRIs and tricyclics (Briley and Moret, 1993), as well as for the pathophysiology of depression.

Forebrain 5-HT projections originate in the DRN (Törk, 1990; Baker et al., 1991). Rodent models further support disruption of the DRN in depression. Genetically introducing serotonin transporter deficiency in the DRN induces depression-like behavior in mice (Lira et al., 2003). Social stress has also been shown to influence serotoninergic neurons in the DRN of rats that adopted a proactive coping strategy against stress (Wood et al., 2013). More recently, the volume of the raphe nuclei, as well as other monoaminergic regions, have been shown to be negatively correlated with social avoidance, which indexes stress susceptibility (Anacker et al., 2016) The DRN cells have inhibitory projections to the cortex, including the cingulate gyrus (Olpe, 1981), which is also implicated in depression (Bae et al., 2006; Wise et al., 2016).

The pathophysiology of Later-Life Depression (LLD) is considered to be in parallel to the pathology of depression in younger ages, though LLD has certain defining characteristics, such as less genetic influence (Brodaty et al., 2001; Alexopoulos, 2005). Antidepressants have been shown to be especially effective with LLD (Salzman et al., 2002; Schneider et al., 2003). Therefore, it can be hypothesized that the role of the DRN is substantial in the pathology of LDD. The role of the DRN in LLD, however, is not clearly understood.

Neuropathological change of the raphe nuclei has been implicated in depression. Neuronal loss in the raphe nucleus of older patients with depression has been found in a postmortem study (Tsopelas et al., 2011). Lesser gray matter concentration of the DRN was found in patients with major depression compared to the healthy control group (Lee et al., 2011). Patients who had transient relapse of depression induced by tryptophan depletion showed greater correlation between habenula-DRN co-activity compared to those patients who did not show relapse (Morris et al., 1999). Recently, studies in the functional connectivity of the DRN in humans have shown positive connectivity to cortical regions, illuminating 5-HT associated regions (Beliveau et al., 2015). Yet, functional connectivity of the DRN in depression or LLD has not been extensively studied. Here, in order to elucidate the functional connectivity of the DRN, we examined the resting state of functional connectivity in LLD in comparison to an age-matched control cohort. We hypothesized that the disrupted DRN connectivity would be found in regions whose connectivity manifests a signature role of the DRN in neuropathophysiology of LLD.

MATERIALS AND METHODS

Participants

We examined a total of 95 individuals, including 33 LLD patients and 62 healthy age-matched participants. All patients met the DSM-IV criteria for major depressive disorder. Mean age of the LLD group was 60.40 (SD = 7.82) years, and healthy group 62.73 (7.43) years. Patients were recruited from Yamaguchi University Hospital; referred by area clinics and hospitals; and diagnosed by clinical interviews performed by senior psychiatrists, case conferences with psychiatrists, and structured interviews using the Mini International Neuropsychiatric Interview (MINI, Japanese version 5.0.0; Otsubo et al., 2005). Patients' clinical demographics were obtained through a clinical interview. Patients with current or a history of substance abuse/dependence or other psychotic illnesses were excluded from the study. Healthy control participants were recruited from the community through local advertisements and word of mouth. Any healthy subject who had psychiatric illness was excluded through the MINI and clinical interviews. Participants with an immediate family member with a psychiatric disorder were also excluded. Exclusion criteria included ambidextrous or left handedness (Oldfield, 1971), MR imaging contraindications, presence of serious medical conditions, and hospitalization in the prior 6 months. Current mood states were assessed using the Structured Interview Guide for the Hamilton Depression Rating Scale (SIGH-D; Williams, 1988). Social functioning was assessed by the Global Assessment of Functioning scale (GAF; American Psychiatric Association, 2000). Participants with scores of 23 or below on the Mini-Mental State Examination were considered demented and excluded (Folstein et al., 1975). Through interviews, blood tests, and physical examinations, subjects with endocrinological disease, head trauma, neurological disease, a family history of hereditary neurological disorders, or other medical conditions (i.e., hypertension, diabetes, active liver disease, kidney problems, or respiratory problems) were also excluded from the study. LLD was defined as depression in patients over 50 years old at the time of study participation. The mean number of depressive episodes was 2.3 (1.8) in patients with LLD. Thirty patients were under medication at the time of study participation. Five patients were treated only with antidepressants; eight with antidepressants and first-generation antipsychotics; 12 with antidepressants and second-generation antipsychotics; two with an antidepressant and a mood stabilizer; with antidepressant, a second-generation antipsychotic, and a mood stabilizer; one with a second-generation antipsychotic; and one was with a mood stabilizer. Among the remaining three patients, one was drug-naïve, and the other two had been medication-free at least for the previous 4 years. The mean imipramine-equivalent dose among all the patients was 174.5 (151.3) mg. Most patients were under one or more antidepressant medications: SSRI-16; SNRI-14; Tricyclics-8; Others (mirtazapine, trazodone and mianserin)-13. This study was conducted in accordance with the latest version of the Declaration of Helsinki. This study was approved by the Yamaguchi University Institutional Review Board and written informed consent was obtained from all study participants.

Clinical Assessments

Current mood states were examined using the SIGH-D (Williams, 1988). To assess social functioning, the GAF (American Psychiatric Association, 2000) was used. Self-reported depression status was measured by the Beck Depression Inventory (BDI; Beck et al., 1961). To uniformly assess various antidepressant dosage Imipramine Equivalent Potency was calculated.

MRI Data Acquisition

A total of 204 echo-planner imaging (EPI) volumes were acquired on a Siemens Magnetom Skyra system (TR = 2500 ms, TE = 30 ms, matrix = 64 $*$ 64, FOV = 220 mm, slice thickness = 4 mm, 34 continuous axial slices) as well as the MPRAGE structural volume (TR = 2300 ms, TE = 2.95 ms, flip angle = 9°, matrix = 256 × 256, FOV = 270 mm, 1.2 mm thick sagittal images).

MRI Data Processing

Script package from the 1000 Functional Connectomes Project[1] (Biswal et al., 2010) was used for preprocessing and seed-voxel correlation matrix production whereby FSL[2] and AFNI[3] are called. Motion correction and spatial smoothing (6-mm FWHM Gaussian kernel) were carried out through preprocessing. Each individual rs-fMRI series was registered and normalized to MNI152 2 mm space via T1 volume. Through this registration, 12 affine parameters were created between rs-fMRI volume and MNI152 2 mm space, so that a seed ROI can be later registered to each individual rs-fMRI space. The rs-fMRI time series were band-pass filtered (between 0.005 Hz and 0.1 Hz). Each resting state volume was regressed by white matter and cerebrospinal fluid signal fluctuations as well as the six motion parameters.

The DRN seed was defined as a 32 mm^3 region centered at [MNI: 0, −27, −9] following the literature (Kranz et al., 2012; Beliveau et al., 2015). From the DRN seed, voxel-wise connectivity analyses were conducted by the "singlesubjectRSFC fcon" script, whereby the time course is spatially averaged within the ROI so that correlations from the ROI to each individual voxel across the brain.

To compare the two groups, a Z statistic image was estimated where clusters were determined by a family-wise, error-corrected cluster significance threshold of $p < 0.01$ assuming a Gaussian random field for the Z-statistics.

In order to examine the association between the functional connectivity differences and status of depression, clusters that showed significant effect of group were tested for further association with depression scales within the LLD group. The mean Z-scores of a cluster were calculated and correlations between the mean score and each of the depression scales was tested.

RESULTS

The LLD group showed significant indications of depression; BDI (control: 7.15 ± 4.71; LDD: 29.53 ± 11.45), GAF (control: 93.02 ± 4.72; LDD: 52.79 ± 6.19), and SIGH-D 17 (control: 0.81 ± 1.07; LDD: 21.87 ± 3.49), as well as their antidepressant medications assessed as imipramine equivalent potency (control: 0 ± 0; LDD: 193.64 ± 145.75).

The LLD group showed significantly lower functional connectivity between the DRN and bilateral posterior cingulate cortex (PCC). There was no other cluster that showed lower functional connectivity in the LLD group. The cluster had 301 voxels and the peak voxel (corrected $p < 0.001$) was at [MNI: −4 −30 26] (**Figure 1**). No region showed greater connectivity in the LLD group than the control group.

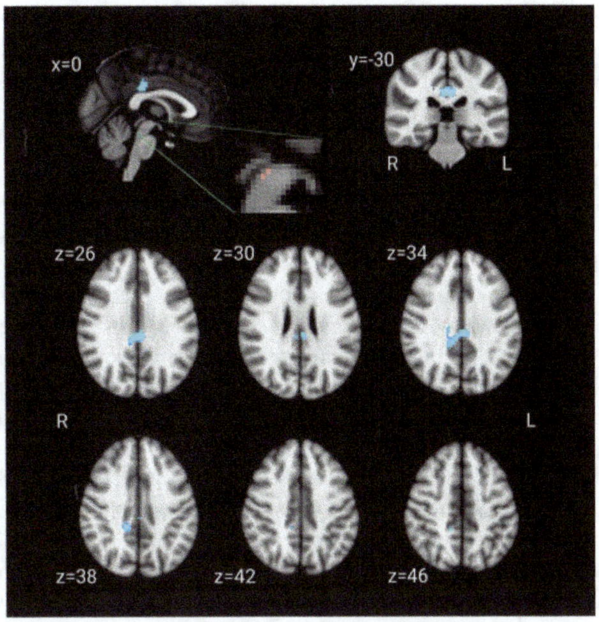

FIGURE 1 | *Pink*: the dorsal raphe nucleus (DRN) ROI. *Blue*: the cluster that showed lesser connectivity with the DRN ROI in patients compared to the control group.

In the LLD group, none of these depression scales (SIGH, BDI and GAF) or imipramine equivalent dose showed significant correlation to the functional connectivity between the DRN and cluster in the posterior cingulate cortices.

DISCUSSION

This study aimed to isolate the functional connectivity patterns of the DRN distinct in LLD. Here, the DRN showed deficient functional connectivity to the PCC in LLD. The results illuminate the serotoninergic dysfunction that may influence LLD pathology, which is independent from the depressive status.

The current results are solely based on the functional connectivity between two distant regions, and therefore does not grant anatomical connections between two regions. However, serotoninergic projections from the DRN to PCC has been well-documented in rodents (Olpe, 1981; Finch et al., 1984; Kosofsky and Molliver, 1987). In humans, depressive symptoms in Parkinson's disease have been found to be associated with 5-HT transporter binding in the raphe nuclei and PCC, as well as other limbic structures (Politis et al., 2010), suggesting the association between depression and raphe-cingulate 5-HT projections. The current findings are consistent with raphe-cingulate serotoninergic projections that have been shown to be anatomically present.

[1] http://www.nitrc.org/projects/fcon_1000
[2] http://www.fmrib.ox.ac.uk
[3] http://afni.nimh.nih.gov/afni

Dysfunctions of the PCC have repeatedly been found in depression (Zhou et al., 2010; Berman et al., 2011; Leech and Sharp, 2014). At the same time, SSRIs have been shown to ameliorate PCC deficits. Sertraline and fluoxetine increase glucose metabolism in the PCC, correlating with clinical improvement (Buchsbaum and Hazlett, 1997; Mayberg et al., 2000). In addition, administration of SSRIs has been found to increase the PCC volume in the non-depressed, healthy population (Kraus et al., 2014). The current results are consistent with the previous PCC findings in depression. In the non-depressed, human population, the PCC has been shown to mediate emotion and memory related processes (Maddock et al., 2003), implicating its importance to mood disorders whereby impacts of emotional input are amplified. The PCC has been suggested to be associated with social/contextual self-reflection, duties or obligations, and autobiographical memory, suggesting PCC's role in self rumination (Johnson et al., 2006, 2009; Svoboda et al., 2006; Herwig et al., 2012). The current results support the understanding that serotoninergic dysfunction at the DRN underlies LLD by showing the disruption of the connectivity between the DRN and PCC in LLD.

The PCC in non-depressed population has also been shown to play critical roles in the default mode network (Fox et al., 2005; Buckner et al., 2008; Fransson and Marrelec, 2008; Uddin et al., 2009). The PCC is one of the regions that is more active at rest than during a task (Buckner et al., 2008). Furthermore, the PCC activity negatively predicts the motor-control network (Uddin et al., 2009), implicating the importance of the PCC during rest. It may imply that the PCC may mediate cognitive process of *rest* through the default mode network. Remarkably, the default mode network has been found to be suppressed in major depressive disorder (Sheline et al., 2009).

The functional connectivity between the DRN and PCC was not significantly associated with any of depression scales or antidepressant dose, while LLD group showed significantly lesser connectivity compared to the control group. It may suggest that the reduced DRN-PCC functional connectivity is a trait characteristic of depression independent from the depressive state. The association between depressive traits and the PCC has previously been implicated. In a task fMRI study, greater activation of the PCC in depression was found during negative rumination tasks, compared to the healthy control group (Cooney et al., 2010). Increased dominance of the default mode network in depression, compared to the task positive network, was associated with higher levels of depressive rumination (Hamilton et al., 2011). Decreased connectivity of the PCC to the default mode network in depression has also been found in a resting state fMRI study and was associated with over general autobiographical memory (Zhu et al., 2012). Taken together, the PCC in depression is associated with negative rumination. Recall that the raphe serotoninergic projection to the PCC is inhibitory (Olpe, 1981). Our results can imply that decreased DRN-PCC connectivity reflect lesser inhibitory inputs to the PCC, which would downregulate negative rumination.

The imprecision of the DRN seed needs to be addressed as the limitation of this study. The DRN seed was defined in 2 mm^3 space, which would not have sufficient resolutions to exclusively isolate the DRN. It should also be recalled that 6 mm smoothing was applied. Therefore, the seed may contain other structures around the DRN. Specifically, the median raphe nucleus (MRN) may not be excluded. In the previous study that differentiated resting state connectivity of DRN and MRN (Beliveau et al., 2015), [^{11}C]DASB PET data were acquired in each subject and the DRN and MRN were localized in each individual brain. As we did not obtain PET data, we have far coarse localization of the DRN. The current finding might not be exclusively attributed to the DRN but it may also include the greater raphe nuclei including MRN. It would be ideal to conduct a similar study with PET data for more precise localization of the DRN.

The MRN also possesses serotoninergic characteristics which implicates an association with depression (Bach-Mizrachi et al., 2008). MRN has also been shown to modulate emotional behaviors (López Hill et al., 2013). The association with the hippocampus has been found more in the MRN than DRN (Jacobs et al., 1974). Also, the MRN has known efferent to the cingulate cortex (Azmitia and Segal, 1978). It might be more appropriate to apprehend the finding as Raphe—PCC disconnectivity in LDD.

There are other limitations of this study that need to be addressed. The relationship between medication and functional connectivity is unclear. The findings may be the effect of medication as opposed to the effect of LLD. Studies examining a non-medicated population could better discriminate these possibilities. Though no association was found between the DRN-PCC connectivity and imipramine equivalent dose, it does not exclude the possibility for the influence of medication. In addition, the experience of being in an MRI scanner may have influenced the groups differently. LLD may trigger differential neuronal activation as a function of the experience.

In conclusion, this study found disconnectivity between the DRN and PCC in the LLD group that is consistent with serotoninergic dysfunction of the DRN in depression.

AUTHOR CONTRIBUTIONS

KM and YW conceived and designed the experiments. KH, MN, TH, NH, FH, KO, TS, TW, TM and HY performed the experiments. TI, KM and KH analyzed the data and wrote the article.

FUNDING

This study was supported, in part, by the "Integrated Research on Neuropsychiatric Disorders" conducted under the Strategic Research Program for Brain Sciences from the MEXT and AMED (HY), Japan Society for the Promotion of Science (JSPS) KAKENHI (16K10189 to HY, 15K09832 to KM), and the GlaxoSmithKline (GSK) Japan Research Grant (to HY).

REFERENCES

Alexopoulos, G. S. (2005). Depression in the elderly. *Lancet* 365, 1961–1970. doi: 10.1016/S0140-6736(05)66665-2

American Psychiatric Association. (2000). *Diagnostic and Statistical Manual of Mental Disorders. Fourth Edition, Text Revision (DSM-IV-TR).* Washington, DC: American Psychiatric Association.

Anacker, C., Scholz, J., O'Donnell, K. J., Allemang-Grand, R., Diorio, J., Bagot, R. C., et al. (2016). Neuroanatomic differences associated with stress susceptibility and resilience. *Biol. Psychiatry* 79, 840–849. doi: 10.1016/j.biopsych.2015.08.009

Azmitia, E. C., and Segal, M. (1978). An autoradiographic analysis of the differential ascending projections of the dorsal and median raphe nuclei in the rat. *J. Comp. Neurol.* 179, 641–667. doi: 10.1002/cne.901790311

Bach-Mizrachi, H., Underwood, M. D., Tin, A., Ellis, S. P., Mann, J. J., and Arango, V. (2008). Elevated expression of tryptophan hydroxylase-2 mRNA at the neuronal level in the dorsal and median raphe nuclei of depressed suicides. *Mol. Psychiatry* 13, 507–513, 465. doi: 10.1038/sj.mp.4002143

Bae, J. N., MacFall, J. R., Krishnan, K. R. R., Payne, M. E., Steffens, D. C., and Taylor, W. D. (2006). Dorsolateral prefrontal cortex and anterior cingulate cortex white matter alterations in late-life depression. *Biol. Psychiatry* 60, 1356–1363. doi: 10.1016/j.biopsych.2006.03.052

Baker, K. G., Halliday, G. M., Hornung, J.-P., Geffen, L. B., Cotton, R. G. H., and Tork, I. (1991). Distribution, morphology and number of monoamine-synthesizing and substance P-containing neurons in the human dorsal raphe nucleus. *Neuroscience* 42, 757–775. doi: 10.1016/0306-4522(91)90043-n

Beck, A. T., Ward, C. H., Mendelson, M. M., Mock, J. J., and Erbaugh, J. J. (1961). An inventory for measuring depression. *Arch. Gen. Psychiatry* 4, 561–571. doi: 10.1001/archpsyc.1961.01710120031004

Beliveau, V., Svarer, C., Frokjaer, V. G., Knudsen, G. M., Greve, D. N., and Fisher, P. M. (2015). Functional connectivity of the dorsal and median raphe nuclei at rest. *Neuroimage* 116, 187–195. doi: 10.1016/j.neuroimage.2015.04.065

Berman, M. G., Peltier, S., Nee, D. E., Kross, E., Deldin, P. J., and Jonides, J. (2011). Depression, rumination and the default network. *Soc. Cogn. Affect. Neurosci.* 6, 548–555. doi: 10.1093/scan/nsq080

Biswal, B. B., Mennes, M., Zuo, X.-N., Gohel, S., Kelly, C., Smith, S. M., et al. (2010). Toward discovery science of human brain function. *Proc. Natl. Acad. Sci. U S A* 107, 4734–4739. doi: 10.1073/pnas.0911855107

Briley, M., and Moret, C. (1993). Neurobiological mechanisms involved in antidepressant therapies. *Clin. Neuropharmacol.* 16, 387–400. doi: 10.1097/00002826-199310000-00002

Brodaty, H., Luscombe, G., Parker, G., Wilhelm, K., Hickie, I., Austin, M.-P., et al. (2001). Early and late onset depression in old age: different aetiologies, same phenomenology. *J. Affect. Disord.* 66, 225–236. doi: 10.1016/s0165-0327(00)00317-7

Buchsbaum, M. S., and Hazlett, E. A. (1997). Functional brain imaging and aging in schizophrenia. *Schizophr. Res.* 27, 129–141. doi: 10.1016/s0920-9964(97)00076-5

Buckner, R. L., Andrews-Hanna, J. R., and Schacter, D. L. (2008). The brain's default network: anatomy, function, and relevance to disease. *Ann. N Y Acad. Sci.* 1124, 1–38. doi: 10.1196/annals.1440.011

Cooney, R. E., Joormann, J., Eugène, F., Dennis, E. L., and Gotlib, I. H. (2010). Neural correlates of rumination in depression. *Cogn. Affect. Behav. Neurosci.* 10, 470–478. doi: 10.3758/CABN.10.4.470

Drevets, W. C., Frank, E., Price, J. C., Kupfer, D. J., Holt, D., Greer, P. J., et al. (1999). Pet imaging of serotonin 1A receptor binding in depression. *Biol. Psychiatry* 46, 1375–1387. doi: 10.1016/s0006-3223(99)00189-4

Finch, D. M., Derian, E. L., and Babb, T. L. (1984). Afferent fibers to rat cingulate cortex. *Exp. Neurol.* 83, 468–485. doi: 10.1016/0014-4886(84)90116-x

Folstein, M. F., Folstein, S. E., and McHugh, P. R. (1975). "Mini-mental state": a practical method for grading the cognitive state of patients for the clinician. *J. Psychiatr. Res.* 12, 189–198. doi: 10.1016/0022-3956(75)90026-6

Fox, M. D., Snyder, A. Z., Vincent, J. L., Corbetta, M., Van Essen, D. C., and Raichle, M. E. (2005). The human brain is intrinsically organized into dynamic, anticorrelated functional networks. *Proc. Natl. Acad. Sci. U S A* 102, 9673–9678. doi: 10.1073/pnas.0504136102

Fransson, P., and Marrelec, G. (2008). The precuneus/posterior cingulate cortex plays a pivotal role in the default mode network: evidence from a partial correlation network analysis. *Neuroimage* 42, 1178–1184. doi: 10.1016/j.neuroimage.2008.05.059

Hahn, A., Haeusler, D., Kraus, C., Höflich, A. S., Kranz, G. S., Baldinger, P., et al. (2014). Attenuated serotonin transporter association between dorsal raphe and ventral striatum in major depression. *Hum. Brain Mapp.* 35, 3857–3866. doi: 10.1002/hbm.22442

Hamilton, J. P., Furman, D. J., Chang, C., Thomason, M. E., Dennis, E., and Gotlib, I. H. (2011). Default-mode and task-positive network activity in major depressive disorder: implications for adaptive and maladaptive rumination. *Biol. Psychiatry* 70, 327–333. doi: 10.1016/j.biopsych.2011.02.003

Herwig, U., Kaffenberger, T., Schell, C., Jäncke, L., and Brühl, A. B. (2012). Neural activity associated with self-reflection. *BMC Neurosci.* 13:52. doi: 10.1186/1471-2202-13-52

Jacobs, B. L., Wise, W. D., and Taylor, K. M. (1974). Differential behavioral and neurochemical effects following lesions of the dorsal or median raphe nuclei in rats. *An. Acad. Bras. Cienc.* 79, 353–361. doi: 10.1016/0006-8993(74)90433-8

Jacobsen, J. P. R., Medvedev, I. O., and Caron, M. G. (2012). The 5-HT deficiency theory of depression: perspectives from a naturalistic 5-HT deficiency model, the tryptophan hydroxylase 2Arg439His knockin mouse. *Philos. Trans. R. Soc. Lond. B Biol. Sci.* 367, 2444–2459. doi: 10.1098/rstb.2012.0109

Johnson, M. K., Nolen-Hoeksema, S., Mitchell, K. J., and Levin, Y. (2009). Medial cortex activity, self-reflection and depression. *Soc. Cogn. Affect. Neurosci.* 4, 313–327. doi: 10.1093/scan/nsp022

Johnson, M. K., Raye, C. L., Mitchell, K. J., Touryan, S. R., Greene, E. J., and Nolen-Hoeksema, S. (2006). Dissociating medial frontal and posterior cingulate activity during self-reflection. *Soc. Cogn. Affect. Neurosci.* 1, 56–64. doi: 10.1093/scan/nsl004

Kato, M., Fukuda, T., Wakeno, M., Okugawa, G., Takekita, Y., Watanabe, S., et al. (2009). Effect of 5-HT1A gene polymorphisms on antidepressant response in major depressive disorder. *Am. J. Med. Genet. B Neuropsychiatr. Genet.* 150B, 115–123. doi: 10.1002/ajmg.b.30783

Kosofsky, B. E., and Molliver, M. E. (1987). The serotoninergic innervation of cerebral cortex: different classes of axon terminals arise from dorsal and median raphe nuclei. *Synapse* 1, 153–168. doi: 10.1002/syn.890010204

Kranz, G. S., Hahn, A., Savli, M., and Lanzenberger, R. (2012). Challenges in the differentiation of midbrain raphe nuclei in neuroimaging research. *Proc. Natl. Acad. Sci. U S A* 109, E2000–E2000. doi: 10.1073/pnas.1206247109

Kraus, C., Ganger, S., Losak, J., Hahn, A., Savli, M., Kranz, G. S., et al. (2014). Gray matter and intrinsic network changes in the posterior cingulate cortex after selective serotonin reuptake inhibitor intake. *Neuroimage* 84, 236–244. doi: 10.1016/j.neuroimage.2013.08.036

Lee, H.-Y., Tae, W. S., Yoon, H.-K., Lee, B.-T., Paik, J.-W., Son, K.-R., et al. (2011). Demonstration of decreased gray matter concentration in the midbrain encompassing the dorsal raphe nucleus and the limbic subcortical regions in major depressive disorder: an optimized voxel-based morphometry study. *J. Affect. Disord.* 133, 128–136. doi: 10.1016/j.jad.2011.04.006

Leech, R., and Sharp, D. J. (2014). The role of the posterior cingulate cortex in cognition and disease. *Brain* 137, 12–32. doi: 10.1093/brain/awt162

Lim, J.-E., Pinsonneault, J., Sadee, W., and Saffen, D. (2006). Tryptophan hydroxylase 2 (TPH2) haplotypes predict levels of TPH2 mRNA expression in human pons. *Mol. Psychiatry* 12, 491–501. doi: 10.1038/sj.mp.4001923

Lira, A., Zhou, M., Castanon, N., Ansorge, M. S., Gordon, J. A., Francis, J. H., et al. (2003). Altered depression-related behaviors and functional changes in the dorsal raphe nucleus of serotonin transporter-deficient mice. *Biol. Psychiatry* 54, 960–971. doi: 10.1016/s0006-3223(03)00696-6

López Hill, X., Pascovich, C., Urbanavicius, J., Torterolo, P., and Scorza, M. C. (2013). The median raphe nucleus participates in the depressive-like behavior induced by MCH: differences with the dorsal raphe nucleus. *Peptides* 50, 96–99. doi: 10.1016/j.peptides.2013.10.002

Maddock, R. J., Garrett, A. S., and Buonocore, M. H. (2003). Posterior cingulate cortex activation by emotional words: fMRI evidence from a valence decision task. *Hum. Brain Mapp.* 18, 30–41. doi: 10.1002/hbm.10075

Matthews, P. R., and Harrison, P. J. (2012). A morphometric, immunohistochemical, and in situ hybridization study of the dorsal raphe nucleus in major depression, bipolar disorder, schizophrenia and suicide. *J. Affect. Disord.* 137, 125–134. doi: 10.1016/j.jad.2011.10.043

Mayberg, H. S., Brannan, S. K., Tekell, J. L., Silva, J. A., Mahurin, R. K., McGinnis, S., et al. (2000). Regional metabolic effects of fluoxetine in major depression: serial changes and relationship to clinical response. *Biol. Psychiatry* 48, 830–843. doi: 10.1016/s0006-3223(00)01036-2

Morris, J. S., Smith, K. A., Cowen, P. J., Friston, K. J., and Dolan, R. J. (1999). Covariation of activity in habenula and dorsal raphé nuclei following tryptophan depletion. *Neuroimage* 10, 163–172. doi: 10.1006/nimg.1999.0455

Oldfield, R. C. (1971). The assessment and analysis of handedness: the Edinburgh inventory. *Neuropsychologia* 9, 97–113. doi: 10.1016/0028-3932(71)90067-4

Olpe, H.-R. (1981). The cortical projection of the dorsal raphe nucleus: some electrophysiological and pharmacological properties. *Brain Res.* 216, 61–71. doi: 10.1016/0006-8993(81)91278-6

Otsubo, T., Tanaka, K., Koba, R., Shinoda, J., Sano, N., Tanaka, S., et al. (2005). Reliability and validity of japanese version of the mini-international neuropsychiatric interview. *Psychiatry Clin. Neurosci.* 59, 517–526. doi: 10.1111/j.1440-1819.2005.01408.x

Politis, M., Wu, K., Loane, C., Turkheimer, F. E., Molloy, S., Brooks, D. J., et al. (2010). Depressive symptoms in PD correlate with higher 5-HTT binding in raphe and limbic structures. *Neurology* 75, 1920–1927. doi: 10.1212/WNL.0b013e3181feb2ab

Salzman, C., Wong, E., and Wright, B. C. (2002). Drug and ECT treatment of depression in the elderly, 1996–2001: a literature review. *Biol. Psychiatry* 52, 265–284. doi: 10.1016/s0006-3223(02)01337-9

Schneider, L. S., Nelson, J. C., Clary, C. M., Newhouse, P., Krishnan, K. R. R., Shiovitz, T., et al. (2003). An 8-week multicenter, parallel-group, double-blind, placebo-controlled study of sertraline in elderly outpatients with major depression. *Am. J. Psychiatry* 160, 1277–1285. doi: 10.1176/appi.ajp.160.7.1277

Serretti, A., Chiesa, A., Porcelli, S., Han, C., Patkar, A. A., Lee, S.-J., et al. (2011). Influence of TPH2 variants on diagnosis and response to treatment in patients with major depression, bipolar disorder and schizophrenia. *Psychiatry Res.* 189, 26–32. doi: 10.1016/j.psychres.2011.02.001

Sheline, Y. I., Barch, D. M., Price, J. L., Rundle, M. M., Vaishnavi, S. N., Snyder, A. Z., et al. (2009). The default mode network and self-referential processes in depression. *Proc. Natl. Acad. Sci. U S A* 106, 1942–1947. doi: 10.1073/pnas.0812686106

Svoboda, E., McKinnon, M. C., and Levine, B. (2006). The functional neuroanatomy of autobiographical memory: a meta-analysis. *Neuropsychologia* 44, 2189–2208. doi: 10.1016/j.neuropsychologia.2006.05.023

Törk, I. (1990). Anatomy of the serotonergic systema. *Ann. N Y Acad. Sci.* 600, 9–34; discussion 34–35. doi: 10.1111/j.1749-6632.1990.tb16870.x

Tsopelas, C., Stewart, R., Savva, G. M., Brayne, C., Ince, P., Thomas, A., et al. (2011). Neuropathological correlates of late-life depression in older people. *Br. J. Psychiatry* 198, 109–114. doi: 10.1192/bjp.bp.110.078816

Uddin, L. Q., Kelly, A. M., Biswal, B. B., Castellanos, F. X., and Milham, M. P. (2009). Functional connectivity of default mode network components: correlation, anticorrelation, and causality. *Hum. Brain Mapp.* 30, 625–637. doi: 10.1002/hbm.20531

Underwood, M. D., Khaibulina, A. A., Ellis, S. P., Moran, A., Rice, P. M., Mann, J. J., et al. (1999). Morphometry of the dorsal raphe nucleus serotonergic neurons in suicide victims. *Biol. Psychiatry* 46, 473–483. doi: 10.1016/s0006-3223(99)00043-8

Williams, J. W. (1988). A structured interview guide for the hamilton depression rating scale. *Arch. Gen. Psychiatry* 45, 742–747. doi: 10.1001/archpsyc.1988.01800320058007

Wise, T., Radua, J., Via, E., Cardoner, N., Abe, O., Adams, T. M., et al. (2016). Common and distinct patterns of grey-matter volume alteration in major depression and bipolar disorder: evidence from voxel-based meta-analysis. *Mol. Psychiatry* doi: 10.1038/mp.2016.72 [Epub ahead of print].

Wood, S. K., Zhang, X.-Y., Reyes, B. A. S., Lee, C. S., Van Bockstaele, E. J., and Valentino, R. J. (2013). Cellular adaptations of dorsal raphe serotonin neurons associated with the development of active coping in response to social stress. *Biol. Psychiatry* 73, 1087–1094. doi: 10.1016/j.biopsych.2013.01.026

Zhou, Y., Yu, C., Zheng, H., Liu, Y., Song, M., Qin, W., et al. (2010). Increased neural resources recruitment in the intrinsic organization in major depression. *J. Affect. Disord.* 121, 220–230. doi: 10.1016/j.jad.2009.05.029

Zhu, X., Wang, X., Xiao, J., Liao, J., Zhong, M., Wang, W., et al. (2012). Evidence of a dissociation pattern in resting-state default mode network connectivity in first-episode, treatment-naive major depression patients. *Biol. Psychiatry* 71, 611–617. doi: 10.1016/j.biopsych.2011.10.035

Zill, P., Baghai, T. C., Zwanzger, P., Schüle, C., Eser, D., Rupprecht, R., et al. (2004). SNP and haplotype analysis of a novel tryptophan hydroxylase isoform (TPH2) gene provide evidence for association with major depression. *Mol. Psychiatry* 9, 1030–1036. doi: 10.1038/sj.mp.4001525

9

Patterns of Longitudinal Neural Activity Linked to Different Cognitive Profiles in Parkinson's Disease

Atsuko Nagano-Saito [1†], Mohamed S. Al-Azzawi [1†], Alexandru Hanganu [2,3], Clotilde Degroot [1], Béatriz Mejia-Constain [1], Christophe Bedetti [1], Anne-Louise Lafontaine [4], Valérie Soland [5], Sylvain Chouinard [5] and Oury Monchi [1,2,3,4]*

[1] Centre de Recherche de l'Institut Universitaire de Gériatrie de Montréal, Montréal, QC, Canada, [2] Departments of Clinical Neurosciences and Radiology, University of Calgary, Calgary, AB, Canada, [3] Hotchkiss Brain Institute, Calgary, AB, Canada, [4] Department of Neurology and Neurosurgery, McGill University, Montreal, QC, Canada, [5] Centre Hospitalier de l'Université de Montréal, Montréal, QC, Canada

***Correspondence:**
Oury Monchi
Oury.Monchi@ucalgary.ca

† These authors have contributed equally to this work

Mild cognitive impairment in Parkinson's disease (PD) has been linked with functional brain changes. Previously, using functional magnetic resonance imaging (fMRI), we reported reduced cortico-striatal activity in patients with PD who also had mild cognitive impairment (MCI) vs. those who did not (non-MCI). We followed up these patients to investigate the longitudinal effect on the neural activity. Twenty-four non-demented patients with Parkinson's disease (non-MCI: 12, MCI: 12) were included in the study. Each participant underwent two fMRIs while performing the Wisconsin Card Sorting Task 20 months apart. The non-MCI patients recruited the usual cognitive corticostriatal loop at the first and second sessions (Time 1 and Time 2, respectively). However, decreased activity was observed in the cerebellum and occipital area and increased activity was observed in the medial prefrontal cortex and parietal lobe during planning set-shift at Time 2. Increased activity in the precuneus was also demonstrated while executing set-shifts at Time 2. The MCI patients revealed more activity in the frontal, parietal and occipital lobes during planning set-shifts, and in the parietal and occipital lobes, precuneus, and cerebellum, during executing set-shift at Time 2. Analysis regrouping of both groups of PD patients revealed that hippocampal and thalamic activity at Time 1 was associated with less cognitive decline over time. Our results reveal that functional alteration along the time-points differed between the non-MCI and MCI patients. They also underline the importance of preserving thalamic and hippocampal function with respect to cognitive decline over time.

Keywords: Parkinson's disease, functional magnetic resonance image, Wisconsin Card Sorting Task, mild cognitive impairment, longitudinal study

INTRODUCTION

In Parkinson's disease (PD), cognitive deficits are frequently present even early in the course of disease development (Foltynie et al., 2004). Mild cognitive impairment (MCI) has been conceptualized as a stage when cognitive deficits don't impede on daily activities (Litvan et al., 2012). The prevalence of MCI in the early stages of PD is estimated to be between 25 and 40%

(Dalrymple-Alford et al., 2011). The evolution of cognitive deficits in PD remain poorly understood and medication treatment of cognitive deficits in PD yields very modest results (Goldman and Holden, 2014). Using functional Magnetic Resonance Imaging (fMRI) we recently studied the effect of MCI in PD on the patterns of fronto-striatal activations while performing the Wisconsin Card Sorting Task (WCST). When planning a set-shift in our WCST PD patients without MCI (PD non-MCI) revealed patterns of activation similar to healthy individuals in our previous studies (Monchi et al., 2004, 2007), with significant activation in the ventrolateral prefrontal cortex (PFC) and caudate nucleus. In contrast, PD patients with MCI (PD-MCI) had no significant activation in these regions (Nagano-Saito et al., 2014). Similar results have been reported by other studies that analyzed resting state networks (Baggio et al., 2015) or fMRI in PD-MCI and PD non-MCI patients while performing a working memory task (Lewis et al., 2003; Ekman et al., 2012; Nagano-Saito et al., 2014), suggesting that PD non-MCI have compensational patterns that allow them to maintain the cognitive function at the same level as healthy individuals, while MCI in PD is associated with the loss of compensational patterns and development of specific functional brain abnormalities in the cognitive cortico-striatal loops with decreased cortico-cortical and cortico-subcortical connectivity compared to PD non-MCI, including the caudate nucleus and the PFC. This hypothesis has been suggested by a previous longitudinal study using Positron Emission Tomography in PD patients while performing a visual sequence learning-task (Carbon et al., 2010). They observed that while hippocampus was not significantly solicited in healthy individuals, the PD patients who did decline in their performance between the baseline and repeated measurement, showed significantly increased regional cerebral blood flow in the hippocampus. In order to confirm whether functional patterns from our previous study are specific for MCI in PD, a longitudinal fMRI study has to be performed, that would help us understand the functional changes in these loops over time.

The aim of the present study was to use fMRI to longitudinally follow up the brain neural activity of non-demented PD patients with and without MCI while they were performing the WCST. We also aimed to find out which patterns of neural activity at Time 1 would be the most predictive of cognitive decline over time. We applied our previously developed WCST fMRI protocol (Monchi et al., 2001, 2004) in PD-MCI and PD non-MCI patients at two time points. We expected to find preserved activation of the cognitive cortico-striatal loop usually associated with planning a set-shift (Monchi et al., 2001, 2007; Nagano-Saito et al., 2014) in the PD non-MCI group over time. By contrast, we expected that PD-MCI patients would show a modification over time of activity beyond the cortico-striatal loops. Based on our previous studies showing that the hippocampus is one key region involved in cognitive function in PD patients (Nagano-Saito et al., 2004, 2005, 2014), we also predicted that recruitment of hippocampus activity at Time 1 would correlate with preserved cognition at Time 2.

MATERIALS AND METHODS

Subjects

Twenty-seven non-demented PD participants at stages I and II of Hoehn and Yahr were recruited for the study. All participants were assessed by the movement disorders neurologists (A-LL., SC., VS.) and diagnosed as PD with the UK brain bank criteria for idiopathic PD (Hughes et al., 1992). All patients were responsive to dopamine medication. Patients with other concurrent major neurological or psychiatric conditions were excluded. The demographic information of the patients is given in **Table 1**. All patients provided written informed consent, which was approved by the Research Ethics Committee of the Regroupement Neuroimagerie Québec.

Participants were studied twice at 19.8 ± 2.7 months apart. In each session (at baseline Time 1 and follow-up at Time 2) they underwent a comprehensive neuropsychological assessment and fMRI during which they performed a computerized version of WCST (Monchi et al., 2001, 2004). Participants were asked not to take any dopaminergic medication at least 12 h prior to the sessions. Based on the neuropsychological assessment, participants were divided into two groups: those with MCI and those cognitively intact (non-MCI) at Time 1. Three patients with non-MCI at Time 1 turned into MCI at Time 2. Therefore, for the analyses to investigate the group difference, 24 subjects (mean age, 60.33 ± 5.8 years; 11 males and 13 females; 12 MCI, and 12 non-MCI) were included. For group-combined analyses, all 27 subjects (mean age 60.3 ± 5.5 years; 12 males and 15 females) were included.

TABLE 1 | PD patient demographics according to cognitive impairment group (MCI).

Demographic data	PD non-MCI	PD with MCI	Difference *p-value*	PD all
TIME 1				
N	12	12	N/A	27
Age	58.2 ± 5.4	62.25 ± 5.6	0.941	60.3 ± 5.5
Male/Female	6/6	8/4	0.248	15/12
Years since diagnosis	3.8 ± 3.4	5.0 ± 3.1	0.343	4.4 ± 3.3
Education	14.6 ± 2.5	13.8 ± 3.2	0.495	14.1 ± 3.0
Hand R/L/A	7/4/1	10/0/2	0.063	19/4/4
MoCA (off medication)	28.4 ± 1.6	27.3 ± 1.0	0.02	27.9 ± 1.8
UPDRS (off medication)	27.2 ± 8.9	26.9 ± 8.3	0.935	26.6 ± 8.1
BDI	6.0 ± 4.2	11.3 ± 6.1	0.046	9.0 ± 5.7
TIME 2				
Age	59.9 ± 5.5	64.0 ± 5.5	0.083	61.9 ± 5.5
Years since diagnosis	5.3 ± 3.6	6.4 ± 3	0.417	6.1 ± 3.4
MoCA (off medication)	29.1 ± 1.2	27 ± 1.3	0.001	28 ± 1.6
UPDRS (off medication)	27.3 ± 6	26.9 ± 8.3	0.918	26.6 ± 7.5
BDI	7.8 ± 3.9	11.3 ± 6.1	0.119	9.3 ± 5.4

The p-values indicate the group difference based on chi-squared test (sex and handedness) or student t-test (others). Legend: MoCA, Montreal cognitive assessment; UPDRS, Unified Parkinson's disease Rating Scale; BDI, Beck Depressive Inventory II. Individual MoCA scores are presented in Supplementary Table 3.

Inclusion criteria for MCI were based on the Movement Disorder Society Task Force guidelines for Parkinson's disease (Level I and II) (Litvan et al., 2012), based on five cognitive domains (Supplementary Table 1) and were the same as our previous study (Nagano-Saito et al., 2014). Objective evidence of cognitive decline was set with performance >1.5 standard deviations below standardized mean of the same age-group on two or more subtests within a cognitive domain.

Demographically, no significant differences were observed between the groups with respect to age and the motor section of the Unified Parkinson's Disease Rating Scale at Time 1 and 2. Group demographic characteristics are listed in detail in **Table 1**.

Neuropsychological Assessment

A screening test, the Montreal Cognitive Assessment (MoCA) (Nasreddine et al., 2005), was administered at the beginning of each scanning session. The same comprehensive neuropsychological battery previously used in Jubault et al. (2009), Hanganu et al. (2013), Nagano-Saito et al. (2014), was performed by a licensed neuropsychologist (Dr. BMC) to assess five domains of cognition, attention and working memory, executive functions, language, memory and visuospatial functions. Details of the tasks used are given in Supplementary Table 1.

Cognitive Task during fMRI

A computerized version of the WCST (Monchi et al., 2001, 2004) was administered using stimulus presentation software. Participants were fully trained on the task prior to the scanning sessions. On each trial of the task, participants were asked to match a new test card to one of the four fixed reference cards based either on the color, shape, or the number of the stimuli in each reference card.

In WCST the classification rule was not given to the participant. Instead, s/he had to find it using the feedback (positive or negative) that followed each trial. On each experimental trial, participants had to find the proper classification rule, and apply it as long as a positive feedback preceded their response. A bright screen indicated a correct classification and a dark screen indicated an incorrect classification. On each control trial, the test card was identical to one of the four reference cards, therefore participants only had to select the twin reference card. On the control trials, the screen maintain its original brightness throughout the feedback period.

The first period of each trial started with the presentation of a new test card, at which point the participant choose one of the four reference cards. Response time was measured for each selection. The second period of each trial started as soon as the subject made a selection and consisted of feedback conveyed through a change in screen brightness lasting 2.3 s.

Each functional MRI run contained blocks of each of the four trial classifications (color, shape, number, and control) presented in random order. In WCST trial blocks, six consecutive correct matching responses were required before a change in classification rule could occur. Control blocks contained eight trials.

To evaluate the pattern of activation during the different stages of the WCST, four experimental and two control time periods were defined as follows: (1) Receiving negative feedback (RNF): the screen darkens indicating an incorrect response: a set-shift is therefore required and must be planned; (2) Matching after negative feedback (MNF): execution of the set-shift; (3) Receiving positive feedback (RPF): the screen brightens indicating a correct response: the current matching criterion must continue; (4) Matching after positive feedback (MPF): selection using the same classification rule as the previous trial; (5) Receiving control feedback (RCF): original screen brightness is maintained; (6) Matching with control feedback (MCF): select reference card identical to test card.

fMRI Scanning

Participants were scanned using the Siemens Tim Trio 3.0 T scanner at the Unité de Neuroimagerie Fonctionnelle of the Centre de Recherche de l'Institut Universitaire de Gériatrie de Montréal. Sessions began with high-resolution, T1-weighted, 3D volume acquisition for anatomical localization with resolution of 1 × 1 × 1 mm, followed by echoplanar T2*-weighted image acquisitions with blood oxygenation level-dependent (BOLD) contrast (echo time 30 ms; flip angle 90°; matrix size, 64 × 64 pixels; voxel size, 3.7 × 3.7 × 3.7 mm^3). Functional images were acquired over five runs in a single session. Volumes were acquired continuously every 2.5 s, for a total 155 volumes within runs, and contained 36 slices.

MRI Data Analysis

Contrast Analyses

As was previously done with the same fMRI task, a General Linear Model data analysis was performed using fmristat (Monchi et al., 2001, 2004; Worsley et al., 2002; Jubault et al., 2009; Nagano-Saito et al., 2014). Briefly, the following contrasts were computed for each subject: 1. RNF vs. RPF: reflecting the planning of the set-shift, 2. MNF vs. MPF: reflecting the execution of the set-shift, 3. RPF vs. RCF: reflecting the maintaining of the set-shift, and 4. MPF vs. MCF: reflecting the matching according to the same rule. Next, the results of each run for each subject, were non-linearly transformed into standard proportional stereotaxic space (ICBM152 template) using anatomical MRI to template transformation parameters (Collins et al., 1994; Zijdenbos et al., 2002). In the second step, runs and subjects were combined using a mixed-effects linear model (Worsley et al., 2002). Both t-maps of inter-group (MCI and non-MCI of each time point) and within-group comparison (Time 1 vs. Time 2 of each group and combined groups) were generated. Statistical maps threshold was set at $p < 0.05$ correcting for multiple comparisons, yielding a threshold of $t > 4.82$ for a single voxel. Predicted peaks reaching $p < 0.0001$ ($t > 3.87$) uncorrected with a cluster size >40 mm^3 assessed on the spatial extent of contiguous voxels are also reported and identified with an asterisk (∗) in the tables. A region was predicted if it had been identified in our previous work using this task (Monchi et al., 2001, 2004; Jubault et al., 2009; Nagano-Saito et al., 2014) For within-group comparisons (Time 1 vs. Time 2), statistical maps threshold was set at $p < 0.0001$

($t > 3.87$) uncorrected with a cluster size >40 mm^3. Predicted peaks reaching $p < 0.001$ ($t > 3.18$) uncorrected with a cluster size >40 mm^3 are reported.

Additionally, in order to evaluate the common neural regions solicited by both groups (PD-MCI and PD non-MCI), we performed a conjunction analysis using a conjunction null hypothesis with a threshold of $p < 0.0001$ for each group.

Correlation Analysis

We wanted to separately address how individual cognitive performance ability affects the patterns of brain activity during the various stages of the WCST. To do this, we performed correlation analyses on the BOLD data while performing the WCST using cognitive scores of MoCA (Nasreddine et al., 2005) at the subject level. Secondly, in order to find which patterns of activity would be predictive of cognitive decline over time we correlated the BOLD data while performing the WCST at Time 1 with the difference of the MoCA scores between Time 1 and Time 2 at the subject level (Nasreddine et al., 2005). These analyses were performed across all participants combined (i.e., both MCI and non-MCI PD patients grouped). Finally, in order to look whether patterns of activity are associated with significant changes in performance of the WCST task, we correlated the BOLD data with the WCST accuracy and the WCST accuracy over time. These analyses were performed across all participants combined (i.e., both MCI and non-MCI PD patients grouped), at Time 1 and Time 2, separately.

Statistical maps threshold was set at $p < 0.0001$ ($t > 3.87$) uncorrected with a cluster size >40 mm^3. Predicted peaks reaching $p < 0.001$ ($t > 3.18$) uncorrected are reported. A region was predicted if it had been identified in our previous work using the WCST. We especially expected involvement of the striatum, the thalamus, the hippocampus, and/or the PFC, because the activation of those regions was correlated with cognitive scores (Nagano-Saito et al., 2014).

RESULTS

General Cognitive Scale Measured by MoCA

The mean of MoCA is shown in the **Table 1**. A mixed-design repeated measures ANOVA (time × group) indicated main effect of group ($F = 9.1$, $p = 0.006$) but no effect of time and time × group interaction ($p > 0.1$).

Performance of WCST

The error rates and reaction times for the task are shown in the **Table 2**. A mixed-design repeated measures ANOVA for the error rate and reaction time (task × time × group) indicated a main effect of task ($F = 98.8$, $p < 0.001$). No other main effects (including the group effect) or interaction was observed ($p > 0.1$). The mean reaction times are shown in **Table 2**. A mixed-design repeated measures ANOVA for the reaction time in control, after positive and after negative feedbacks (task × time × group) indicated a main effect of task ($F = 29.9$, $p < 0.001$), and time ($F = 4.70$, $p = 0.041$). A trend of interaction was observed for the time × task × group ($F = 3.0$, $p = 0.059$). No other significant effect was observed ($p > 0.1$).

Imaging Analysis

Our previous study at Time 1 indicated no significant difference of other contrasts in the intergroup comparison. Thus, we selectively reported the comparison RNF vs. RPF (planning the set shift) and MNF vs. MPF (executing the set-shift), because our previous study at Time 1 indicated no significant difference of other contrasts in the intergroup comparison (Nagano-Saito et al., 2014).

Planning the Set-Shift

Similar to our previous study (Nagano-Saito et al., 2014), when planning the set shift at Time 1, the PD non-MCI group demonstrated significant activation in the PFC, precuneus, parietal cortex, occipital cortex and cerebellum (**Table 3**). Activation was also observed in the caudate when a lower threshold was used ($p < 0.001$ uncorrected). At Time 2, this group demonstrated significant activations in the posterior PFC, ventrolateral PFC, medial PFC, occipital, and parietal cortices. Activation was again observed in the caudate when a lower threshold was used ($p < 0.001$ uncorrected). Longitudinal comparison (Time 1 vs. Time 2) indicated decreased activity at Time 2 in the occipital area and cerebellum hemisphere, and increased activity at Time 2 in the right parietal lobe and the posterior prefrontal frontal cortex (Supplementary Table 2).

By contrast, the PD-MCI group demonstrated significant activation peaks in the dorsolateral PFC, posterior PFC, and the occipital cortex. At Time 2, PD-MCI revealed significant activation peaks in the dorsolateral PFC, ventrolateral PFC, medial PFC, posterior PFC, posterior parietal cortex, and visual occipital area (**Table 3**). Longitudinal analyses showed decreased

TABLE 2 | Performance level of WCST.

		PD non-MCI		PD-MCI	
		Time 1	Time 2	Time 1	Time 2
Error rate (%)	Control	2.7±3.0	3.2±2.7	2.8±4.3	4.5±4.2
	WCST	13.3±6.5	13.8±8.9	19.2±6.9	15.9±7.1
Reaction time (sec)	Control	2.45±0.76	2.58±0.73	2.50±0.56	3.17±1.25
	After positive feedback	2.64±0.64	2.89±0.74	2.88±0.55	3.16±1.15
	After negative feedback	3.05±0.53	3.39±0.81	3.41±0.86	3.85±1.80

TABLE 3 | Significant activations in the contrasts for RNF minus RPF, and MNF minus MPF.

Anatomical Area		Non-MCI				MCI				Non-MCI and MCI (conjunction)			
		Time 1		Time 2		Time 1		Time 2		Time 1		Time 2	
		XYZ	*t*	XYZ	*t*	XYZ	*t*	XYZ	*t*	XYZ	*t*	XYZ	*t*
RNF–RPF													
DLPFC	L	−40, 38, 8	3.95*										
	R					40, 28, 18	4.49*	42, 24, 18	4.46*				
								44, 34, 14	4.34*				
VLPFC	L	−32, 26, 0	5.01										
	R	32, 24, 2	4.82	30, 26, −6	4.71*			32, 28, −2	4.36*			20, 28, −4	7.92
mPFC	L			−6, 28, 40	4.19*			−8, 26, 40	4.29*			−6, 26, 42	8.38
	R			6, 24, 36	4.12*								
pPFC	L	−42, 6, 32	4.69*	−40, 12, 24	4.64*			−42, 10, 28	4.52*	−38, 10, 26	4.98	−40, 10, 30	7.35
	R	44, 8, 20	4,37*	38, 6, 24	5.11	44, 8, 24	4.28*	44, 14, 30	4.8*	40, 14, 24	6.07	44, 10, 28	8.34
		40, 14, 24	4.26*			38, 18, 22	4.45*						
Parietal	L	−30, −70, 28	5.77	−32, −60, 38	4.67*								
	R	32, −74, 20	5.38	32, −60, 50	4.17			30, −70, 32	5.34				
								26, −64, 56	3.99*				
Precuneus	L	−10, −74, 48	4.29*										
Occipital	L	−22, −82, −14	6.98	−24, −78, −8	4.34*								
				−40, −84, 14	4.5*								
	R	40, −82, 6	4.11*	36, −84, 12	5.35	42, −80, 12	4.01*	40, −84, 12	5.28	40, −82, 12	5.33	38, −84, 12	9.71
		30, −60, −12	6.73					20, −66, 26	4.58*			26, −60, −12	7.39
Cerebellum	L	−10, −80, −28	4.99										
		−32, −66, −32	4.62*										
	R	8, −80, −26	4.42*										
		30, −70, −30	4.31*										
Caudate	L	−14, 20, −4	3.77**										
	R			16, 16, −6	3.48**								
MNF–MPF													
DLPFC	L	−46, 40, 28	5.23	−46, 30, 34	5.01								
	R	42, 40, 32	4.74*	42, 30, 36	4.54*								
				46, 40, 22	5.2								
PMC	L	−26, 30, 58	4.08*										
	R	24, 24, 58	4.78*										
VLPFC	L	−32, 26, −8	4.64*										
	R	32, 26, −8	4.04*										
mPFC	L			−2, 16, 50	3.95*								
	R	0, 28, 44	5.63	6, 24, 44	4.62*								
aPFC	L	−36, 54, 12	5.02			−32, 52, 8	4.4*			−32, 52, 8	6.33		
	R	38, 56, 18	4.5*	32, 60, 6	4.15*								
		38, 50, 6	4.21*										
		42, 52, 14	4.03*										

(Continued)

TABLE 3 | Continued

Anatomical Area		Non-MCI				MCI				Non-MCI and MCI (conjunction)			
		Time 1		Time 2		Time 1		Time 2		Time 1		Time 2	
		XYZ	*t*	XYZ	*t*	XYZ	*t*	XYZ	*t*	XYZ	*t*	XYZ	*t*
Parietal	L	−34, −54, 40	4.84*	−34, −62, 38	5.44			−30, −54, 44	4.33*			−32, −56, 40	6.01
								−62, −66, 30	4.24*				
	R	36, −62, 60	4.69*	22, −70, 60	4.23*								
		50, −44, 54	4.35*	46, −62, 52	4.1*								
Precuneus	L			−4, −76, 48	4.33*			−12, −74, 56	4.82*			−4, −78, 50	5.98
	R	2, −68, 44	4.48*	14, −78, 56	4.31*								
Occipital	L	−26, −96, 0	5.5	−30, −84, −12	4.05*								
	R	34, −92, 0	5.75			−28, −84, 34	5.06	28, −80, −18	4.13*				
								32, −74, 24	4.13*				
Cerebellum	L	−40, −76, −46	4.37*					−32, −76, −16	4.46*				
								−6, −78, −26	4.29*				
								−18, −84, −22	4.1*				
	R	24, −86, −20	4.74*			30, −64, −32	4.76*						

*Legend. Results presented at $t > 4.82$; $p < 0.05$ corrected for multiple comparisons. *predicted regions ($t > 3.87$; $p < 0.0001$). **trends ($t > 3.18$; $p < 0.001$). t, t-value; L, left; R, right; DLPFC, dorsolateral prefrontal cortex (BA 46, 9/46); pPFC, posterior PFC (BA 6, 8, 44); VLPFC, ventrolateral prefrontal cortex and insula (BA 47/12/13); aPFC, anterior prefrontal cortex (BA 10); mPFC, medial prefrontal cortex (BA 6, 8, 32); Parietal, parietal cortex (BA 40, 7); Precuneus, precuneus cortex (BA 40, 7); Occipital, occipital or striate/ extrastriate cortices (BA 17, 18, 19); PMC, premotor area (BA 6).*

activity at Time 2 in the cerebellum and increased activity at Time 2 in the visual occipital cortex (Supplementary Table 2).

Conjunction analysis over both groups revealed significant activations in the posterior PFC and occipital cortex at Time 1, as well as significant activation in the ventrolateral PFC, posterior PFC and occipital cortex at Time 2 (**Table 2**, RNF-RPF).

The localisation of the observed peaks are shown in **Figure 1A**. The results of the longitudinal comparison (Time 1 vs. Time 2) with all the subjects ($n = 27$) is also shown in the Supplementary Table 2.

Executing the Set-Shift

When executing the set-shift, the non-MCI group at Time 1 revealed significant activations in the dorsolateral PFC, premotor cortex, ventrolateral PFC, medial PFC, anterior PFC, parietal cortex, precuneus, the visual occipital areas, and cerebellum (**Table 3**). The pattern was similar to our previous study (Nagano-Saito et al., 2014). At Time 2, the PD non-MCI group revealed significant activation in the dorsolateral PFC, medial PFC, anterior PFC, parietal cortex bilaterally, precuneus and occipital visual area (**Table 3**). Longitudinally, there was reduced activation in the cerebellum and increased activity in the precuneus at Time 2 compared to Time 1 (Supplementary Table 2).

By contrast, the PD-MCI group demonstrated activation peaks in the middle occipital cortex, occipital cortex and cerebellum at Time 1, while at Time 2, positive significant activations were revealed in the parietal lobe, precuneus, visual occipital areas and cerebellum (**Table 3**). Longitudinally there were no significant differences between Time 1 and Time 2 in the PD-MCI group (Supplementary Table 2).

Conjunction analysis over both groups revealed significant activations in the anterior PFC at Time 1 and activations in the parietal cortex and precuneus at Time 2 (**Table 2**, MNF-MPF).

The localisation of the observed peaks are shown in **Figure 1B**. The results of the longitudinal comparison (Time 1 vs. Time 2) with all the subjects ($n = 27$) is also shown in the Supplementary Table 2.

Correlation Analysis

When planning the set-shift, no significant correlation was observed with the MoCA scores at Time 1. A significantly positive correlation was observed in the medial PFC at Time 2, overlapping with the more activated area at Time 2 (**Table 4**). When executing the set-shift, significant correlation was observed in the striatum and the left thalamus at Time 1 as well as with the precuneus at Time 2.

When we added the MoCA decline across the time points as a confounder, significant negative correlations were observed in the internal capsule, thalamus, and hippocampus during planning the set-shift (**Table 4**, **Figure 2**). During executing the set-shift, significant negative correlations were observed in the medial PFC (**Table 4**). They indicate that less cognitive decline occurs as more of these regions are solicited.

Correlations with WCST accuracy were also depicted. Planning the set-shift showed significant correlations with the ventral striatum, ventrolateral PFC and occipital area at Time 1, as well as with ventrolateral PFC, premotor cortex, parietal, and caudate at Time 2. Executing the set-shift showed significant

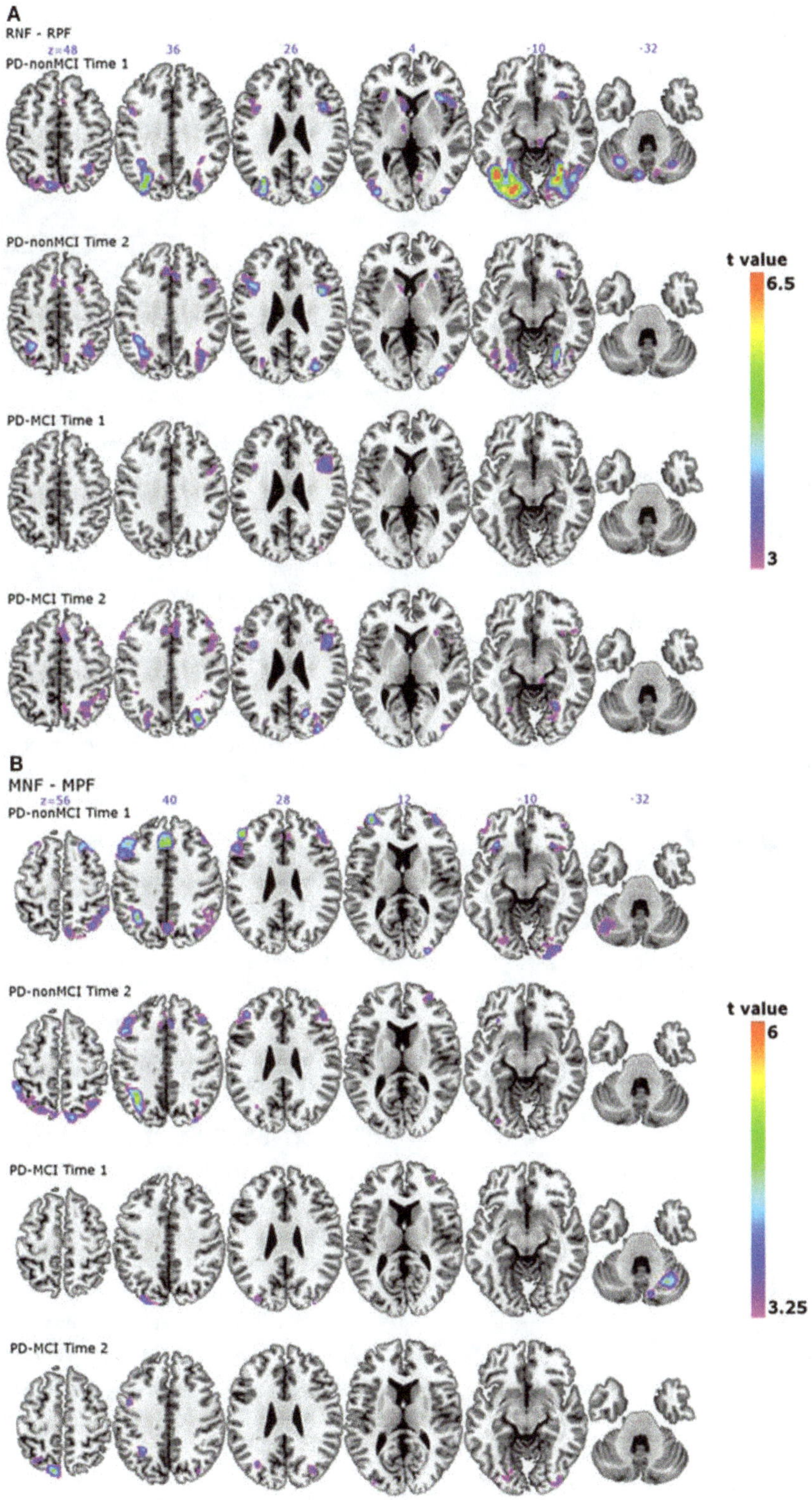

FIGURE 1 | Patterns of activation in PD-nonMCI and PD-MCI at time 1 and time 2 separately. (A) The contrast receiving negative feedback vs. receiving positive feedback, corresponding to planning the set-shift, is shown. For each group at each time point, slices are shown at ICBM co-ordinates $Z = 48$, $Z = 36$, $Z = 26$, $Z = 4$, $Z = -10$, and $Z = -32$. **(B)** The contrast matching following negative feedback vs. matching following positive feedback, corresponding to executing the set-shift is shown. For each group at each time point, slices are shown at ICBM co-ordinates $Z = 56$, $Z = 40$, $Z = 28$, $Z = 12$, $Z = -10$, and $Z = -32$.

TABLE 4 | Correlation between regions in all PD patients with MoCA score and WCST accuracy (Time 1 vs. Time 2).

Anatomical Area		XYZ	*t*
CORRELATION BETWEEN REGIONS AND THE MOCA SCORE			
MoCA score and fMRI Time 1			
MNF–MPF			
Thalamus	L	−18, −20, 10	3.61*
Striatal	L	−8, −54, 0	5.16
MoCA score and fMRI Time 2			
RNF–RPF			
mPFC	L	−6, 38, 34	3.99
MNF–MPF			
Precuneus	L	−6, −82, 46	4.63
MoCA score over time, fMRI Time 1			
RNF-RPF			
Internal Capsule	R	28, −22, 6	4.56
Thalamus	L	−12, −24, 8	4.57
	R	16, −26, 8	4.31
Hippocampus	L	−34, −32, −10	3.48*
	R	36, −30, −12	3.54*
MNF-MPF			
mPFC	R	4, 34, 48	3.25*
CORRELATION BETWEEN REGIONS AND THE WCST ACCURACY			
Accuracy and fMRI Time 1			
RNF–RPF			
Ventral striatum	L	−20, 14, −8	5.49
	R	20, 14, −6	4.35
VLPFC	L	−30, 26, 0	3.7*
Occipital	L	−46, −62, −10	4.5
MNF–MPF			
mPFC	L	−8, 24, 38	4.41
	R	8, 36, 34	5.14
DLPFC	L	42, 18, 26	3.57*
	R	40, 22, 40	3.9
Caudate	R	12, 2, 16	3.49*
Hippocampus	R	24, −22, −16	3.31*
Accuracy and fMRI Time 2			
RNF–RPF			
VLPFC	R	32, 22, 8	3.66*
PMC	L	−46, 6, 22	3.25*
Parietal	R	36, −48, 36	4.08
Caudate	L	−16, 16, 8	3.44*
Accuracy over Time, fMRI Time 1			
RNF-RPF			
aPFC	L	−28, 52, −4	4.43
MNF-MPF			
DLPFC	R	38, 18, 32	3.54*
mPFC	L	−10, 20, 32	4.11
Occipital	L	−58, −58, 12	5.84
Parietal	L	−46, −64, 35	4.19
Precuneus	L	−6, −42, 36	5.29
Hippocampus	R	22, −20, −14	3.91

*Legend. Results presented at $t > 3.87$; $p < 0.0001$, uncorrected; *indicates predicted regions ($t > 3.18$; $p < 0.001$ uncorrected). t, t-value; L, left; R, right; DLPFC, dorsolateral prefrontal cortex (BA 46, 9/46); VLPFC, ventrolateral prefrontal cortex and insula (BA 47/12/13); aPFC, anterior prefrontal cortex (BA 10); mPFC, medial prefrontal cortex (BA 6, 8, 32); Parietal, parietal cortex (BA 40, 7); Precuneus, precuneus cortex (BA 40, 7); Occipital, occipital or striate/ extrastriate cortices (BA 17, 18, 19); PMC, premotor area (BA 6).*

correlations between the WCST accuracy and activations in the medial PFC, dorsolateral PFC, caudate, hippocampus at Time 1, but no correlation were shown at Time 2.

When WCST accuracy over time was correlated with BOLD at Time 1, planning the set-shift showed significant correlations with the anterior PFC, while executing the set-shift showed correlations with dorsolateral PFC, medial PFC, occipital cortex, parietal, precuneus, and hippocampus, indicating that greater activity in these regions at Time 1 is indicative of preserved performance on the WCST over time.

DISCUSSION

We longitudinally followed up the brain neural activation of non-demented PD patients undergoing an fMRI session while performing the WCST with different levels of cognitive impairment. As predicted, the PD non-MCI and PD-MCI groups were different in their patterns of activity-change over time when performing the WCST.

PD Non-MCI Patterns over Time

Patterns of Preserved Activity

At both time points, significant activation was observed in the frontal and parietal cortex, with a trend in the caudate, during planning the set-shift. Fronto-striatal activation in the cognitive loop has been reported to be preserved in non-MCI PD patients, but affected in MCI patients (Lewis et al., 2003; Ekman et al., 2012; Nagano-Saito et al., 2014: **Table 3**). Thus, our observation may indicate relatively preserved function in the cognitive loop at Time 2 in the non-MCI PD patients. This is in agreement with another longitudinal study showing stable activity across time-points in non-MCI patients with the n-back working memory task (Ekman et al., 2014). During the execution of the set-shift, significant activation was also preserved in the frontal and parietal cortex (**Table 3**). However, overall, the activation was relatively weak at Time 2, and intra-group comparison did not reach significance. Considering the fact that the activated regions during this period could correspond to the motor-loop (Monchi et al., 2004, 2007) this relatively weak activation may reflect the

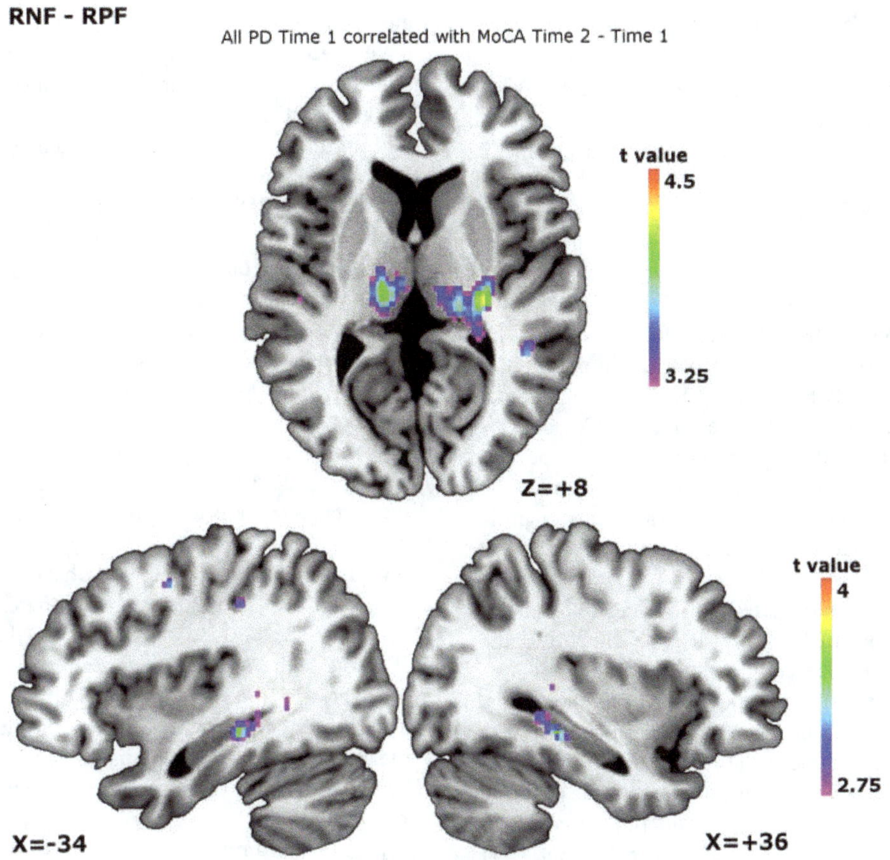

FIGURE 2 | Patterns of activity over all participants at time 1 correlating with MoCA evolution Time 2 vs. Time 1. The correlation patterns are shown for the contrast receiving negative feedback vs. receiving positive feedback, corresponding to planning the set-shift. The higher the peaks, the less MoCA decline. This was observed in the thalamus, show on the slice at ICBM co-ordinate $Z = +8$, the left hippocampus, shown on the slice at ICBM co-ordinate $X = -34$, and the right hippocampus, shown on the slice at ICBM co-ordinate $X = +36$.

disease progress affecting more motor-related function in non-MCI PD patients. Actually, slower RT was observed at Time 2 in non-MCI PD patients (**Table 2**), without a change in accuracy in the performance of the WCST.

Regions with Decreased Patterns of Activity over Time

Activation in the occipital visual cortex during planning the set-shift and the cerebellum during planning and executing the set-shift, was reduced during the time course, between Time 1 and Time 2 (Supplementary Table 2). It has been reported in non-demented PD patients that lowered regional cerebral metabolic rates in the occipital area correlate with the motor dysfunction (Bohnen et al., 1999) We also previously reported lower regional cerebral metabolic rates for glucose in the occipital area accompanied by dopaminergic availability in the striatum, along with motor dysfunction in non-demented PD patients (Nagano-Saito et al., 2004) Simultaneously, cerebellar activity is likely to contribute to pathophysiological change underlying PD (Martinu and Monchi, 2013) Thus, the reduced activation in the occipital area and cerebellum may reflect remote effects of the progress of the disease on dopamine projections in the striatum. However, they might also reflect a learning effect with reduction of visual attention and motor effort at Time 2. A longitudinal study with healthy volunteers would help to understand these observations.

PD-MCI Patterns over Time

Patterns of Increased Activity

During planning the set-shift, PD-MCI revealed significantly increased activation in the frontal, parietal and occipital areas at Time 2 (**Table 3**). These regions were overlapped with the activation pattern of PD non-MCI. PD patients have been reported to often have fluctuations in non-motor functions (Witjas et al., 2002) This might explain the relatively higher performance at Time 2 observed in this group of patients. Actually, the error rate was smaller with MCI patients across time, although it did not reach significance. Nevertheless, RT became slower at Time 2. This may indicate that the relay of information from the cognitive loop to motor loop could not be recovered.

During executing the set-shift, more activation was observed in the parietal areas, precuneus and cerebellum, but not in the frontal regions at Time 2 (**Table 4**). Thus, the recovered activation is not likely to be supported by the cortico-striatal loops, but by alternative brain circuit.

Medial PFC and Precuneus Patterns of Activation in Both Groups

We observed significant activation in the medial PFC during planning the set-shift in both groups and in the conjunction analyses only at Time 2 (**Table 3**). Moreover, in the group of all patients during planning a set-shift, the activity in the medial PFC showed a positive correlation with the MoCA scores at Time 2 and preserved WCST accuracy score over time (**Table 4**). In addition, when executing the set-shift, increased activity in the medial PFC correlated with preserved cognition over time (as measured by the MoCA), with WCST accuracy at Time 1 and with preserved WCST accuracy score over time (**Table 4**). The mPFC is considered to play an important role in learning association between events and in linking adaptive responses (Euston et al., 2012). The medial PFC activates both during externally guided and internally guided decision making tasks (Nakao et al., 2012). The recovery of the mPFC activity at Time 2 could therefore help in relating the cognitive processes required to select a response to the actual motor selection.

Another region that was recruited during executing the set-shift at Time 1 in PD non-MCI only and at Time 2 in both groups which was confirmed by the conjunction analyses at Time 2 (**Table 3**) was the precuneus. In the all patients group the strength of the activation in the precuneus during executing the set-shift showed a significantly positive correlation with the MoCA scores at Time 2 and the preserved WCST accuracy over time (**Table 4**). This shows the importance of this region's function for cognition. The precuneus, as a part of the parietal cortex (Vogt et al., 2001), functionally connects to the medial PFC and superior frontal cortex (Laird et al., 2009; Margulies et al., 2009), and is considered to be involved in reaching to visual targets (Bernier and Grafton, 2010). More generally, precuneus and medial PFC are components of the dorsomedial motor stream. (Rizzolatti and Matelli, 2003; Binkofski and Buxbaum, 2013) Interestingly, in PD non-MCI the posterior PFC, which is considered as a part of the dorsomedial motor stream, was higher at Time 2, compared to Time 1, although the more anterior PFC showed tendency of decreasing of activity. Previous studies reported decreased resting state connectivity in bilateral PFC (as part of the dorsomedial motor network) and fronto-parietal areas in PD-MCI patients (Amboni et al., 2015; Baggio et al., 2015), along with a ordered connectivity reduction (HC > PD, non-MCI > PD-MCI). Thus, our results for the precunes and the medial PFC activation may reflect increased recruitment of the dorsomedial motor stream, compensating the cortico-striatal loop, and allowing a better performance as shown by the correlations with WCST accuracy.

Patterns of Activity Predictive of Cognitive Evolution

When planning the set-shift, increased activity in the thalamus and the hippocampus correlated with preserved cognition over time as measured by the MoCA (**Table 4, Figure 2**). Furthermore, when executing the set-shift the increased activity in the hippocampus correlated with preserved WCST performance over time (**Table 4**).

We recently reported that cortical thinning occurs significantly faster overtime in the medial temporal lobe in PD-MCI vs. PD non-MCI, suggesting that temporal lobe atrophy could be used as a predictor of dementia in PD (Hanganu et al., 2014). Carbon et al. (2010), performed a longitudinal PET study in PD patients and controls, where participants performed a visual sequence-learning task (Carbon et al., 2010). The researchers observed that while the hippocampus was not significantly solicited in controls during the task, the PD patients whose performance did not decline between the two time points (i.e., the best performers) showed significant increase in rCBF in the hippocampus over time, as compared to the lower performers. They suggested that a compensatory hippocampal activation response may be a specific functional indicator of incipient cognitive decline in non-demented PD patients at early disease stages. Our present results are in agreement with this notion.

We have observed decreased thalamus activity in PD vs. controls in the context of two different set-shifting tasks (Monchi et al., 2001, 2007) hence, the thalamus activity level correlating with preserved cognition may reflect the importance of the preserved function of cognitive cortico-striatal loop. Furthermore, connectivity between the hippocampus and the posterior parts of the thalamus has been observed in animals (Herkenham, 1978; Wouterlood et al., 1990; Vertes et al., 2006) and in humans (Behrens et al., 2003). Our previous fMRI study, which examined the same task in healthy volunteers, showed that hippocampal deactivation was less accompanied by extensive activation in the thalamus during a set-shift, when dopamine was lowered (Nagano-Saito et al., 2008). A recent voxel based morphometry study reported reduced thalamic and hippocampal gray matter intensity in PD-MCI vs. PD non-MCI (Chen et al., 2016). Thus, the functional integrity of the thalamus, possibly connecting to the hippocampus, might be an important marker of cognitive preservation in PD.

CONCLUSION

In conclusion, our results show differential neural changes in PD-MCI patients as compared with the PD non-MCI group over time. They indicate that, as long as the cognitive cortico-striatal loops are preserved, the circuit seems to be recruited. However, when the cortico-striatal loops cannot perform the demanded functional task, the extra circuits, including the mPFC, and the precuneus, could be recruited. Moreover, hippocampal compensation is used to maintain cognitive abilities over time. More work in this area is warranted to determine the precise phenotypes of such sub-groups of patients.

AUTHOR CONTRIBUTIONS

Research project: Conception: OM. Organization: BM, CB, AL, VS, and SC. Execution: CD, BM, AH, CB, AL, VS, and SC.

Statistical Analysis: Design: OM and AN. Execution: MA and AN. Review and Critique: OM and AN. Manuscript: Writing of the first draft: MA and AN. Review and Critique: OM, AN, and AH.

FUNDING

This work was supported by a Canadian Institutes of Health Research grant (MOP-81114), a psychosocial grant from the Parkinson Society Canada, the Canada Research Chair in non-motor symptoms of Parkinson's disease, and the Tourmaline Oil Chair in Parkinson's disease to OM.

ACKNOWLEDGMENTS

The authors would like to thank Holly Breton for thoroughly proof-reading the manuscript, all the participants for taking part in the study, as well as the Functional Neuroimaging Unit team of the Institut de Gériatrie de Montréal.

REFERENCES

Amboni, M., Tessitore, A., Esposito, F., Santangelo, G., Picillo, M., Vitale, C., et al. (2015). Resting-state functional connectivity associated with mild cognitive impairment in Parkinson's disease. *J. Neurol.* 262, 425–434. doi: 10.1007/s00415-014-7591-5

Baggio, H. C., Segura, B., Sala-Llonch, R., Marti, M. J., Valldeoriola, F., Compta, Y., et al. (2015). Cognitive impairment and resting-state network connectivity in Parkinson's disease. *Hum. Brain Mapp.* 36, 199–212. doi: 10.1002/hbm.22622

Behrens, T. E., Johansen-Berg, H., Woolrich, M. W., Smith, S. M., Wheeler-Kingshott, C. A., Boulby, P. A., et al. (2003). Non-invasive mapping of connections between human thalamus and cortex using diffusion imaging. *Nat. Neurosci.* 6, 750–757. doi: 10.1038/nn1075

Bernier, P. M., and Grafton, S. T. (2010). Human posterior parietal cortex flexibly determines reference frames for reaching based on sensory context. *Neuron* 68, 776–788. doi: 10.1016/j.neuron.2010.11.002

Binkofski, F., and Buxbaum, L. J. (2013). Two action systems in the human brain. *Brain Lang.* 127, 222–229. doi: 10.1016/j.bandl.2012.07.007

Bohnen, N. I., Minoshima, S., Giordani, B., Frey, K. A., and Kuhl, D. E. (1999). Motor correlates of occipital glucose hypometabolism in Parkinson's disease without dementia. *Neurology* 52:541. doi: 10.1212/WNL.52.3.541

Burgess, P. W., and Shallice, T. (1997). *The Hayling and Brixton Tests. Test Manual.* Bury St. Edmunds: Thames Valley Test Company.

Carbon, M., Reetz, K., Ghilardi, M. F., Dhawan, V., and Eidelberg, D. (2010). Early Parkinson's disease: longitudinal changes in brain activity during sequence learning. *Neurobiol. Dis.* 37, 455–460. doi: 10.1016/j.nbd.2009.10.025

Chen, F. X., Kang, D. Z., Chen, F. Y., Liu, Y., Wu, G., Li, X., et al. (2016). Gray matter atrophy associated with mild cognitive impairment in Parkinson's disease. *Neurosci. Lett.* 617, 160–165. doi: 10.1016/j.neulet.2015.12.055

Collins, D. L., Neelin, P., Peters, T. M., and Evans, A. C. (1994). Automatic 3D intersubject registration of MR volumetric data in standardized Talairach space. *J. Comput. Assist. Tomogr.* 18, 192–205. doi: 10.1097/00004728-199403000-00005

Culbertson, C. W., and Zillmer, E. A. (2005). *Tower of London Drexel University (TOL DX).* North Tonawanda, NY: Multi-Health Systems Incorporated (MHS).

Dalrymple-Alford, J. C., Livingston, L., Macaskill, M. R., Graham, C., Melzer, T. R., Porter, R. J., et al. (2011). Characterizing mild cognitive impairment in Parkinson's disease. *Mov. Disord.* 26, 629–636. doi: 10.1002/mds.23592

Ekman, U., Eriksson, J., Forsgren, L., Domellöf, M. E., Elgh, E., Lundquist, A., et al. (2014). Longitudinal changes in task-evoked brain responses in Parkinson's disease patients with and without mild cognitive impairment. *Front. Neurosci.* 8:207. doi: 10.3389/fnins.2014.00207

Ekman, U., Eriksson, J., Forsgren, L., Mo, S. J., Riklund, K., and Nyberg, L. (2012). Functional brain activity and presynaptic dopamine uptake in patients with Parkinson's disease and mild cognitive impairment: a cross-sectional study. *Lancet Neurol.* 11, 679–687. doi: 10.1016/S1474-4422(12)70138-2

Euston, D. R., Gruber, A. J., and Mcnaughton, B. L. (2012). The role of medial prefrontal cortex in memory and decision making. *Neuron* 76, 1057–1070. doi: 10.1016/j.neuron.2012.12.002

Foltynie, T., Brayne, C. E., Robbins, T. W., and Barker, R. A. (2004). The cognitive ability of an incident cohort of Parkinson's patients in the UK. The CamPaIGN study. *Brain* 127, 550–560. doi: 10.1093/brain/awh067

Golden, C. J., and Freshwater, S. M. (1998). *Stroop Color and Word Test: A Manual for Clinical and Experimental Uses.* Wood Dale, IL: Stoelting Co.

Goldman, J. G., and Holden, S. (2014). Treatment of psychosis and dementia in Parkinson's disease. *Curr. Treat. Options Neurol.* 16, 1–18. doi: 10.1007/s11940-013-0281-2

Hanganu, A., Bedetti, C., Degroot, C., Mejia-Constain, B., Lafontaine, A. L., Soland, V., et al. (2014). Mild cognitive impairment is linked with faster rate of cortical thinning in patients with Parkinson's disease longitudinally. *Brain* 137, 1120–1129. doi: 10.1093/brain/awu036

Hanganu, A., Bedetti, C., Jubault, T., Gagnon, J. F., Mejia-Constain, B., Degroot, C., et al. (2013). Mild cognitive impairment in patients with Parkinson's disease is associated with increased cortical degeneration. *Mov. Disord.* 28, 1360–1369. doi: 10.1002/mds.25541

Herkenham, M. (1978). The connections of the nucleus reuniens thalami: evidence for a direct thalamo-hippocampal pathway in the rat. *J. Comp. Neurol.* 177, 589–610. doi: 10.1002/cne.901770405

Hooper, H. E. (1958). *The Hooper Visual Organization Test.* Los Angeles, CA: Western Psychological Services.

Hughes, A. J., Daniel, S. E., Kilford, L., and Lees, A. J. (1992). Accuracy of clinical diagnosis of idiopathic Parkinson's disease: a clinico-pathological study of 100 cases. *J. Neurol. Neurosurg. Psychiatry* 55, 181–184. doi: 10.1136/jnnp.55.3.181

Joanette, Y., Ska, B., and Côté, H. (2004). *Protocole Montréal D'évaluation de la Communication (Protocole MEC).* Isbergues: Ortho Édition.

Jubault, T., Brambati, S. M., Degroot, C., Kullmann, B., Strafella, A. P., Lafontaine, A. L., et al. (2009). Regional brain stem atrophy in idiopathic Parkinson's disease detected by anatomical MRI. *PLoS ONE* 4:e8247. doi: 10.1371/journal.pone.0008247

Kaplan, E., Goodglass, H., and Weintraub, S. (1983). *Boston Naming Test.* Philadelphia, PA: Lea & Febiger.

Laird, A. R., Eickhoff, S. B., Li, K., Robin, D. A., Glahn, D. C., and Fox, P. T. (2009). Investigating the functional heterogeneity of the default mode network using coordinate-based meta-analytic modeling. *J. Neurosci.* 29, 14496–14505. doi: 10.1523/JNEUROSCI.4004-09.2009

Lewis, S. J., Dove, A., Robbins, T. W., Barker, R. A., and Owen, A. M. (2003). Cognitive impairments in early Parkinson's disease are accompanied by reductions in activity in frontostriatal neural circuitry. *J. Neurosci.* 23, 6351–6356.

Litvan, I., Goldman, J. G., Tröster, A. I., Schmand, B. A., Weintraub, D., Petersen, R. C., et al. (2012). Diagnostic criteria for mild cognitive impairment in Parkinson's disease: movement disorder society task force guidelines. *Mov. Disord.* 27, 349–356. doi: 10.1002/mds.24893

Margulies, D. S., Vincent, J. L., Kelly, C., Lohmann, G., Uddin, L. Q., Biswal, B. B., et al. (2009). Precuneus shares intrinsic functional architecture in humans and monkeys. *Proc. Natl. Acad. Sci. U.S.A.* 106, 20069–20074. doi: 10.1073/pnas.0905314106

Martinu, K., and Monchi, O. (2013). Cortico-basal ganglia and cortico-cerebellar circuits in Parkinson's disease: pathophysiology or compensation? *Behav. Neurosci.* 127, 222–236. doi: 10.1037/a0031226

Monchi, O., Petrides, M., Doyon, J., Postuma, R. B., Worsley, K., and Dagher, A. (2004). Neural bases of set-shifting deficits in Parkinson's disease. *J. Neurosci.* 24, 702–710. doi: 10.1523/JNEUROSCI.4860-03.2004

Monchi, O., Petrides, M., Mejia-Constain, B., and Strafella, A. P. (2007). Cortical activity in Parkinson's disease during executive processing depends on striatal involvement. *Brain* 130, 233–244. doi: 10.1093/brain/awl326

Monchi, O., Petrides, M., Petre, V., Worsley, K., and Dagher, A. (2001). Wisconsin card sorting revisited: distinct neural circuits participating in different stages of the task identified by event-related functional magnetic resonance imaging. *J. Neurosci.* 21, 7733–7741.

Nagano-Saito, A., Habak, C., Mejía-Constaín, B., Degroot, C., Monetta, L., Jubault, T., et al. (2014). Effect of mild cognitive impairment on the patterns of neural activity in early Parkinson's disease. *Neurobiol. Aging* 35, 223–231. doi: 10.1016/j.neurobiolaging.2013.06.025

Nagano-Saito, A., Kato, T., Arahata, Y., Washimi, Y., Nakamura, A., Abe, Y., et al. (2004). Cognitive- and motor-related regions in Parkinson's disease: FDOPA and FDG PET studies. *Neuroimage* 22, 553–561. doi: 10.1016/j.neuroimage.2004.01.030

Nagano-Saito, A., Leyton, M., Monchi, O., Goldberg, Y. K., He, Y., and Dagher, A. (2008). Dopamine depletion impairs frontostriatal functional connectivity during a set-shifting task. *J. Neurosci.* 28, 3697–3706. doi: 10.1523/JNEUROSCI.3921-07.2008

Nagano-Saito, A., Washimi, Y., Arahata, Y., Kachi, T., Lerch, J. P., Evans, A. C., et al. (2005). Cerebral atrophy and its relation to cognitive impairment in Parkinson disease. *Neurology* 64, 224–229. doi: 10.1212/01.WNL.0000149510.41793.50

Nakao, T., Ohira, H., and Northoff, G. (2012). Distinction between externally vs. internally guided decision-making: operational differences, meta-analytical comparisons and their theoretical implications. *Front. Neurosci.* 6:31. doi: 10.3389/fnins.2012.0003

Nasreddine, Z. S., Phillips, N. A., Bédirian, V., Charbonneau, S., Whitehead, V., Collin, I., et al. (2005). The Montreal Cognitive Assessment, MoCA: a brief screening tool for mild cognitive impairment. *J. Am. Geriatr. Soc.* 53, 695–699. doi: 10.1111/j.1532-5415.2005.53221.x

Reitan, R. M., and Wolfson, D. (1985). *The Halstead-Reitan Neuropsychological Test Battery: Theory and Clinical Interpretation.* Tucson, AZ: Neuropsychology Press.

Rizzolatti, G., and Matelli, M. (2003). Two different streams form the dorsal visual system: anatomy and functions. *Exp. Brain Res.* 153, 146–157. doi: 10.1007/s00221-003-1588-0

Schmidt, M. (1996). *Rey Auditory Verbal Learning Test: A Handbook.* Los Angeles, CA: Western Psychological Services.

Shulman, K. I. (2000). Clock-drawing: is it the ideal cognitive screening test? *Int. J. Geriatr. Psychiatry* 15, 548–561. doi: 10.1002/1099-1166(200006)15:6<548::aid-gps242>3.0.co;2-u

Shulman, K. I., Pushkar Gold, D., Cohen, C. A., and Zucchero, C. A. (1993). Clock-drawing and dementia in the community: a longitudinal study. *Int. J. Geriatr. Psychiatry* 8, 487–496. doi: 10.1002/gps.930080606

Vertes, R. P., Hoover, W. B., Do Valle, A. C., Sherman, A., and Rodriguez, J. J. (2006). Efferent projections of reuniens and rhomboid nuclei of the thalamus in the rat. *J. Comp. Neurol.* 499, 768–796. doi: 10.1002/cne.21135

Vogt, B. A., Vogt, L. J., Perl, D. P., and Hof, P. R. (2001). Cytology of human caudomedial cingulate, retrosplenial, and caudal parahippocampal cortices. *J. Comp. Neurol.* 438, 353–376. doi: 10.1002/cne.1320

Wechsler, D. (1997). *Wechsler Adult Intelligence Scale-III (WAIS-III).* New York, NY: Psychological Corporation.

Wechsler, D. (1999). *Wechsler Abbreviated scale of Intelligence (WASI).* San Antonio, TX: Psychological Corporation.

Witjas, T., Kaphan, E., Azulay, J., Blin, O., Ceccaldi, M., Pouget, J., et al. (2002). Nonmotor fluctuations in Parkinson's disease frequent and disabling. *Neurology* 59, 408–413. doi: 10.1212/WNL.59.3.408

Worsley, K. J., Liao, C. H., Aston, J., Petre, V., Duncan, G. H., Morales, F., et al. (2002). A General Statistical Analysis for fMRI Data. *Neuroimage* 15, 1–15. doi: 10.1006/nimg.2001.0933

Wouterlood, F. G., Saldana, E., and Witter, M. P. (1990). Projection from the nucleus reuniens thalami to the hippocampal region: light and electron microscopic tracing study in the rat with the anterograde tracer Phaseolus vulgaris-leucoagglutinin. *J. Comp. Neurol.* 296, 179–203. doi: 10.1002/cne.902960202

Zijdenbos, A. P., Forghani, R., and Evans, A. C. (2002). Automatic "pipeline" analysis of 3-D MRI data for clinical trials: application to multiple sclerosis. *Med. Imaging IEEE Trans.* 21, 1280–1291. doi: 10.1109/TMI.2002.806283

10

Attentional Orienting and Dorsal Visual Stream Decline: Review of Behavioral and EEG Studies

Evatte T. Sciberras-Lim and Anthony J. Lambert*

Department of Psychology, University of Auckland, Auckland, New Zealand

***Correspondence:**
Evatte T. Sciberras-Lim
esci911@aucklanduni.ac.nz

Every day we are faced with an overwhelming influx of visual information. Visual attention acts as the filtering mechanism that enables us to focus our limited neural resources, by selectively processing only the most relevant and/or salient aspects of our visual environment. The ability to shift attention to the most behaviorally relevant items enables us to successfully navigate and interact with our surroundings. The dorsal visual stream is important for the rapid and efficient visuospatial orienting of attention. Unfortunately, recent evidence suggests that the dorsal visual stream may be especially vulnerable to age-related decline, with significant deterioration becoming evident quite early in the aging process. Yet, despite the significant age-related declines to the dorsal visual stream, the visuospatial orienting of attention appears relatively well preserved in older adults, at least in the early stages of aging. The maintenance of visuospatial orienting of attention in older adults appears to be facilitated by the engagement of compensatory neural mechanisms. In particular, older adults demonstrate heightened activity in the frontal regions to compensate for the reduced activity in the posterior sensory regions. These findings suggest that older adults are more reliant on control processes mediated by the anterior regions of the frontoparietal attention network to compensate for less efficient sensory processing within the posterior sensory cortices.

Keywords: aging, visuospatial orienting of attention, compensation, dorsal visual stream, magnocellular pathway

INTRODUCTION

Everything from playing tennis to simply walking down the street require the successful orienting of attention from one location to the next. This process of shifting attention is referred to as the visuospatial orienting of attention. A process which relies on an interacting network of structures, which include regions of the lateral prefrontal cortex (Corbetta and Shulman, 2002, 2011; Corbetta et al., 2008; Schall, 2009; Vandenberghe and Gillebert, 2009; Asplund et al., 2010), working in conjunction with the dorsal visual stream (Siegel et al., 2008; Lambert and Shin, 2010; Marrett et al., 2011; Capilla et al., 2014) to guide the deployment of attentional resources. The involvement of dorsal visual stream processing in visuospatial orienting is consistent with both Goodale and Milner's (1992) duplex model of vision which suggests that the dorsal visual stream is responsible for visually guided actions (including eye movements; Milner and Goodale, 2008), and with the premotor theory of attention which suggests that there is considerable overlap in the neural mechanisms responsible for the overt and covert orienting of attention (Rizzolatti et al., 1987). Unfortunately, recent evidence suggests that the dorsal visual stream may be vulnerable to age-related declines from relatively early on in the aging process (Langrová et al., 2006). This mini-review article examines the impact of these age-related declines on the visuospatial orienting of attention.

AGE-RELATED DECLINE OF THE DORSAL VISUAL STREAM

Recent studies suggest that the dorsal visual stream may be vulnerable to age-related atrophy and decline due to its cellular composition. The dorsal visual stream which extends from area V1 to the dorsolateral occipital cortex (Maunsell, 1987), and regions of the posterior parietal cortex (Kravitz et al., 2011), receives input primarily from the magnocellular layers of the lateral geniculate nucleus (LGN; Celesia and DeMarco, 1994; Grill-Spector and Malach, 2004). In contrast, the ventral visual stream which extends from area V1 to the inferior temporal cortex (Kravitz et al., 2011), receives input from both the magnocelluar and parvocellular layers (Celesia and DeMarco, 1994; Grill-Spector and Malach, 2004) of the LGN. Braddick et al.'s (2003) dorsal stream vulnerability hypothesis argues that, since magno cells are larger than parvo cells, and neurons with larger cell bodies and axon diameters are more susceptible to damage, magno cells are more susceptible to degeneration. In addition, losses in the magnocellular pathway may be more readily apparent as there are far fewer magno cells than parvo cells (Skottun, 2000). Thus, even when similar numbers of neurons are lost in both the magnocellular and parvocellular pathways, functional declines may be more apparent in the magnocellular pathway. Since the dorsal visual stream's primary input comes from magno cells (Celesia and DeMarco, 1994), the dorsal visual stream is in turn, more susceptible to degeneration (Braddick and Atkinson, 2011). Although Braddick's proposal of dorsal visual stream vulnerability was based on an examination of dorsal visual stream deficits in early childhood development; it does highlight the possibility that the dorsal visual stream may be more susceptible to decline in general.

Evidence of age-related dorsal visual stream declines has come from studies examining the age-related declines to neural structures. In a study by Ziegler et al. (2012), 547 participants between the ages of 19–86 years old were recruited, to perform a large-sample cross-sectional voxel-based morphometry (VBM) study to examine reductions in gray matter volume with advancing age. The results revealed that the dorsal visual stream exhibited substantially larger reductions in gray matter volume, compared to the ventral visual stream and the primary visual areas. These declines have been localized to the superior parietal cortex (Driscoll et al., 2009), as well as, the superior and inferior parietal gyri (Crivello et al., 2014; Fjell et al., 2014), all of which are crucial for the visuospatial orienting of attention (Corbetta and Shulman, 2002). Moreover, in elderly subjects, neural declines in the parietal regions (Resnick et al., 2003; Driscoll et al., 2009; Thambisetty et al., 2010; Crivello et al., 2014; Fjell et al., 2014) are compounded by a reduction in cerebral blood flow to the region (Martin et al., 1991), resulting in less efficient processing within the dorsal visual stream.

IMPACT OF DORSAL VISUAL STREAM DECLINES (BEHAVIORAL)

This mini-review article will focus primarily on the impact of these declines on the age-related changes to performance within the spatial cueing paradigm. In these studies, a cue elicits a shift of attention to its location (in the case of a peripheral cue; Eriksen and Hoffman, 1974; Theeuwes, 1991; Rafal and Henik, 1994; Yantis and Hillstrom, 1994; Oonk and Abrams, 1998), or to the location signaled by the cue stimulus (in the case of a central cue; Jonides, 1981; Shepherd and Müller, 1989; Cheal and Lyon, 1991; Theeuwes, 1991; Friesen et al., 2004). Subsequently, a target appears in either the location signaled by the cue stimulus (valid trial), or at an un-cued location (invalid trial). Participants are tasked with making a response to the onset of the target stimulus. The cueing benefit is indexed by a decrease in reaction times when targets appear in the location signaled by the cue stimulus and is believed to reflect the engagement of attentional resources at the target location (e.g., Jonides, 1981; Shepherd and Müller, 1989; Theeuwes, 1991; Yantis and Hillstrom, 1994; Friesen et al., 2004). Conversely, the cueing cost is indexed by an increase in reaction times when the target appears at an un-cued location, and is believed to reflect the disengagement and shifting of attentional resources from the invalidly cued location to the target location (Posner, 1980).

It appears that despite the declines to the dorsal visual stream, the visuospatial orienting of attention appears relatively well-preserved in older adults (Nissen and Corkin, 1985; Hartley et al., 1990). In spite of the slower reaction times seen in older adults, the magnitude of cueing benefit for both peripherally (Folk and Hoyer, 1992, Experiment 1; Greenwood et al., 1993; Olk and Kingstone, 2009) and centrally (Greenwood et al., 1993; Lincourt et al., 1997; Curran et al., 2001; Lorenzo-López et al., 2002; Olk and Kingstone, 2009) presented cues is similar for both younger and older adults. However, some studies have noted an increase in cueing costs following invalidly cued targets (Hartley et al., 1990; Greenwood and Parasuraman, 1994). Taken together, these results suggest that aging may be selectively associated with reduced efficiency in disengaging and shifting attentional resources from one location to the next, while the ability to effectively utilize the cues to guide the deployment of attentional resources remains intact.

One potential shortcoming of the aforementioned studies is that in these studies participants are required to make a detection or discrimination response to a target in an otherwise empty screen. In contrast, visual scenes are typically cluttered and we need to be able to rapidly identify a relevant item (target) from surrounding items (distractors). A process which has typically been studied using the visual search paradigm (Treisman and Gelade, 1980). In these studies, participants are required to identify a target that differs from surrounding items by a single feature (feature search) or by a conjunction of features (conjunction search; Treisman and Gelade, 1980). Results indicate that aging appears to selectively impair conjunction search while feature search remains intact (Plude and Doussard-Roosevelt, 1989). An elegant study by Greenwood and Parasuraman (1999) examined if the selective age-related impairment in conjunction search could in part be accounted for by an age-related reduction in the ability to flexibly expand and contract the focus of attention. To do so, they employed the use of precues that indicated the location of an upcoming target with a varying degree of precision (element-size precue: highlights a single possible location; column-size precue: highlights a column of possible locations; array-size precue: highlights a whole array of potential locations). The results indicated that age-related impairments in conjunction search can be alleviated by the use of precise and valid precues. Although this benefit was somewhat smaller in the oldest group of participants (above 76 years old). They suggest that aging impairs the ability to flexibly expand and contract the focus of attention and that elderly participants are more reliant on the precues to adjust the scale of their attention. But in the oldest participants the ability to utilize the precues to adjust the scale of attention is reduced. These findings suggest that although the visuospatial orienting of attention remains relatively well preserved in older adults, its flexibility is somewhat reduced.

IMPACT OF DORSAL VISUAL STREAM DECLINES (EEG)

Additionally, some studies have also employed the use of electroencephalographic (EEG) recordings in order to examine the electrophysiological correlates of attention shifts. These event-related potential (ERP) studies have most commonly focused on the P1 (80–130 ms) and the N1 (140–200 ms) components in relation to processing of target stimuli (Mangun and Hillyard, 1991; Wright et al., 1995). These studies demonstrate that shifting attention to a particular location of the visual field, increases the amplitude of P1 and N1 components (Mangun and Hillyard, 1991; Eimer, 1994; Luck et al., 1994; Mangun, 1995; Anllo-Vento et al., 1998) evoked by stimuli within the attended location. The amplification of these components appears to involve a selective enhancement of the signal to noise ratio of stimuli within the attended area, thereby strengthening the perceptual representation of stimuli located within that region (see Carrasco, 2011, for review; Heinze et al., 1990, 1994). Consequently, stimuli within the attended area are more rapidly detected; giving rise to more rapid response times when targets appear at the cued location (valid trials) compared to when targets appear at un-cued locations (invalid trials). Results from ERP studies examining the age-related changes to the underlying neural substrates of visuospatial orienting closely parallel the results of behavioral studies. These studies demonstrate that despite delayed latency of the P1 (80–130 ms) and N1 (140–200 ms) components, the augmentation of these early components elicited by attended relative to unattended targets is similar across both younger and older adults (Yamaguchi et al., 1995; Curran et al., 2001; Nagamatsu et al., 2011). With some studies showing linear correlations between the latency of ERP components and the mean reaction times of elderly participants (Li et al., 2013), which further bolsters the proposal that reductions in transmission efficiency of neural signals may account for slowed visuospatial orienting in elderly subjects (Hong and Rebec, 2012).

More recently, researchers have begun to focus on the neural activity elicited during the cue-target interval; much of this work has focused upon examining the modulation of prestimulus alpha activity along the fronto-occipital axis during the cue-target interval (Foxe et al., 1998; Worden et al., 2000; Babiloni et al., 2006; Rihs et al., 2009; Foxe and Snyder, 2011). Alpha-band desynchronization of the contralateral fronto-occipital axis appears to increase perceptual sensitivity by causing a baseline shift in the sensitivity of the neurons representing the to-be-attended location (Sauseng et al., 2005; Rihs et al., 2007; Siegel et al., 2008; Capotosto et al., 2009; Kelly et al., 2009; Capilla et al., 2014), while a concurrent alpha-band synchronization of the ipsilateral fronto-occipital axis inhibits processing of unattended regions (Kelly et al., 2006; Klimesch et al., 2007; Rihs et al., 2007, 2009; Capotosto et al., 2009; Foxe and Snyder, 2011; Bengson et al., 2012). The lateralization of prestimulus alpha reflects the top-down attentional modulation of neural processing in the visual cortices, and is referred to as proactive attentional control (Braver, 2012). It is termed proactive as it reflects the ability of the attentional system to bias perceptual processing in favor of an upcoming target before it is presented. In contrast, reactive attentional control refers to resolving interference between target and potentially distracting information at later stages of the processing hierarchy (Geerligs et al., 2014).

Recent studies indicate that the level of alpha power lateralization during the cue-target interval is significantly reduced in older adults (Vaden et al., 2012; Hong et al., 2015; Li and Zhao, 2015), and this reduction is most prominent along parietal-occipital regions (Zanto et al., 2011; Deiber et al., 2013). Specifically, older adults showed significant reductions in the level of event-related synchronization of prestimulus alpha (ipsilaterally) along these sites (Karrasch et al., 2004; Deiber et al., 2010; Vaden et al., 2012), which is consistent with earlier reports suggesting that older adults face significant difficulty with distractor suppression (Gazzaley et al., 2008; Schmitz et al., 2010; Haring et al., 2013). The decreased modulation of prestimulus alpha is proposed to be the result of the overall decline in alpha power in older adults, which renders the modulation of prestimulus alpha a less efficient means of attentional control (Vaden et al., 2012; Deiber et al., 2013; Hong et al., 2015; Li and Zhao, 2015). Older adults may compensate for this deficit with stronger early engagement of motor areas (Deiber et al., 2013), and an increase in reactive control (Paxton et al., 2008; Geerligs et al., 2014) mediated by the anterior nodes of the frontoparietal attention network (De Fockert et al., 2009; Schmitz et al., 2010; Haring et al., 2013; Li et al., 2013; Geerligs et al., 2014). These findings suggest that the age-related deterioration of parietal-occipital regions impairs elderly participants' ability to engage in the proactive attentional biasing of early sensory regions and leads to an increased reliance on more reactive control strategies.

Additionally, while the majority of research into the patterns of age-related cerebral reorganization have centered on intra-hemispheric patterns of reorganization, there is also extensive evidence to support inter-hemispheric patterns of reorganization (Cabeza et al., 1997; Madden et al., 1999; Tulving et al., 1994; Reuter-Lorenz et al., 2000; Cappell et al., 2010). It has been proposed that with the progressive age-related deterioration of specialized neural networks, the high metabolic costs of inter-hemispheric communication (Bullmore and Sporns, 2012; Liang et al., 2013) are outweighed by the benefits to behavioral performance (Banich, 1998; Cabeza, 2002). Although most studies of age-related asymmetry reduction have focused predominantly on the bilateral recruitment of the prefrontal cortices (Madden et al., 1999; Reuter-Lorenz et al., 2000), there is also evidence for age-related asymmetry reduction within the parietal cortices (Garavan et al., 1999). This implies that while the control of spatial attention may be strongly right lateralized in young adults (Corbetta et al., 1993; Foxe et al., 2003; Thiebaut de Schotten et al., 2011), older adults may maintain their performance on visuospatial orienting tasks by the bilateral recruitment of the posterior parietal cortex. Evidence for the hemispheric asymmetry reduction in visuospatial attention comes from studies demonstrating age-related attenuation of pseudoneglect in healthy older adults (Schmitz and Peigneux, 2011; Benwell et al., 2014; Learmonth et al., 2017). Pseudoneglect refers to the consistent attentional bias to the left visual field that is typically observed in healthy young adults (Bowers and Heilman, 1980; Voyer et al., 2012), and is believed to be due to the right hemisphere dominance for visuospatial processing (Waberski et al., 2008; Cavézian et al., 2012). Learmonth et al. (2017) demonstrated the typical leftward attentional bias in young adults was coupled with greater activity over the right parieto-occipital regions, and this lateralization was absent in older adults (whom also failed to show a leftward attentional bias). These results suggest that in older adults' deterioration of parieto-occipital regions may lead to compensatory increases in activity from homologous regions within the opposite hemisphere.

CONCLUSION

In summary, these studies suggest that in spite of the early age-related declines of the dorsal visual stream the visuospatial orienting of attention remains relatively well preserved, at least in the earlier stages of aging. This maintenance appears to be facilitated by the engagement of compensatory neural mechanisms; which is consistent with both the compensation-related utilization of neural circuits hypothesis (CRUNCH; Reuter-Lorenz and Cappell, 2008), and the scaffolding theory of aging and cognition (STAC; Park and Reuter-Lorenz, 2009), which propose that the age-related deterioration of the frontoparietal attention network will result in the engagement of compensatory neural mechanisms to support the performance of visual attention tasks. Although the engagement of compensatory neural mechanisms enables older adults to shift attention in the face of widespread structural deterioration (Schneider-Garces et al., 2010; Vallesi et al., 2011; Shafto et al., 2012; Meunier et al., 2014), it results in slower and less efficient task performance (Park and Reuter-Lorenz, 2009; Meunier et al., 2014; Reuter-Lorenz and Park, 2014). Furthermore, progressive deterioration of the frontoparietal network will result in an increased reliance on compensatory neural mechanisms, but at the same time increasing levels of atrophy and structural deterioration also limits the brain's capacity for reorganization (Burke and Barnes, 2006). As age-related atrophy proceeds, the brain will eventually reach its limits for functional reorganization and result in the more apparent attentional declines seen in the later stages of old age (80 years and above; Daffner et al., 2011).

AUTHOR CONTRIBUTIONS

The mini review was written by ETS-L with assistance and feedback from AJL.

FUNDING

Funding Body: Marsden Fund of New Zealand. Project Number: 3711736. Project Title: Sight unseen: penetrating the enigma of unconscious vision.

REFERENCES

Anllo-Vento, L., Luck, S. J., and Hillyard, S. A. (1998). Spatio-temporal dynamics of attention to color: evidence from human electrophysiology. *Hum. Brain Mapp.* 6, 216–238. doi: 10.1002/(sici)1097-0193(1998)6:4<216::aid-hbm3>3.0.co;2-6

Asplund, C. L., Todd, J. J., Snyder, A. P., and Marois, R. (2010). A central role for the lateral prefrontal cortex in goal-directed and stimulus-driven attention. *Nat. Neurosci.* 13, 507–512. doi: 10.1038/nn.2509

Babiloni, C., Vecchio, F., Bultrini, A., Luca Romani, G., and Rossini, P. M. (2006). Pre- and poststimulus alpha rhythms are related to conscious visual perception: a high-resolution EEG study. *Cereb. Cortex* 16, 1690–1700. doi: 10.1093/cercor/bhj104

Banich, M. T. (1998). The missing link: the role of interhemispheric interaction in attentional processing. *Brain Cogn.* 36, 128–157. doi: 10.1006/brcg.1997.0950

Bengson, J. J., Mangun, G. R., and Mazaheri, A. (2012). The neural markers of an imminent failure of response inhibition. *Neuroimage* 59, 1534–1539. doi: 10.1016/j.neuroimage.2011.08.034

Benwell, C. S. Y., Thut, G., Grant, A., and Harvey, M. (2014). A rightward shift in the visuospatial attention vector with healthy aging. *Front. Aging Neurosci.* 6:113. doi: 10.3389/fnagi.2014.00113

Bowers, D., and Heilman, K. M. (1980). Pseduneglect: effects of hemispace on tactile line bisection task. *Neuropsychologia* 18, 491–498. doi: 10.1016/0028-3932(80)90151-7

Braddick, O., and Atkinson, J. (2011). Development of human visual function. *Vision Res.* 51, 1588–1609. doi: 10.1016/j.visres.2011.02.018

Braddick, O., Atkinson, J., and Wattam-Bell, J. (2003). Normal and anomalous development of visual motion processing: motion coherence and 'dorsal-stream vulnerability'. *Neuropsychologia* 41, 1769–1784. doi: 10.1016/s0028-3932(03)00178-7

Braver, T. S. (2012). The variable nature of cognitive control: a dual mechanisms framework. *Trends Cogn. Sci.* 16, 106–113. doi: 10.1016/j.tics.2011.12.010

Bullmore, E., and Sporns, O. (2012). The economy of brain network organization. *Nat. Rev. Neurosci.* 13, 336–349. doi: 10.1038/nrn3214

Burke, S. N., and Barnes, C. A. (2006). Neural plasticity in the ageing brain. *Nat. Rev. Neurosci.* 7, 30–40. doi: 10.1038/nrn1809

Cabeza, R. (2002). Hemispheric asymmetry reduction in older adults: the Harold model. *Psychol. Aging* 17, 85–100. doi: 10.1037//0882-7974.17.1.85

Cabeza, R., Grady, C. L., Nyberg, L., McIntosh, A. R., Tulving, E., Kapur, S., et al. (1997). Age-related differences in neural activity during memory encoding and retrieval: a positron emission tomography study. *J. Neurosci.* 17, 391–400.

Capilla, A., Schoffelen, J. M., Paterson, G., Thut, G., and Gross, J. (2014). Dissociated α-band modulations in the dorsal and ventral visual pathways in visuospatial attention and perception. *Cereb. Cortex* 24, 550–561. doi: 10.1093/cercor/bhs343

Capotosto, P., Babiloni, C., Romani, G., and Corbetta, M. (2009). Frontoparietal cortex control spatial attention through modulation of anticipatory alpha rhythms. *J. Neurosci.* 29, 5863–5872. doi: 10.1523/JNEUROSCI.0539-09.2009

Cappell, K. A., Gmeindl, L., and Reuter-Lorenz, P. A. (2010). Age differences in prefontal recruitment during verbal working memory maintenance depend on memory load. *Cortex* 46, 462–473. doi: 10.1016/j.cortex.2009.11.009

Carrasco, M. (2011). Visual attention: the past 25 years. *Vision Res.* 51, 1484–1525. doi: 10.1016/j.visres.2011.04.012

Cavézian, C., Valadao, D., Hurwitz, M., Saoud, M., and Danckert, J. (2012). Finding centre: ocular and fMRI investigations of bisection and landmark task performance. *Brain Res.* 1437, 89–1103. doi: 10.1016/j.brainres.2011.12.002

Celesia, G. G., and DeMarco, P. J. Jr. (1994). Anatomy and physiology of the visual system. *J. Clin. Neurophysiol.* 11, 482–492.

Cheal, M., and Lyon, D. R. (1991). Central and peripheral precuing of forced-choice discrimination. *Q. J. Exp. Psychol. A.* 43, 859–880. doi: 10.1080/14640749108400960

Corbetta, M., Miezin, F. M., Shulman, G. L., and Petersen, S. E. (1993). A PET study of visuospatial attention. *J. Neurosci.* 13, 1202–1226.

Corbetta, M., Patel, G., and Shulman, G. L. (2008). The reorienting system of the human brain: from environment to theory of mind. *Neuron* 58, 306–324. doi: 10.1016/j.neuron.2008.04.017

Corbetta, M., and Shulman, G. L. (2002). Control of goal-directed and stimulus-driven attention in the brain. *Nat. Rev. Neurosci.* 3, 201–215. doi: 10.1038/nrn755

Corbetta, M., and Shulman, G. L. (2011). Spatial neglect and attention networks. *Annu. Rev. Neurosci.* 34, 569–599. doi: 10.1146/annurev-neuro-061010-113731

Crivello, F., Tzourio-Mazoyer, N., Tzourio, C., and Mazoyer, B. (2014). Longitudinal assessment of global and regional rate of grey matter atrophy in 1,172 healthy older adults: modulation by sex and age. *PLoS One* 9:e114478. doi: 10.1371/journal.pone.0114478

Curran, T., Hills, A., Patterson, M. B., and Strauss, M. E. (2001). Effects of aging on visuospatial attention: an ERP study. *Neuropsychologia* 39, 288–301. doi: 10.1016/s0028-3932(00)00112-3

Daffner, K. R., Sun, X., Tarbi, E. C., Rentz, D. M., Holcomb, P. J., and Riis, J. L. (2011). Does compensatory neural activity survive old age? *Neuroimage* 54, 427–438. doi: 10.1016/j.neuroimage.2010.08.006

De Fockert, J. W., Ramchurn, A., van Velzen, J., Bergström, Z., and Bunce, D. (2009). Behavioral and ERP evidence of greater distractor processing in old age. *Brain Res.* 1282, 67–73. doi: 10.1016/j.brainres.2009.05.060

Deiber, M., Ibañez, V., Missonnier, P., Rodriguez, C., and Giannakopoulos, P. (2013). Age-associated modulations of cerebral oscillatory patterns related to attentional control. *Neuroimage* 82, 531–546. doi: 10.1016/j.neuroimage.2013.06.037

Deiber, M. P., Rodriguez, C., Jaques, D., Missonnier, P., Emch, J., Millet, P., et al. (2010). Aging effects on selective attention-related electroencephalographic patterns during face encoding. *Neuroscience* 171, 173–186. doi: 10.1016/j.neuroscience.2010.08.051

Driscoll, I., Davatzikos, C., An, Y., Wu, X., Shen, D., Kraut, M., et al. (2009). Longitudinal pattern of regional brain volume change differentiates normal aging from MCI. *Neurology* 72, 1906–1913. doi: 10.1212/wnl.0b013e3181a82634

Eimer, M. (1994). An ERP study on visual spatial priming with peripheral onsets. *Psychophysiology* 31, 154–163. doi: 10.1111/j.1469-8986.1994.tb01035.x

Eriksen, C. W., and Hoffman, J. E. (1974). Selective attention: noise suppression or signal enhancement? *Bull. Psychon. Soc.* 4, 587–589. doi: 10.3758/bf03334301

Fjell, A. M., Westlye, L. T., Grydeland, H., Amlien, I., Espeseth, T., Reinvang, I., et al. (2014). Accelerating cortical thinning: unique to dementia or universal in aging? *Cereb. Cortex* 24, 919–934. doi: 10.1093/cercor/bhs379

Folk, C. L., and Hoyer, W. J. (1992). Aging and shifts of visual spatial attention. *Psychol. Aging* 7, 453–465. doi: 10.1037//0882-7974.7.3.453

Foxe, J. J., McCourt, M. E., and Javitt, D. C. (2003). Right hemisphere control of visuospatial attention: line-bisection judgements evaluated with high-density electrical mapping and source analysis. *Neuroimage* 19, 710–726. doi: 10.1016/s1053-8119(03)00057-0

Foxe, J. J., Simpson, G. V., and Ahlfors, S. P. (1998). Parietal-occipital 10 Hz activity reflects anticipatory state of visual attention mechanisms. *Neuroreport* 9, 3929–3933. doi: 10.1097/00001756-199812010-00030

Foxe, J. J., and Snyder, A. C. (2011). The role of alpha-band brain oscillations as a sensory suppression mechanism during selective attention. *Front. Psychol.* 2:154. doi: 10.3389/fpsyg.2011.00154

Friesen, C. K., Ristic, J., and Kingstone, A. (2004). Attentional effects of counter predictive gaze and arrow cues. *J. Exp. Psychol. Hum. Percept. Perform* 30, 319–329. doi: 10.1037/0096-1523.30.2.319

Garavan, H., Ross, T. J., and Stein, E. A. (1999). Right hemispheric dominance of inhibitory control: an event-related functional MRI study. *Proc. Natl. Acad. Sci. U S A* 96, 8301–8306. doi: 10.1073/pnas.96.14.8301

Gazzaley, A., Clapp, W., Kelley, J., McEvoy, K., Knight, R. T., and D'Esposito, M. (2008). Age-related top-down suppression deficit in the early stages of cortical visual memory processing. *Proc. Natl. Acad. Sci. U S A* 105, 13122–13126. doi: 10.1073/pnas.0806074105

Geerligs, L., Saliasi, E., Maurits, N. M., Renken, R. J., and Lorist, M. M. (2014). Brain mechanisms underlying the effects of aging on different aspects of selective attention. *Neuroimage* 91, 52–62. doi: 10.1016/j.neuroimage.2014.01.029

Goodale, M. A., and Milner, A. D. (1992). Separate visual pathways for perception and action. *Trends. Neurosci.* 15, 20–25. doi: 10.1016/0166-2236(92)90344-8

Greenwood, P. M., and Parasuraman, R. (1994). Attentional disengagement deficit in nondemented elderly over 75 years of age. *Aging Cogn.* 1, 188–202. doi: 10.1080/13825589408256576

Greenwood, P. M., and Parasuraman, R. (1999). Scale of attentional focus in visual search. *Percept. Psychophys.* 61, 837–859. doi: 10.3758/bf03206901

Greenwood, P. M., Parasuraman, R., and Haxby, J. V. (1993). Changes in visuospatial attention over the adult lifespan. *Neuropsychologia* 31, 471–485. doi: 10.1016/0028-3932(93)90061-4

Grill-Spector, K., and Malach, R. (2004). The human visual cortex. *Annu. Rev. Neurosci.* 27, 649–677. doi: 10.1146/annurev.neuro.27.070203.144220

Haring, A. E., Zhuravleva, T. Y., Alperin, B. R., Rentz, D. M., Holcomb, P. J., and Daffner, K. R. (2013). Age-related differences in enhancement and suppression of neural activity underlying selective attention in matched young and old adults. *Brain Res.* 1499, 69–79. doi: 10.1016/j.brainres.2013.01.003

Hartley, A. A., Kieley, J. M., and Slabach, E. H. (1990). Age differences and similarities in the effects of cues and prompts. *J. Exp. Psychol. Hum. Percept. Perform.* 16, 523–537. doi: 10.1037//0096-1523.16.3.523

Heinze, H. J., Luck, S. J., Mangun, G. R., and Hillyard, S. A. (1990). Visual event-related potentials index focused attention within bilateral stimulus arrays. I. Evidence for early selection. *Electroencephalogr. Clin. Neurophysiol.* 75, 511–527. doi: 10.1016/0013-4694(90)90138-a

Heinze, H. J., Mangun, G. R., Burchert, W., Hinrichs, H., Scholz, M., Münte, T. F., et al. (1994). Combined spatial and temporal imaging of brain activity during visual selective attention in humans. *Nature* 372, 543–546. doi: 10.1038/372543a0

Hong, S. L., and Rebec, G. V. (2012). A new perspective on behavioral inconsistency and neural noise in aging: compensatory speeding of neural communication. *Front. Aging Neurosci.* 4:27. doi: 10.3389/fnagi.2012.00027

Hong, X., Sun, J., Bengson, J. J., Mangun, G. R., and Tong, S. (2015). Normal aging selectively diminishes alpha lateralization in visual spatial attention. *Neuroimage* 106, 353–363. doi: 10.1016/j.neuroimage.2014.11.019

Jonides, J. (1981). "Voluntary versus automatic control over the mind's eye's movement," in *Attention and Performance IX*, eds J. B. Long and A. D. Baddeley (Hillsdale, NJ: Erlbaum), 187–203.

Karrasch, M., Laine, M., Rapinoja, P., and Krause, C. M. (2004). Effects of normal aging on event-related desynchronization/synchronization during a memory task in humans. *Neurosci. Lett.* 366, 18–23. doi: 10.1016/j.neulet.2004.05.010

Kelly, S. P., Gomez-Ramirez, M., and Foxe, J. J. (2009). The strength of anticipatory spatial biasing predicts target discrimination at attended locations: a high-density EEG study. *Eur. J. Neurosci.* 30, 2224–2234. doi: 10.1111/j.1460-9568.2009.06980.x

Kelly, S. P., Lalor, E. C., Reilly, R. B., and Foxe, J. J. (2006). Increases in alpha oscillatory power reflect an active retinotopic mechanism for distracter suppression during sustained visuospatial attention. *J. Neurophysiol.* 95, 3844–3851. doi: 10.1152/jn.01234.2005

Klimesch, W., Sauseng, P., and Hanslmayr, S. (2007). EEG alpha oscillations: the inhibition–timing hypothesis. *Brain Res. Rev.* 53, 63–88. doi: 10.1016/j.brainresrev.2006.06.003

Kravitz, D. J., Saleem, K. S., Baker, C. I., and Mishkin, M. (2011). A new neural framework for visuospatial processing. *Nat. Rev. Neurosci.* 12, 217–230. doi: 10.1038/nrn3008

Lambert, A. J., and Shin, M. J. (2010). The hare and the snail: dissociating visual orienting from conscious perception. *Vis. Cogn.* 18, 829–838. doi: 10.1080/13506281003693569

Langrová, J., Kuba, M., Kremlácek, J., Kubová, Z., and Vit, F. (2006). Motion-onset VEPs reflect long maturation and early ageing of visual motion processing system. *Vision Res.* 46, 536–544. doi: 10.1016/j.visres.2005.06.024

Learmonth, G., Benwell, C. S. Y., Thut, G., and Harvey, M. (2017). Age-related reduction of hemispheric lateralisation for spatial attention: an EEG study. *Neuroimage* 153, 139–151. doi: 10.1016/j.neuroimage.2017.03.050

Li, L., Gratton, C., Fabiani, M., and Knight, R. T. (2013). Age-related frontoparietal changes during the control of bottom-up and top-down attention: an ERP study. *Neurobiol. Aging* 34, 477–488. doi: 10.1016/j.neurobiolaging.2012.02.025

Li, L., and Zhao, D. (2015). Age-related inter-region EEG coupling changes during the control of bottom-up and top-down attention. *Front. Aging Neurosci.* 7:223. doi: 10.3389/fnagi.2015.00223

Liang, X., Zou, Q., He, Y., and Yang, Y. (2013). Coupling of functional connectivity and regional cerebral blood flow reveals a physiological basis for network hubs of the brain. *Proc. Natl. Acad. Sci. U S A* 110, 1929–1934. doi: 10.1073/pnas.1214900110

Lincourt, A. E., Folk, C. L., and Hoyer, W. J. (1997). Effects of aging on voluntary and involuntary shifts of attention. *Aging Neuropsychol. Cogn.* 4, 290–303. doi: 10.1080/13825589708256654

Lorenzo-López, L., Doallo, S., Vizoso, C., Amenedo, E., Holguín, S. R., and Cadaveira, F. (2002). Covert orienting of visuospatial attention in the early stages of aging. *Neuroreport* 13, 1459–1462. doi: 10.1097/00001756-200208070-00022

Luck, S. J., Hillyard, S. A., Mangun, G. R., and Gazzaniga, M. S. (1994). Independent attentional scanning in the separated hemispheres of split-brain patients. *J. Cogn. Neurosci.* 6, 84–91. doi: 10.1162/jocn.1994.6.1.84

Madden, D. J., Turkington, T. G., Provenzale, J. M., Denny, L. L., Hawk, T. C., Gottlob, L. R., et al. (1999). Adult age differences in functional neuroanatomy of verbal recognition memory. *Hum. Brain Mapp.* 7, 115–135. doi: 10.1002/(sici)1097-0193(1999)7:2<115::aid-hbm5>3.0.co;2-n

Mangun, G. R. (1995). Neural mechanisms of visual selective attention. *Psychophysiology* 32, 4–18. doi: 10.1111/j.1469-8986.1995.tb03400.x

Mangun, G. R., and Hillyard, S. A. (1991). Modulations of sensory-evoked brain potentials indicate changes in perceptual processing during visual-spatial priming. *J. Exp. Psychol. Hum. Percept. Perform.* 17, 1057–1074. doi: 10.1037//0096-1523.17.4.1057

Marrett, N. E., de-Wit, L. H., Roser, M., Kentridge, R. W., Milner, A. D., and Lambert, A. J. (2011). Testing the dorsal stream attention hypothesis: electrophysiological correlates and the effects of ventral stream damage. *Vis. Cogn.* 19, 1089–1121. doi: 10.1080/13506285.2011.622729

Martin, J., Friston, K. J., Colebatch, J. G., and Frackowiak, R. S. J. (1991). Decreases in regional cerebral blood flow with normal aging. *J. Cereb. Blood Flow Metab.* 11, 684–689. doi: 10.1038/jcbfm.1991.121

Maunsell, J. H. R. (1987). "Physiological evidence for two visual subsystems," in *Matters of Intelligence*, ed. L. M. Vaina (Netherlands: Reidel Dordrecht), 59–87.

Meunier, D., Stamatakis, E. A., and Tyler, L. K. (2014). Age-related functional reorganization, structural changes, and preserved cognition. *Neurobiol. Aging* 35, 42–54. doi: 10.1016/j.neurobiolaging.2013.07.003

Milner, A. D., and Goodale, M. A. (2008). Two visual systems re-viewed. *Neuropsychologia* 46, 774–785. doi: 10.1016/j.neuropsychologia.2007.10.005

Nagamatsu, L. S., Carolan, P., Liu-Ambrose, T. Y., and Handy, T. C. (2011). Age-related changes in the attentional control of visual cortex: a selective problem in the left visual hemifield. *Neuropsychologia* 49, 1670–1678. doi: 10.1016/j.neuropsychologia.2011.02.040

Nissen, M. J., and Corkin, S. (1985). Effectiveness of attentional cueing in older and younger adults. *J. Gerontol.* 40, 185–191. doi: 10.1093/geronj/40.2.185

Olk, B., and Kingstone, A. (2009). A new look at aging and performance in the antisaccade task: the impact of response selection. *Eur. J. Cogn. Psychol.* 21, 406–427. doi: 10.1080/09541440802333190

Oonk, H. M., and Abrams, R. A. (1998). New perceptual objects that capture attention produced inhibition of return. *Psychon. B. Rev.* 5, 510–515.

Park, D. C., and Reuter-Lorenz, P. (2009). The adaptive brain: aging and neurocognitive scaffolding. *Annu. Rev. Psychol.* 60, 173–196. doi: 10.1146/annurev.psych.59.103006.093656

Paxton, J. L., Barch, D. M., Racine, C. A., and Braver, T. S. (2008). Cognitive control, goal maintenance, and prefrontal function in healthy aging. *Cereb. Cortex* 18, 1010–1028. doi: 10.1093/cercor/bhm135

Plude, D. J., and Doussard-Roosevelt, J. A. (1989). Aging, selective attention and feature integration. *Psychol. Aging* 4, 98–105. doi: 10.1037//0882-7974.4.1.98

Posner, M. I. (1980). Orienting of attention. *Q. J. Exp. Psychol.* 32, 3–25. doi: 10.1080/00335558008248231

Rafal, R., and Henik, A. (1994). "The neurology of inhibition: integrating controlled and automatic processes," in *Inhibitory Processes in Attention, Memory, and Language*, eds D. Dagenbach and T. H. Carr (San Diego, CA: Academic Press), 1–51.

Resnick, S. M., Pham, D. L., Kraut, M. A., Zonderman, A. B., and Davatzikos, C. (2003). Longitudinal magnetic resonance imaging studies of older adults: a shrinkingbrain. *J. Neurosci.* 23, 3295–3301.

Reuter-Lorenz, P. A., and Cappell, K. A. (2008). Neurocognitive aging and the compensation hypothesis. *Curr. Dir. Psychol. Sci.* 17, 177–182. doi: 10.1111/j.1467-8721.2008.00570.x

Reuter-Lorenz, P. A., Jonides, J., Smith, E. E., Hartley, A., Miller, A., Marshuetz, C., et al. (2000). Age differences in the frontal lateralization of verbal and spatial working memory revealed by PET. *J. Cogn. Neurosci.* 12, 174–187. doi: 10.1162/089892900561814

Reuter-Lorenz, P., and Park, D. C. (2014). How does it STAC up? Revisiting the scaffolding theory of aging and cognition. *Neuropsychol. Rev.* 24, 355–370. doi: 10.1007/s11065-014-9270-9

Rihs, T. A., Michel, C. M., and Thut, G. (2007). Mechanisms of selective inhibition in visual spatial attention are indexed by α-band EEG synchronization. *Eur. J. Neurosci.* 25, 603–610. doi: 10.1111/j.1460-9568.2007.05278.x

Rihs, T. A., Michel, C. M., and Thut, G. (2009). A bias for posterior α-band power suppression versus enhancement during shifting versus maintenance of spatial attention. *Neuroimage* 44, 190–199. doi: 10.1016/j.neuroimage.2008.08.022

Rizzolatti, G., Riggio, L., Dascola, I., and Umiltá, C. (1987). Reorienting attention across the horizontal and vertical meridians: evidence in favour of a premotor theory of attention. *Neuropsychologia* 25, 31–40. doi: 10.1016/0028-3932(87)90041-8

Sauseng, P., Klimesch, W., Stadler, W., Schabus, M., Doppelmayr, M., Hanslmayr, S., et al. (2005). A shift of visual spatial attention is selectively associated with human EEG alpha activity. *Eur. J. Neurosci.* 22, 2917–2926. doi: 10.1111/j.1460-9568.2005.04482.x

Schall, J. D. (2009). "Frontal eye fields," in *Encyclopedia of Neuroscience*, eds M. D. Binder, N. Hirokawa and U. Windhorst (Berlin: Springer-Verlag GmbH), 1635–1638.

Schmitz, T. W., Cheng, F. H. T., and De Rosa, E. (2010). Failing to ignore: paradoxical neural effects of perceptual load on early attentional selection in normal aging. *J. Neurosci.* 30, 14750–14758. doi: 10.1523/JNEUROSCI.2687-10.2010

Schmitz, R., and Peigneux, P. (2011). Age-related changes in visual pseudoneglect. *Brain Cogn.* 76, 382–389. doi: 10.1016/j.bandc.2011.04.002

Schneider-Garces, N. J., Gordon, B. A., Brumback-Peltz, C. R., Shin, E., Lee, Y., Sutton, B. P., et al. (2010). Span, CRUNCH, and beyond: working memory capacity and the aging brain. *J. Cogn. Neurosci.* 22, 655–669. doi: 10.1162/jocn.2009.21230

Shafto, M., Randall, B., Stamatakis, E. A., Wright, P., and Tyler, L. K. (2012). Age-related neural reorganization during spoken word recognition: the interaction of form and meaning. *J. Cogn. Neurosci.* 24, 1434–1446. doi: 10.1162/jocn_a_00218

Shepherd, M., and Müller, H. J. (1989). Movement versus focusing of visual attention. *Percept. Psychophys.* 46, 146–154. doi: 10.3758/bf03204974

Siegel, M., Donner, T. H., Oostenveld, R., Fries, P., and Engel, A. K. (2008). Neuronal synchronization along the dorsal visual pathway reflects the focus of spatial attention. *Neuron* 60, 709–719. doi: 10.1016/j.neuron.2008.09.010

Skottun, B. C. (2000). The magnocellular deficit theory of dyslexia: the evidence from contrast sensitivity. *Vision Res.* 40, 111–127. doi: 10.1016/s0042-6989(99)00170-4

Thambisetty, M., Wan, J., Carass, A., An, Y., Prince, J. L., and Resnick, S. M. (2010). Longitudinal changes in cortical thickness associated with normal aging. *Neuroimage* 52, 1215–1223. doi: 10.1016/j.neuroimage.2010.04.258

Thiebaut de Schotten, M., Dell'Acqua, F., Forkel, S. J., Simmons, A., Vergani, F., Murphy, D. G. M., et al. (2011). A lateralized brain network for visuospatial attention. *Nat. Neurosci.* 14, 1245–1246. doi: 10.1038/nn.2905

Theeuwes, J. (1991). Exogenous and endogenous control of attention: the effects of visual onsets and offsets. *Percept. Psychophys.* 49, 83–90. doi: 10.3758/bf03211619

Treisman, A., and Gelade, G. (1980). A feature-integration theory of attention. *Cogn. Psychol.* 12, 97–136. doi: 10.1016/0010-0285(80)90005-5

Tulving, E., Kapur, S., Craik, F. I., Moscovitch, M., and Houle, S. (1994). Hemispheric encoding/retrieval asymmetry in episodic memory: positron emission tomography findings. *Proc. Natl. Acad. Sci. U S A* 91, 2016–2020.

Vaden, R. J., Hutcheson, N. L., McCollum, L. A., Kentros, J., and Visscher, K. M. (2012). Older adults, unlike younger adults, do not modulate alpha power to suppress irrelevant information. *Neuroimage* 63, 1127–1133. doi: 10.1016/j.neuroimage.2012.07.050

Vallesi, A., McIntosh, A. R., and Stuss, D. T. (2011). Overrecruitment in the aging brain as a function of task demands: evidence for a compensatory view. *J. Cogn. Neurosci.* 23, 801–815. doi: 10.1162/jocn.2010.21490

Vandenberghe, R., and Gillebert, C. R. (2009). Parcellation of parietal cortex: convergence between lesion-symptom mapping and mapping of the intact functioning brain. *Behav. Brain Res.* 199, 171–182. doi: 10.1016/j.bbr.2008.12.005

Voyer, D., Voyer, S. D., and Tramonte, L. (2012). Free-viewing laterality tasks: a multi-level meta-analysis. *Neuropsychology* 26, 551–567.doi: 10.1037/a0028631

Waberski, T. D., Gobbelé, R., Lamberty, K., Buchner, H., Marshall, J. C., and Fink, G. R. (2008). Timing of visuo-spatial information processing: electrical source imaging related to line bisection judgements. *Neuropsychologia* 46, 1201–1210. doi: 10.1016/j.neuropsychologia.2007.10.024

Worden, M. S., Foxe, J. J., Wang, N., and Simpson, G. V. (2000). Anticipatory biasing of visuospatial attention indexed by retinotopically specific alpha-band electroencephalography increases over occipital cortex. *J. Neurosci.* 20:RC63.

Wright, M. J., Geffen, G. M., and Geffen, L. B. (1995). Event related potentials during covert orientation of visual attention: effects of cue validity and directionality. *Biol. Psychol.* 41, 183–202. doi: 10.1016/0301-0511(95)05128-7

Yamaguchi, S., Tsuchiya, H., and Kobayashi, S. (1995). Electrophysiologic correlates of age effects on visuospatial attention shift. *Cogn. Brain Res.* 3, 41–49. doi: 10.1016/0926-6410(95)00017-8

Yantis, S., and Hillstrom, A. P. (1994). Stimulus-driven attentional capture: evidence from equiluminant visual objects. *J. Exp. Psychol. Hum. Percept. Perform.* 20, 95–107.

Zanto, T. P., Pan, P., Liu, H., Bollinger, J., Nobre, A. C., and Gazzaley, A. (2011). Age-related changes in orienting attention in time. *J. Neurosci.* 31, 12461–12470. doi: 10.1523/JNEUROSCI.1149-11.2011

Ziegler, G., Dahnke, R., Jäncke, L., Yotter, R. A., May, A., and Gaser, C. (2012). Brain structural trajectories over the adult lifespan. *Hum. Brain Mapp.* 33, 2377–2389. doi: 10.1002/hbm.21374

11

Biosystems Study of the Molecular Networks Underlying Hippocampal Aging Progression and Anti-Aging Treatment in Mice

Jiao Wang[1], Qian Li[1], Yanyan Kong[2], Fangfang Zhou[1], Jie Li[1], Weihao Li[1], Kai Wang[3], Ting Wu[4], Yihui Guan[2], Jiang Xie[5] and Tieqiao Wen[1]**

[1] Laboratory of Molecular Neural Biology, School of Life Sciences, Shanghai University, Shanghai, China, [2] Position Emission Computed Tomography Center, Huashan Hospital, Fudan University, Shanghai, China, [3] Shanghai Key Laboratory of Molecular Andrology, Institute of Biochemistry and Cell Biology, Shanghai Institutes for Biological Sciences, Chinese Academy of Sciences, Shanghai, China, [4] Shanghai Stem Cell Group, Shanghai, China, [5] School of Computer Engineering and Science, Shanghai University, Shanghai, China

***Correspondence:**
Tieqiao Wen
wtq@shu.edu.cn
Jiang Xie
jiangx@shu.edu.cn

Aging progression is a process that an individual encounters as they become older, and usually results from a series of normal physiological changes over time. The hippocampus, which contributes to the loss of spatial and episodic memory and learning in older people, is closely related to the detrimental effects of aging at the morphological and molecular levels. However, age-related genetic changes in hippocampal molecular mechanisms are not yet well-established. To provide additional insight into the aging process, differentially-expressed genes of 3- versus 24- and 29-month old mice were re-analyzed. The results revealed that a large number of immune and inflammatory response-related genes were up-regulated in the aged hippocampus, and membrane receptor-associated genes were down-regulated. The down-regulation of transmembrane receptors may indicate the weaker perception of environmental exposure in older people, since many transmembrane proteins participate in signal transduction. In addition, molecular interaction analysis of the up-regulated immune genes indicated that the hub gene, *Ywhae*, may play essential roles in immune and inflammatory responses during aging progression, as well as during hippocampal development. Our biological experiments confirmed the conserved roles of *Ywhae* and its partners between human and mouse. Furthermore, comparison of microarray data between advanced-age mice treated with human umbilical cord blood plasma protein and the phosphate-buffered saline control showed that the genes that contribute to the revitalization of advanced-age mice are different from the genes induced by aging. These results implied that the revitalization of advanced-age mice is not a simple reverse process of normal aging progression. Our data assigned novel roles of genes during aging progression and provided further theoretic evidence for future studies exploring the underlying mechanisms of aging and anti-aging-related disease therapy.

Keywords: aging, immune response, hippocampal development, umbilical cord blood, molecular interaction network

---

Abbreviations: BioGRID, The Biological General Repository for Interaction Datasets; DAVID, The Database for Annotation, Visualization and Integrated Discovery; DEG, differentially-expressed gene; GFAP, glial fibrillary acidic protein; HSCs, hematopoietic stem cells; PBS, phosphate-buffered saline; qPCR, real-time quantitative polymerase chain reaction.

INTRODUCTION

Aging is the process of an organism, particularly mammals, becoming older and characterized by a progressive loss of physiological integrity (Lopez-Otin et al., 2013). It is the result of a series of normal changes in gene regulatory networks over time, and is usually reflected by physiological changes (Lopez-Otin et al., 2013). The hippocampus aging, which contributes to the loss of spatial and episodic memory and learning in aging people, is closely related to the detrimental effects of aging at the morphological and molecular levels (Castellano et al., 2017).

The aged hippocampus may impair neural and cognitive function and lead to many neurological disorders such as Alzheimer's disease (Stilling et al., 2014; Castellano et al., 2017), aphasia, agnosia, and Parkinson's disease (Ghika, 2008). The aging hippocampus seems to suffer a generalized loss of synapses (Miller and O'Callaghan, 2003), which influence spatial memory and plasticity functions in multiple species (Moser and Moser, 1998; Hampson et al., 1999; Burke and Barnes, 2006). Moreover, a decrease in neuronal density (Mani et al., 1986; Keuker et al., 2003) and hippocampal volume (Driscoll et al., 2003) were found in the aging hippocampus, and these age-related losses occur in some degenerative conditions (West et al., 1994). Certain genes were predicted, for instance, a deubiquitinating enzyme- UCHL5 hub protein (Kikuchi et al., 2013), and neuropeptide arginine-vasopressin $_{(4-8)}$ (AVP_{4-8}) (Xiong et al., 2000) may be potential candidates for treating age-related disease. The increasing elderly population has increased labor costs and financial burden for both families and governments, thus, delaying or even partially reversing the aging process is of great interest (Castellano et al., 2017). However, due to the limited knowledge regarding aging, there are still numerous difficulties with different treatments for degenerative diseases linked to aging.

The most common theories for aging include telomere attrition, endocrine disorders, and oxidative stress (Patel et al., 2015). It has been suggested that low-grade inflammation, which is characterized by increased levels of inflammatory cytokines in response to environmental signals, contributes to aging processes (Nikodemova et al., 2016). The chronic inflammation eventually initiates immune-senescence in both the immune and central nervous system, resulting in the functional decline of the immune system with age (Regulski, 2017). Recently, advances in knowledge regarding neuroinflammation and immunity to brain aging have been reviewed (Di Benedetto et al., 2017). Since a plethora of research has been conducted in the exploration of aging mechanisms, recent research has been dedicated to elucidating ways in which to cease aging (Loffredo et al., 2013; Katsimpardi et al., 2014; Sinha et al., 2014; Castellano et al., 2017). GDF11 has been identified as a circulating factor in young mice that declines with age, and subsequently, GDF11 has been shown to be a rejuvenating factor for skeletal muscle (Sinha et al., 2014) and the brain (Katsimpardi et al., 2014). Furthermore, recent research has shown that tissue inhibitor of metalloproteinases 2, an umbilical cord plasma protein, provides a reservoir for the neuroplasticity-promoting process (Di Benedetto et al., 2017). Despite these research efforts, the molecular mechanisms underlying the progression of biological aging have not yet been established, likely due to the complexity of chronic aging progressions.

In the present paper, we aim to explore the molecular interaction mechanisms underlying aging using a biological systems approach that integrates computational and experimental methods. We assume that DEGs between advanced-age and young mice likely contribute to aging progression via certain mechanisms. Investigation into the molecular interactions of the genes identified potential aging regulators (or hub genes of the network). The key candidate genes inferred from network analysis were validated using qPCR. Our present study provides a more comprehensive analysis of the mechanisms underlying the aging process, and has laid the foundation for the exploration of genetic changes involved in the promotion of rejuvenation from advanced-age to young individuals.

MATERIALS AND METHODS

Mice

Specific pathogen free C57BL/6 wild-type mice were fed under a controlled temperature (23°C) and kept on a 12 h light/dark cycle with food and water provided *ad libitum*. 3–4 mice were kept in individually ventilated cages. Littermate male mice (4 and 20 months old) were used, and three different tissue samples for RNA extraction were obtained per strain. All animal handling protocols were approved by the Animal Ethics Committee of Shanghai University.

RNA Extraction and RT-PCR

Hippocampus was rapidly dissected in 0°C PBS and placed in RNA extraction solution (Promega, United States). RNA extraction was carried out in accordance with the manufacturer's protocol. 2 μg total RNA and 4 μl 5X RT Master Mix (TaKaRa, Japan) were added to RNA-free water to a final reaction volume of 20 μl for cDNA synthesis under different temperature of 25°C for 5 min, 37°C for 30 min, 85°C for 10 s, and 12°C for 10 min. The target genes were quantified by real-time PCR using qPCR SYBR Green Master Mix (Yeasen, China). Each reaction contained 1 μl cDNA sample (100–200 ng/μl), 10 μl qPCR SYBR Green Master Mix, 0.8 μl (10 μM) designated primers, and RNA-free water to a final volume of 20 μl. The PCR conditions were as follows: 95°C for 30 s, 55°C for 20 s, 72°C for 30 s, 40 thermal cycles. The mRNA expression was normalized to GAPDH. The primers of each gene were shown in **Table 1**.

Identification of DEGs and Function Annotation

For comparison of gene expression in the hippocampus of 3-, 24-, and 29 month-old mice, the following methods were used. Raw RNA-Seq reads of the gene expression series GSE61915 were downloaded from the NCBI Gene Expression Omnibus database (Stilling et al., 2014). Low quality bases and 5′ and 3′ ($Q20 \leq 20$) ends of each read were trimmed using a locally developed Perl script, and adapters were removed by trimmomatic (version 0.36)

TABLE 1 | Primers used in qPCR.

Gene name		Primer sequence (5′–3′)
YWHAE	Forward	GATTCGGGAATATCGGCAAATGG
	Reverse	GCTGGAATGAGGTGTTTGTCC
EZH2	Forward	AATCAGAGTACATGCGACTGAGA
	Reverse	GCTGTATCCTTCGCTGTTTCC
RARA	Forward	AAGCCCGAGTGCTCTGAGA
	Reverse	TTCGTAGTGTATTTGCCCAGC
HDAC1	Forward	AGTCTGTTACTACTACGACGGG
	Reverse	TGAGCAGCAAATTGTGAGTCAT
DCLK2	Forward	CCAAGAAGGCGCGGTTCTA
	Reverse	TGGGGCAGGTTCACATTGTC
TGM1	Forward	GCAATGAGATCTACATCCTCTTC
	Reverse	GAAGAGGATGTAGATCTCATTGC
CD74	Forward	TCACCTCCCAGAACCTGCA
	Reverse	TGCATCACATGGTCCT
VIM	Forward	GAGAAATTGCAGGAGGAGATGC
	Reverse	CAAGGTCAAGACGTGCCAGAGA
RBM3	Forward	CTTCGTAGGAGGGCTCAACTT
	Reverse	CAACAACCACCTCAGAGATAGG
C4B	Forward	GCTGAGGGGAAGTGCCCTCG
	Reverse	TGCAGGACTTGGGTGATCTTGG
SFTPC	Forward	AGCAAAGAGGTCCTGATGGAGAG
	Reverse	ACCACCACCACAACCACGAT
RET	Forward	GCATGTCAGACCCGAACTGG
	Reverse	CGCTGAGGGTGAAACCATCC
GAPDH	Forward	TCACCACCATGGAGAAGGC
	Reverse	GCTAAGCAGTTGGTGGTGCA
β-ACTIN	Forward	CATGTACGTTGCTATCCAGGC
	Reverse	CTCCTTAATGTCACGCACGAT

(Bolger et al., 2014). The clear reads were mapped against mouse genes (GRCm38.p5) using HISAT2 (version 2.0.5) (Kim et al., 2015). The read counts were generated by BEDTools (Quinlan, 2014) and expression values were calculated using the RPKM (Reads per Kilobase per Million mapped reads) method. DEGs were obtained using the fold change of $\geq$1.50 or $\leq$0.67, and a t-test p-value of $\leq$0.05 was also required.

For comparison of gene expression in the hippocampus of mice treated with PBS or human cord plasma protein, human young plasma, and human advanced-age plasma, the processed data from GSE75416 were used directly (Castellano et al., 2017). DEGs were obtained using the fold change of $\geq$1.2 or $\leq$0.83, as well as a t-test p-value of $\leq$0.05.

Enriched functions of significantly changed genes were generated using DAVID 6.8 (Huang da et al., 2009).

Molecular Interaction Network Construction

Human and mouse molecular interactions were collected from the BioGRID (version 3.4.153) (Chatr-Aryamontri et al., 2017) and IntAct (release 2017/9/2) (Orchard et al., 2014) databases, respectively. The BioGRID and IntAct databases contain various experimentally validated interactions, such as: two-hybrid, affinity capture, co-localization, far-western blotting, proximity label-MS, phage display, coimmunoprecipitation, pull-down, x-ray crystallography, and cross-linking. We were especially interested in the genes that directly interacted with the DEGs of special functions. All the interactions were collected from published literature, and could be retrieved from the original paper via the PubMed IDs. Thus, these data are more reliable than other computationally predicted interactions. All interactions were represented by gene symbol pairs, the BioGRID and IntAct dataset were merged based on these gene symbol pairs. Only human–human or mouse–mouse interactions were retained. For molecular interaction network construction, the first neighbors (most of which represents more reliable and usually direct interactions) of the genes related to the immune response (**Figure 2A**) were selected, and the interactions were displayed using Cytoscape 3.5.1 (Shannon et al., 2003).

The gene functions in hippocampal development were collected from Uniprot (Boutet et al., 2016) according to their GO annotation. The hippocampal development (Supplementary Table S1)-associated network was constructed using the same method. A slight difference was that all genes that interacted with hippocampal development-associated genes were DEGs, while the immune response-related genes were DEGs in the above network.

The human and mouse networks were constructed.

Plasmid Construction

PsiRNA-YWHAE was constructed for the intracellular silence of *YWHAE* expression. The hairpin sequence containing *YWHAE* (*YWHAE*-for 5′- TCC CAG CTA ACA CTG GCG AGT CCA AGG TTT CAA GAG AAA ACC TTG GAC TCG CCA GTG TTA GCT T -3′ and *YWHAE*-rev 5′- CAA AAA GCT AAC ACT GGC GAG TCC AAG GTT TTC TCT TGA AAC CTT GGA CTC GCC AGT GTT AGC T -3′) was inserted into the psiRNA-hH1neo vector at two restriction enzyme sites (Bpi I). The negative control (psiRNA-control) with a random sequence (non-targeting siRNA) was also constructed in the same way (**Supplementary Figure S1**).

Cell Culture and Transfection

HEK293T, an inbreeding of HEK293 (Human embryonic kidney cells 293) cells, were cultured in DMEM (Invitrogen, United States) containing 10% fetal bovine serum (Invitrogen, United States), at 37°C with 5% CO_2. Cells were plated on 6-well plates at a density of 5 × 10^5/ml, and the following day transfected with 4 μg psiRNA-YWHAE or psiRNA-control as a negative control and cultured for 36 h. Transfection was carried out using Lipofectamine2000 (Invitrogen, United States), according to the manufacturer's protocol.

Immunofluorescence

The human brain sections (provided by Huashan Hospital, Fudan University, Shanghai, China) were washed three times with PBS, treated with 0.2% Triton X-100 (diluted with PBS) for 30 min, and then blocked in 5% albumin from bovine serum for 60 min. Next, the sections were incubated with an YWHAE antibody at room temperature overnight. The following day, the sections were washed three times with PBS (5 min per wash) and then incubated with a secondary antibody for 1.5 h. Finally, the sections were stained with 4′,6-diamidino-2-phenylindole for 20 min. The expression of YWHAE was detected by confocal microscopy. The experiment protocols were approved by the Human Ethic Committee of Huashan Hospital (Fudan University, Shanghai, China), and Shanghai University Ethics Committee.

RESULTS

DEGs in the Hippocampus between Young and Advanced-Age Mice

To determine the difference at the molecular level during the hippocampal aging process, we compared the gene expression in the hippocampus between young (3 months) and advanced-age (24 and 29 months) mice (Stilling et al., 2014). In comparison with 3 month-age mice, 29 month-age mice showed a larger difference than that of 24 month-age mice, as can be seen from the greater discrete degree in the scatter plot (**Figure 1A**). These DEGs were subsequently classified into two categories, which included 510 up-regulated and 132 down-regulated genes (**Figure 1B**). Specifically, 378 and 271 genes were up-regulated by at least 1.5-fold (t-test p-value $\leq$ 0.05) in the 24- and 29 month-age mice respectively and 139 genes were consistently up-regulated (**Figure 1B**). 44 and 99 genes, respectively, were down-regulated by at least 1.5-fold, and 11 genes were collectively down-regulated (**Figure 1B**). The small overlap between the up and down regulated genes of the 24 and 29 months old mice is due to the variable gene expressions between these stages, indicating the aging is a dynamically changing process. It can be inferred that there are more genes up-regulated than those down-regulated. Moreover, the number of overlapping genes in the up-regulated group (139) is substantially larger than in the down-regulated group (11), illustrating that these common genes may play a general role during the process of hippocampal aging. Furthermore, DAVID (Huang da et al., 2009) functional annotation shows that the majority of the up-regulated genes are associated with the innate and inflammatory immune responses (**Figure 1C**). Interestingly, the immune response-related functions were also found to have significant changes during aging (High, 2004; Weinberger et al., 2008; Balivada et al., 2017), indicating that immune response-related genes may play important roles during the hippocampal aging process.

Immune Response-Associated Molecular Interaction Network during Hippocampal Aging

The above analysis demonstrates the importance of the immune response (**Figure 1C**) in hippocampal aging, however, the underlying mechanism of this genes network is still unknown. Thus, we investigated the molecular interactions (see section "Materials and Methods") of these genes in the BioGRID (Chatr-Aryamontri et al., 2017) and IntAct (Orchard et al., 2014) databases. The molecular interactions formed a network (**Figures 2A,B**) that included 97 nodes and 78 edges, with 24 immune response-related genes being up-regulated (indicated in red nodes) and interacted with its partners. Meanwhile, there are 12 single genes without interactions to others. Through interaction with these 24 genes, their partner genes (green nodes) may indirectly participate in the aging-related immune response. Notably, *Ywhae* is shown to be linked to many immune response-related genes (**Table 2**), forming a hub in the network (**Figure 2B**). Considering its connection to many immune response genes (**Figure 2B**), it can be speculated that *Ywhae* may not only have an influence in the nervous system (Baxter et al., 2002; Toyo-oka et al., 2003) but also in the immune response during the aging process.

We also investigated the interactions in human. The hub gene *Ywhae* of the above immune response associated molecular interaction network in mice was not observed in human (**Supplementary Figure S2**). However, this does not mean the immune response associated molecular interaction network is not conserved between human and mouse, since the interaction dataset of both human and mouse were incomplete, the overlapped interactions were limited.

Membrane Receptors Are Down-Regulated during the Hippocampal Aging Process

In addition to the 139 up-regulated genes (**Figure 1B**), 11 down-regulated genes were also observed, as shown in **Figure 3**. The majority of these genes, including *Ret*, *Sftpc*, *Gpr17*, *Tpsb2*, and *Glp1r* are associated with disulfide bonds that are crucial to protein structure (Butera et al., 2014), it has been reported that disulfide bonds may influence the function of proteins in the blood (Butera et al., 2014). In addition to disulfide bonds, cell membrane and receptor-associated genes were also observed, including *Ret*, *Lims2*, *Gpr17* and *Glp1r*. Membrane receptors embedded in the plasma membrane bind extracellular molecules and allow communication between the extracellular and intracellular space, meaning that environmental exposure may influence aging through transmembrane receptors (Bettio et al., 2017). As shown in **Figure 3**, *Sftpc*, for example, encodes the membrane protein surfactant-associated protein C (SP-C) (Glasser et al., 2013). It has been reported that *Sftpc* plays an important role in innate host defense, enhancing macrophage-mediated phagocytosis and clearing, and limiting inflammatory responses (Glasser et al., 2008), which are all important during aging (**Figure 1C**). Further, GPR17 is a marker for progenitor progression within the oligodendroglia lineage (Boda et al., 2011) and is expressed in all regions of the brain, indicating that downregulation of GPR17 in our network may interfere with normal brain function and lead to aging. In conclusion, these down-regulated genes take part in many different regulatory pathways together with the up-regulated genes. The current results demonstrate that the identified genes have important biological significance in hippocampal aging research.

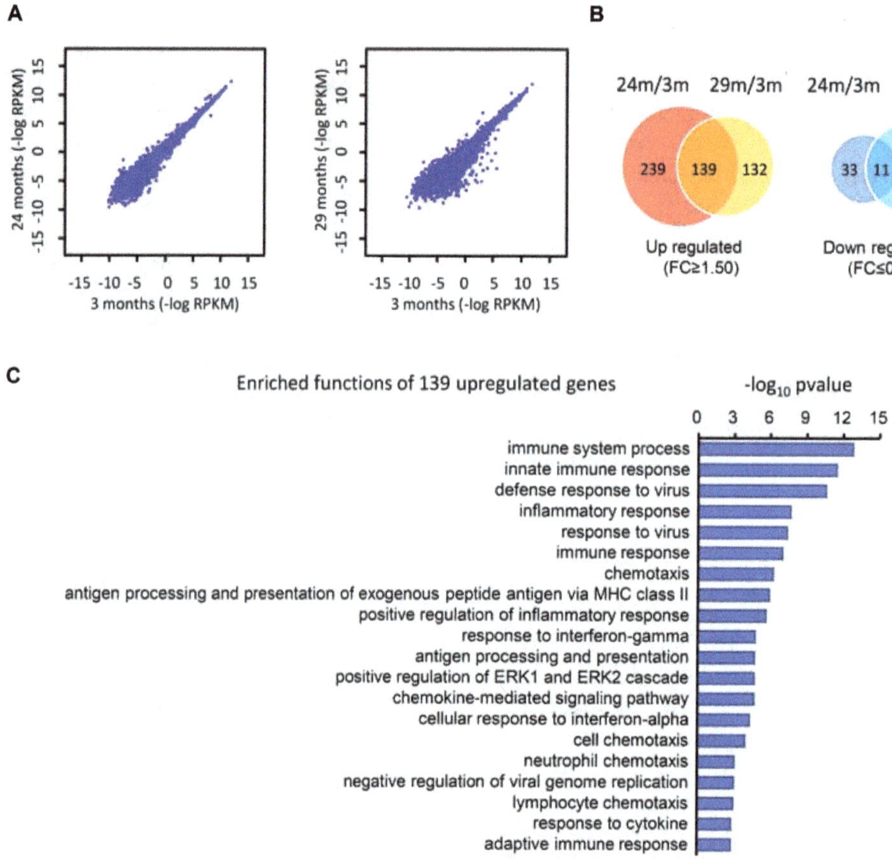

FIGURE 1 | Identification of the DEGs in the hippocampus of advanced-age mice (comparison of 3-, 24-, and 29-month-old mice). **(A)** The distribution of genes in 3 month- (3M) vs. 24 month- (24M, left panel) and 3M- vs. 29 month- (29M, right panel) old mice. Each dot in the diagrams corresponds to one gene. Compared with the left panel (24 month vs. 3 month), the right panel (29 month vs. 3 month) shows a greater degree of dispersion. **(B)** Venn diagrams show the overlap of up-regulated and down-regulated genes in the 24M/3M and 29M/3M groups, respectively. **(C)** The gene function enrichment analysis of 139 up-regulated genes using the DAVID platform.

DEGs during Hippocampal Aging Are Closely Related to Hippocampal Development

It has been reported that a change in hippocampal volume and structure is observed with age-related decline in learning and memory (Verbitsky et al., 2004; Arias-Cavieres et al., 2017; Bettio et al., 2017; Moret-Tatay et al., 2017). Additionally, in the aging hippocampus, neurobiological alterations have been clearly observed including those that alter intracellular signaling and gene expression, and cause neuroinflammation response (Bettio et al., 2017). In recent years, studies regarding of the age-related hippocampus have focused on cognitive decline and impaired memory (Arias-Cavieres et al., 2017; Bettio et al., 2017; Moret-Tatay et al., 2017). Several studies revealed the DEGs in hippocampus between young and the aging mice linked to the cognitive deficient (Xiong et al., 2000; Cheng et al., 2007; Thomas et al., 2014), synaptic plasticity (Dempsey and Ali, 2014) and various dysregulated pathways related to immune and inflammatory response (Landel et al., 2016). In order to understand how significantly up- and down-regulated genes are involved in hippocampal function during aging, their interactions were investigated using public databases and established a network using the privous methods (von Mering et al., 2003; Liu and Zhao, 2004). Interestingly, most of these genes interact with *Ywhae* (**Figure 4**), which is the hub gene in the immune response network during hippocampal aging (**Figure 2B**). Nucleotide polymorphisms in *Ywhae* would lead to abnormal hippocampal development (Kido et al., 2014), implying that *Ywhae* maybe influence the function of hippocampus during aging through certain signaling pathway. As shown in **Figure 4**, YWHAE interacts with VIM, which is an integral regulator of cell adhesion (Dave and Bayless, 2014), neurite extension (Dave and Bayless, 2014), and myelination (Triolo et al., 2012), suggesting that *Ywhae* may be involved in the regulation of neural function through *Vim* during aging. Furthermore, GFAP, which is expressed in astrocytes of the central nervous system (Eng and Ghirnikar, 1994), is the partner of YWHAE (**Figure 4**) and is important for the brain to accommodate

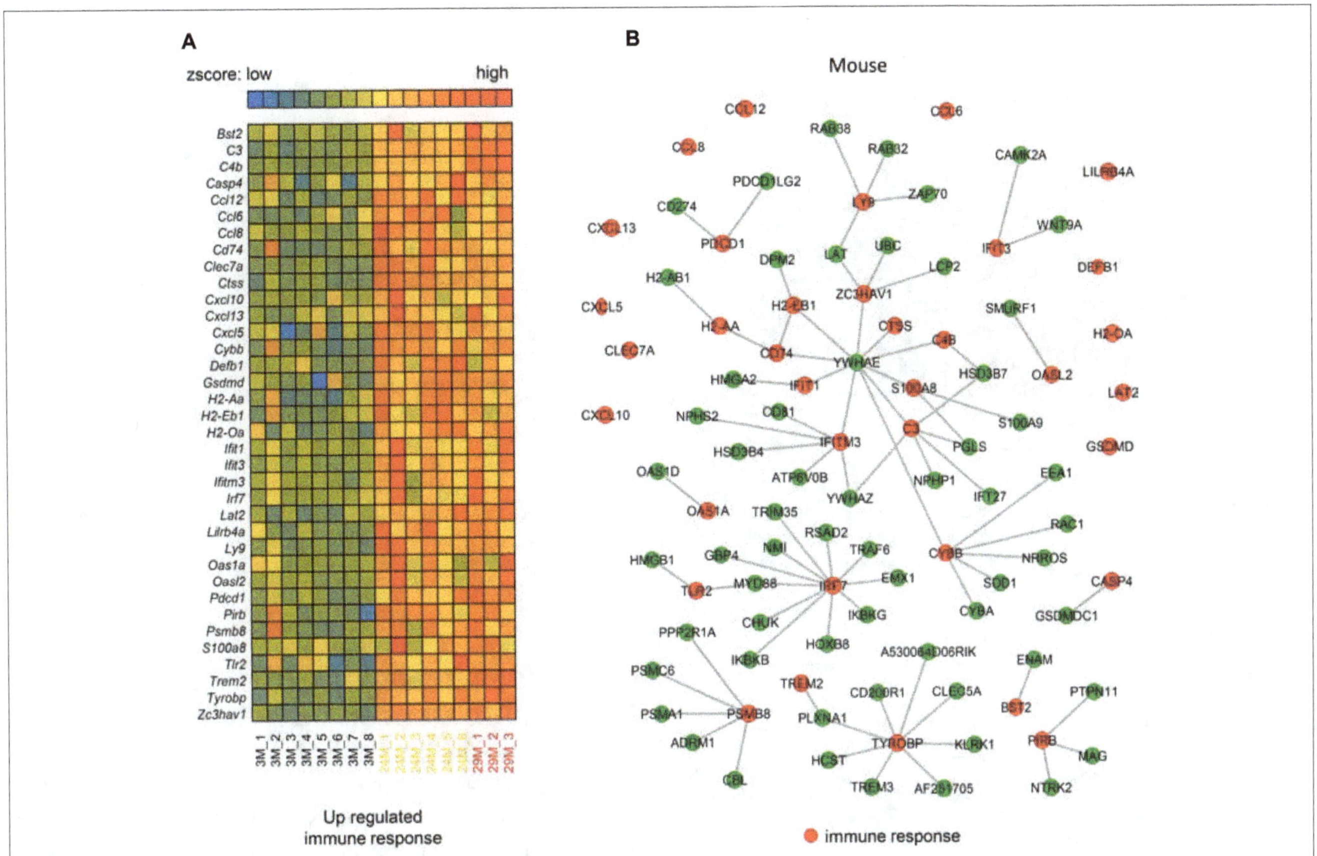

FIGURE 2 | The molecular interaction network of up-regulated genes that are associated with the immune response in mice. **(A)** Heatmap of up-regulated immune response-related genes in the 3 age groups of mice (3M, $n = 8$; 24M, $n = 6$; 29M, $n = 3$). Red represents genes with high expression and blue represents those with low expression. **(B)** The molecular interaction network related to the immune response (red nodes) and their partner genes (green nodes; 61). A gray line represents an interaction between two nodes.

neural activities or changes during development (Kim et al., 2011). Moreover, GFAP also plays a crucial role in neuroinflammation of central nervous system injury (Otani et al., 2003), which is consistent with the speculation that *Ywahe* is involved in the immune response (**Figure 2B**) together with GFAP. In conclusion, the interaction between YWHAE and its partners is obviously important for hippocampal development in the nervous system, implying an important function of these genes in the aging process. Interestingly, YWHAE interacts with C4B, which is up-regulated in aging mice and may influence the autoimmune process in diseases (Paul et al., 2002) or modulate interstitial inflammation (Welch et al., 2001), participating in the immune response. Moreover, C4B is also associated with ITGB2, which regulates the lineage distribution of hematopoietic cells in the blood and bone marrow (Gomez and Doerschuk, 2010), implying that *Ywhae* may be involved in different signaling pathways contributing to the aging process. Essentially, aging is a slow and complicated process that is accompanied by numerous changes in gene expression, especially those related to hippocampal development. This also partially explains why these genes influence hippocampal development and impair memory and learning ability, accelerating aging.

TABLE 2 | The up-regulated immune response-related genes that interacted with *Ywhae*.

Index	Gene symbol	Gene name
1	*Cybb*	Cytochrome b-245, beta polypeptide
2	*Ifit1*	Interferon-induced protein with tetratricopeptide repeats 1
3	*Ctss*	Cathepsin S
4	*Ifitm3*	Interferon induced transmembrane protein 3
5	*H2-Eb1*	Histocompatibility 2, class II antigen E beta
6	*Cd74*	CD74 antigen
7	*C4b*	Complement component 4B
8	*C3*	Complement component 3
9	*S100a8*	S100 calcium binding protein A8
10	*Zc3hav1*	Zinc finger CCCH type, antiviral 1

Verification of Gene Expression in the Interaction Network by QPCR

In order to further verify the expression of the genes in our current research (**Figure 4**), a number of genes in the network were randomly chosen and their expression was evaluated by qPCR in advanced-age and young mice. Hippocampal tissues were extracted from 4- and 20 month-old male mice and the

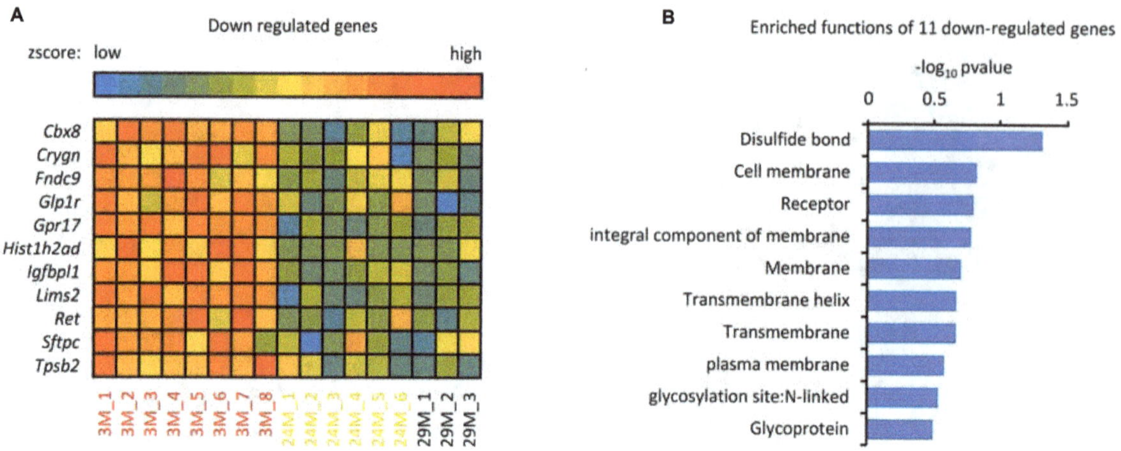

FIGURE 3 | The analysis of down-regulated genes in the hippocampus of advanced-age mice. **(A)** Heatmap of the 11 down-regulated genes in mice of different ages. The red and blue color spectrum represents high and low expressed genes, respectively (3M, $n = 8$; 24M, $n = 6$; 29M, $n = 3$). **(B)** Function enrichment analysis of 11 down-regulated genes. The DAVID platform was used for analysis; the 11 down-regulated genes have 10 functions exhibited in the column diagram. The majority of the genes were enriched in disulfide bonds.

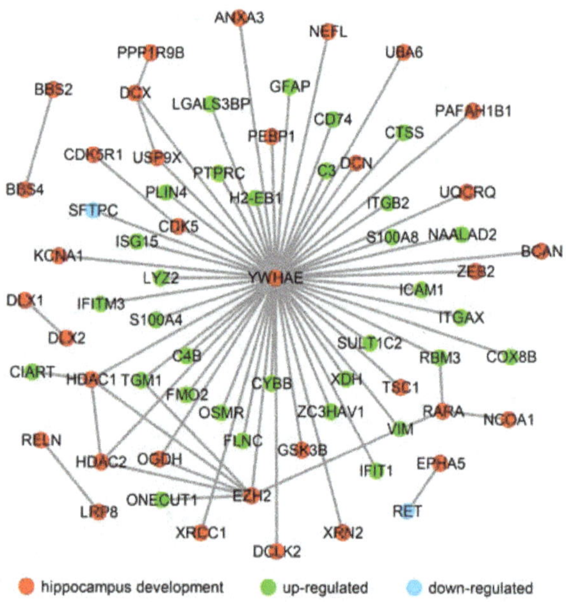

FIGURE 4 | The molecular interaction network revealed the up- and down-regulated genes that are strongly associated with hippocampal development. Hippocampal development genes (34) are marked with red nodes, and the 32 green nodes refer to the up-regulated genes in advanced-age compared with young mice. The down-regulated genes (*Sftpc* and *Ret*) are labeled with blue nodes.

mRNA amplified and compared with that of 4 month-old mice as a control. As shown in **Figure 5**, the majority of hippocampal development genes (*Dclk2*, *Rara*, *Hdac1*, and *Ezh2*) were up-regulated, with the exception of *Ywhae*. Moreover, *Tgm1*, *Cd74*, *Rbm3*, and *C4b* were also up-regulated compared with the young mice group, which is consistent with the network shown in **Figure 4**.

Interactions between YWHAE and Its Partners Are Conserved between Humans and Mice

In order to further explore the expression pattern of YWHAE (**Figure 4**) in humans, the expression of YWHAE was evaluated in human brain (**Figure 6A**). It was found that compared with the young human brain (15- and 25-years-old), YWHAE is down-regulated in the older human brain (69-year-old). These results are consistent with those seen in mice (**Figures 5A,B**). Furthermore, to evaluate whether the interaction network of YWHAE in mice is conserved in humans, qPCR was carried out to detect the mRNA expression in HEK293T cells after silencing *YWHAE*. The psiRNA-YWHAE vector was constructed to silence it in HEK293T cells. As shown in **Figures 6B,C**, with the obvious down-regulated expression of YWHAE, the mRNA levels of DCLK2, RARA, HDAC1, CD74, and RBM3 were significantly increased in HEK293T cells, which is consistent with the results observed in mice (**Figure 5A**). However, due to the diversity of gene expression in different species, not all genes exhibit the same expression pattern (**Figure 5A**). For instance, there is no significant difference in the expression of EZH2, TGM1, or C4B at the mRNA level. In conclusion, the gene expression pattern in humans is consistent with that in mice, indicating that the interaction network of YWHAE is conserved between humans and mice.

The Genes That Contribute to the Revitalization of Advanced-Age Mice Are Different from the Genes Which Are Induced by Aging

It has been reported that human umbilical cord plasma proteins can revitalize hippocampal function in advanced-age mice (Castellano et al., 2017), and that tissue inhibitor of metalloproteinases 2, which is an umbilical cord plasma

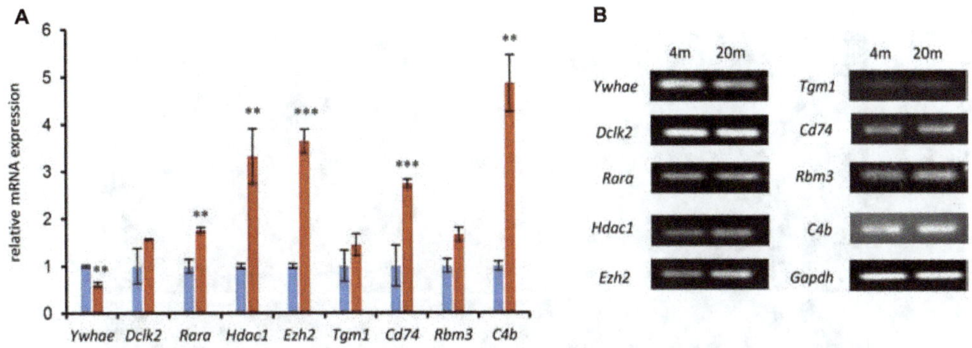

FIGURE 5 | The expression of nine randomly selected genes was identified by qPCR in the 4- and 20-month-old hippocampus. **(A)** The relative genes were randomly selected from the network in **Figure 4** and confirmed by qPCR. The blue columns refer to mRNA levels of these genes in 4-month-old mice, and the red columns represent those in the 20-month-old mice. The 4M mice are regarded as a control (***$p \le 0.001$; **$p \le 0.05$; two-sided t-test; $n \ge 3$). **(B)** QPCR products were mixed with DNA loading buffer and separated on a 1% agarose gel, detected using ethidium bromide staining, and visualized on a gel imaging system. GAPDH was used as control in each mRNA transcript. Data are represented as the mean ± SEM, $n \ge 3$. *$p \le 0.05$; **$p \le 0.01$; ***$p \le 0.001$.

protein, provides a reservoir for the neuroplasticity-promoting process. In order to gain more information regarding this process, microarray data from mice treated with human cord plasma (Castellano et al., 2017) were re-analyzed (**Figure 7**). In comparison with the PBS control, a total of 148 up-regulated and 190 down-regulated genes (up- or down-regulated by least 1.2-fold, p-value ≤ 0.05) were observed in the samples treated with human cord plasma (**Figure 7A**). Function enrichment analysis indicates that these genes exhibit functions including sensory perception, skeletal muscle cell differentiation, G protein-coupled receptor signaling, and detection of chemical, amino acid, hormone stimuli (**Figures 7B,C**). The hypothesis exists that changes in textural perception (Conroy et al., 2017) and loss of skeletal muscle stem cells with age may drive the degeneration of age-related neuromuscular junctions (Liu et al., 2017), indicating that genes with these functions (**Figures 7B,C**) may participate in aging progression or the revitalization progress. Interestingly, certain inflammatory- and immune response-related genes were also observed among those genes that were down-regulated (**Figure 7D**). However, no overlapping genes (**Figure 7E**) were found between those up-regulated during hippocampal aging (**Figure 2A**) and those down-regulated following treatment with human cord plasma (**Figure 7D**), indicating that mice adopt a different process to become younger after human umbilical cord plasma treatment. Our current data suggest that advanced-age mice do indeed benefit from these DEGs; however, it is noteworthy that this appears not to be a reverse process from advanced-age to young mice following treatment with umbilical cord plasma. In other words, the genes which contribute to the revitalization of advanced-age mice are different from the genes which are induced by aging during the normal hippocampal aging process.

DISCUSSION

In the present study, we identified DEGs between young and advanced-age mice, and found that the majority of the up-regulated genes in DEGs were enriched in the immune response process (**Figure 1**). Moreover, membrane receptor-associated genes were down-regulated (**Figure 3**). The analysis of the molecular interaction network indicated that *Ywhae* plays important roles during hippocampal aging (**Figure 2B**). Subsequently, we found that the interactions between YWHAE and its partners are conserved between humans and mice (**Figures 5, 6**). Furthermore, our results also showed that the genes that contribute to the revitalization of advanced-age mice are different from the genes induced by aging (**Figure 7**). Our data assigned novel roles for genes during hippocampal aging progression and provided further theoretical evidence for future studies exploring the underlying mechanisms of hippocampal aging and anti-aging-related disease therapy.

The progression of aging is complex. In order to explore the mystery of aging, many researchers have used microarray-related approaches to perform aging-related research (Bishop et al., 2010; Stilling et al., 2014). In addition, transcriptional profiles were focused on (Pawlowski et al., 2009; Bishop et al., 2010; Stilling et al., 2014) with different research purposes. In our current research, this common approach was also used to analyze DEGs associated with hippocampal aging progression. Some researchers have revealed that DEGs are closely linked to synaptic plasticity (Dempsey and Ali, 2014), cognitive impairment (Cheng et al., 2007; Park et al., 2015), age-associated spatial learning impairment (ASLI) (Uddin and Singh, 2013), degenerative diseases (Xiong et al., 2000; Kikuchi et al., 2013) and even various dysregulated pathways (Landel et al., 2016). In addition, it has been reported that the immune system is dysregulated in the aging brain (Patterson, 2015), which was consistent with our results that the majority of up-regulated genes were enriched in the immune response-related process (**Figure 1C**).

In order to build a reliable network, we collected interaction data from the BioGRID (Chatr-Aryamontri et al., 2017) and IntAct (Orchard et al., 2014) databases. These databases contain various experimentally validated interactions curated from published literature. Moreover, the networks we built were

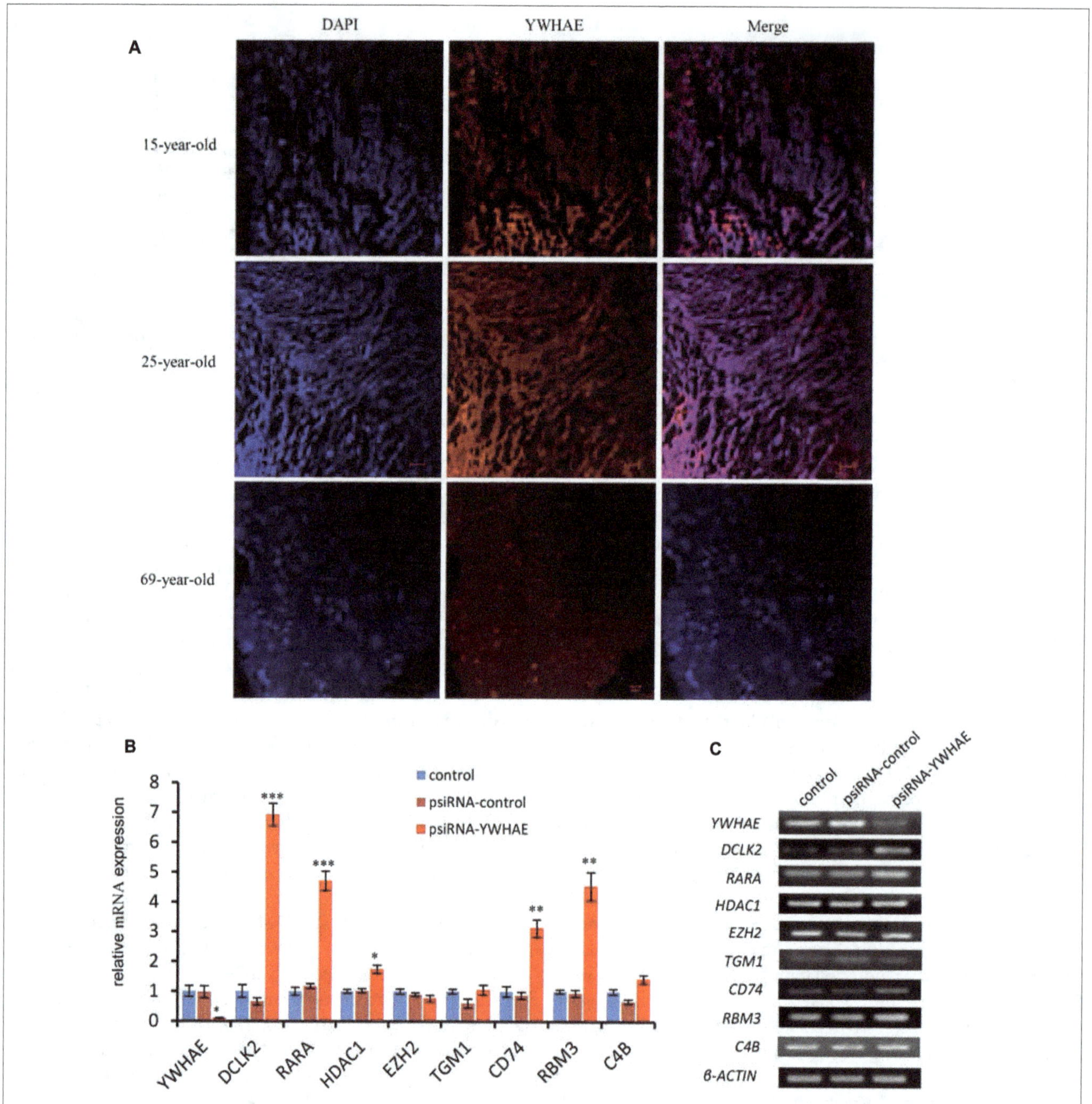

FIGURE 6 | The expression of *YWHAE* and its partner genes in the human brain and HEK293T cells. **(A)** Immunofluorescence staining showing the low expression of YWHAE in the aged human brain compared with young human brain (red:YWHAE, blue:nuclei). **(B)** QPCR of gene expression in HEK293T cells after silencing of the expression of *YWHAE*. The eight genes were assessed by qPCR in the control group, vehicle group (transfected with psiRNA-control), and silencing group (transfected with psiRNA-YWHAE), in HEK293T cells. **(C)** QPCR products were mixed with DNA loading buffer and separated on 2% agarose gels, detected using ethidium bromide staining, and visualized on a gel imaging system. β-actin was used as a loading control for each mRNA transcript. Data are represented as the mean ± SEM, $n \geq 3$. $^{*}p \leq 0.05$; $^{**}p \leq 0.01$; $^{***}p \leq 0.001$.

first-neighbor networks, since the first neighbors represent the most reliable interactions. The second-neighbor network may contain many genes and interactions that are directly linked to the first neighbors but not the genes that we are interested in (immune response or hippocampal development), thus, the center of the network may be shifted. However, we also constructed a second-neighbor network for mice based on the immune response-related genes (**Supplementary Figure S3**). We found that the network is huge, containing 5,283 genes and 19,641 interactions. Link degree analysis of each node in

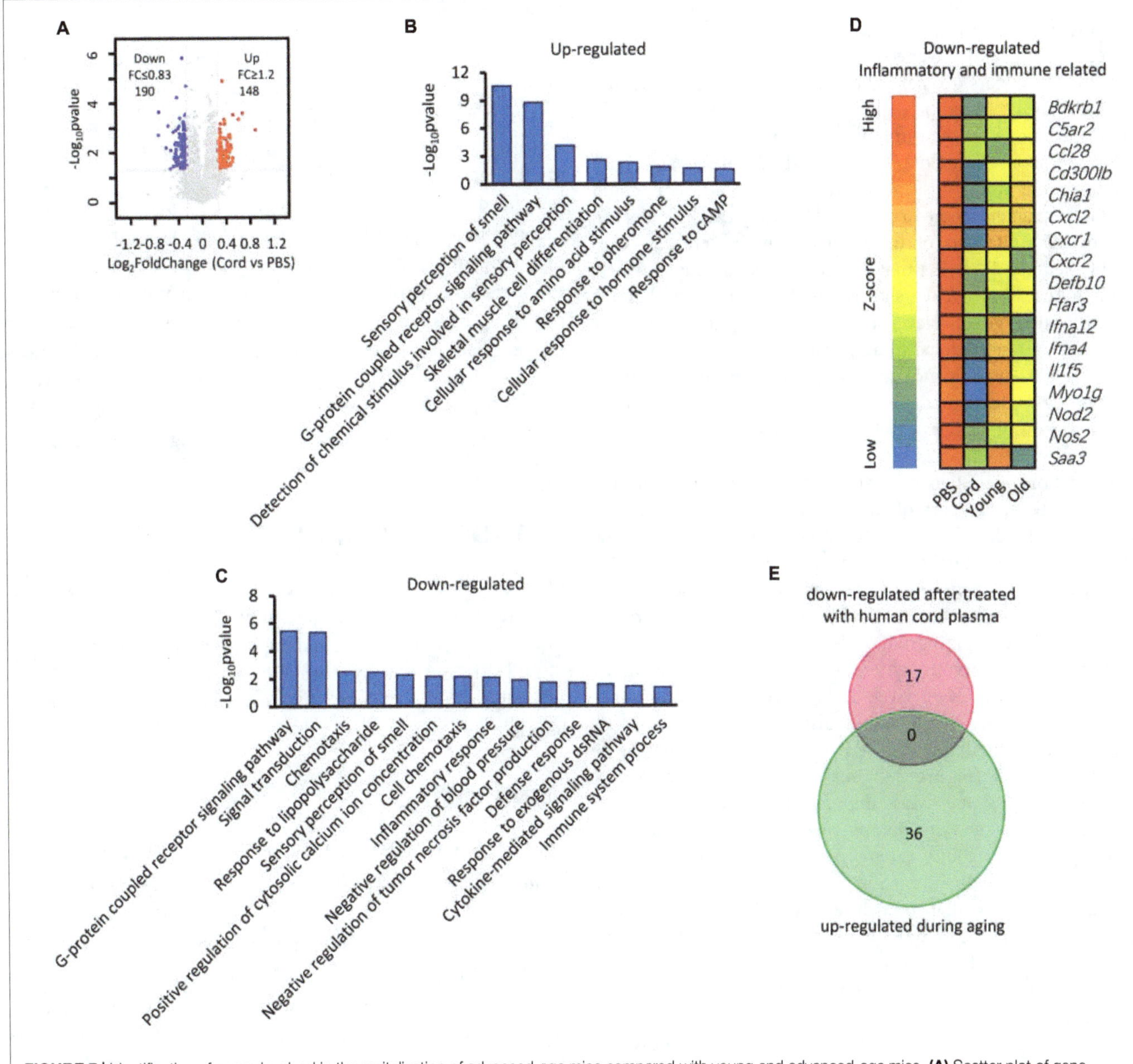

FIGURE 7 | Identification of genes involved in the revitalization of advanced-age mice compared with young and advanced-age mice. **(A)** Scatter plot of gene expression following treatment with umbilical cord blood protein or PBS. Each point refers to one gene. **(B,C)** The DAVID platform was used to analyze the function of DEGs. **(D)** Heatmap of down-regulated genes related to inflammatory and immune responses. The first group is treated with PBS and regarded as a control, the second is treated with human umbilical cord protein, and the remaining two groups are the young and the advanced-age group, respectively. **(E)** Venn diagrams show the overlap of inflammatory and immune response-related genes that up-regulated during aging and those down-regulated following treatment with human cord plasma.

the network indicated that *Ywhae, Eed, Ywhaz, Ubc, Hsd3b4, Pgls, Hsd3b7, Ywhab, Hmga2,* and *Dlg4* were the top 10 genes with the most interactions with other genes. YWHAE still had the most links with other genes, which is the similar phenomenon as seen in **Figure 2B**. Most interestingly, YWHAE, YWHAZ, and YWHAB belong to the 14-3-3 protein family, which mediate signal transduction by binding to phosphoserine-containing proteins (Conklin et al., 1995). These results implied that the 14-3-3 protein family has a potential role during the hippocampal aging process. We also checked the conversation of the hippocampus development associated network in human and mice (**Supplementary Figure S4** and **Figure 4**). In mice, *Ywhae* was linked to many up-regulated DEGs (**Figure 4**, green nodes), indicating *Ywhae* may be involved in the regulation of those genes (green nodes) during hippocampus development. However, the same situation was not observed in human (**Supplementary Figure S4**). Considering the incompletion of the interaction data deposited in both BioGRID and IntAct, this may be due to the largely un-delineated overlapping of the two datasets.

Consistent with the previous studies (Stilling et al., 2014), the constructed network implied that the up-regulated DEGs between young and advanced-age mice (**Figure 2A**) interact with their partners to participate in the immune response and facilitate hippocampal aging progression (**Figure 2B**). As people become older, their immune systems become weaker and antibody responses are slow (Montecino-Rodriguez et al., 2013), which induces many dysfunctions (Weigle, 1989). This could explain why older people are more likely to get sick. However, due to the limitations of the database, there were 12 genes (Supplementary Table S2) that did not appear in this network, meaning that these genes showed no functional associations with the other genes. Nevertheless, this does not mean that these genes are not related to hippocampal aging. For instance, CXCL5, a CXC-type chemokine, has been reported to be secreted by aging prostate stroma, implying its important function in aging progression (Begley et al., 2008). As shown in **Figure 3**, five down-regulated genes are associated with disulfide bonds, and oxidation of protein sulfhydryl groups to disulfide groups occurs as a normal part of human aging (Takemoto, 1996), indicating that disulfide bonds play an important unclarified role in aging, and further research is needed to explore the underlying mechanisms. In addition, cell membrane and receptor were also enriched in **Figure 3B**. For instance, *Ret* is a crucial gene that plays an important role in the development and function of the nervous system (Gabreski et al., 2016), as well as driving HSCs survival. Ablation of *Ret* cannot only impair the number of HSCs but also influences its normal differentiation potential (Fonseca-Pereira et al., 2014). The down-regulation of *Ret* (**Figure 3A**) implies that HSC function is impaired during aging. Most importantly, the enrichment of many down-regulated membrane proteins may also indicate weaker perception ability to environmental exposure of older people, since many membrane proteins participate in different signaling pathways that transduce extracellular information across the plasma membrane. In conclusion, this indicates that these genes, although enriched in different functions, may work together to promote hippocampal aging through regulating cell communication.

Our results also showed that no overlapping genes (**Figure 7E**) were found between those up-regulated during hippocampal aging (**Figure 2A**) and those down-regulated following treatment with human cord plasma (**Figure 7D**), indicating that the revitalization induced by the treatment of human umbilical cord blood plasma protein is not a simple reverse process of natural aging progression. We noticed that the mice strains from the other research studies are different. Immuno-deficient (NSG) mice were chosen for the injection experiment, since the mice can receive intravenous injection of human plasma without an adverse immune response (Castellano et al., 2017), while, C57BL/6J mice were used for detecting gene expression differences in the other research. This likely provides an explanation for the lack of overlap in gene expression. Another possibility for our results could be that the mice treated with PBS and human cord plasma was 14-months-old rather than 24- or 29-months-old. The distance in age of the mice may have led to differences in gene expression.

CONCLUSION

The present study provides a more comprehensive analysis of aging and anti-aging treatment using a biological systems approach. Our data suggested that a large number of immune and inflammatory response-related genes were up-regulated in the aged hippocampus, and that membrane receptor-associated genes were down-regulated. Moreover, *Ywhae* in the predicted network may be assigned novel roles during hippocampal aging progression. The results also implied that the revitalization of advanced-age mice may be not a simple reverse process of normal aging progression. Considering the association of aging-related diseases such as Alzheimer's disease, hypertension, and cancer, our study provides further theoretic evidence for future studies exploring the underlying mechanisms of aging and anti-aging-related disease therapy.

AUTHOR CONTRIBUTIONS

JW and TW contributed to the design, analysis, and interpretation of data for the study. JW and QL drafted the work, interpreted the data and conducted the experiments. QL, FZ, JL, WL, and KW conducted the experiments. YK, TW, and YG collected data. JX and TQW finally approved the version to be published.

FUNDING

This work was sponsored by the National Natural Science Foundation of China (Grant Number: 31500827), Young Eastern Scholar (Grant Number: QD2015033), the Natural Science Foundation of Shanghai (Grant Number: 14ZR1414400, 17ZR1409900), the National Natural Science Foundation of China (81571345; 81471162; 31601163), the Science and Technology Commission of Shanghai (Grant Number: 14JC1402400), and China Postdoctoral Science Foundation (Grant Number: 2016M601661).

ACKNOWLEDGMENT

The authors would like to thank Dr. Natalie Ward (Medical College of Wisconsin, Wauwatosa, WI, United States) for editing this manuscript.

SUPPLEMENTARY MATERIAL

FIGURE S1 | The interfere fragment of *YWHAE* was successfully inserted into the vector of psiRNA-hH1neo. **(A)** The diagram of plasmids construction. The sequence of YWHAE was marked in yellow. **(B)** The plasmids of psiRNA-hH1neo and psiRNA-YWHAE were identified by 0.6% agarose gels. The arrow shows the recombinant plasmid. **(C)** The product of plasmids that were cut by single enzyme

(Xba I) was identified by 0.6% agarose gels. The arrows shows the sequence was successfully inserted into psiRNA-hH1neo.

FIGURE S2 | The molecular interaction network related to the immune response in human. Red nodes represent the immune responds genes. A gray line represents an interaction between two nodes.

FIGURE S3 | The second neighbor molecular interaction network related to the immune response in mice.

FIGURE S4 | The human molecular interaction network involved in hippocampus development. Hippocampus development associate genes (37) are marked with red nodes. The 13 green nodes refer to the homologous DEGs in the mice.

REFERENCES

Arias-Cavieres, A., Adasme, T., Sanchez, G., Munoz, P., and Hidalgo, C. (2017). Aging impairs hippocampal- dependent recognition memory and LTP and prevents the associated RyR up-regulation. *Front. Aging Neurosci.* 9:111. doi: 10.3389/fnagi.2017.00111

Balivada, S., Ganta, C. K., Zhang, Y., Pawar, H. N., Ortiz, R. J., Becker, K. G., et al. (2017). Microarray analysis of aging-associated immune system alterations in the rostral ventrolateral medulla of F344 rats. *Physiol. Genomics* 49, 400–415. doi: 10.1152/physiolgenomics.00131.2016

Baxter, H. C., Liu, W. G., Forster, J. L., Aitken, A., and Fraser, J. R. (2002). Immunolocalisation of 14-3-3 isoforms in normal and scrapie-infected murine brain. *Neuroscience* 109, 5–14. doi: 10.1016/S0306-4522(01)00492-4

Begley, L. A., Kasina, S., MacDonald, J., and Macoska, J. A. (2008). The inflammatory microenvironment of the aging prostate facilitates cellular proliferation and hypertrophy. *Cytokine* 43, 194–199. doi: 10.1016/j.cyto.2008.05.012

Bettio, L. E. B., Rajendran, L., and Gil-Mohapel, J. (2017). The effects of aging in the hippocampus and cognitive decline. *Neurosci. Biobehav. Rev.* 79, 66–86. doi: 10.1016/j.neubiorev.2017.04.030

Bishop, N. A., Lu, T., and Yankner, B. A. (2010). Neural mechanisms of ageing and cognitive decline. *Nature* 464, 529–535. doi: 10.1038/nature08983

Boda, E., Vigano, F., Rosa, P., Fumagalli, M., Labat-Gest, V., Tempia, F., et al. (2011). The GPR17 receptor in NG2 expressing cells: focus on in vivo cell maturation and participation in acute trauma and chronic damage. *Glia* 59, 1958–1973. doi: 10.1002/glia.21237

Bolger, A. M., Lohse, M., and Usadel, B. (2014). Trimmomatic: a flexible trimmer for Illumina sequence data. *Bioinformatics* 30, 2114–2120. doi: 10.1093/bioinformatics/btu170

Boutet, E., Lieberherr, D., Tognolli, M., Schneider, M., Bansal, P., Bridge, A. J., et al. (2016). UniProtKB/Swiss-Prot, the manually annotated section of the UniProt knowledgebase: how to use the entry view. *Methods Mol. Biol.* 1374, 23–54. doi: 10.1007/978-1-4939-3167-5_2

Burke, S. N., and Barnes, C. A. (2006). Neural plasticity in the ageing brain. *Nat. Rev. Neurosci.* 7, 30–40. doi: 10.1038/nrn1809

Butera, D., Cook, K. M., Chiu, J., Wong, J. W., and Hogg, P. J. (2014). Control of blood proteins by functional disulfide bonds. *Blood* 123, 2000–2007. doi: 10.1182/blood-2014-01-549816

Castellano, J. M., Mosher, K. I., Abbey, R. J., McBride, A. A., James, M. L., Berdnik, D., et al. (2017). Human umbilical cord plasma proteins revitalize hippocampal function in aged mice. *Nature* 544, 488–492. doi: 10.1038/nature22067

Chatr-Aryamontri, A., Oughtred, R., Boucher, L., Rust, J., Chang, C., Kolas, N., et al. (2017). The BioGRID interaction database: 2017 update. *Nucleic Acids Res.* 45, D369–D379. doi: 10.1093/nar/gkw1102

Cheng, X. R., Zhou, W. X., Zhang, Y. X., Zhou, D. S., Yang, R. F., and Chen, L. F. (2007). Differential gene expression profiles in the hippocampus of senescence-accelerated mouse. *Neurobiol. Aging* 28, 497–506. doi: 10.1016/j.neurobiolaging.2006.02.004

Conklin, D. S., Galaktionov, K., and Beach, D. (1995). 14-3-3 proteins associate with cdc25 phosphatases. *Proc. Natl. Acad. Sci. U.S.A.* 92, 7892–7896. doi: 10.1073/pnas.92.17.7892

Conroy, P. M., Sullivan, M. G., Hamill, R. M., and Kerry, J. P. (2017). Sensory capability of young, middle-aged and elderly Irish assessors to identify beef steaks of varying texture. *Meat Sci.* 132, 125–130. doi: 10.1016/j.meatsci.2017.05.020

Dave, J. M., and Bayless, K. J. (2014). Vimentin as an integral regulator of cell adhesion and endothelial sprouting. *Microcirculation* 21, 333–344. doi: 10.1111/micc.12111

Dempsey, K. M., and Ali, H. H. (2014). Identifying aging-related genes in mouse hippocampus using gateway nodes. *BMC Syst. Biol.* 8:62. doi: 10.1186/1752-0509-8-62

Di Benedetto, S., Muller, L., Wenger, E., Duzel, S., and Pawelec, G. (2017). Contribution of neuroinflammation and immunity to brain aging and the mitigating effects of physical and cognitive interventions. *Neurosci. Biobehav. Rev.* 75, 114–128. doi: 10.1016/j.neubiorev.2017.01.044

Driscoll, I., Hamilton, D. A., Petropoulos, H., Yeo, R. A., Brooks, W. M., Baumgartner, R. N., et al. (2003). The aging hippocampus: cognitive, biochemical and structural findings. *Cereb. Cortex* 13, 1344–1351. doi: 10.1093/cercor/bhg081

Eng, L. F., and Ghirnikar, R. S. (1994). GFAP and astrogliosis. *Brain Pathol.* 4, 229–237. doi: 10.1111/j.1750-3639.1994.tb00838.x

Fonseca-Pereira, D., Arroz-Madeira, S., Rodrigues-Campos, M., Barbosa, I. A., Domingues, R. G., Bento, T., et al. (2014). The neurotrophic factor receptor RET drives haematopoietic stem cell survival and function. *Nature* 514, 98–101. doi: 10.1038/nature13498

Gabreski, N. A., Vaghasia, J. K., Novakova, S. S., McDonald, N. Q., and Pierchala, B. A. (2016). Exon skipping in the RET gene encodes novel isoforms that differentially regulate RET protein signal transduction. *J. Biol. Chem.* 291, 16249–16262. doi: 10.1074/jbc.M115.709675

Ghika, J. (2008). Paleoneurology: neurodegenerative diseases are age-related diseases of specific brain regions recently developed by Homo sapiens. *Med. Hypotheses* 71, 788–801. doi: 10.1016/j.mehy.2008.05.034

Glasser, S. W., Maxfield, M. D., Ruetschilling, T. L., Akinbi, H. T., Baatz, J. E., Kitzmiller, J. A., et al. (2013). Persistence of LPS-induced lung inflammation in surfactant protein-C-deficient mice. *Am. J. Respir. Cell Mol. Biol.* 49, 845–854. doi: 10.1165/rcmb.2012-0374OC

Glasser, S. W., Senft, A. P., Whitsett, J. A., Maxfield, M. D., Ross, G. F., Richardson, T. R., et al. (2008). Macrophage dysfunction and susceptibility to pulmonary *Pseudomonas aeruginosa* infection in surfactant protein C-deficient mice. *J. Immunol.* 181, 621–628. doi: 10.4049/jimmunol.181.1.621

Gomez, J. C., and Doerschuk, C. M. (2010). The role of CD18 in the production and release of neutrophils from the bone marrow. *Lab. Invest.* 90, 599–610. doi: 10.1038/labinvest.2010.4

Hampson, R. E., Simeral, J. D., and Deadwyler, S. A. (1999). Distribution of spatial and nonspatial information in dorsal hippocampus. *Nature* 402, 610–614. doi: 10.1038/45154

High, K. P. (2004). Infection as a cause of age-related morbidity and mortality. *Ageing Res. Rev.* 3, 1–14. doi: 10.1016/j.arr.2003.08.001

Huang da, W., Sherman, B. T., and Lempicki, R. A. (2009). Systematic and integrative analysis of large gene lists using DAVID bioinformatics resources. *Nat. Protoc.* 4, 44–57. doi: 10.1038/nprot.2008.211

Katsimpardi, L., Litterman, N. K., Schein, P. A., Miller, C. M., Loffredo, F. S., Wojtkiewicz, G. R., et al. (2014). Vascular and neurogenic rejuvenation of the aging mouse brain by young systemic factors. *Science* 344, 630–634. doi: 10.1126/science.1251141

Keuker, J. I., Luiten, P. G., and Fuchs, E. (2003). Preservation of hippocampal neuron numbers in aged rhesus monkeys. *Neurobiol. Aging* 24, 157–165. doi: 10.1016/S0197-4580(02)00062-3

Kido, M., Nakamura, Y., Nemoto, K., Takahashi, T., Aleksic, B., Furuichi, A., et al. (2014). The polymorphism of YWHAE, a gene encoding 14-3-3epsilon, and brain morphology in schizophrenia: a voxel-based morphometric study. *PLOS ONE* 9:e103571. doi: 10.1371/journal.pone.0103571

Kikuchi, M., Ogishima, S., Miyamoto, T., Miyashita, A., Kuwano, R., Nakaya, J., et al. (2013). Identification of unstable network modules reveals disease modules associated with the progression of Alzheimer's disease. *PLOS ONE* 8:e76162. doi: 10.1371/journal.pone.0076162

Kim, D., Langmead, B., and Salzberg, S. L. (2015). HISAT: a fast spliced aligner with low memory requirements. *Nat. Methods* 12, 357–360. doi: 10.1038/nmeth.3317

Kim, J. S., Kim, J., Kim, Y., Yang, M., Jang, H., Kang, S., et al. (2011). Differential patterns of nestin and glial fibrillary acidic protein expression in mouse hippocampus during postnatal development. *J. Vet. Sci.* 12, 1–6. doi: 10.4142/jvs.2011.12.1.1

Landel, V., Millet, P., Baranger, K., Loriod, B., and Feron, F. (2016). Vitamin D interacts with Esr1 and Igf1 to regulate molecular pathways relevant to Alzheimer's disease. *Mol. Neurodegener.* 11, 22. doi: 10.1186/s13024-016-0087-2

Liu, W., Klose, A., Forman, S., Paris, N. D., Wei-LaPierre, L., Cortes-Lopez, M., et al. (2017). Loss of adult skeletal muscle stem cells drives age-related neuromuscular junction degeneration. *Elife* 6, 1–15. doi: 10.7554/eLife.26464

Liu, Y., and Zhao, H. (2004). A computational approach for ordering signal transduction pathway components from genomics and proteomics Data. *BMC Bioinformatics* 5:158.

Loffredo, F. S., Steinhauser, M. L., Jay, S. M., Gannon, J., Pancoast, J. R., Yalamanchi, P., et al. (2013). Growth differentiation factor 11 is a circulating factor that reverses age-related cardiac hypertrophy. *Cell* 153, 828–839. doi: 10.1016/j.cell.2013.04.015

Lopez-Otin, C., Blasco, M. A., Partridge, L., Serrano, M., and Kroemer, G. (2013). The hallmarks of aging. *Cell* 153, 1194–1217. doi: 10.1016/j.cell.2013.05.039

Mani, R. B., Lohr, J. B., and Jeste, D. V. (1986). Hippocampal pyramidal cells and aging in the human: a quantitative study of neuronal loss in sectors CA1 to CA4. *Exp. Neurol.* 94, 29–40. doi: 10.1016/0014-4886(86)90269-4

Miller, D. B., and O'Callaghan, J. O. (2003). Effects of aging and stress on hippocampal structure and function. *Metabolism* 52(10 Suppl. 2), 17–21. doi: 10.1016/S0026-0495(03)00296-8

Montecino-Rodriguez, E., Berent-Maoz, B., and Dorshkind, K. (2013). Causes, consequences, and reversal of immune system aging. *J. Clin. Invest.* 123, 958–965. doi: 10.1172/JCI64096

Moret-Tatay, C., Lemus- Zuniga, L. G., Tortosa, D. A., Gamermann, D., Vazquez-Martinez, A., Navarro-Pardo, E., et al. (2017). Age slowing down in detection and visual discrimination under varying presentation times. *Scand. J. Psychol.* 58, 304–311. doi: 10.1111/sjop.12372

Moser, M. B., and Moser, E. I. (1998). Functional differentiation in the hippocampus. *Hippocampus* 8, 608–619. doi: 10.1002/(SICI)1098-1063(1998)8:6<608::AID-HIPO3>3.0.CO;2-7

Nikodemova, M., Small, A. L., Kimyon, R. S., and Watters, J. J. (2016). Age-dependent differences in microglial responses to systemic inflammation are evident as early as middle age. *Physiol. Genomics* 48, 336–344. doi: 10.1152/physiolgenomics.00129.2015

Orchard, S., Ammari, M., Aranda, B., Breuza, L., Briganti, L., Broackes-Carter, F., et al. (2014). The MIntAct project–IntAct as a common curation platform for 11 molecular interaction databases. *Nucleic Acids Res.* 42, D358–D363. doi: 10.1093/nar/gkt1115

Otani, N., Nawashiro, H., Nomura, N., Fukui, S., Tsuzuki, N., Ishihara, S., et al. (2003). A role of glial fibrillary acidic protein in hippocampal degeneration after cerebral trauma or kainate-induced seizure. *Acta Neurochir. Suppl.* 86, 267–269. doi: 10.1007/978-3-7091-0651-8_58

Park, C. S., Valomon, A., and Welzl, H. (2015). Integrative transcriptome profiling of cognitive aging and its preservation through Ser/Thr protein phosphatase regulation. *PLOS ONE* 10:e0130891. doi: 10.1371/journal.pone.0130891

Patel, P., Lockey, R. F., and Kolliputi, N. (2015). Can inflammation regulate systemic aging? *Exp. Gerontol.* 67, 1–2. doi: 10.1016/j.exger.2015.04.011

Patterson, S. L. (2015). Immune dysregulation and cognitive vulnerability in the aging brain: interactions of microglia, IL-1β, BDNF and synaptic plasticity. *Neuropharmacology* 96(Pt A), 11–18. doi: 10.1016/j.neuropharm.2014.12.020

Paul, E., Pozdnyakova, O. O., Mitchell, E., and Carroll, M. C. (2002). Anti-DNA autoreactivity in C4-deficient mice. *Eur. J. Immunol.* 32, 2672–2679. doi: 10.1002/1521-4141(200209)32:9<2672::AID-IMMU2672>3.0.CO;2-X

Pawlowski, T. L., Bellush, L. L., Wright, A. W., Walker, J. P., Colvin, R. A., and Huentelman, M. J. (2009). Hippocampal gene expression changes during age-related cognitive decline. *Brain Res.* 1256, 101–110. doi: 10.1016/j.brainres.2008.12.039

Quinlan, A. R. (2014). BEDTools: the swiss-army tool for genome feature analysis. *Curr. Protoc. Bioinformatics* 47, 11.12.1–11.12.34. doi: 10.1002/0471250953.bi1112s47

Regulski, M. J. (2017). Cellular senescence: What, Why, and How. *Wounds* 29, 168–174.

Shannon, P., Markiel, A., Ozier, O., Baliga, N. S., Wang, J. T., Ramage, D., et al. (2003). Cytoscape: a software environment for integrated models of biomolecular interaction networks. *Genome Res.* 13, 2498–2504. doi: 10.1101/gr.1239303

Sinha, M., Jang, Y. C., Oh, J., Khong, D., Wu, E. Y., Manohar, R., et al. (2014). Restoring systemic GDF11 levels reverses age-related dysfunction in mouse skeletal muscle. *Science* 344, 649–652. doi: 10.1126/science.1251152

Stilling, R. M., Benito, E., Gertig, M., Barth, J., Capece, V., Burkhardt, S., et al. (2014). De-regulation of gene expression and alternative splicing affects distinct cellular pathways in the aging hippocampus. *Front. Cell Neurosci.* 8:373. doi: 10.3389/fncel.2014.00373

Takemoto, L. (1996). Increase in the intramolecular disulfide bonding of alpha-A crystallin during aging of the human lens. *Exp. Eye Res.* 63, 585–590. doi: 10.1006/exer.1996.0149

Thomas, J., Garg, M. L., and Smith, D. W. (2014). Dietary resveratrol supplementation normalizes gene expression in the hippocampus of streptozotocin-induced diabetic C57Bl/6 mice. *J. Nutr. Biochem.* 25, 313–318. doi: 10.1016/j.jnutbio.2013.11.005

Toyo-oka, K., Shionoya, A., Gambello, M. J., Cardoso, C., Leventer, R., Ward, H. L., et al. (2003). 14-3-3epsilon is important for neuronal migration by binding to NUDEL: a molecular explanation for Miller-Dieker syndrome. *Nat. Genet.* 34, 274–285. doi: 10.1038/ng1169

Triolo, D., Dina, G., Taveggia, C., Vaccari, I., Porrello, E., Rivellini, C., et al. (2012). Vimentin regulates peripheral nerve myelination. *Development* 139, 1359–1367. doi: 10.1242/dev.072371

Uddin, R. K., and Singh, S. M. (2013). Hippocampal gene expression meta-analysis identifies aging and age-associated spatial learning impairment (ASLI) genes and pathways. *PLOS ONE* 8:e69768. doi: 10.1371/journal.pone.0069768

Verbitsky, M., Yonan, A. L., Malleret, G., Kandel, E. R., Gilliam, T. C., and Pavlidis, P. (2004). Altered hippocampal transcript profile accompanies an age-related spatial memory deficit in mice. *Learn. Mem.* 11, 253–260. doi: 10.1101/lm.68204

von Mering, C., Huynen, M., Jaeggi, D., Schmidt, S., Bork, P., and Snel, B. (2003). STRING: a database of predicted functional associations between proteins. *Nucleic Acids Res.* 31, 258–261. doi: 10.1093/nar/gkg034

Weigle, W. O. (1989). Effects of aging on the immune system. *Hosp. Pract. (Off Ed).* 24, 112–119. doi: 10.1080/21548331.1989.11703827

Weinberger, B., Herndler-Brandstetter, D., Schwanninger, A., Weiskopf, D., and Grubeck-Loebenstein, B. (2008). Biology of immune responses to vaccines in elderly persons. *Clin. Infect. Dis.* 46, 1078–1084. doi: 10.1086/529197

Welch, T. R., Frenzke, M., Carroll, M. C., and Witte, D. P. (2001). Evidence of a role for C4 in modulating interstitial inflammation in experimental glomerulonephritis. *Clin. Immunol.* 101, 366–370. doi: 10.1006/clim.2001.5125

West, M. J., Coleman, P. D., Flood, D. G., and Troncoso, J. C. (1994). Differences in the pattern of hippocampal neuronal loss in normal ageing and Alzheimer's disease. *Lancet* 344, 769–772. doi: 10.1016/S0140-6736(94)92338-8

Xiong, Y., Liu, X., Wang, Y., and Du, Y. (2000). Cloning of cytidine triphosphate: phosphocholine cytidylyltransferase mRNA upregulated by a neuropeptide arginine-vasopressin((4-8)) in rat hippocampus. *Neurosci. Lett.* 283, 129–132. doi: 10.1016/S0304-3940(00)00929-0

12

White Matter Deterioration may Foreshadow Impairment of Emotional Valence Determination in Early-Stage Dementia of the Alzheimer Type

Ravi Rajmohan[1], Ronald C. Anderson[2], Dan Fang[3], Austin G. Meyer[4], Pavis Laengvejkal[5], Parunyou Julayanont[5], Greg Hannabas[6], Kitten Linton[7], John Culberson[7], Hafiz M. R. Khan[6], John De Toledo[5], P. Hemachandra Reddy[1,8,9,10] and Michael O'Boyle[1,3]*

[1]Department of Pharmacology and Neuroscience, Texas Tech University Health Sciences Center, Lubbock, TX, USA, [2]Department of Electrical and Computer Engineering, Texas Tech University, Lubbock, TX, USA, [3]Department of Human Development and Family Studies, Texas Tech University, Lubbock, TX, USA, [4]School of Medicine, Texas Tech University Health Sciences Center, Lubbock, TX, USA, [5]Department of Neurology, Texas Tech University Health Sciences Center, Lubbock, TX, USA, [6]Department of Public Health, Texas Tech University Health Sciences Center, Lubbock, TX, USA, [7]Department of Family Medicine, Texas Tech University Health Sciences Center, Lubbock, TX, USA, [8]Garrison Institute on Aging, Texas Tech University Health Sciences Center, Lubbock, TX, USA, [9]Cell Biology and Biochemistry, Texas Tech University Health Sciences Center, Lubbock, TX, USA, [10]Speech, Language and Hearing Sciences, Texas Tech University Health Sciences Center, Lubbock, TX, USA

***Correspondence:**
Ravi Rajmohan
ravi.rajmohan@ttuhsc.edu

In Alzheimer Disease (AD), non-verbal skills often remain intact for far longer than verbally mediated processes. Four (1 female, 3 males) participants with early-stage Clinically Diagnosed Dementia of the Alzheimer Type (CDDAT) and eight neurotypicals (NTs; 4 females, 4 males) completed the emotional valence determination test (EVDT) while undergoing BOLD functional magnetic resonance imaging (fMRI). We expected CDDAT participants to perform just as well as NTs on the EVDT, and to display increased activity within the bilateral amygdala and right anterior cingulate cortex (r-ACC). We hypothesized that such activity would reflect an increased reliance on these structures to compensate for on-going neuronal loss in frontoparietal regions due to the disease. We used diffusion tensor imaging (DTI) to determine if white matter (WM) damage had occurred in frontoparietal regions as well. CDDAT participants had similar behavioral performance and no differences were observed in brain activity or connectivity patterns within the amygdalae or r-ACC. Decreased fractional anisotropy (FA) values were noted, however, for the bilateral superior longitudinal fasciculi and posterior cingulate cortex (PCC). We interpret these findings to suggest that emotional valence determination and non-verbal skill sets are largely intact at this stage of the disease, but signs foreshadowing future decline were revealed by possible WM deterioration. Understanding how non-verbal skill sets are altered, while remaining largely intact, offers new insights into how non-verbal communication may be more successfully implemented in the care of AD patients and highlights the potential role of DTI as a presymptomatic biomarker.

Keywords: Alzheimer, chimeric faces, brain networks, DTI, fMRI, emotional valence

INTRODUCTION

Alzheimer disease (AD) is marked by a progressive decline in cognitive functions. As this occurs, the affected individual becomes less capable of understanding the world around them. This occurs in part due to a loss of ability to interpret the body language and facial expressions of others. Face-processing represents a group of complex cognitive operations in which information is extracted from facial features in such a way that the observer is able to perceive pertinent information about the person they are viewing. Previous studies of moderate-stage AD patients showed that their ability to interpret basic emotional cues from faces is largely intact (Roudier et al., 1998; Luzzi et al., 2007). However, dysfunctions are detectable (Albert et al., 1991; Cadieux and Greve, 1997; Hargrave et al., 2002). Luzzi et al. (2007) showed that the ability to interpret emotional cues directly correlated to participants' performance on constructional praxis and visuospatial memory tasks, which are examples of non-verbally-mediated skills, in early-moderate-stage AD.

These findings, combined with the observation that stroke participants' performance on certain visuospatial tests correlates with the degree of localization of damage to the right parietal lobe (Luzzi et al., 1998), suggest that activity of the right parietal lobe is directly related to the interpretation of emotional cues. This concurs with both the current clinical and pathological picture of AD, which shows that non-verbal memory loss, as well as damage to the right parietal lobe, is a late-stage finding (Braak et al., 2006; Ally et al., 2009).

We attempted to correlate the non-verbal skills of participants with early-stage Clinically Diagnosed Dementia of the Alzheimer Type (CDDAT) with findings from both functional magnetic resonance imaging (fMRI) and diffusion tensor imaging (DTI) measures during a non-verbally mediated face-processing task. Participants underwent a well-established, standardized, non-verbal skill test (the Rey-Osterrieth Complex figure B, visuospatial memory test (ROCFB-VMT); Luzzi et al., 2007) before entering the scanner to establish their visuospatial memory baseline. Participants then performed a variation of the Chimeric Face Test (CFT; Levy et al., 1983) that we created called the "emotional valence determination task (EVDT)" while in the scanner.

CDDAT patients were expected to perform as well as or slightly worse than neurotypicals (NTs) on the EVDT. Neuroimaging data was expected to show functional under-activation within the frontal (inferior frontal; left middle frontal) and parietal lobes (bilateral supramarginal gyri and left precuneus), given their association with non-verbal emotional processing, as well as increased activation of the bilateral amygdala and right anterior cingulate cortex (r-ACC), reflecting a greater reliance on these structures, during the EVDT (Nakamura et al., 1999; Fusar-Poli et al., 2009). Likewise, we hypothesized that DTI may show some deterioration of white matter (WM) tracts within frontoparietal connections, but not within amygdaloidal or cingulate tracts. Performance on the EVDT was expected to correlate to ROCFB-VMT performance. We hypothesized that this represents a relationship between emotional valence determination and visuospatial memory. By investigating the potential association of early-stage AD neuroimaging findings and non-verbal skill performance, we assessed the usefulness of these tests as cost effective supportive diagnostic markers of AD.

As may be expected, most task-related studies of AD focused on memory and displayed a pattern of early compensation followed by decreased activity. Pariente et al. (2005) noted increased activation during episodic memory encoding and recall in the posterior cingulate cortex (PCC), precuneus, parietal lobe and frontal lobe in early-stage AD patients with a mean Mini Mental State Exam (MMSE) score of 25 $\pm$ 1.8. Grady et al. (2003), Dickerson et al. (2005), Celone et al. (2006) and Zhou et al. (2008), on the other hand, observed decreased or even absent activation relative to NTs in the same regions in early-stage AD patients with mean MMSE scores of 21.1 $\pm$ 3.1, 22 $\pm$ 5, 21.3 $\pm$ 2.7, respectively. These findings support the assertion of Risacher and Saykin (2013) that increased activation occurs early on in an attempt to compensate, but ultimately leads to decreased activation once the disease burden is too great. We reasoned that this pattern of initially increased activation leading to decreased activation could be demonstrated for other cognitive domains as well because it represents a fundamental mechanism of the energetics of neurodegeneration. For a comprehensive review of AD discoveries through neuroimaging see Risacher and Saykin (2013).

Of equal importance is the understanding of how WM tracts are affected by the disease. WM alterations appear to parallel gray matter (GM) changes in that cortical abnormalities are greater in posterior brain regions relative to anterior regions at the early-stages of AD (Arnold et al., 1991; Braak and Braak, 1995). When the disease progresses, the neurofibrillary pathology advances from limbic to frontal structures, into higher-order association cortices, and finally into primary sensorimotor areas, which correlates with the clinical manifestations of AD (Braak and Braak, 1995). DTI-based tractography studies (Fellgiebel et al., 2005) and whole-brain DTI studies (Medina et al., 2006; Rose et al., 2006; Zhang et al., 2007) have consistently shown that fibers located deep in the posterior WM (e.g., the superior longitudinal fasciculus (SLF) and the posterior cingulum bundle (PCB)) are affected in patients with AD and mild cognitive impairment (MCI), a common precursor to AD. Bartzokis et al. (2003, 2004) have proposed that this may occur because as brain development takes place, later myelinated regions (cortical association areas) have fewer oligodendrocytes supporting greater numbers of axons (Bartzokis, 2004). DTI findings of decreased WM integrity in later myelinated regions at the onset of AD support this "reversed demyelination" construct (Medina and Gaviria, 2008). Furthermore, Huang et al. (2007) delineated a neuroanatomical pattern of functional alterations showing that changes in WM diffusion in parietal lobes correlated with scores of visuospatial skills.

Research on amnestic type MCI (aMCI) populations using neuropsychological tests of declarative memory extend this trend as they have demonstrated significant correlations between declining performance and decreases in posterior WM fractional anisotropy (FA), particularly in the PCB (Fellgiebel et al., 2005, 2008, Rose et al., 2006). Recalling the proposal of

Bartzokis et al. (2004), disruptions in transcortical connectivity may serve as early contributors to the pathophysiology of dementia, as the observed WM deteriorations were embedded beneath cortical GM that is often affected early within the disease course. For a more in-depth review of DTI findings in AD, see Medina and Gaviria (2008).

Although memory deficits are a hallmark characteristic of AD, there may be little to gain from testing face-processing related to familiarity that isn't already known (Sperling et al., 2003; Golby et al., 2005; Winchester, 2009; Donix et al., 2013). On the other hand, the fundamentals of face-processing (e.g., emotional valence) have received little attention (Job, 2012) and warrant further investigation. The use of neuropsychological tests in combination with neuroimaging techniques stresses the importance of attempting to integrate pathological observations with clinical symptoms. In doing so, we are able to reinforce findings from either end of the spectrum to more efficiently develop our understanding of the disease. In order to investigate a cognitive operation as complex as face-processing, it will be necessary to use appropriate tests that can isolate its specific subdivisions. This is particularly important when performing an fMRI investigation, as some studies suggest that face-processing and recognition occurs in fractions of a second (Vuilleumier and Schwartz, 2001; Batty and Taylor, 2003). If such factors are not properly accounted for, it would be very difficult to remove these confounds from the fMRI data as the canonical hemodynamic response curve peaks between 4–6 s after the presented stimuli, making it far too slow to tease out these processes (Poldrack et al., 2011).

To this end, the EVDT was of particular value since it is a variation of the CFT. The CFT was originally developed by Levy et al. (1983) "to index functional cerebral asymmetry for processing facial characteristics." It was shown to be highly reliable in detecting differences between right- and left-handers as well as being stable with regard to individual differences in perceptual asymmetries (Levy et al., 1983).

CFTs have previously been used to investigate asymmetries in the processing of emotions from facial expressions. Early works by Albert et al. (1991) and Cadieux and Greve (1997) suggested that by the moderate-stage, AD patients were impaired in recognizing emotions, but the authors noted that they could not rule out confounds "due to the deficits in recognizing non-emotional facial features and in verbal processing". Roudier et al. (1998) demonstrated that moderate-stage AD patients could accurately recognize when different emotions were displayed using the same human face. Hargrave et al. (2002) reconciled this difference through the use of a "same-different" emotion differentiation task in which participants were presented with a pair of photographs of different people and were asked to state if the two photographs in the pair were depicting the same or different emotions. From this, it was determined that moderate-stage AD patients do, in fact, have difficulty differentiating emotions independent of verbally-mediated and non-emotional facial features. Indersmitten and Gur (2003) then determined that two separate circuits likely underlie emotional processing in facial asymmetries and, while the left hemiface/right cerebral hemisphere circuit was dominant for expressions of sad, fearful and happy, the right hemiface/left cerebral hemisphere proved to be more efficient on task performance in NTs.

Then, Luzzi et al. (2007) used a variation of the CFT called the Mona Lisa test (MLT) wherein they determined that when using a cartoon face, emotional valence determination was impaired in some participants with moderate-stage AD, but not significantly across the entire cohort. Luzzi et al. (2007) found that in those with impaired recognition of facial emotions, the impairment correlated to poor performance on constructional praxis and non-verbal memory test, but not to the verbal fluency test (VFT) or MMSE score. Therefore, the ability to recognize facial emotions correlated to non-verbal performance. Finally, a fMRI meta-analysis by Fusar-Poli et al. (2009) discovered that the processing of facial expressions for emotional valence was associated with neural activation in the parietal and frontal cortices in NTs, thereby making these ideal regions of interest for investigation of the emotional subdivision of face-processing.

All things considered, we chose to use a "same-different" task similar to Hargrave et al. (2002) to observe changes in brain activity and connectivity in early-stage CDDAT patients as it represents the most clinically relevant task given its translatability to real life scenarios. Their work did not incorporate neuroimaging techniques, however, representing a gap in knowledge which we intended to fill with the current study. The works of Roudier et al. (1998), Indersmitten and Gur (2003), Luzzi et al. (2007) and Fusar-Poli et al. (2009) established crucial observations that were necessary to proceed in such a manner as without them there would be too many potential confounds to consider using depictions of actual human faces, let alone a series of different faces, to assess emotional processing through neuroimaging. Additionally, by using non-chimeric variations of faces based on the Mattingley et al. (1993) chimeric faces, we more directly assessed the emotional valence components of face-processing than we could through the original CFT.

The ROCFB served as an ideal cognitive test for investigating the non-verbal underpinnings of emotional valence determination because it had been described by Luzzi et al. (2011) to be "a valid instrument to assess non-verbal memory in adults and in the elderly". Building upon the findings of Luzzi et al. (2007), we investigated the relationship between the ROCFB-VMT and the EVDT. We assessed the potential relationship between visuospatial memory (as measured by the ROCFB-VMT) and the EVDT to determine if the ability to discern emotional states from facial expressions is rooted in the brain's ability to recognize and retain visuospatial relations between shapes.

MATERIALS AND METHODS

Participant Identification and Selection

The University Medical Center Departments of Neurology, Family Medicine, and Geriatrics saw 171 patients for complaints of "memory problems" or "dementia" spanning a 6-month period (November 2015–April 2016). Potential participants were identified and classified into their respective categories by physician assessment. Of that, 100 were determined to have AD or its precursor, aMCI, in accordance with the guidelines outlined by McKhann et al. (2011) for "dementia due to AD" or "MCI due to AD" (Albert et al., 2011). Those in the possible early-stage AD category were selected based on an MMSE score (Folstein et al., 1975) of 26–21 in accordance with National Institute for health Care and Excellence guidelines (National Institute for Health and Care Excellence, 2011). Twenty of these patients were determined to fit our inclusion/exclusion criteria, four of whom agreed to participate. All CDDAT participants had an existing medical MRI scan interpreted by a radiologist within the last 5 years prior to the study. These individuals were grouped into the CDDAT group. Detailed inclusion/exclusion criteria for the CDDAT group are listed below:

Inclusion criteria

- The diagnosis of AD was made in line with international diagnostic criteria (Albert et al., 2011; McKhann et al., 2011) on the basis of clinical history, neurologic, psychiatric, neuropsychological evaluation and hematologic screening for dementia (including liver and kidney function, thyroid function, folic acid and B12 vitamin levels, neoplastic markers), electroencephalogram, carotid ultrasonography, and neuroimaging studies (computed tomography and/or magnetic resonance) as determined by the attending physician.
- Mean general cognitive decline was evaluated with the MMSE (Folstein et al., 1975).
- All participants gave their informed consent to participate in the study.

Exclusion criteria

- Inability to understand the instructions from the principal investigator (PI) or research conductors.
- History of substance abuse.
- History of neurological deficits not related to AD.
- Inability or refusal to give informed consent.
- Motor, visual, or hearing impairment that precluded ability to perform cognitive testing assessments.
- Failure to pass the MRI safety checklist guidelines.

Ten age-matched cognitively normal participants (5 males, 5 females) were recruited from a nearby senior living center and were grouped into the NT group. NTs were required to have an MMSE score >27 and meet all inclusion and exclusion criteria stated above, except for that concerning the existence of Alzheimer-related pathology. One male participant was retroactively removed after receiving a diagnosis of normal pressure hydrocephalus. One female participant from the NT group was removed due to a scanner script runtime error that prevented the EVDT from being run. Therefore, there were 4 CDDAT (1 female, 3 males) and 8 NT (4 females, 4 males) participants in this study. All participants were right-handed, except for 1 non-right-hand-dominant NT female, as confirmed by the Edinburgh Handedness Inventory-revised (EHI-r; Williams, 1986). The non-right-hand-dominant NT female that was kept in the study was kept because the participant was shown to have no significant difference in either their accuracy, reaction time (RT), or within-group contrast mapping for either fMRI or DTI measures when compared to the rest of the control group.

Participants were informed that their participation was voluntary and they may withdraw from the study at any time and that their refusal to participate would have no impact on their level of care. This study was carried out in accordance with the recommendations of Texas Tech University Human Protections Internal Review Board with written informed consent from all subjects. All subjects gave written informed consent in accordance with the Declaration of Helsinki. The protocol study was approved by the Texas Tech University Human Protections Internal Review Board.

Sample Size

A 2004 meta-analysis by Henry et al. (2004) demonstrated an effect size of $r = 0.73$ for a test of semantic fluency in patients with Dementia of the Alzheimer Type (DAT). From this it was determined that an assumed effect size of $r = 0.8$ would achieve 80% power with a minimum sample size of 4. Our behavioral analyses, therefore, seek to determine if an impairment on either the EVDT or ROCFB-VMT is greater than or equal to the known deficit of verbal fluency, as this currently represents the most consistent and pronounced clinical manifestation of the disease at this stage. Effect size for each test was calculated using Cohen's *d* and converted to its r-equivalent (Cohen, 1992).

The number of necessary participants was based on the Desmond and Glover (2002) report that single voxel-level power of 80%, corrected for multiple comparisons can be achieved with a sample size of 24 per group. According to Desmond and Glover (2002), "Sample size increases power because the standard error of the mean decreases by the square root of *N*" (N = the number of subjects). In our study, we had a minimum of four subjects within each group. Therefore, we may expect to reach of 32.7% power at the single voxel level (i.e., since we have 1/6 of the number of subjects we will reach 41% of the power achieved by having 24 per group or 33% overall; the square root of $4/24 = 0.41*0.8 = 0.328$). As such, even by the most conservative of estimates (assuming a power of 10 exponential) our minimum detection for 80% power is 316 voxels ($80\%/32\% = 2.5$; $10^{2.5} = 316$). Given that this is a region-of-interest-based investigation (ROI) >1000 voxels, however, we may reasonably expect to surpass 80% power for each ROI with a sample size of ≥ 4 per group.

Participant Demographics

Participant demographics are summarized in **Table 1**. We recruited four right-handed Caucasian patients (3 males, 1 female) with a diagnosis of aMCI or early-stage AD between the ages of 73–93 (median age 83.5 ± 8.4) with MMSE scores between 26–23 (median of 24.5 ± 1.3). Two of the males (MMSE scores of 26 and 25) had an existing diagnosis of "MCI due to AD" (Albert et al., 2011). The remaining male and female had an existing diagnosis of "dementia due to AD" (MMSE scores of 24 and 23, respectively; McKhann et al., 2011). Eight (7 right-handed and 1 non-right-hand-dominant) cognitively

TABLE 1 | Participant demographics.

Group	Age (median ± stdev)	Sex	Handedness	Race	MMSE (median ± stdev)
CDDAT (n = 4)	83 ± 8	1 F, 3 M	4 R	4 CA	24.5 ± 1.3
NT (n = 8)	80 ± 4	4 F, 4 M	7 R, 1 nR	8 CA	30 ± 0

CDDAT, clinically diagnosed dementia of the Alzheimer type; NT, neurotypical; F, female; M, male; R, right-handed; nR, non-right-handed; CA, Caucasian.

normal Caucasian participants (4 males, 4 females; all with MMSE scores of 30) between the ages of 79–91 (median age 80 ± 4.0) also participated. Handedness was determined using the EHI-r (Williams, 1986).

There was no significant difference in median age (p = 0.561), but there was an observable difference in median MMSE score for the two groups (p = 0.014). While there may be some concern given our lack of equal sex-distribution (1 female and 3 males) within the CDDAT group, no differences in performance were discernable based on sex within our NT group (4 females, 4 males) across either cognitive test (ROCFB-VMT or EVDT) for either accuracy or RT (data not shown) nor for within-group sex-based contrast mapping for fMRI or DTI (data not shown).

Administration of Rey Osterrieth Complex Figure B Visuospatial Memory Test

Participants were first asked to copy the ROCFB as accurately as possible, without tracing it, on a different sheet of paper that had the same dimensions as the paper containing the figure. The size of the model was 5.5 cm × 8 cm, and the sheet of paper on which it was printed was half the size of an 8.5″ × 11″ sheet. Participants were then asked to reproduce the ROCFB from memory on a different sheet of paper after an interval of 5 min, during which they were engaged with the VFT (Luzzi et al., 2007). The rate of retention was calculated as a percentage of the score obtained on reproduction from memory compared to the original figure-copying score. Digital photographs were taken of the drawings produced by participants to ensure accuracy of scoring. The test was administered and scored following the protocol detailed in Luzzi et al. (2011).

Imaging Methodology and Analyses

Stimulus Presentation and Participant Response

After completing the ROCFB-VMT, all participants were briefly trained on the EVDT before entering the scanner to ensure task comprehension by allowing them to practice on a single example trial of each condition type. Pairs of faces based on the chimeric faces of Mattingley et al. (1993) were presented in an event-related design for the EVDT using Eprime 2.0. Presentation order was counterbalanced across participants using a Latin square design. The question "Are the emotions the same?" was displayed upon the screen for 4 s inside the scanner. A set of 40 trails were randomized and displayed for 4 s (s) each with a jittered inter-stimulus interval (ISI) randomized for five time points between 800–1200 ms, by 100 ms apiece. Participants responded using a fiber optic controller held in the right hand where button 1 was pressed by the index finger and button 2 was pressed by the middle finger. Participants pressed one of two buttons to indicate Yes (button 1) or No (button 2) in response to the question. An example of this test is given in **Figure 1**.

Scanning Parameters

All images were acquired with a 3T Siemens MR system (Skyra, Germany) at the Texas Tech Neuroimaging Institute. The T1 anatomic scan parameters were: TR: 1900 ms; TE: 2.49 ms; FOV: 240; Flip angle: 9, Voxel size = 0.9 × 0.9 × 0.9 mm; slice number: 192. The fMRI parameters were: TR: 2500 ms; TE: 20.0 ms; FOV: 231; Flip angle: 75, Voxel size = 2.5 × 2.5 × 3.0 mm; slice number: 41. In each fMRI dataset, there are 80 volumes. The DTI parameters were: TR: 5000 ms; TE: 95 ms; FOV: 220; B/W: 1562, Voxel size = 1.7 × 1.7 × 4.0 mm; slice number: 32. There were 64 directions for DTI.

Image Preprocessing

fMRI

Image preprocessing steps included removing non-brain structures by Brain Extraction Tool (BET), motion correction by using Motion Correction for FSL Linear Registration Tool (MCFLIRT), temporal high-pass filtering with a cutoff period of 24 s, spatial smoothing with a 5 mm Gaussian full width, half maximum (FWHM) algorithm, and co-registering of the functional images to the high resolution T1 structure images in their native space using boundary border registration (BBR) and FSL Linear Registration Tool (FLIRT; Jenkinson and Smith, 2001; Jenkinson et al., 2002) at 12 degrees of freedom to the Korean Normal Elderly (KNE96; Lee et al., 2016) standard brain space.

DTI

FSL Diffusion Toolbox 3.0 (FDT) from FMRIB Software Library (FSL 5.0.5) was used to complete the construction of and preprocessing for all anatomical brain networks for all subjects. It processed DICOM/NIfTI files into diffusion metrics (e.g., FA) that were ready for statistical analysis at the voxel-level after performing corrections for image alignment and artifact clean-up (Top-Up) and local field distortions (eddy current correction; Smith et al., 2004).

Image Processing

fMRI

fMRI data processing was carried out using FMRI Expert Analysis Tool (FEAT) Version 6.00, part of FSL[1] (Worsley, 2001). The time series for the behavioral events of the EVDT were analyzed for the following conditions:

[1]www.fmrib.ox.ac.uk/fsl

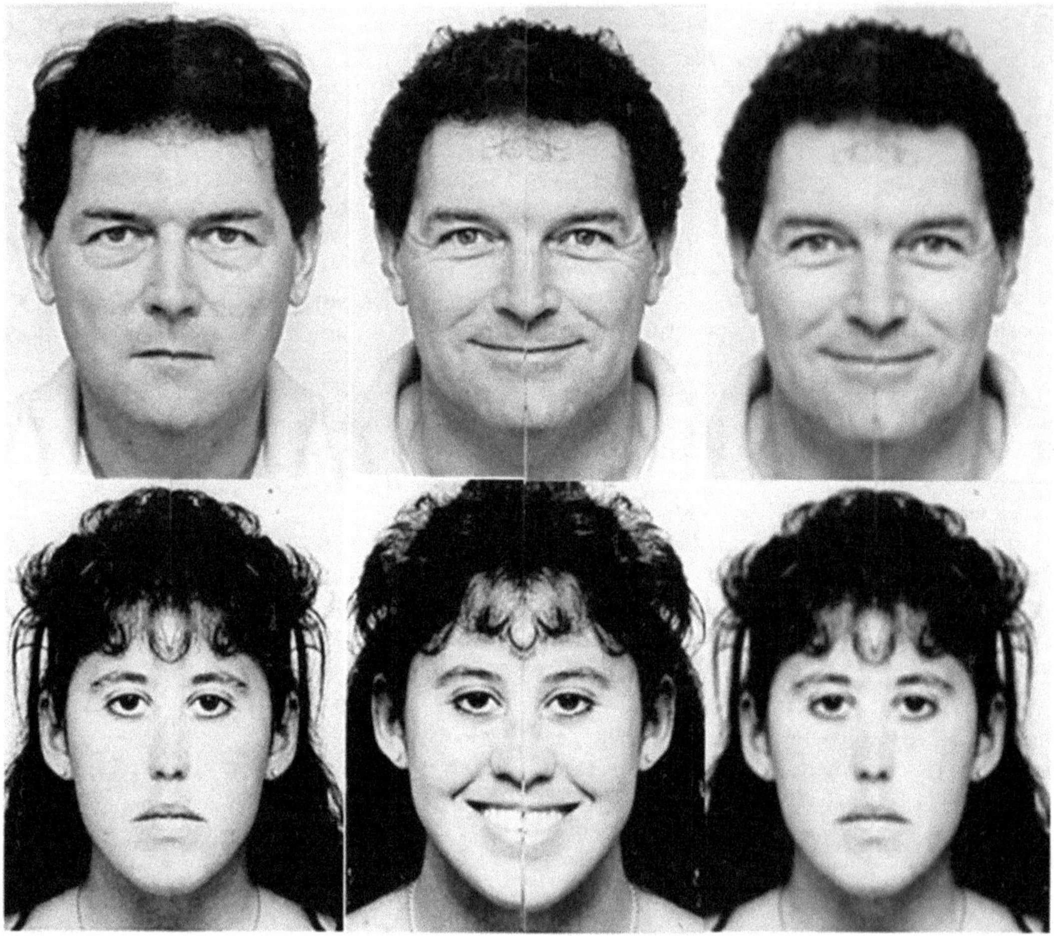

FIGURE 1 | Examples of the emotional valence determination test (EVDT). EVDT examples in response to the question: "Are the emotions the same?" (left) "yes"; two neutral faces. (center) "yes"; two happy faces. (right) "no"; happy (top) and neutral (bottom).

For "presentation of stimuli scenarios" (i.e., when the participant was shown two happy faces, two neutral faces, or one of each)—brain activity from the first 2 s following the presentation of a stimulus was recorded for each trial. In the event a participant responded within <2 s, the interval between the presentation of the stimulus and 250 ms before the response was used for the recording interval. This was done to avoid brain activity artifacts related to the button press. Instances where a participant made no response before the presentation of the next stimulus were discarded.

For "participant response" scenarios (i.e., when the participant chose "yes" (y) or "no" (n) in response to the question: "Are the emotions the same?")—brain activity from the first 2 s following the press of a button was recorded for each trial. In the event a participant responded within <2 s before the presentation of the next stimulus, that interval was used for the recoding time. Instances where a participant made no response before the presentation of the next stimulus were discarded.

A summary of fMRI contrasts is given in **Table 2**. A total of five subject-level contrast maps were created for all subjects using threshold free cluster enhancement (TFCE) of $z > 2.3$ and a cluster corrected significance threshold of $p < 0.05$. These modeled time series were convolved with the double gamma hemodynamic response function (dg-HRF), which was modeled from a combination of Gaussian functions. Group-level contrast maps were created using FMRIB's Local Analysis of Mixed Effects (FLAME1). The thresholds for group level activation maps were created using TFCE of $z > 1.5$ and a cluster-corrected significance threshold of $p < 0.05$. The exact regions of brain activity were determined using the KNE96 coordinate space and Harvard-Oxford cortical and subcortical structural atlases.

TABLE 2 | Summary of functional magnetic resonance imaging (fMRI) contrasts.

Task type	Option 1	Option 2	Option 3
EVDT-presentation of stimuli:	Two happy faces	Two neutral faces	One of each
EVDT-choice of the participant:	Yes	No	–

A total of five subject-level contrast maps were created for all subjects. EVDT, emotional valence determination test.

DTI

Voxel-based group differences were calculated for the *FA* images using Tract-Based Spatial Statistics (TBSS; Smith et al., 2006; Smith and Nichols, 2009; Cheon et al., 2011). TBSS linearly registered individual *FA* images in native space and then to the *FA* template via the FLIRT command of FSL. The resultant warping transformations were then used to convert images of diffusion (i.e., *FA*) to Montreal Neuroimaging Institute (MNI152) space with a spatial resolution of 1 × 1 × 1 mm. For statistical inference, including correction for multiple comparisons, permutation testing was used (Nichols and Holmes, 2002; Cheon et al., 2011) as implemented by RANDOMISE of the FSL software package. Five hundred permutations were performed for significant group differences at a threshold of 0.2; corresponding to $p < 0.05$, corrected for multiple comparisons using TFCE (Smith and Nichols, 2009; Cheon et al., 2011). WM tracts were identified using the Johns-Hopkins University ICBM-DTI-81 WM labels and probabilities of tract accuracy were assessed using the Johns-Hopkins University WM Tractography atlas.

Behavioral Methodology and Analyses

All statistical calculations for behavioral analyses were performed using Rstudio Desktop (version 0.99.896, Rstudio, Inc., Boston, MA, USA).

Comparison of Test Performance Amongst Study Groups

Mann-Whitney U-tests with false discovery rate corrections of $\alpha = 0.05$ for multiple comparisons to reach significance at $p < 0.05$ were used to evaluate differences in test performance between the study groups. A one-sample *t*-test with mu = 30 and two-sample U-test were used to calculate the group difference in MMSE score given that the variance for the NT group was zero. Both tests revealed a significant result. Additionally, the zero variance for the NT group on the MMSE is within reason for cognitively normal elderly individuals, as persons without cognitive deficits may be expected to receive a perfect score (30/30) as was seen here (Folstein et al., 1975).

Correlation of CFTs to Cognitive Test Performance

Pearson correlation coefficients, with false discovery rate corrections of $\alpha = 0.05$ for multiple comparisons to reach significance at $p < 0.05$, were used to correlate CFT performance to performance on their respective cognitive tests.

Assessing Tests as Classifiers

Fischer Exact test, with corrections for multiple comparisons of $\alpha = 0.05$ to reach significance at $p < 0.05$, were used to determine strength of each test as a classifier between CDDAT and NT.

RESULTS

Behavioral Data

We found no significant difference in median ROCFB-VMT or EVDT score for the two groups (NT = 58 ± 26.2 vs. CDDAT = 41 ± 23.6; Cohen's $d = -0.196$, r-equivalent effect size = −0.0975, $p = 0.555$, NT = 85 ± 8.8 vs. CDDAT = 87 ± 13; Cohen's $d = 0.671$, r-equivalent effect size = 0.318, $p = 0.969$, respectively). There was also no significant different RT for the EVDT (CDDAT = 2166 ± 461 ms vs. NT = 2084 ± 493 ms, not shown). Therefore, neither ROCFB-VMT nor EVDT function as a potential classifier between NT and CDDAT given their nearly identical overlap. All of these findings suggest that no observable difference in either emotional valence determination or visuospatial ability exists between these two groups at this stage of the disease. Additionally, we found no correlation between the ROCFB-VMT and EVDT performance ($R^2 = 0.022$, $p = 0.648$). Thus, at this stage of the disease there appeared to be no connection between emotional valence determination ability and visuospatial memory decline; this finding, however, may be the result of a ceiling effect in participant performance. Behavioral results are summarized in **Figure 2**.

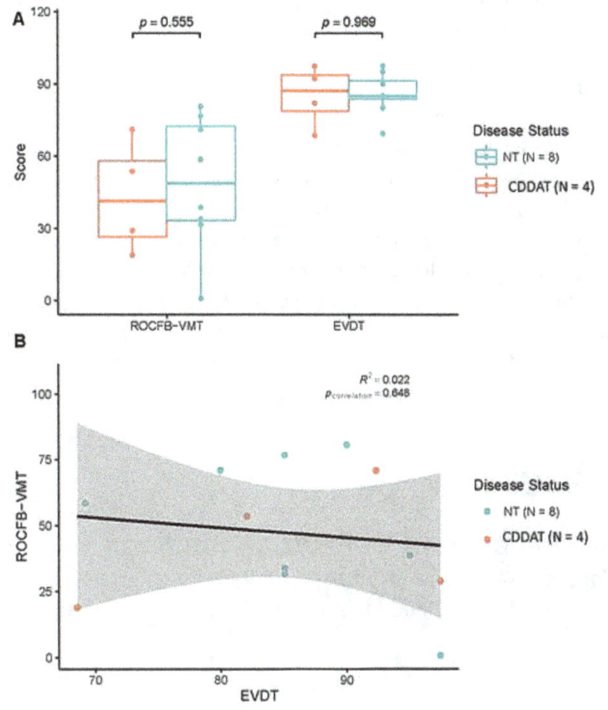

FIGURE 2 | (A) Results of Rey-Osterrieth Complex Figure B-Visuospatial Memory Test (ROCFB-VMT) and EVDT. **(B)** ROCFB-VMT and EVDT performance were not correlated Pearson Correlation $r = 0.022$, $p_{correlation} = 0.648$. NT, Neurotypicals; CDDAT, Clinically diagnosed dementia of the Alzheimer Type.

Imaging Results

fMRI Results

There were no significant differences in areas of activation between groups upon stimulus presentation regardless of the emotional pairing displayed (data not shown). Furthermore, no differences in areas of activation were observed between groups with relation to when they chose "yes" or "no" in response to the question: "Are the emotions the same?", thus indicating no fundamental difference in perception or processing of the faces (data not shown).

DTI Results

CDDAT did not show higher *FA* values in any areas. NTs showed higher *FA* values than CDDATS in the right inferior longitudinal fasciculus (r-ILF), right posterior thalamic radiations (r-PTR) and the bilateral PCC (b-PCC) and superior longitudinal fasciculi (b-SLF). For the SLF, the differences between NTs and CDDATs were greater in the left than the right hemisphere, suggesting WM deterioration has occurred in the CDDAT group. No significant differences were observed in any of the three major amygdala connection pathways: the amygdalofugal, the stria terminalis, or the anterior commissure. Imaging results are summarized in **Figure 3**.

DISCUSSION

Significance of Behavioral Findings

Consistent with our hypothesis and the previous findings of Albert et al. (1991) and Luzzi et al. (2007), CDDAT participants displayed no difference in accuracy or RT for either the ROCFB-VMT or the EVDT. These findings support the notion that non-verbal abilities, as measured by the ROCFB-VMT, and emotional valence determination, as measured by the EVDT, are largely intact in early-stage AD patients.

All of the subjects were combined together when analyzing the correlation of CFTs to cognitive test performance. Although it would be possible to add a categorical variable representing disease/no disease to the model to generate a multivariate linear model that controls for disease status, that would be ideal if the goal was to produce the most predictive model or if we were trying to demonstrate the causal dependence of the dependent variable on the independent variable.

However, there are several reasons we chose not to control for disease status. First, in principle, people who might apply these tests would likely not know disease status prior to administration. Thus, a model that controls for a variable that they don't have available might confuse its application. Second, we are not proposing that CFT is causing cognitive test performance so much as they are simply correlated; that is, our goal is not necessarily to construct the most explanatory possible model. Controlling for disease status makes that impossible.

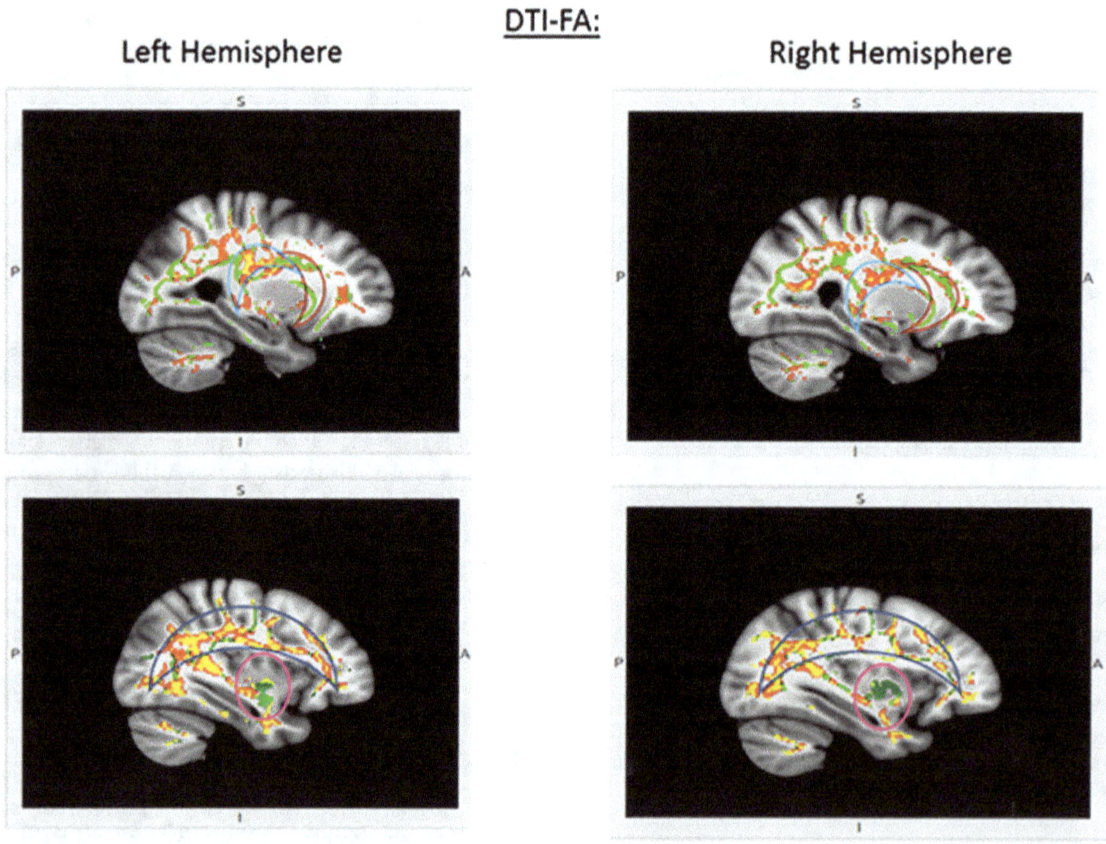

FIGURE 3 | Pertinent diffusion tensor imaging (DTI) results for the EVDT. Significant differences were seen in the posterior cingulate cortex (PCC; light blue crescent, top) and superior longitudinal fasciculi (blue crescent, bottom), but not anterior cingulate (red crescent, top) or amygdaloidal connections (pink circle, bottom). Areas where NT > CDDAT for fractional anisotropy (FA) measures are shown in red. Green lines represent the FA skeleton. NT, Neurotypicals; CDDAT, Clinically Diagnosed Dementia of the Alzheimer Type.

Significance of fMRI Findings

Further support for our hypothesis comes from the fMRI results. We hypothesized that, in the absence of differences in behavioral performance, there would likely be no difference in brain activity. We also hypothesized that, if such a difference were seen, it would occur within the parietal lobes, amygdalae, or r-ACC based on fMRI findings in NTs reported by Fusar-Poli et al. (2009). The lack of differences between the brain activity patterns of the two groups upon stimulus presentation and during the selection of a response suggests that early-stage AD patients perceive the stimuli and choose a response in a fundamentally similar way to NTs, thereby strengthening the notion that these processes are not yet demonstrably affected by the disease.

Significance of DTI Findings

Although our behavioral and functional imaging results seem promising with regard to the retention of non-verbal skill sets, a more concerning observation was made through DTI. Consistent with our hypothesis, we saw lower *FA* values in the b-SLF, especially within the left hemisphere, and b-PCC, but no differences in the amygdalae or r-ACC. While there were no significant differences in the major amygdala or anterior cingulate connection pathways, the changes in the SLF and the PCC are consistent with both the pathological progression of WM deterioration in AD (Braak and Braak, 1997; Bartzokis, 2004; Leech and Sharp, 2014) and proposed mechanisms of emotional valance (Maddock et al., 2003; Fusar-Poli et al., 2009).

In congruence with Indersmitten and Gur (2003), we propose the greater deterioration of the left-SLF tracts observed herein suggests a decline in processing efficiency for emotion, but a retention of the dominant circuit, which is served by tracts of the right-SLF. Finally, Kosaka et al. (2003) determined that the PCC plays an important role in face-processing for the transition of a face from being unrecognized to being acknowledged as familiar in NTs. Therefore, the early deterioration of PCC connecting fibers may play a significant role in AD patients' impaired ability to recognize loved ones independent of semantic memory loss. Taken together, our findings further support the reverse demyelination hypothesis, proposed by Medina and Gaviria (2008), and Bartzokis's (2004) assertion of the role of myelin damage predating neuronal loss and its possible role in exacerbating the progression of AD.

Limitations

We acknowledge that the instances in which our behavioral analyses did not find a significant difference between our NT and CDDAT groups does not necessarily mean that impairments are not present at this time. Instead, it indicates that such deficits, if they exist, are less severe than those of semantic verbal fluency, which currently represents the most consistent and pronounced clinical manifestation of this disease at this stage (Henry et al., 2004). Additionally, the perfect score with zero variance obtained on the MMSE by our control group makes them an idealized group for comparison, but it also makes them less representative of the NT geriatric population as a whole. It is important to note, however, that they were not intentionally selected to obtain a perfect score and that this is an incidental result.

As previously mentioned, the inability to directly correlate ROCFB-VMT: EVDT performance may be due to a ceiling effect. Replicating this experiment with a more difficult visuospatial test, such as the Rey Osterrieth Complex figure A (ROCFA) may result in an observable difference between NTs and early-stage CDDAT, but given that a similar correlation has been established for the MLT and ROCFB in moderate-stage AD by Luzzi et al. (2007) such an observation may be more academic than clinically relevant.

It is important to note, however, that since the etiology of AD is unknown and requires post mortem confirmation it is possible that our findings may not extend to all individuals affected with the ailment. Other potential cofounders could be differences in the demographics and comorbidities in the two groups. Due to restrictions related to the approved Human Protections Board protocol, we do not have any additional medical or demographic information (e.g., marital status, list of medications or medical comorbidities that are not of a neurologic or psychiatric nature) on our participants than what is currently described. An alternative interpretation is that although there is significant structural damage, the lack of functional differences between the groups may represent a type of structural compensation independent of reverse demyelination. Conversely, these observations may be rooted in fundamental issues of neurodegeneration and may therefore extend to other neurodegenerative diseases making these findings simultaneously of larger interest to the field as a whole, but less exclusive to AD. Additional investigations will be necessary to access the reproducibility of these findings in other populations as well as their specificity to AD.

CONCLUSION

While we observed that both groups performed similarly on both skill sets, we found no correlation between the two, due in part to the massive variations in ROCFB-VMT scores. Yet, since both groups scored within normative ranges after adjusting for age and education (Becker et al., 1987), we conclude that both skill sets are intact within these participants at this stage of the disease. Furthermore, there were no significant differences in BOLD fMRI activation with regard to either stimulus presentation or participant response, strengthening our assertion that these skill sets are, as of yet, unaffected. Lastly, these findings are consistent with the previous work by Luzzi et al. (2007). The deterioration of WM tracts within the b-SLF and b-PCC may foreshadow the impending decline of these functions, as would be consistent with clinical observations (Moore and Wyke, 1984; Haupt et al., 1991; Liu et al., 1991) and autopsy findings (Braak and Braak, 1997) for the progression of the disease.

In conclusion, our discoveries highlight the potential of WM tractography as a presymptomatic biomarker for AD. Based on our observations we suggest that when caring for patients with suspected early-stage AD, use direct/pronounced body language and facial expressions over verbal commands whenever possible. Emphasizing non-verbally mediated social cues has the added benefit of strengthening social interaction, which may help slow the progression of symptoms (Bennett et al., 2006) and reduce the risk of depression (Yaffe et al., 1999).

AUTHOR CONTRIBUTIONS

RR created and executed the project, analyzed and interpreted the data, and wrote the manuscript. RCA and DF assisted in the neuroimaging experimental design and analyses. AGM and HMRK assisted in experimental design and statistical analyses and interpretation. PL, PJ, GH, KL, JC and JT determined participant eligibility and consulted on medical interpretation and significance. PHR and MB provided consultation on experimental design and interpretation.

ACKNOWLEDGMENTS

Funding for this research was provided by the I. Wylie Briscoe College of Human Sciences Endowment for Alzheimer Research. PHR is supported by NIH grants (AG042178, AG047812) and the Garrison Family Foundation. This study was completed in agreement with the Alzheimer Disease Neuroimaging Initiative Image and Data Archive (ADNI LONI IDA) data sharing policy. Raw and preprocessed images are available at http://adni.loni.usc.edu/data-samples/access-data/. Portions of this article are taken from the dissertation (Rajmohan, 2016) in compliance with Frontiers in Aging Neuroscience's rules and regulations.

REFERENCES

Albert, M. S., Cohen, C., and Koff, E. (1991). Perception of affect in patients with dementia of the Alzheimer type. *Arch. Neurol.* 48, 791–795. doi: 10.1001/archneur.1991.00530200027013

Albert, M. S., DeKosky, S. T., Dickson, D., Dubois, B., Feldman, H. H., Fox, N. C., et al. (2011). The diagnosis of mild cognitive impairment due to Alzheimer disease: recommendations from the National institute on aging-Alzheimer's association workgroups on diagnostic guidelines for Alzheimer disease. *Alzheimers Dement.* 7, 270–279. doi: 10.1016/j.jalz.2011.03.008

Ally, B. A., Gold, C. A., and Budson, A. E. (2009). The picture superiority effect in patients with Alzheimer's disease and mild cognitive impairment. *Neuropsychologia* 47, 595–598. doi: 10.1016/j.neuropsychologia.2008.10.010

Arnold, S. E., Hyman, B. T., Flory, J., Damasio, A. R., and Van Hoesen, G. W. (1991). The topographical and neuroanatomical distribution of neurofibrillary tangles and neuritic plaques in the cerebral cortex of patients with Alzheimer's disease. *Cereb. Cortex* 1, 103–116. doi: 10.1093/cercor/1.1.103

Bartzokis, G. (2004). Age-related myelin breakdown: a developmental model of cognitive decline and Alzheimer's disease. *Neurobiol. Aging* 25, 5–18. doi: 10.1016/j.neurobiolaging.2003.03.001

Bartzokis, G., Cummings, J. L., Sultzer, D., Henderson, V. W., Nuechterlein, K. H., and Mintz, J. (2003). White matter structural integrity in healthy aging adults and patients with Alzheimer disease: a magnetic resonance imaging study. *Arch. Neurol.* 60, 393–398. doi: 10.1001/archneur.60.3.393

Bartzokis, G., Sultzer, D., Lu, P. H., Nuechterlein, K. H., Mintz, J., and Cummings, J. L. (2004). Heterogenous age related breakdown of white matter structural integrity: implications for cortical "disconnection" in aging and Alzheimer's disease. *Neurobiol. Aging* 25, 843–851. doi: 10.1016/j.neurobiolaging.2003.09.005

Batty, M., and Taylor, M. J. (2003). Early processing of the six basic facial emotional expressions. *Cogn. Brain Res.* 17, 613–620. doi: 10.1016/s0926-6410(03)00174-5

Becker, J. T., Boller, F., Saxton, J., and McGonigle-Gibson, K. L. (1987). Normal rates of forgetting of verbal and non-verbal material in Alzheimer's disease. *Cortex* 23, 59–72. doi: 10.1016/s0010-9452(87)80019-9

Bennett, D. A., Schneider, J. A., Tang, Y., Arnold, S. E., and Wilson, R. S. (2006). The effect of social networks on the relation between Alzheimer's disease pathology and level of cognitive function in old people: a longitudinal cohort study. *Lancet Neurol.* 5, 406–412. doi: 10.1016/s1474-4422(06)70417-3

Braak, H., Alafuzoff, I., Arzberger, T., Kretzschmar, H., and Del Tredici, K. (2006). Staging of Alzheimer disease-associated neurofibrillary pathology using paraffin sections and immunocytochemistry. *Acta Neuropathol.* 112, 389–404. doi: 10.1007/s00401-006-0127-z

Braak, H., and Braak, E. (1995). Staging of Alzheimer's disease-related neurofibrillary changes. *Neurobiol. Aging* 16, 271–278. doi: 10.1016/0197-4580(95)00021-6

Braak, H., and Braak, E. (1997). Frequency of stages of Alzheimer-related lesions in different age categories. *Neurobiol. Aging* 18, 351–357. doi: 10.1016/s0197-4580(97)00056-0

Cadieux, N. L., and Greve, K. W. (1997). Emotion processing in Alzheimer's disease. *J. Int. Neuropsychol. Soc.* 3, 411–419.

Celone, K. A., Calhoun, V. D., Dickerson, B. C., Atri, A., Chua, E. F., Miller, S. L., et al. (2006). Alterations in memory networks in mild cognitive impairment and Alzheimer's disease: an independent component analysis. *J. Neurosci.* 26, 10222–10231. doi: 10.1523/JNEUROSCI.2250-06.2006

Cheon, K. A., Kim, Y. S., Oh, S. H., Park, S. Y., Yoon, H. W., Herrington, J., et al. (2011). Involvement of the anterior thalamic radiation in boys with high functioning autism spectrum disorders: a diffusion tensor imaging study. *Brain Res.* 1417, 77–86. doi: 10.1016/j.brainres.2011.08.020

Cohen, J. (1992). A power primer. *Psychol. Bull.* 112, 155–159. doi: 10.1037/0033-2909.112.1.155

Desmond, J. E., and Glover, G. H. (2002). Estimating sample size in functional MRI (fMRI) neuroimaging studies: statistical power analyses. *J. Neurosci. Methods* 118, 115–128. doi: 10.1016/s0165-0270(02)00121-8

Dickerson, B. C., Salat, D. H., Greve, D. N., Chua, E. F., Rand-Giovannetti, E., Rentz, D. M., et al. (2005). Increased hippocampal activation in mild cognitive impairment compared to normal aging and AD. *Neurology* 65, 404–411. doi: 10.1212/01.wnl.0000171450.97464.49

Donix, M., Jurjanz, L., Meyer, S., Amanatidis, E. C., Baeumler, D., Huebner, T., et al. (2013). Functional imaging during recognition of personally familiar faces and places in Alzheimer's disease. *Arch. Clin. Neuropsychol.* 28, 72–80. doi: 10.1093/arclin/acs093

Fellgiebel, A., Müller, M. J., Wille, P., Dellani, P. R., Scheurich, A., Schmidt, L. G., et al. (2005). Color-coded diffusion-tensor-imaging of posterior cingulate fiber tracts in mild cognitive impairment. *Neurobiol. Aging* 26, 1193–1198. doi: 10.1016/j.neurobiolaging.2004.11.006

Fellgiebel, A., Schermuly, I., Gerhard, A., Keller, I., Albrecht, J., Weibrich, C., et al. (2008). Functional relevant loss of long association fibre tracts integrity in early Alzheimer's disease. *Neuropsychologia* 46, 1698–1706. doi: 10.1016/j.neuropsychologia.2007.12.010

Folstein, M. F., Folstein, S. E., and McHugh, P. R. (1975). "Mini-mental state". A practical method for grading the cognitive state of patients for the clinician. *J. Psychiatr. Res.* 12, 189–198. doi: 10.1016/0022-3956(75)90026-6

Fusar-Poli, P., Placentino, A., Carletti, F., Landi, P., Allen, P., Surguladze, S., et al. (2009). Functional atlas of emotional faces processing: a voxel-based meta-analysis of 105 functional magnetic resonance imaging studies. *J. Psychiatry Neurosci.* 34, 418–432.

Golby, A., Silverberg, G., Race, E., Gabrieli, S., O'Shea, J., Knierim, K., et al. (2005). Memory encoding in Alzheimer's disease: an fMRI study of explicit and implicit memory. *Brain* 128, 773–787. doi: 10.1093/brain/awh400

Grady, C. L., McIntosh, A. R., Beig, S., Keightley, M. L., Burian, H., and Black, S. E. (2003). Evidence from functional neuroimaging of a compensatory prefrontal network in Alzheimer's disease. *J. Neurosci.* 23, 986–993.

Hargrave, R., Maddock, R. J., and Stone, V. (2002). Impaired recognition of facial expressions of emotion in Alzheimer's disease. *J. Neuropsychiatry Clin. Neurosci.* 14, 64–71. doi: 10.1176/jnp.14.1.64

Haupt, M., Pollman, S., and Kurz, A. (1991). Disoriented behavior in familiar surroundings is strongly associated with perceptual impairment in mild Alzheimer's disease. *Dement. Geriatr. Cogn. Disord.* 2, 259–261. doi: 10.1159/000107213

Henry, J. D., Crawford, J. R., and Phillips, L. H. (2004). Verbal fluency performance in dementia of the Alzheimer's type: a meta-analysis. *Neuropsychologia* 42, 1212–1222. doi: 10.1016/j.neuropsychologia.2004.02.001

Huang, J., Friedland, R. P., and Auchus, A. P. (2007). Diffusion tensor imaging of normal-appearing white matter in mild cognitive impairment and early Alzheimer disease: preliminary evidence of axonal degeneration in the temporal lobe. *AJNR Am. J. Neuroradiol.* 28, 1943–1948. doi: 10.3174/ajnr.a0700

Indersmitten, T., and Gur, R. C. (2003). Emotion processing in chimeric faces: hemispheric asymmetries in expression and recognition of emotions. *J. Neurosci.* 23, 3820–3825.

Jenkinson, M., Bannister, P., Brady, M., and Smith, S. (2002). Improved optimization for the robust and accurate linear registration and motion correction of brain images. *Neuroimage* 17, 825–841. doi: 10.1016/s1053-8119(02)91132-8

Jenkinson, M., and Smith, S. (2001). A global optimisation method for robust affine registration of brain images. *Med. Image Anal.* 5, 143–156. doi: 10.1016/s1361-8415(01)00036-6

Job, R. (2012). Final activity and management report summary—FMRI IN AD (A functional neuroimaging study of face-processing in early Alzheimer's disease). European Commission Community Research and Development Information Services. Project reference: 46512. Record Number: 52155

Kosaka, H., Omori, M., Iidaka, T., Murata, T., Shimoyama, T., Okada, T., et al. (2003). Neural substrates participating in acquisition of facial familiarity: an fMRI study. *Neuroimage* 20, 1734–1742. doi: 10.1016/s1053-8119(03)00447-6

Lee, H., Yoo, B. I., Han, J. W., Lee, J. J., Oh, S. Y. W., Lee, E. Y., et al. (2016). Construction and validation of brain MRI templates from a Korean normal elderly population. *Psychiatry Investig.* 13, 135–145. doi: 10.4306/pi.2016.13.1.135

Leech, R., and Sharp, D. J. (2014). The role of the posterior cingulate cortex in cognition and disease. *Brain* 137, 12–32. doi: 10.1093/brain/awt162

Levy, J., Heller, W., Banich, M. T., and Burton, L. A. (1983). Asymmetry of perception in free viewing of chimeric faces. *Brain Cogn.* 2, 404–419. doi: 10.1016/0278-2626(83)90021-0

Liu, L., Gauthier, L., and Gauthier, S. (1991). Spatial disorientation in persons with early senile dementia of the Alzheimer type. *Am. J. Occup. Ther.* 45, 67–74. doi: 10.5014/ajot.45.1.67

Luzzi, S., Monacelli, E., Cantoni, C., Frizza, S., Stracci, F., Sciarma, T., et al. (1998). Valutazione neuropsicologica del sistema emozionale in pazienti cerebrolesi destri. *Riv Neurolobiol.* 44, 417–423.

Luzzi, S., Pesallaccia, M., Fabi, K., Muti, M., Viticchi, G., Provinciali, L., et al. (2011). Non-verbal memory measured by Rey-Osterrieth complex figure B: normative data. *Neurol. Sci.* 32, 1081–1089. doi: 10.1007/s10072-011-0641-1

Luzzi, S., Piccirilli, M., and Provinciali, L. (2007). Perception of emotions on happy/sad chimeric faces in Alzheimer disease: relationship with cognitive functions. *Alzheimer Dis. Assoc. Disord.* 21, 130–135. doi: 10.1097/wad.0b013e318064f445

Maddock, R. J., Garrett, A. S., and Buonocore, M. H. (2003). Posterior cingulate cortex activation by emotional words: fMRI evidence from a valence decision task. *Hum. Brain Mapp.* 18, 30–41. doi: 10.1002/hbm.10075

Mattingley, J. B., Bradshaw, J. L., Phillips, J. G., and Bradshaw, J. A. (1993). Reversed perceptual asymmetry for faces in left unilateral neglect. *Brain Cogn.* 23, 145–165. doi: 10.1006/brcg.1993.1052

McKhann, G. M., Knopman, D. S., Chertkow, H., Hyman, B. T., Jack, C. R., Kawas, C. H., et al. (2011). The diagnosis of dementia due to Alzheimer's disease: recommendations from the National institute on aging-Alzheimer's association workgroups on diagnostic guidelines for Alzheimer's disease. *Alzheimers Dement.* 7, 263–269. doi: 10.1016/j.jalz.2011.03.005

Medina, D., deToledo-Morrell, L., Urresta, F., Gabrieli, J. D. E., Moseley, M., Fleischman, D., et al. (2006). White matter changes in mild cognitive impairment and AD: a diffusion tensor imaging study. *Neurobiol. Aging* 27, 663–672. doi: 10.1016/j.neurobiolaging.2005.03.026

Medina, D. A., and Gaviria, M. (2008). Diffusion tensor imaging investigations in Alzheimer's disease: the resurgence of white matter compromise in the cortical dysfunction of the aging brain. *Neuropsychiatr. Dis. Treat.* 4, 737–742. doi: 10.2147/ndt.s3381

Moore, V., and Wyke, M. A. (1984). Drawing disability in patients with senile dementia. *Psychol. Med.* 14, 97–105. doi: 10.1017/s003329170000310x

Nakamura, K., Kawashima, R., Ito, K., Sugiura, M., Kato, T., Nakamura, A., et al. (1999). Activation of the right inferior frontal cortex during assessment of facial emotion. *J. Neurophysiol.* 82, 1610–1614.

National Institute for Health and Care Excellence. (2011). Donepezil, galantamine, rivastigmine and memantine for the treatment of Alzheimer's disease. Available online at: https://www.nice.org.uk/guidance/ta217

Nichols, T. E., and Holmes, A. P. (2002). Nonparametric permutation tests for functional neuroimaging: a primer with examples. *Hum. Brain Mapp.* 15, 1–25. doi: 10.1002/hbm.1058

Pariente, J., Cole, S., Henson, R., Clare, L., Kennedy, A., Rossor, M., et al. (2005). Alzheimer's patients engage an alternative network during a memory task. *Ann. Neurol.* 58, 870–879. doi: 10.1002/ana.20653

Poldrack, R. A., Mumford, J. A., and Nichols, T. E. (2011). *Handbook of Functional MRI Data Analysis.* Cambridge, MA: Cambridge University Press.

Rajmohan, R. (2016). *Neuroimaging of Face-Processing in Clinically Diagnosed Early-Stage Dementia of the Alzheimer Type.* [Dissertation] Lubbock, TX: Texas Tech University Health Sciences Center.

Risacher, S. L., and Saykin, A. J. (2013). Neuroimaging and other biomarkers for Alzheimer's disease: the changing landscape of early detection. *Annu. Rev. Clin. Psychol.* 9, 621–648. doi: 10.1146/annurev-clinpsy-050212-185535

Rose, S. E., McMahon, K. L., Janke, A. L., O'Dowd, B., de Zubicaray, G., Strudwick, M. W., et al. (2006). Diffusion indices on magnetic resonance imaging and neuropsychological performance in amnestic mild cognitive impairment. *J. Neurol. Neurosurg. Psychiatry* 77, 1122–1128. doi: 10.1136/jnnp.2005.074336

Roudier, M., Marcie, P., Grancher, A. S., Tzortzis, C., Starkstein, S., and Boller, F. (1998). Discrimination of facial identity and of emotions in Alzheimer's disease. *J. Neurol. Sci.* 154, 151–158. doi: 10.1016/s0022-510x(97)00222-0

Smith, S. M., Jenkinson, M., Johansen-Berg, H., Rueckert, D., Nichols, T. E., Mackay, C. E., et al. (2006). Tract-based spatial statistics: voxelwise analysis of multi-subject diffusion data. *Neuroimage* 31, 1487–1505. doi: 10.1016/j.neuroimage.2006.02.024

Smith, S. M., Jenkinson, M., Woolrich, M. W., Beckmann, C. F., Behrens, T. E., Johansen-Berg, H., et al. (2004). Advances in functional and structural MR image analysis and implementation as FSL. *Neuroimage* 23, S208–S219. doi: 10.1016/j.neuroimage.2004.07.051

Smith, S. M., and Nichols, T. E. (2009). Threshold-free cluster enhancement: addressing problems of smoothing, threshold dependence and localisation in cluster inference. *Neuroimage* 44, 83–98. doi: 10.1016/j.neuroimage.2008.03.061

Sperling, R., Chua, E., Cocchiarella, A., Rand-Giovannetti, E., Poldrack, R., Schacter, D. L., et al. (2003). Putting names to faces:: successful encoding of associative memories activates the anterior hippocampal formation. *Neuroimage* 20, 1400–1410. doi: 10.1016/S1053-8119(03)00391-4

Vuilleumier, P., and Schwartz, S. (2001). Beware and be aware: capture of spatial attention by fear-related stimuli in neglect. *Neuroreport* 12, 1119–1122. doi: 10.1097/00001756-200105080-00014

Williams, S. M. (1986). Factor analysis of the Edinburgh Handedness inventory. *Cortex* 22, 325–326. doi: 10.1016/s0010-9452(86)80058-2

Winchester, J. (2009). *Face-Processing in Persons With and Without Alzheimer's Disease.* Boca Raton, FL: Florida Atlantic University.

Worsley, K. J. (2001). "Chapter 14 Statistical analysis of activation images," in *Functional MRI: An Introduction to Methods*, eds P. Jezzard, P. M. Matthews and S. M. Smith (New York, NY: Oxford University Press), 251–270.

Yaffe, K., Blackwell, T., Gore, R., Sands, L., Reus, V., and Browner, W. S. (1999). Depressive symptoms and cognitive decline in nondemented elderly women: a prospective study. *Arch. Gen. Psychiatry* 56, 425–430. doi: 10.1001/archpsyc.56.5.425

Zhang, Y., Schuff, N., Jahng, G.-H., Bayne, W., Mori, S., Schad, L., et al. (2007). Diffusion tensor imaging of cingulum fibers in mild cognitive impairment and Alzheimer disease. *Neurology* 68, 13–19. doi: 10.1212/01.wnl.0000250326.77323.01

Zhou, Y., Dougherty, J. H., Hubner, K. F., Bai, B., Cannon, R. L., and Hutson, R. K. (2008). Abnormal connectivity in the posterior cingulate and hippocampus in early Alzheimer's disease and mild cognitive impairment. *Alzheimers Dement.* 4, 265–270. doi: 10.1016/j.jalz.2008.04.006

13

The Aerobic and Cognitive Exercise Study (ACES) for Community-Dwelling Older Adults with or At-Risk for Mild Cognitive Impairment (MCI): Neuropsychological, Neurobiological and Neuroimaging Outcomes of a Randomized Clinical Trial

Cay Anderson-Hanley[1], Nicole M. Barcelos[1], Earl A. Zimmerman[2], Robert W. Gillen[3], Mina Dunnam[4], Brian D. Cohen[5], Vadim Yerokhin[6], Kenneth E. Miller[7], David J. Hayes[1], Paul J. Arciero[8], Molly Maloney[1] and Arthur F. Kramer[9]*

[1] The Healthy Aging and Neuropsychology Lab, Union College, Schenectady, NY, United States, [2] Alzheimer's Disease Center, Albany Medical Center, Albany, NY, United States, [3] Sunnyview Rehabilitation Hospital, Schenectady, NY, United States, [4] Stratton VA Medical Center, Albany, NY, United States, [5] Department of Biology, Union College, Schenectady, NY, United States, [6] Biomedical Sciences Department, Oklahoma State University, Tulsa, OK, United States, [7] Department of Anatomy and Cell Biology, Oklahoma State University, Tulsa, OK, United States, [8] Department of Health & Human Physiological Sciences, Skidmore College, Saratoga Springs, NY, United States, [9] Beckman Institute, University of Illinois, Urbana-Champaign, Champaign, IL, United States

***Correspondence:**
Cay Anderson-Hanley
andersoc@union.edu

Prior research has found that cognitive benefits of physical exercise and brain health in older adults may be enhanced when mental exercise is interactive simultaneously, as in exergaming. It is unclear whether the cognitive benefit can be maximized by increasing the degree of mental challenge during exercise. This randomized clinical trial (RCT), the Aerobic and Cognitive Exercise Study (ACES) sought to replicate and extend prior findings of added cognitive benefit from exergaming to those with or at risk for mild cognitive impairment (MCI). ACES compares the effects of 6 months of an *exer-tour* (virtual reality bike rides) with the effects of a more effortful *exer-score* (pedaling through a videogame to score points). Fourteen community-dwelling older adults meeting screening criteria for MCI (sMCI) were adherent to their assigned exercise for 6 months. The primary outcome was executive function, while secondary outcomes included memory and everyday cognitive function. Exer-tour and exer-score yielded significant moderate effects on executive function (Stroop A/C; d's = 0.51 and 0.47); there was no significant interaction effect. However, after 3 months the exer-tour revealed a significant and moderate effect, while exer-score showed little impact, as did a game-only condition. Both exer-tour and exer-score conditions also resulted in significant improvements in verbal memory. Effects appear to generalize to self-reported everyday cognitive function. Pilot data, including salivary biomarkers and structural MRI, were gathered at baseline and 6 months; exercise dose was associated with increased BDNF as well as increased gray matter volume in the PFC and ACC. Improvement in memory was associated with an increase in the DLPFC. Improved executive function was associated with increased expression of exosomal miRNA-9. Interactive physical and cognitive exercise (both high and low mental challenge) yielded similarly significant cognitive benefit for adherent sMCI exercisers over 6 months. A larger RCT is needed to confirm these findings. Further innovation and clinical trial data are needed to develop accessible, yet engaging and effective interventions to combat cognitive decline for the growing MCI population.

ClinicalTrials.gov ID: NCT02237560

Keywords: cognitive, exercise, aging, MCI, dementia, neuropsychological, exergame, Alzheimer's disease

INTRODUCTION

Annual diagnoses of dementia, such as due to Alzheimer's disease (AD), are expected to approach 1 million in 2050, more than double the new cases diagnosed in 2000 (Alzheimer's Association, 2014). Lacking a cure for any of the many causes of this devastating decline in cognitive function and loss of independence, a rising public health outcry has helped spark initiatives like the National Alzheimer's Project Act (2011) and the Healthy Brain Initiative (Alzheimer's Association and Centers for Disease Control Prevention, 2013). Research continues to press on, seeking innovative and empirically-validated ways to prevent or ameliorate cognitive decline and impairment.

While behavioral interventions are unlikely to completely prevent or halt dementia, there is the potential for physical exercise to reduce the risk of dementia onset (Heyn et al., 2004; Hillman et al., 2008) or slow progression (Larson, 2010). It has been estimated that if the onset of dementia could be delayed a few years, the impact on the population over time could be dramatic, decreasing prevalence by 1 million cases after 10 years in the United States alone. By also delaying progression for 2 years this could reduce dementia incidence by an astonishing 18 million cases globally per year (Sano et al., 1997; Brookmeyer et al., 1998). Interventions that reach patients before they have declined into diagnosable dementia can have the greatest impact. Thus, it is especially desirable to develop interventions that target those who may be at an intermediate stage, perhaps diagnosed with or at risk for mild cognitive impairment (MCI; per DSM-IV in 1994; Jak et al., 2009) also known more recently as mild neurocognitive disorder (mNCD per DSM-V in 2013; henceforth MCI will be used for simplicity; Roberts and Knopman, 2013; Jak et al., 2016).

Neuropsychological Effects of Physical and Cognitive Exercise

Researchers have been investigating a variety of behavioral interventions, including exercise, to improve cognitive function and decrease risk of progression to dementia among individuals with MCI (e.g., Kramer et al., 1999; Colcombe and Kramer, 2003; Studenski et al., 2006; Angevaren et al., 2008; Baker et al., 2010; Geda et al., 2010; Martin et al., 2011). Physical exercise has garnered significant support in the literature for its potency in effecting cognitive benefits (e.g., Colcombe and Kramer, 2003). While the literature examining the relationship between physical exercise and cognitive benefit is not without issues (e.g., recent Cochrane Reviews; Forbes et al., 2015; Young et al., 2015, which focused on dementia and normative older adults, respectively), it is widely accepted that exercise benefits cognition, particularly executive function among symptomatic individuals, that are yet early in their cognitive decline (e.g., MCI), the very population on which this study focused (e.g., Colcombe and Kramer, 2003; Etnier and Chang, 2009; Geda et al., 2010; Gates, 2013; Hess et al., 2014; Zheng et al., 2016). Indeed, pre-clinical persons, ranging from asymptomatic older adults to those with early MCI, may experience the greatest benefit from exercise, due to the relatively preserved brain structures and functions (in contrast with more progressed dementia) that can support and supply components needed to realize neuroplasticity as triggered by exercise (e.g., Colcombe et al., 2004; Kramer and Erickson, 2007; Ahlskog et al., 2011; Teixeira et al., 2016). However, knowing that physical exercise may be good for one's body and brain may not be enough to induce regular practice of exercise. Most older adults do not meet the guideline from the American College of Sports Medicine (ACSM) which now recommends 45 min per day, 5–7 days per week, including vigorous exercise (Chodzko-Zajko et al., 2009).

In a previous randomized clinical trial (Anderson-Hanley et al., 2012), we aimed to induce a thorough dose of exercise (Vidoni et al., 2015) by assigning older adults to an exergame[1]. We expected that the engagement of a stimulating exergame would motivate regular exercise, therefore allowing older adults to achieve maximum cognitive benefit. Three months of pedaling a virtual-reality-enhanced stationary ergometer, displaying scenic bike tours which we referred to as a "cybercycle" (see **Figure 1**), was compared with a traditional stationary bike. In the end, the cybercycle condition yielded significantly greater cognitive benefit, as hypothesized. However, surprisingly, it was not due to a difference in dose; we found instead that both the cybercycle and traditional cyclists has been similarly adherent (e.g., no significant difference between groups in miles, minutes, power, heart rate, etc.).

This unexpected finding raised the possibility that the screen display was providing benefit, beyond that of basic entertainment

[1]Exergaming is a subset of health games, sometimes referred to as active games, that combine physical exercise with interactive gaming features, often through a virtual reality-type platform (Van Schaik et al., 2008; Read and Shortell, 2011; Stanmore et al., 2017).

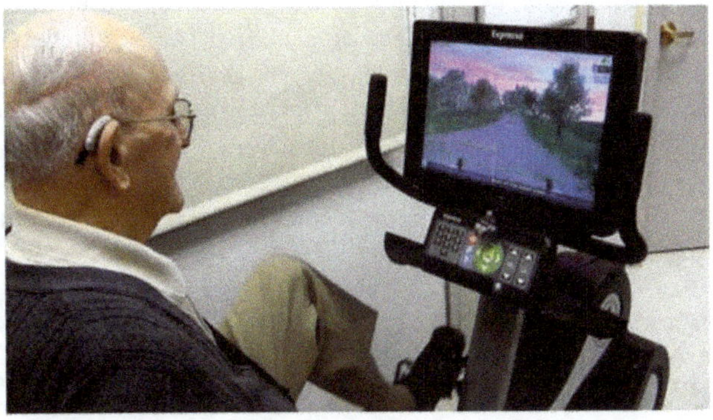

FIGURE 1 | Stationary bike equipped with virtual reality display (aka "cybercycle" so named in our previous RCT; Anderson-Hanley et al., 2012). Former study participant demonstrating use of a cybercycle exergame; used with permission.

or motivation. We theorized the enhanced form of exercise was yielding findings much like those of the environmental enrichment literature (e.g., animals provided with greater physical and mental stimulation experience enhanced brain function; Pusic et al., 2016); thus it seems more (even two types at once) is generally better, although to a point. In humans the complexity of experience and the diversity of type, timing and compounding of "enrichment" makes this considerably challenging to study as a unique phenomenon. It seemed that for our participants, by interacting with the tour stimuli on screen (e.g., changing pedaling speed yielded a change in speed of scenery moving by), they were certainlyengaged in some additional amount of cognitive processing beyond the control condition. This layered cognitive stimulation may have combined with the physical exercise required of the exergame to create a "two-for-one" impact that resulted in the observed additional cognitive benefit for participants. Hence, we hypothesized that participants experienced better neuropsychological outcomes because of the potentially synergistic phenomena created by combining a type of "mental exercise" that was interactive with physical exercise (Anderson-Hanley et al., 2012; Frantzidis et al., 2014).

Several areas of the research literature speak to the possible validity of this hypothesized compounding or synergistic effect. As previously mentioned, there is a robust literature documenting the cognitive benefits of physical exercise. There is also a growing literature on cognitive training that purports significant effects (Willis et al., 2006; Karr et al., 2014; Toril et al., 2014; Wang et al., 2014; Huntley et al., 2015; Train the Brain Consortium, 2017). However, in our view, the claims are less convincing due to problems with reporting, limited generalizability, and other reasons that have been cited in various critiques of the literature and related "brain training" industry (e.g., Owen et al., 2010; Muijden et al., 2012; Redick et al., 2013; Boot and Kramer, 2014; Simons et al., 2016; Zokaei et al., 2016). Indeed, a Cochrane Review of 11 RCTs concluded there was "no indication of any significant benefits from cognitive training" (Bahar-Fuchs et al., 2013, p. 1). Nevertheless, considering some "mixed" results on the potential benefits of cognitive training, and as well as the animal literature on neurobiological impact of cognitive enrichments (reviewed below), there is potential for mental challenge to have its own benefit on cognition. Although perhaps it is most effectively implemented as part of a more naturalistic intervention, as when integrated with physical activity that taps additional neural mechanisms.

One way to examine this possibility further is to evaluate the body of literature that encompasses the cognitive effects of interventions with multiple components (e.g., cognitive training and physical exercise). Often these are referred to as:

- "combined" interventions, wherein the components are administered sequentially/in tandem (e.g., Barnes et al., 2013; Fiatarone et al., 2014; Law et al., 2014; Wang et al., 2014; Rahe et al., 2015; Karssemeijer et al., 2017; Lipardo et al., 2017),which can be contrasted with:
- "dual-task" interventions, wherein components are administered simultaneously, but typically are separate tasks (e.g., reciting numbers backwards while walking; Schaefer and Schumacher, 2011; Coelho et al., 2013b; Forte et al., 2013; Theill et al., 2013; Bherer, 2015; Eggenberger et al., 2015; Yokoyama et al., 2015; Desjardins-Crépeau et al., 2016), which can be further contrasted with:
- interactive interventions, as in exergaming, in which the actions in one realm affect the other (e.g., pedaling and steering controls progress in a virtual world and attainment of goals; Anderson-Hanley et al., 2012; Maillot et al., 2012; González-Palau et al., 2014; Schoene et al., 2014; Bamidis et al., 2015; Styliadis et al., 2015; Eggenberger et al., 2016; Lauenroth et al., 2016; Wang et al., 2016; Stanmore et al., 2017).

Indeed, there is a vast literature on "dual-task" experiments and interventions (Kramer et al., 1985; Hiyamizu et al., 2012; Kramer and Wong et al., 2015; Hosseini et al., 2017), which sometimes focus on the limitations of human abilities to manage two separate (non-interactive tasks) at once (e.g., walking and counting numbers backwards). Traditionally, the aim of dual-task training might focus on interference effects (Al-Yahya et al., 2011) and improving physical outcomes (e.g., decreasing falls) for impaired individuals (e.g., post-stroke), especially while managing dual tasks. More recently, studies have examined cognitive outcomes in dual tasks wherein there is more naturalistic interactivity (as in the cybercycle scenario above; Anderson-Hanley et al., 2012; as well as other interactive modalities such as dance: Foster, 2013; Kattenstroth et al., 2013; Dhami et al., 2015; Schoene et al., 2015; Burzynska et al., 2017; Marquez et al., 2017; Müller et al., 2017; Rehfeld et al., 2017). These recent studies seem to be converging on a similar cognitive-enhancing phenomenon that lends empirical support to the synergistic hypothesis outlined above and in part, elsewhere (Fissler et al., 2013). Recent reviews of the literature on the cognitive benefits of exergaming for older adults conclude the preliminary evidence is promising (Smith et al., 2010; Schoene et al., 2013; Bamidis et al., 2014; Barry et al., 2014; Chao et al., 2014; Ogawa et al., 2016; Zhu et al., 2016; Zilidou et al., 2016), but further research of the effects of these interactive interventions and the impact of specific components (e.g., passive stimulation vs. active cognitive training, aerobic vs. non-aerobic activity, etc.) is necessary.

We have previously hypothesized that the benefits of interactive physical and cognitive exercise may increase with increased mental effort and our lab published a pilot trial as a precursor to this present RCT, the Aerobic and Cognitive Exercise Study pilot (ACES-pilot; Barcelos et al., 2015). The ACES-pilot sought to investigate whether greater cognitive challenge while exergaming would yield differential outcomes in executive function and generalize to everyday functioning. Sixty-four community-dwelling older adults (mean age = 82) were randomly assigned to pedal a stationary bike, while interactively engaging on-screen with: (1) a low cognitive demand task (pedaling a steering along a virtual bike tour, referred to as *exer-tour*), or (2) a high cognitive demand task (pedaling and steering to chase dragons and score points in a 3D video game, referred to as *exer-score*). Executive function (indices from Trails, Stroop and Digit Span) was assessed before and after a single-bout and 3-month exercise intervention. A significant group × time interaction after 3 months of exergaming (Stroop; among 20 adherents). Those in the high cognitive demand group performed better than those in the low cognitive dose condition. Self-reported everyday function improved across both exercise conditions. These pilot data indicated that for older adults, cognitive benefit while exergaming increased concomitantly with higher doses of interactive mental challenge (Barcelos et al., 2015). The present study aims to replicate and extend that finding to MCI.

Neurobiological and Neuroimaging Effects of Physical and Cognitive Exercise

It is our hypothesis that interactivity can produce greater cognitive effects due to synergistic processes that compound or magnify the benefit in a non-linear way, perhaps by activation and utilization of neurobiological substrate of the mind-body interface that is evolutionarily adapted for success in naturalistic tasks (in this case, goal-directed motion through 3D space). While theory and research connecting cognitive processes to neurobiological pathways triggered by exercise in humans is expanding rapidly, there are indications of important links with various biomarkers (e.g., brain-derived neurotrophic factor [BDNF], insulin-like growth factor [IFG-1]; Cotman et al., 2007; Knaepen et al., 2010), including expression of microRNA (miRNA) in circulating exosomes (Pusic et al., 2016; Bertoldi et al., 2017), and brain structure and function (e.g., gray and white matter regions: Colcombe et al., 2006; hippocampus; Thomas et al., 2012; Erickson et al., 2015; Sexton et al., 2016). Animal models have more plainly linked certain differential, compounding or synergistic cognitive benefits with neurobiological phenomenon when both physical and mental exercise are provided (e.g., in laboratory mice exposed to enriched environments with physical and/or cognitive challenges; Greenough et al., 1999; Churchill et al., 2002; Olson et al., 2006; Galvan and Bredesen, 2007; Fabel et al., 2009; Voss et al., 2013; Jessberger and Gage, 2014). These studies and others, detail a variety of mechanisms and impacts linking mental and physical exercise to improved neuronal and brain health (e.g., via increased cerebral perfusion, neurogenesis, angiogensis, synaptogenesis; Greenough et al., 1999; Gage, 2002; Trachtenberg et al., 2002; Tsai et al., 2016; Kleemeyer et al., 2017), even detailing specific differential benefits (Black et al., 1990; Olson et al., 2006; Suo et al., 2016) such as cell proliferation with physical exercise, and cell survival with mental exercise (Van Praag et al., 2005; van Praag, 2008).

The Present Research

Since only a tiny fraction of older adults exercise at levels recommended by the ACSM and American Heart Association (AHA; Chodzko-Zajko et al., 2009), and physician recommendation appears to do little to change sedentary behaviors (Grandes et al., 2009), the novel exergame utilized in this study holds the promise of increasing compliance by virtue of the distracting components of the virtual reality environment and the interactive and challenging features of the videogame. Besides being a potentially effective way of engaging older adults in exercise, the present RCT augments prior research by exploring the neuropsychological benefits of interactive cognitive and physical training combined, rather than focusing on either alone (Colcombe and Kramer, 2003; Anguera et al., 2013), or in tandem, but lacking interactivity (Fabre et al., 2002; Oswald et al., 2006; Kraft, 2012; Suzuki et al., 2012; Hotting and Roder, 2013; Shatil, 2013; González-Palau et al., 2014; Satoh et al., 2014; Shah et al., 2014; Suo et al., 2016). By examining the neuropsychological effects some of the components separately (e.g., physical exercise and mental exercise alone), this study attempts to tease apart the unique contributions of each component to any benefit to cognition, as well as the potentially differential effect of low- vs. high-cognitive demands. The present research specifically examines the benefits of these behavioral interventions for community-dwelling older adults with or at risk for MCI and thus, attempts to extend previous findings to this more vulnerable population.

Finally, this RCT examines potential underlying mechanisms of effects of combined physical and mental exercise on cognition through the collection of neurobiological and neuroimaging data. Prior research has begun to clarify the role a number of biomarkers (primarily from serum, CNS, or saliva) that change in accord with exercise interventions and appear to be linked improvements in brain health that and/or promote improvements in cognition. For example, exercise has been shown to yield: increases in Brain-Derived Neurotrophic Factor (BDNF; Cotman et al., 2007; Coelho et al., 2013a; Leckie et al., 2014; Vaughan et al., 2014; Dinoff et al., 2016; Maass et al., 2016) and variable responses of insulin-like growth factor 1 (IGF-1; Lorens-Martín et al., 2009). Research linking traditional physical exercise and cognition in older adults has identified BDNF and IGF-1 as biomarkers linking cognitive function and healthy aging (Voss et al., 2010; Bellar et al., 2011; Erickson et al., 2012; Hotting and Roder, 2013; Phillips et al., 2014; Szuhany et al., 2014; Geerlings et al., 2015; Lara et al., 2015; Maass et al., 2016). BDNF plays an important role in neuronal growth and survival, it modulates neurotransmitters, and is involved in the cascade to promote neuronal plasticity, while IGF-1 has also been implicated as a mechanism in exercise-induced neuronal plasticity (Voss et al., 2010; Brown et al., 2013; Phillips et al., 2015; Maass et al., 2016). Cotman et al. (2007) has presented a model in which exercise induces activity of BDNF and IGF-1 in multiple pathways that facilitate: (a) learning, (b) neurogenesis, and (c) angiogenesis. Furthermore, some research has found increases in vascular endothelial growth factor with exercise (VEGF; Vital et al., 2014). While growth factors are typically said to increase with exercise, there are number of reports of decreases in inflammatory markers: C-reactive protein and Interleukin-6 (CRP and IL6; Thielen et al., 2016; Monteiro-Junior et al., 2017). Additionally, recent progressive research has also been examining the potential for circulating exosomes to serve as early markers of neuropathology, such as AD, to act as delivery vehicles for potentially reparative miRNA expressions, and even to play a positive role the neurbiological effects of exercise (e.g., Zhang et al., 2014; Kumar and Reddy, 2016; Pusic et al., 2016; Batistela et al., 2017; Bertoldi et al., 2017). Some promising research has pointed to miRNA-9 and miRNA-193 as linked to benefit in neurobiological processes such that they play a therapeutic role in dementia (e.g., Russell et al., 2013; Párrizas et al., 2015; Li et al., 2016; Riancho et al., 2017).

In sum, exercise appears to be able to trigger or enhance the function of complex cascades of neurobiological processes that have sometimes been linked to cognitive benefits or other expressions of brain or CNS health. It is likely that a number of those processes act on neurophysiological substrate to foster improved brain health that leads to improved cognition; some of those mediating phenonmena may even be visible through structural imaging.

Structural changes in certain regions of the brain have been found to follow exercise and are often linked to concomitant changes in cognition; for example, increases in the hippocampus (Lorens-Martín et al., 2009; Erickson et al., 2011), as well as the anterior cingulate cortex, dorsal lateral prefrontal cortex, and more broadly the prefrontal cortex (ACC, DLPC, and PFC; Gordon et al., 2008; Erickson et al., 2011; Weinstein et al., 2012; Curlik and Shors, 2013; Hayes et al., 2013; Nishiguchi et al., 2015; ten Brinke et al., 2015; Jonasson et al., 2017; Li et al., 2017). While the body of research has been growing with respect to linking physical exercise and cognition via biomarkers, scant literature has yet explored how these indicators and mechanisms react in the case of combined or interactive mental and physical exercise interventions in humans, wherein there might be somewhat differential or compounding beneficial effects given a two-for-one intervention (for a promising exception, see Eggenberger et al., 2016). The present study aims to address a number of these gaps and replicate or extend other findings in the literature.

Hypotheses

This study is a partial replication and extension of the ACES-pilot (Barcelos et al., 2015) and it was hypothesized that, similar to that which was found in that prior pilot study: physical exercise interactive with effortful cognitive challenge (exer-score; **Figure 2**), would produce greater cognitive benefit than physical exercise that was interactive with relatively passive cognitive processing (exer-tour). We expected this previously observed phenomenon to extend to MCI specifically. The primary aim of the trial was for community-dwelling older adults with or at risk for MCI to engage their assigned intervention regularly for 6 months (longer than the ACES-pilot, which extended only to 3 months). Baseline to 6-month intervention (exer-tour vs. exer-score) were hypothesized to yield these effects:

1. executive function would increase significantly after either exer-score and exer-tour (within subjects main effect)
2. executive function would increase significantly more for exer-score (high mental challenge) than for exer-tour (low mental challenge; between subjects interaction effect)
3. effects of either exer-score or exer-tour would exceed that of game-only
   a. additionally, a comparison would be made with archival/normative exercise-only data (available only for a 3-month window, this trial's midpoint)
4. salivary biomarker changes expected to be correlated with improved cognition and exercise dose included:
   a. increased growth factors: BDNF, IGF-1, and VEGF
   b. decreased inflammatory markers: CRP and IL-6
   c. increased exosomal expression of miRNA-193 and miRNA-9
5. neuroimaging changes expected to be associated with improved cognition and exercise dose included:
   a. increased gray matter volume in the ACC, DLPFC, hippocampus, and PFC.

METHODS

Participants

All study procedures were approved by the appropriate Institutional Review Boards (i.e., including the PI's institution and the three medical centers where the study was conducted; see section Author Notes). Older adults with a diagnosis of MCI were initially sought via referrals from neurology and neuropsychology at three medical centers in a specific region of upstate New York where participants were to exercise (using a cybercyle placed at each center's physical therapy clinic). However, given difficulties enrolling patients (especially due to travel requirements, but also due to challenges targeting patients with MCI before progression to dementia), further IRB approval was obtained to expand recruitment by locating additional cybercycles at several more locations around the region (e.g., retirement communities, YMCAs, etc.) for a total of 14 sites. Enrollment was thus expanded to include self-referred community-dwelling older adults, aiming to include especially those that might be undiagnosed (because symptoms had not affected function), but yet who might meet criteria for, or could be said to be at risk for MCI (e.g., thus those that would meet screening criteria for MCI, herein referred to as "screened as MCI" or sMCI[2]). Participants were recruited using fliers,

[2]Screened as MCI (sMCI) based on a MoCA cut-off score for MCI of <26 (Nasreddine et al., 2005). This screening approach was utilized after initial planned attempts to enroll clinically diagnosed patients with MCI (e.g., recruited from neurologists, neuropsychologists, and geriatricians, yielded patients that had often

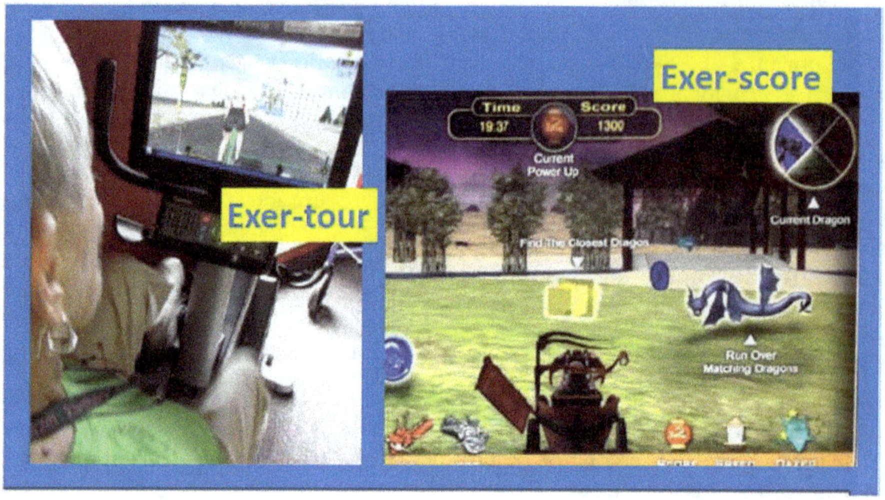

FIGURE 2 | Exer-tour (relatively cognitively passive) vs. Exer-score (cognitively effortful). Exer-tour (pedaling controls speed on screen and progress along scenic bike paths; involves steering, but relatively passive compared to exer-score; for example, can't leave road or crash into anything or any rider which one can steer through; could cease steering without consequence other than tilted view, bike will follow curb). Exer-score (requires navigating in 360° radius to locate colored coins and matching colored dragons of varying speed/difficulty to steer through; the goal is to score points and strategy may be employed to avoid losing points by avoiding hazards, while also seeking out bonus points available via tagging specialized objects one can choose to explore). Former study participant demonstrating exer-tour condition; used with permission.

newspaper ads, and information sessions. The timeline for the conduct of the study was 2014–2016. Volunteers (n = 220; see CONSORT **Figure 3** for details) were screened by phone and were excluded if they had known neurologic disorders (e.g., Alzheimer's, Parkinson's, or seizures) or functional limitations that would restrict participation in cognitive testing or exercise. After reviewing the informed consent form (ICF) and answering all questions, a signed document was obtained from all participants and their surrogate, if appropriate, based on the Impaired Decision Making Capacity screen (IDMC; Karlawish, 2008). Physician approval (PCP and if applicable, cardiologist) was obtained for all participants to engage in exercise as assigned. Enrollees (n = 111) were community-dwelling older adults with a mean age of 78.1 (SD = 9.9), who were predominantly female (66%), well educated (average years of education = 16.2, SD = 2.4) Causasians (three individuals self-reported minority ethnic/racial status). Participants scored on average 23.7 (SD = 3.1) on the Montreal Cognitive Assessment (MoCA; 30-point multidimensional scale, with higher scores indicative of better global cognitive function; Nasreddine et al., 2005; Freitas et al., 2012; Julayanont et al., 2014), such that 75% of enrollees were categorized at meeting screening criteria for sMCI ("screened as MCI" based on MoCA < 26; Nasreddine et al., 2005).

To provide an additional point of comparison of the relative effect of physical exercise alone vs. interactively combined with mental exercise, archival data was culled from our prior Cybercycle Study. In that study, 33 participants were randomly assigned to a traditional exercise or "pedal-only" condition in which participants pedaled a stationary bike (in many cases the same model as used in the present study), but without the virtual reality display (see below for between group comparisons at baseline; for additional details see Anderson-Hanley et al., 2012, 2014; Dimitrova et al., 2016).

Baseline Comparisons Between Groups

Between the three randomly assigned groups in the present study (exer-tour, exer-score, and game-only; n = 46, 45, 20, respectively), cognitive measures revealed that the groups were comparable (no significant differences) on: overall cognitive function (MoCA), rate of sMCI, and performance on individual tests of cognition including: executive function, visual spatial skill, and memory (verbal, nonverbal, list, story, immediate or delayed).

On behavioral measures, those who were in the game-only condition were somewhat less motivated to be in the study, were not as ready for exercise, and reported they were more sedentary (recall that some participants were randomly assigned to game-only, but others were recruited specifically to the condition, including with remuneration, due to a high dropout rate once randomly assigned participants learned they would not be engaging in a physical exercise component). However, self-reported cognitive engagement (both recent and lifetime), was similar across all three groups.

Baseline comparisons between the four groups, including the above three, but also a pedal-only condition (archival control group data from our prior study noted above; n = 33), revealed that all four groups were similar (no significant differences) on: the three primary outcome measures of executive function to be the focus of our study (i.e., ratio scores for Digits, Trails,

already progressed in their decline toward dementia). Indeed, by the time some patients had been referred for clinical evaluations, received a formal diagnosis and subsequently were referred to our study, their disease had progressed such that they no longer fit our target population of MCI. As a result, attempts to enroll such referrals led to exclusion as the patient sometimes would be unable to understand or participate in the research and/or complex intervention procedures.

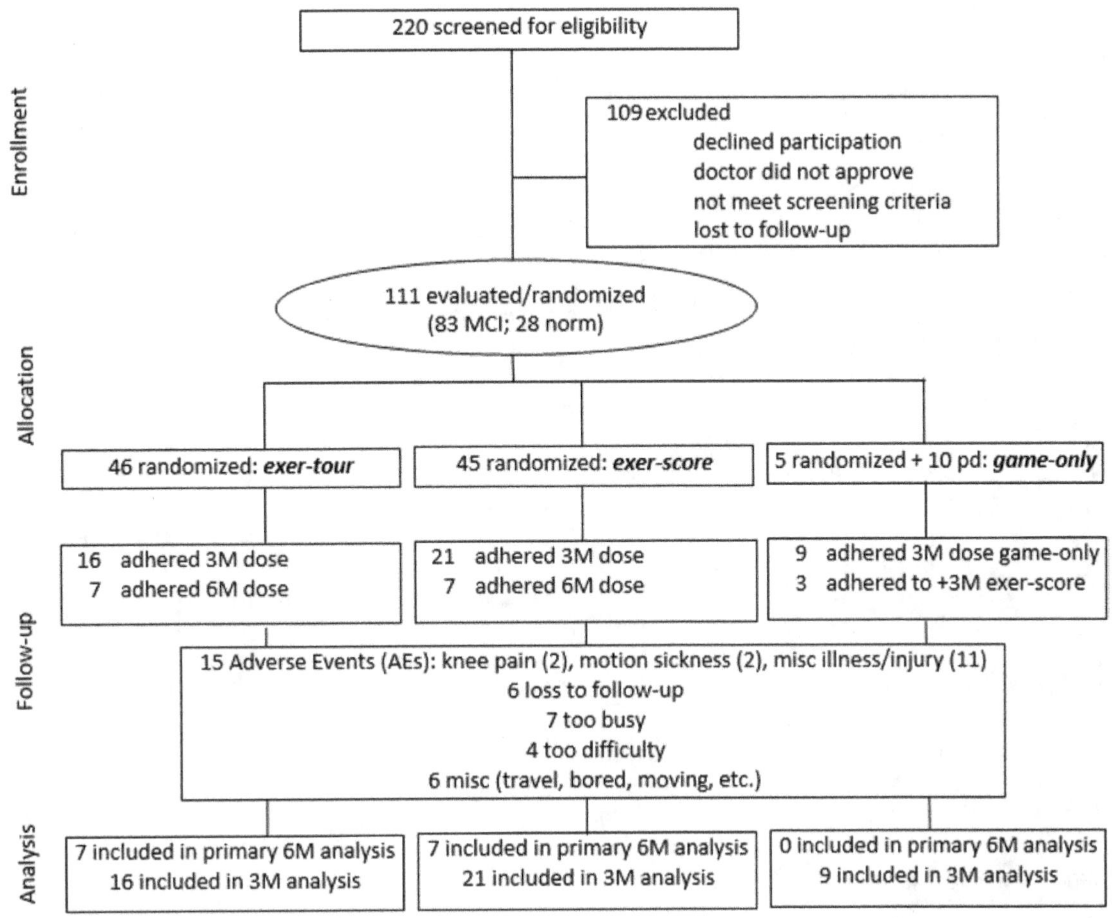

FIGURE 3 | CONSORT flow diagram showing participant enrollment, randomization, and status in trial and analysis.

and Stroop; see below for details). The four groups were also comparable in proportion of men and women and BMI, but the pedal-only condition was significantly older and had fewer years of education[3] (confirming use of age and education covariates in statistical analyses).

Procedures

Participants were initially randomly assigned to one of three conditions for 6 months: (1) exer-tour: physical exercise interactive with relatively passive, low cognitive load, virtual scenic bike tour; or (2) exer-score: physical exercise interactive with a relatively effortful, high cognitive demand, videogame (see **Figure 2** for sample screen shots); or (3) game-only: the same videogame operated by a joystick or keyboard (no physical exercise was required). Exercise participants pedaled a virtual reality enhanced, recumbent stationary bike (Expresso S3R, from Interactive Fitness Holdings, LLC). Individuals in the exer-tour condition pedaled through various virtual scenic bike tours while steering along the path (but without significant consequence for not steering; that is the bike would coast along the curb and one could pass through other riders fluidly). Those in the exer-score condition pedaled through a scenic landscape where the goal was to score points by collecting different colored coins and corresponding colored dragons. Throughout the videogame (either exer-score or game-only), participants could navigate through bonus items to increase their speed and score, while avoiding penalties (e.g., steering into water). The exer-tour condition was presumed to require less mental engagement than the videogame conditions, as the game called for scoring and thus, potentially effortful planning, tracking, multi-tasking, and strategizing (a validity check of this assumption was confirmed by those in the exer-score condition who reported expending significantly greater "mental effort" than those in the exer-score condition; see **Table 1**). Participants were provided "thank you gifts" (e.g., water- bottle, mug, etc.) at each of evaluation (baseline, 3-month, and 6-month).

Given difficulty retaining participants in the game-only condition (due to preference for active/physical exercise, boredom once started, etc.), the protocol was again adjusted, with IRB approval, to allow randomly assigned game-only participants to switch to the exer-score condition at the 3-month

[3]This difference is surmised to be likely due to differences in recruitment as the prior, Cybercycle Study, only included participants exercising at their residential facility, whereas the present study included those that could travel to exercise equipment, often at locations across town.

TABLE 1 | Exer-tour vs. exer-score baseline demographics for adherent completers (0–6M).

	MCI adherents to prescribed dose of 6-month intervention														MCI
	Exer-tour			Exer-score			ANOVA	Combined adherents			Non-adherents			ANOVA
	Ave	SD	n	Ave	SD	n	p[a]	Ave	SD	n	Ave	SD	n	p[a]
DEMOGRAPHICS														
Age	80.9	12.3	7	75.4	9.83	7	0.38	78.1	11.0	14	80.9	8.2	54	0.31
Education (yrs)	14.9	2.3	7	16.6	2.76	7	0.23	15.7	2.6	14	16.1	2.5	52	0.61
Sex (% female)	57%			43%			0.63	50%			69%			0.20
Est IQ (NAART)	128.5	11.9	7	136.8	5.26	7	0.12	132.7	9.8	14	134.3	7.3	54	0.49
Cog fn (MoCA)	21.6	2.7	7	22.0	3.21	7	0.79	21.8	2.9	14	22.6	2.0	54	0.20
Retired	100%		7	100%		7	ns	100%			86%			0.15
BMI	24.8	3.9	7	26.3	2.73	7	0.43	25.6	3.3	14	26.9	3.7	54	0.24
Cog activities (CAS)	17.9	4.5	7	20.1	3.98	7	0.34	19.0	4.3	14	19.3	8.3	54	0.89
Experience bike	2.4	0.79	7	2.3	0.76	7	0.74	2.4	0.74	14	2.1	0.84	52	0.39
Experience computers	2.1	1.1	7	3.1	1.07	7	0.11	2.6	1.2	14	2.6	1.2	52	0.98
Experience videogames	0.43	0.79	7	1.3	0.76	7	0.06	0.9	0.86	14	0.69	0.85	52	0.52
Motivated	2.6	0.53	7	2.4	0.53	7	0.63	2.5	0.52	14	2.7	0.47	51	0.20
PAR	0.86	0.69	7	0.86	0.69	7	1.00	0.9	0.66	14	1.1	1.0	50	0.31
Physical activity level (SRPA)	2.9	1.3	7	3.6	0.98	7	0.28	3.2	1.2	14	2.9	1.2	47	0.43
Functional disability (FAQ)	8.1	9.0	7	1.6	1.81	7	0.08	4.9	7.1	14	2.8	4.7	49	0.06
VALIDITY CHECKS														
Average num rides/wk	3.9	1.2	7	4.0	1.1	7	0.86							
HR average	102.9	13.6	7	108.2	22.1	7	0.60							
Mental effort (self-report)	1.8	0.75	6	3.1	0.69	7	**0.007**							

[a]*Comparison between groups.*
[b]*Comparison with baseline.*
[c]*Repeated meas ANCOVA controlling for age and education.*
Bold value indicate statistically significant ($p \leq 0.05$).

mid-point evaluation. Additionally, game-only participants were also recruited separately with modest periodic remuneration provided. Upon enrollment, participants were phone screened for eligibility and administered the Impaired Decision-Making Capacity structured interview (IDMC; Veterans Administration Medical Center (VAMC), 2007) and provided informed consent (co-signed by a surrogate or legally-authorized representative as applicable and/or per the IDMC). Once scheduled for an initial evaluation, participants were mailed the ICF, demographic, health and fitness history questionnaires. If they were willing, an MRI (3T) of the brain was scheduled. At the baseline evaluation, a saliva sample was collected (passive drool), and they were administered a neuropsychological test battery (specified below). Individuals were trained in the use of the equipment for their assigned condition and underwent a single bout of exercise for 20 min. Participants were asked to maintain a target heart rate level, which was calculated using the Karvonen equation (McAuley et al., 2011) and measured via steering hand-grips built into the cybercycle (displayed on screen for participant monitoring and captured by onboard computer for later data extraction and analysis). Post-testing was conducted following the single bout[4] (SB) of exercise.

Following the baseline (BL) evaluation, individuals were instructed to exercise for at least 20 min at least twice a week, and to gradually increase exercise duration to 45 min and frequency to at least three to five times per week until the 3-month (3M) mid-point evaluation, and then maintain that pattern though a 6-month (6M) final evaluation. Participants were instructed to aim toward their individualized specific target heart rate (per above) throughout the intervention period. Participants were also asked to document their exercise sessions on log pages provided in a binder and used to calculate adherence statistics (e.g., frequency, heart rate average, etc.); additionally, the computer onboard the cybercycle captured similar data which was used for spot verification. A final evaluation, including repeat

[4]single-bout results are not reported herein in part due to space constraints, but also given the focus of the RCT on long-term intervention results which necessarily analyzes a different/smaller sample of those adherent for 6-months; furthermore the single-bout was not a part of a priori hypotheses in the study design, but rather included to accompany the training session and provide a repeat testing experience/familiarization with tests before the follow-up evaluations (3 M and 6 M) which would partly help "wash out"/reach sooner the plateau of practice/learning effects and thus more plainly isolate intervention effects at the follow-up evaluations; finally, the single-bout assessment provides a consistent pattern with our prior RCTs (the Cybercycle Study and the ACES-pilot) in which similarly a second round of testing before the long-term outcome for similar reasons, as such this increases comparability of our data across trials and time-points (both in terms of amount of familiarization with testing and matching of alternate forms at each time-point).

neuropsychological, biomarker, and neuroimaging assessments, was conducted at the end of the 6-month intervention period.

MEASURES

Primary Measures

Cognitive Function

Paper and pencil tests comprised the battery and alternate forms of cognitive tests were utilized at each evaluation to minimize practice/learning effects from serial testing. Cognitive testing was done at baseline (BL) before starting the intervention, after the 20-min training single-bout session, at a 3-month (3M) mid-point, and after concluding the 6-month (6M) intervention period.

Executive Function (Primary Outcome)

Three tests were selected to assess aspects of executive function, which has been shown to be a complex, yet overarching domain of cognitive function. The following three tests were chosen as they are thought to tap overlapping, yet distinct components of executive function, particularly mental flexibility (i.e., Stroop for inhibition, Trails for set shifting, and Digit Span for working memory; Wecker et al., 2000; Strauss et al., 2006). Executive function is critical cognitive function for maintaining independence in later life and thus an important focus of this study's intervention efforts (Pereira et al., 2008; Marshall et al., 2011).

Stroop (Van der Elst et al., 2006)

A short, 40-item version of Stroop was administered. Colored squares (red, green, blue) were presented in rows first (Stroop A), followed by those color words typed in black ink (Stroop B), followed by incongruent color words (Stroop C; in which participants were asked to name the color of the ink while ignoring the written word). A ratio was computed to isolate the executive function component of the task (Stroop A/C; Lansbergen et al., 2007). Among older adults, the ratio score has reasonable test-retest reliability (0.68) over 1–2 months (Ettenhofer et al., 2006) and strong test-retest reliability (0.80) over 2 weeks using the shortened version used herein (Houx et al., 2002). Higher ratios indicate better executive function.

Color trails (D'Elia et al., 1996)

Color Trails 1, requires participants to connect numbered circles in ascending order. Color Trails 2, requires individuals to connect numbered circles in consecutive order while also alternating the color of the circle (pink or yellow). Following the pattern set by Lansbergen et al. (2007) above of isolating the executive function component by dividing basic and faster processing speed by the slower interference trial, a ratio score (Trails1/2) was computed. Reliability and validity are adequate (D'Elia et al., 1996). Higher ratios represent better executive function.

Digit span (Strauss et al., 2006)

Digit Span Forward requires participants to first listen to a list of numbers and repeat them, with the string length increasing to the maximum of their ability. Digit Span Backward, requires repeating a string of numbers in reverse order. Continuing the pattern above to isolate the executive function component, the ratio of the typically smaller sum of correct interference trials on Digit Span Backward, divided by the typically greater sum of correct basic attention trials on Digit Span Forward (DigitsB/F). Good reliability and validity have been reported for Digit Span (Strauss et al., 2006). An increase in the ratio was the desired outcome.

Secondary Measures (Characterization of Sample and Possible Additional Outcomes)

Montreal Cognitive Assessment (MoCA; Nasreddine et al., 2005)

The MoCA was administered at baseline to characterize the sample as either normative aging or "screened as MCI" (sMCI; see details above). The MoCA consists of eight different subtests to assess overall cognitive impairment. Scores below 26 out of 30 were used to categorize sMCI (Nasreddine et al., 2005).

Ecological Validity (EV; Self-Reported Cognitive Function; Klusmann et al., 2010)

In an attempt to measure any generalized, clinically relevant, effects of the interventions (beyond any training to the tests that might occur when using standardized, serial testing), a participant self-report of perceived cognitive function was utilized. Participants were asked about their self-perceptions and beliefs related to their everyday functioning in regards to their cognitive functioning (e.g., memory and concentration). The Ecological Validity Questionnaire (Klusmann et al., 2010) was administered at BL, 3M and 6M. This measure consists of eleven statements that ask about participants perceptions of memory, concentration, and everyday function. Using a 5-point Likert scale (1 = absolutely wrong / bad to 5 = absolutely true / good), participants rated how much each of the statements described their behavior over the past 2 weeks. The total score can range from 11 to 55, with higher scores representing perceptions of better cognitive functioning.

Verbal Memory (Alzheimer's Disease Assessment Scale; ADAS Word List—Immediate and Delayed Recall; Harrison et al., 2007; Podhorna et al., 2016).

Participants are shown a list of 11 words on cards and they recall as many as they are able immediately and also after a delay interval. The number of errors/omissions comprises the score, so lower scores are better.

Get-up-and-go Test (Podsiadlo and Richardson, 1991)

Participants rise from sitting, walk 10 feet, turn around and return to sitting position. The time it takes to complete the task is the score. Lower scores are better.

Other Measures Include

The Physical Activity Readiness Questionnaire (PAR-Q; 0–7, higher scores indicates barriers to readiness; NASM) and Self-reported Physical Activity (SRPA); mental and physical effort thermometers; Exercise Induced Feeling Inventory (EIFI); the Confusion and Vigor subscales of the Brunel Mood Scale (Terry et al., 2003); experience of Flow (Payne et al., 2011), and other neuropsychological measures (e.g., Rey-O, NAART, etc.) not expected to be affected by the intervention, but included for separate use in full characterization of enrollees for later cross-sectional analyses. Due to the focus of this report on a priori hypotheses, and that the small adherent sample available for final analysis and circumscribes statistical power, some of these measures will be reported separately in cross-sectional or other limited analysis.

Exploratory Measures

The following biomarker and neuroimaging data were collected from some willing and able participants, who comprised a small subset of the enrolled participants. Due to the small and incomplete sample, we report these as pilot data to examine comparisons that were planned a priori and provide tentative findings, which may be useful in directing future research.

Biomarkers

Saliva samples (passive drool per Salimetrics protocol) were collected at: BL, SB, 3M, and 6M from willing and able participants. Samples were centrifuged, with a portion reserved for protein analyses and a portion further processed for exosome analyses. Exosomes were isolated from whole saliva via differential ultracentrifugation as described in previously published protocols (Thery et al., 2006; Gallo and Alevizos, 2013; Witwer et al., 2013). Briefly, whole saliva was subjected to differential centrifugation steps at 300 × g, 1,500 × g, 17,000 × g, and 160,000 × g. The exosome pellet was suspended in 1X PBS. All samples were stored at −80°C until analyses were conducted.

Protein Assays

Frozen samples were shipped overnight on dry ice for analysis (to RayBiotech, Inc., Norcross, GA). Protein concentrations of BDNF, CRP, IGF-1, IL-6, and VGEF were obtained via ELISAs (e.g., Mandel et al., 2011). Each patient sample was run in duplicate using 100 ml of plasma diluted by a factor of 2. A commercial multiplexed sandwich ELSIA-based array was used (Quantibody custom array, RayBiotech Inc., Norcross, GA, USA). All of the samples were tested using a panel of cytokines per above. The antibody array is a glass-chip-based multiplexed sandwich ELISA system designed to determine the concentrations all cytokines simultaneously. One standard glass slide was spotted with 16 wells of identical biomarker antibody arrays. Each antibody, together with the positive and negative control, was arrayed in quadruplicate. The samples and standards were added to the wells of the chip array and incubated for 3 h at 4 uC. This was followed by three to four washing steps and the addition of primary antibody and HRP-conjugated streptavidin to the wells. The signals (Cy3 wavelengths: 555 nm excitation, 655 nm emission) were scanned and extracted with an Innopsys laser scanner (Innopsys, Carbonne France), and quantified using Quantibody Analyzer software (Ray Biotech Inc). Each signal was identified by its spot location. The scanner software calculated background signals automatically. Concentration levels, expressed in picograms per milliliter (pg/ml), were calculated against a standard curve set for each biomarker from the positive and negative controls.

Exosome Analyses

Frozen samples were shipped overnight on dry ice for analysis (to VY at Oklahoma State University). The exosome/PBS solution was lyophilized for 9 h and RNA extraction was performed using Trizol™ reagent (Life Technologies®, catalog # 15596026.PPS) following the manufacturer's protocol. A fixed volume of 1,000 ng RNA was reverse-transcribed using the High Capacity cDNA Reverse Transcription Kit (Appled Biosystems, catalog #: 4368814). PCR forward and reverse primers for the human miRNA-193 (forward: CTTTTGGAG GCTGTGGTCTCAGAATC; reverse: CCAGTTGGATAAAAC ATAAACTCATCTCGCC) and miRNA-9 (forward: AGGCGGG GTTGGTTGTTATCTTTG; reverse: CTAGCTTTATGAAGACT CCACACCACTCATAC) were used for real-time quantitative RT-PCR (qRT-PCR) amplification. miRNA-193 and miRNA-9 expression was normalized against the U6 housekeeping miRNA (forward: GTGCCTGCTTCGGCAGC; reverse: TATGGAACGC TTCACGAATTTGCGTG).

The real-time qRT-PCR was performed using SYBR® Select Master Mix (ThermoFisher, cat #: 4472919). 100 ng of cDNA was loaded per well and amplified for 45 cycles using Opticon® 2 real-time PCR instrument (Biorad, model #: CFB-3220) operated by Opticon Monitor 3 software. All samples and references were run in triplicate and each well contained 20 μL total volume. Raw florescence readings were directly imported into, and baseline corrected with, LinregPCR software package (Version 2016.1). Linear regression was performed on the baseline-corrected data to calculate efficiency using a common window-of-linearity for each primer pair (Ruijter et al., 2009). Between-session variations were estimated using a maximum likelihood approach (Ruijter et al., 2006) and inter-plate variability was minimized using factor correction calculated using Factor qPCR software (Version 2016.0). Taking into account the reaction efficiency of each primer set, we used REST 2009 software package (Version 2.0.13, QIAGEN, Valencia, CA, USA) to calculate the relative RNA expression ratios in samples by a Pair Wise Fixed Reallocation Randomization model with 8000 iterations and a combination of randomization and bootstrapping techniques (Pfaffl et al., 2002).

Neuroimaging

Brain imaging T1-weighted 3D MP-RAGE axial images were acquired with a Siemens MAGNETOM Verio 3T MRI scanner running syngo MR B19 software, using an 32-channel bodycoil using the following parameters: 0.5 × 0.5 × 1.3 mm^3 voxel size; 256 × 256 matrix; 25 cm field of view; flip angle = 8°; echo time = 2.9 ms; repetition time = 1,640 ms; inversion time = 828 ms. Gray matter (GM) volume was analyzed using FreeSurfer software v. 5.3.0[5] (Fischl et al., 2002), in a Linux environment, as described in detail previously (Destrieux et al., 2010). Briefly, cortical reconstruction and volumetric segmentation require the initial motion correction and averaging of T1 images, signal intensity normalization, the removal of non-brain tissue, automated Talairach transformation and segmentation of gray and white matter[6], and the parcellation

[5]http://surfer.nmr.mgh.harvard.edu/

[6]total gray matter volumes were the focus of this study (white matter not considered herein)

of the cortex into well-described units, using gyral and sulcal landmarks for automatic differentiation. Each segmented brain volume was then inspected visually for processing errors which can occur during automation, and these were corrected using manual edits and re-processed. The Longitudinal Stream pipeline, available in Freesurfer v.5.3.0 (see website[7]), was used to create an unbiased within-subject template for the two timepoints in the present study (Reuter et al., 2012). Moreover, we expect good reliability and a minimal risk of bias-introduction with the automated pipeline, given that the within-subject scans took place in the same scanner using the same parameters and our focus was on cortical ROIs, which show somewhat better scan-rescan reliability than subcortical structures (e.g., Mills and Tamnes, 2014).

Given the literature cited above and a prioi hypotheses, the regions-of-interest (ROIs) included: hippocampus, dorsolateral prefrontal cortex (DLPFC), prefrontal cortex (PFC) and anterior cingulate cortex (ACC)[8]. Freesurfer does not directly extract these ROIs as they are not singular regions of the brain (see discussion above as to why they are structurally and functionally significant in the present context). As such, we defined our ROIs by combining the following Freesurfer labels: DLPFC = frontal middle gyrus and sulcus from the Destrieux et al. (2010) atlas; ACC = rostral and caudal anterior cingulate cortices from the Desikan et al. (2006) atlas; PFC = ACC + medial orbitofrontal and transverse frontopolar regions (Domenech and Koechlin, 2015). The DLPFC ROI that was chosen is one of the most conservative and non-controversial groupings, although some others have included more medial and/or caudal regions in their work (Vijayakumar et al., 2014; Jonasson et al., 2017). The volumes extracted are a measure of total gray matter only (white matter was parcellated separately and excluded). For the final analysis, GM volumes of each region were extracted and considered as a ratio to total intracranial volume to account for variations in brain size. Given the small sample size, volumetric ratios were used in parametric partial correlations with cognitive outcomes (controlling for age and sex).

Statistical Analyses

Data were analyzed using SPSS version 23 for Windows (IBM Corporation). The primary goal of the RCT was to examine, for those with sMCI, the possible differential effects (via neuropsychological, neurobiological, and neuroimaging measures) of long-term use of different combinations of physical and cognitive exercise (exer-tour vs. exer-score). Analyses focused on those sMCI participants that adhered to the protocol (approximating the minimum prescribed dose by averaging 3×/wk for 6 months, allowing for 2 weeks of vacation, illness, or equipment failure, in each of the 3-month evaluation windows). Given the small sample of completers, there was concern about insufficient power since a priori power analysis suggested a larger sample was indicated (Faul et al., 2007). Additionally, small samples often violate assumptions of standard parametric tests. However, the data for the primary outcome variables was found to be normally distributed (Shapiro-Wilk tests for StroopA/C, Trails1/2, and DigF/B were 0.52, 0.71, 0.16, respectively; Normal Q-Q plots were also reviewed which appeared to be normally distributed, with data following a linear pattern) and error variances were consistent with parametric assumptions (Levine's tests were not significant). Furthermore, given the importance of covariates (more readily implemented in parametric tests), along with the possibility that effects could be magnified in the sMCI sample, and following guidance in the literature on statistical strength of ANCOVA above nonparametric approach, especially in clinical trials (wherein a focus on change from baseline facilitates a trend toward normality; Vickers, 2005), it was decided to proceed with standard parametric analyses. Repeated measure ANOVAs, controlling for age and education were used to examine group (exer-tour vs. exer-score) × time (BL vs. 3M and 6M) interaction effects on the primary outcome measures of executive function. Covariates entered into the repeated measures analyses included: age and education, due to links to outcomes noted in the theoretical and empirical literature (Hannay and Lezak, 2004; Lam et al., 2013). Paired *t*-tests were used to evaluate within group change from baseline to the 3-month mid-point, and baseline to conclusion of the 6-month intervention.

Partial correlations, controlling for age and sex (based on prior literature demonstrating links to secondary outcomes; e.g., BNDF decreases with age: Lommatzsch et al., 2005; brain region variability with sex: Ruigrok et al., 2014), were conducted to explore the relationship between cognitive change and possible corresponding change in biomarkers (proteins and exosomes) and neuroimaging regions of interest, per above hypotheses. Further correlations were conducted to explore relationships between baseline memory and exercise dose as represented by ride frequency.

RESULTS

Effect on Primary Outcome: Executive Function

Full (6-Month) Intervention (Exer-Tour vs. Exer-Score)

Fourteen participants who met criteria for sMCI (MoCA < 26) were adherent to the protocol approximating the minimum assigned weekly average of 3×/week over 6 months. Half had been randomized to exer-tour and half to exer-score. After 6 months of interactive physical and cognitive exercise, the repeated measures ANCOVA omnibus test of executive function measures revealed a non-significant group x time interaction effect, $F_{(3, 7)} = 0.85$, $p = 0.51$, $\eta_p^2 = 0.27$. Univariate tests for StroopA/C, Trails1/2, and DigB/F were also not significant (p = 0.82, 0.11, 0.99, respectively). Paired *t*-tests were conducted to examine the change within groups over 6 months and StroopA/C improved significantly in both the exer-tour, $t_{(1, 5)} = -2.6$, $p = 0.049$, and exer-score conditions; $t_{(1, 6)} = -5.5$; $p = 0.001$ (**Figure 4**); Trails1/2 and DigB/F did not change significantly in either group (**Table 2**). Paired *t*-tests of the

[7]https://surfer.nmr.mgh.harvard.edu/fswiki/LongitudinalProcessing

[8]While the PFC and ACC overlap, they are reported separately here, in an attempt to replicate prior reports in the literature which identified change after exercise in each ROI.

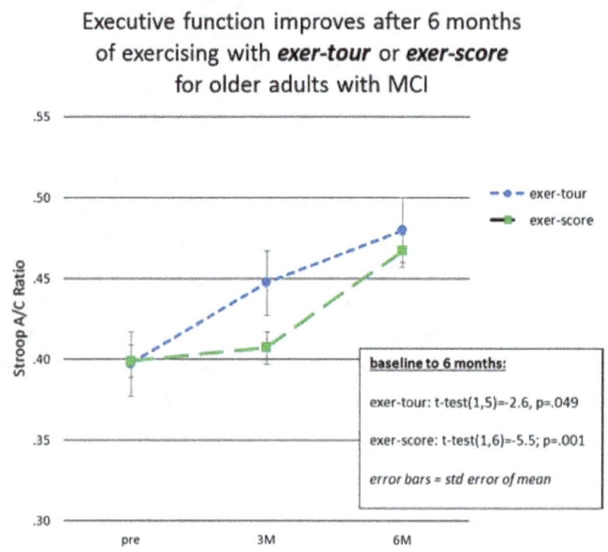

FIGURE 4 | Exer-tour vs. exer-score for sMCI adherents 0–6M.

change from baseline to the mid-point (3M) evaluation revealed no significant differences between the exer-tour and exer-score conditions at that point among sMCI participants ($n = 14$) that were adherent through 6 months (**Table 2**). sMCI participants who had been assigned to either exer-tour or exer-score and were not adherent over 6 months ($n = 54$) did not differ significantly from adherent sMCI participants ($n = 14$) on any baseline variables (including demographics, cognitive, physiological and functional variables; **Table 1**).

Mid-point (3-Month) Intervention (Exer-Tour vs. Exer-Score vs. Game-Only vs. Pedal-Only)

Given the high level of attrition from the game-only condition, as noted above, a mid-course adjustment was made to enroll game-only participants into a 3M-only intervention window. Doing so provided some comparative data regarding the possible relative effect of the mental exercise component separate from physical exercise (videogame practice only). Additionally, we were able to extract comparative 3M control data from our prior Cybercycle Study regarding the effect of a pedal-only condition for older adults. These 3M analyses utilized all older adults (sMCI + normative[9]) that were adherent through 3M in their assigned condition (thus the n's for exer-tour, exer-score, game-only, and pedal-only were: 15, 19, 8, 31, respectively). Paired *t*-tests were conducted and revealed significant gains on StroopA/C by 3M for exer-tour and pedal-only, with statistically significant moderate effects ($d = 0.49$ and 0.35, respectively; **Figure 5**), while exer-score and game-only yielded non-significant small effects ($d = 0.14$ and 0.13, respectively). TrailsA/B and DigF/B did not change significantly. The 6M effect sizes for the two conditions that progressed to 6M (exer-score and exer-tour) are also included in **Figure 4** and reveal that both the exer-tour and exer-score conditions yielded statistically significant moderate effects by 6M ($d = 0.52$ and 0.47, respectively); thus, the exer-score group seems to "catch up" to the exer-tour from 3 to 6M.

Effect on Secondary Outcomes

Full (6-Month) Intervention (Exer-Tour vs. Exer-Score)

There were significant group x time interactions among the 14 sMCI adherents for: (1) immediate verbal memory (exer-tour improved significantly more than exer-score; $p = 0.018$), (2) self-report of everyday cognitive function (as assessed on the Ecological Validity Questionnaire), with exer-tour reporting significantly more improvement while exer-score reported decline; $p = 0.046$), and (3) physical ability (exer-tour increased significantly more than exer-score; $p = 0.001$; see **Table 3**).

Biomarkers[10]

Biomarker samples were sought from all participants, but not all were willing or able to provide saliva samples (data from completers was available from a maximum of $n = 16$ for analysis). Target analytes included: BDNF, CRP, IGF-1, IL-6, and VEGF. Due to low concentrations of IGF-1 in the samples collected, the assay results were below the limit of detection on too many samples and this assay was excluded from analyses. Partial correlations (controlling for age and sex; **Table 4**) were conducted to examine the change from baseline to 6M in biomarkers related to change in the primary outcome measure, executive function (StroopA/C) which, per above, changed significantly with the intervention. Similarly, change in biomarkers were correlated with a secondary outcome that was impacted significantly by both interventions, was verbal memory, and we chose to focus on delayed verbal memory specifically (ADAS errors), since one of the more salient cognitive functions to impact for MCI patients. Finally, the exercise dose, based on average number of rides, was examined for association with the biomarkers change to evaluated the possibility of a dose effect. Exercise dose (rides) was found to correlate significantly with an increase in BDNF ($r = 0.50$, $p = 0.04$). Delayed recall errors showed a trend toward a moderate inverse correlation with increased VEGF such that better memory performance tended to coincide with increasing VEGF ($r = -0.42$, $p = 0.08$). Exosome analyses revealed a significant positive correlation between miRNA-9 expression with improved StroopA/C performance ($r = 0.98$, $p = 0.002$).

Neuroimaging[7]

Neuroimaging (3T structural MRI) was grant-funded and sought from all participants, but not all were willing or able to undergo imaging (data from completers was available from a maximum

[9]The 3M analyses were not limited to sMCI, because added comparison of the fourth group at 3M (the pedal-only condition from the archival dataset; Anderson-Hanley et al., 2012), could not be sorted by the same sMCI criteria used in the present study (MoCA scores were not available for pedal-only participants). Thus, the decision was made to utilize all adherents (normative + sMCI) at 3M from the four groups to retain comparability within the 3M comparisons.

[10]Results for bioassay and neuroimaging data analyses are to be interpreted tentatively as exploratory pilot results, given the small sample sizes even with collapsing across conditions.

TABLE 2 | Exer-tour vs. exer-score for primary neuropsychological outcomes (0–3M–6M).

	MCI adherents to prescribed dose of 6-month intervention												MCI			ANOVA
	Exer-tour				Exer-score			ANOVA	Combined adherents				Non-adherents			
	Ave	*SD*	*n*		Ave	*SD*	*n*	p^a	Ave	*SD*	*n*		Ave	*SD*	*n*	p^a
PRIMARY OUTCOME																
Baseline executive function[a]																
Color Trails ½	0.49	0.17	7		0.47	0.10	7	0.85	0.48	0.13	14		0.48	0.21	54	
Stroop A/C	0.40	0.12	7		0.40	0.14	7	0.98	0.40	0.12	14		0.44	0.12	54	
Digits B/F	0.53	0.13	7		0.59	0.21	7	0.56	0.56	0.17	14		0.61	0.16	54	
				***t*-test**				***t*-test**				***t*-test**				**(grp × time)**[c]
3-Month executive function				p^b				p^b				p^b				***P***
Color Trails ½	0.44	0.11	7	0.41	0.44	0.07	7	0.34	0.44	0.09	14	0.20				0.89
Stroop A/C	0.45	0.06	7	0.25	0.41	0.15	7	0.68	0.43	0.11	14	0.21				0.46
Digits B/F	0.53	0.23	7	0.97	0.61	0.12	7	0.65	0.57	0.18	14	0.77				0.93
6-Month executive function																
Color Trails 1/2	0.38	0.12	6	0.10	0.48	0.17	7	0.83	0.44	0.15	13	0.32				0.11
Stroop A/C	0.48	0.11	6	**0.049**	0.47	0.15	7	**0.001**	0.47	0.13	13	**0.0002**				0.82
Digits B/F	0.60	0.15	6	.38	0.64	0.16	7	0.50	0.62	0.15	13	0.26				0.99

[a]*Comparison between groups.*
[b]*Comparison with baseline.*
[c]*Repeated meas ANCOVA controlling for age and education.*
Bold values indicates statistically significant ($p \leq 0.05$).

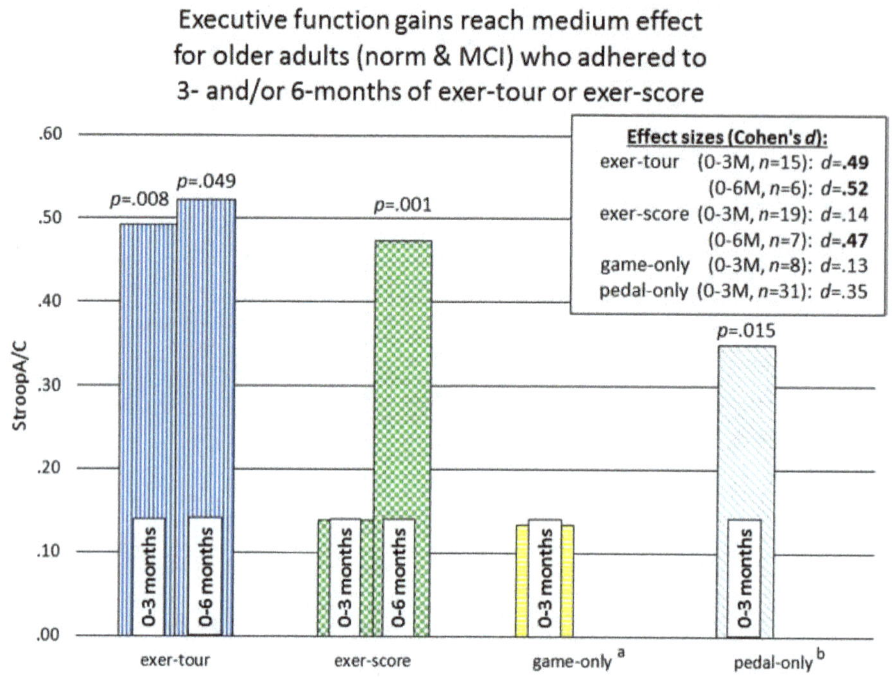

FIGURE 5 | Comparison of effect sizes of components of interactive physical and cognitive exercise across four intervention conditions for 0–3M adherents. *p*-values represent significant change over time within-group (paired) *t*-tests. [a]the game-only condition was initially randomly assigned, but subsequently recruited separately due to challenges with enrollment and retention (see section Methods for further details). [b]the pedal-only comparison data is archival/perviously reported from our lab and was obtained during the Cybercycle Study (Anderson-Hanley et al., 2012), which examined only a 3-month interval and was collected from older adults in the same region, from many of the same retirement communities, and with the same measures of executive function; this data is included here as a point of comparaitve reference, illustrating the magnitude of effect from physical exercise alone.

of $n = 8$ for analysis). Partial correlations, just as described above, are reported in **Table 5**. Greater exercise dose (number of rides over 6M) was positively correlated with increasing PFC ($r = 0.80$, $p = 0.003$) and ACC (right; $r = 0.70$, $p = 0.05$; **Figure 6**). Verbal memory (delayed recall) errors were inversely related to increasing DLPFC, such that improvement in memory corresponded to increasing volume ($r = -0.80$, $p = 0.01$; **Figure 6**).

DISCUSSION

This RCT was an attempt to replicate and extend findings of prior research, which found greater cognitive benefit for older adults engaged in interactive mental and physical exercise (i.e., while exergaming using a cybercycle; Anderson-Hanley et al., 2012) and furthermore, given pilot data which suggested greater mental challenge may increase cognitive benefit of exergaming (Barcelos et al., 2015). This RCT examined whether similar effects would be found among community-dwelling older adults with or at risk for MCI (screened as MCI; sMCI). We hypothesized that a more mentally challenging exergame would yield greater benefit to executive function than a more passive exergame. Community dwelling older adults, with a focus on those with sMCI, were randomly assigned to: exer-tour (pedaling along a virtual bike path), exer-score (pedaling to score points by navigating an interactive videogame), or a game-only condition (the latter having to be adapted due to issues with participant adherence, resulting in a shorter and remunerated, quasi-experimental arm).

Fourteen older adults with sMCI were adherent to the minimum assigned dose (average 3×/wk of exercise) for 6 months. Both conditions were found to yield significant improvement on one of three measures of executive function (Stroop A/C), producing similar moderate effect sizes at 6 months ($d = 0.52$ and 0.47, respectively). There was no interaction effect; however, from informal examination of the graph of the data (**Figure 4**), it appears that the exer-score condition did not produce incremental gains at the mid-point (3M), while the exer-tour condition did appear to yield benefit sooner, although by 6 months the exer-score and exer-tour gains were similar. It is hypothesized that since the exer-score condition does require significant mental effort to play, it may have taken longer for exer-score participants (with sMCI) to master the interactive pedaling and game-play. Thus, there may have been delay in triggering the synergistic effects of the interactive exercise that would lead to a neurobiological cascade of events ultimately linked to any cognitive benefit. Furthermore, it may be different brain networks are activated by various aspects of the interactive physical and mental tasks in each condition, thus resulting in differential enhancement of network functions; for example, the effect on Stroop herein is consistent with activation of

TABLE 3 | Exer-tour vs. exer-score for secondary outcomes: memory, everyday function (self-reported cognition and physical ability (0–6M).

	MCI adherents to prescribed dose of 6-month intervention												MCI			ANOVA
	Exer-tour				Exer-score			ANOVA	Combined adherents				Non-adherents			
	Ave	*SD*	*n*		Ave	*SD*	*n*	p^a	Ave	*SD*	*n*		Ave	*SD*	*n*	p^a
SECONDARY OUTCOMES								***t*-test**								
Baseline								p^a								
Verbal Mem Immed (errors)	15.71	4.39	7		14.43	5.50	7	0.64	15.1	4.8	14		11.96	3.62	54	
Verbal Mem Delay (errors)	6.0	2.8	7		6.6	2.8	7	0.71	6.3	2.7	14		5.2	2.3	54	
Ecological Validity	35.5	7.9	7		40.2	9.8	7	0.34	37.8	8.9	14		41.6	7.9	50	
Physical ability (GUG)	12.7	2.2	7		10.3	1.7	7	**0.039**	11.5	2.3	14		12.7	3.5	54	
				***t*-test**				***t*-test**								**(grp × time)[c]**
6-month				p^b				p^b								***P***
Verbal Mem Immed (errors)	11.17	4.49	6	**0.003**	12.71	4.31	7	0.10	12.0	4.3	13	**0.001**				**0.018**
Verbal Mem Delay (errors)	5.5	3.0	6	0.53	5.1	2.9	7	**0.047**	5.3	2.8	13	**0.040**				0.15
Ecological Validity	41.3	7.3	6	0.20	36.6	7.2	7	0.12	38.8	7.3	13	0.84				**0.046**
Physical ability (GUG)	14.0	1.5	6	**0.009**	11.0	2.0	6	0.46	12.5	2.3	12	**0.013**				**0.001**

[a]*Comparison between groups.*
[b]*Comparison with baseline.*
[c]*Repeated meas ANCOVA controlling for age and education.*
Bold values indicates statistically significant ($p \leq 0.05$).

TABLE 4 | Neurobiological change (0–6M) correlates with exercise dose/effort and change in cognitive function for participants in exer-tour and exer-score: Exploratory pilot data.

Biomarker	Partial correlation[a]	Exercise effort (rides)	Executive function (StroopA/C)	Memory delayed (ADAS errors)
BDNF	*r*	0.50	0.20	0.21
	p	**0.04**	0.42	0.39
	df	15	16	16
CRP	*r*	0.00	0.16	−0.34
	p	0.99	0.53	0.16
	df	15	16	16
IL-6	*r*	0.03	0.15	−0.06
	p	0.91	0.54	0.82
	df	15	16	16
VEGF	*r*	−0.30	−0.05	−0.42
	p	0.25	0.84	0.08
	df	15	16	16
Exosome (miR-9_N0_Rel_U6)	*r*	−0.394	0.984	−0.815
	p	0.51	**0.002**	0.09
	df	3	3	3

[a]*Controlling for age and sex.*
Bold values indicates statistically significant ($p \leq 0.05$).

the fronto-parietal network used in inhibition and switching and the fact that the volume of the ACC as shown on MRI imaging was enlarged proportionally to exercise dose further lends support to the impact on that specific network (Grandjean et al., 2012).

The differential relative impact of the two forms of interactive physical and cognitive exercise, exer-tour and exer-score, was apparent when comparing mid-point (3M) moderate effect with small effect ($d = 0.52$ and 0.14, respectively), while the game-only condition showed little impact (i.e., of cognitive training; $d = 0.13$). By contrast, the pedal-only condition by 3M was more consistent with the literature on the benefits of physical exercise alone for cognition as it yielded a significant within-group improvement (Colcombe and Kramer, 2003), although it was a more modest effect ($d = 0.35$) than the exer-tour, which is also consistent with past research in which the cybercycle effect exceeded exercise alone (Anderson-Hanley et al., 2012). It may be that the measures of executive function that were chosen were not as sensitive to the particular impact of each of the conditions as they could be; while Stroop A/C revealed an effect, Trails 2/1 and Digit Span B/F did not, perhaps because the components of executive function were not particularly enhanced (e.g., task switching and working memory, respectively). Future research, could strategically select measures that might better detect change in selective attention or inhibitory control which arguably might be more affected by repeated use of the exer-score condition in which one is chasing dragons while scanning the horizon for additional opportunities and avoiding pitfalls, and so forth (e.g., Flanker or Go/no-Go tasks might have greater sensitivity to detect for specific and relevant changes in executive function; Diamond, 2013).

Analysis of secondary outcomes from the present study yielded promising indications that this type of exergaming

TABLE 5 | Neuroimaging change (0–6M) correlations with exercise dose/effort and changes in cognitive function (0–6M) for participants in exer-tour and exer-score: Exploratory pilot data.

MRI ROI	Partial correlation[a]	Exercise effort (rides)	Executive function (StroopA/C)	Memory delayed (ADAS errors)
Hippocampus (left)	*r*	0.07	0.22	0.02
	p	0.86	0.55	0.95
	df	6	8	8
Hippocampus (right)	*r*	0.14	0.14	0.08
	p	0.74	0.69	0.83
	df	6	8	8
DLPFC	*r*	−0.10	0.19	−0.80
	p	0.84	0.62	**0.01**
	df	5	7	7
PFC	*r*	0.89	0.51	0.07
	p	**0.003**	0.13	0.85
	df	6	8	8
ACC (left)	*r*	−0.42	−0.36	−0.43
	p	0.30	0.30	0.21
	df	6	8	8
ACC (right)	*r*	0.70	−0.14	0.00
	p	**0.05**	0.70	1.00
	df	6	8	8

[a]*Controlling for age and sex.*
Bold values indicates statistically significant ($p \leq 0.05$).

activity can yield cognitive gains in other realms of cognition[11] (e.g., verbal memory) among individuals with sMCI (with exer-tour outperforming exer-score). Moreover, these effects seem to generalize beyond standardized tests of cognition, to self-reported perceptions of everyday cognitive function and also vigor[12] (again, with exer-tour outperforming exer-score). The latter finding may benefit from further probing, perhaps via focused exit interview questions regarding possible reasons for this curious finding. Perhaps the regular practice of a mentally challenging videogame led participants in that condition to subjectively feel less capable (even though by 6M the gains exer-score made in executive function matched that of exer-tour). It is also likely that there would be individual variability in response to the gaming scenarios (e.g., prior research has found that one's trait competitiveness can interact with benefit from presumably facilitative features of an exergame, such as the presence or absence of an avatar (Snyder et al., 2012). Indeed in conduct of this trial, anecdotally, it was noted that some individuals were keenly enthused by and motivated to keep track of their score, while others were lackadaisical in their approach to pedaling around for exercise but without much care for scoring. Indeed, research shows the salience to the individual of the storyboard of a videogame, as well as other features may affect enjoyment or persistence, and can facilitate or limit use (Wang and Goh, 2017); all relevant issues to consider when designing and planning a long-term clinical trial with a goal of ensuring a thorough dose, via consistent adherence.

These findings of significant effects with both types of exergaming: exer-tour (low mental challenge) and exer-score (high mental challenge) on executive function and memory, mirrors one of the few similar studies, by Eggenberger et al. (2015), who reported similar trends when comparing an interactive dance exergame, with dual-task walking (non-interactive), and physical exercise alone. It is interesting to note that effect sizes were larger in our study and thus reached statistical significance, while the trial above had a much larger sample, but the effects were smaller leading to marginal results, despite having exergaming conditions that were in many ways similar. Perhaps this was due to the fact that the sample herein was sMCI, specifically, while the Eggenberger study utilized normative older adults. It seems likely that general, MCI participants have already begun some cognitive decline and so they may have more room to grow, so to speak, or at least more distance from the ceiling on cognitive tests to reveal change when attempting to attenuate the anticipated downward slope of cognitive decline, and thus the effect may be more readily apparent. Future research could further evaluate the possibilities by enrolling and comparing effects of both normative and MCI participants, with care taken to avoid possible ceiling effects on baseline assessments.

Finally, possible mechanisms linking exercise to enhanced cognition via presumed improved brain health were explored with promising findings from pilot data sampled from willing participants. Biomarker changes (e.g., BDNF and exosomes) were found to correspond to improvements in cognition and dose of exercise, each consistent with prior research (e.g., BDNF has been found to promote the differentiation of new neurons and synapses, and therefore, has been proposed to be a mediator of adult neuroplasticity; Huang and Reichardt, 2001; Leßmann and Brigadski, 2009; Flöel et al., 2010; Park and Poo, 2013; Edelmann et al., 2014). Furthermore, neuroimaging revealed promising gains in key ROIs (e.g., DLPFC and ACC) that corresponded with improvements in cognition and dose of exercise, again consistent with reports in the literature (Burdette et al., 2010; Weinstein et al., 2012; Chapman et al., 2013, 2016; Hayes et al., 2013; Ehlers et al., 2017; Li et al., 2017). While we retain a cautious stance for interpreting these findings given the limitations already noted, we are heartened that changes found are largely consistent with changes in gray matter volume that have been noted in other studies of learning and physical training. Some of which have reported statistically significant changes as early as 1–2 weeks (e.g., Ceccarelli et al., 2009; Zatorre et al., 2012) and specifically regarding training-induced changes in older adults before the 6-month time point (e.g., Boyke et al., 2008).

Strengths of this RCT include a study design crafted to clarify whether cognitive benefit could be maximized with a more challenging videogame component integrated with the physical exercise. In contrast to the findings of the ACES-pilot study (Barcelos et al., 2015), which found that after just three months

[11]Additional cognitive domains that might be sensible to assess in a follow-up study, might include visuospatial skills, given the integration and regular use of visuospatial tracking in the conditions with virtual reality screens.

[12]The two mood subscales (vigor and confusion from the BMS) were probed retrospectively on suggestion of an anonymous reviewer and the ex-tour reported a significantly greater sense of vigor at 6M, than exer-score.

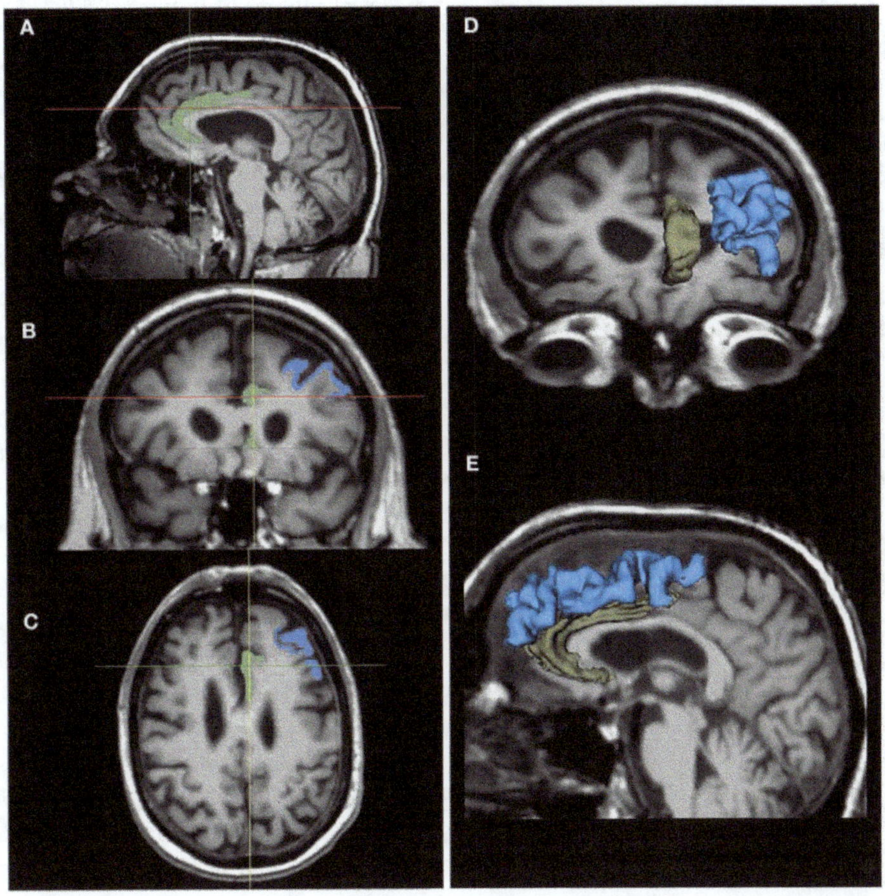

FIGURE 6 | Neuroimaging correlates with exercise and cognition[13]: MRI of ACC and DLPFC. Notes: Illustration of regions-of-interest (ROI): ACC (increased with exercise dose) and DLPFC (increased with improvement in verbal memory); shown here in one individual and in one hemisphere for ease of presentation. Images of ACC (green) and DLPFC (blue) in 3 sagittal **(A),** coronal **(B)**, and axial **(C)** images aligned by crosshairs. ROI 3D model reconstructions give a sense of their structure in 3D space, as seen from the anterior **(D)** and left **(E)** sides.

of exer-score resulted in greater cognitive benefit than the exer-tour. The present findings suggest that for a more impaired MCI population the benefit of exer-tour shows up by three months, but it may be necessary for participants to stick with the interactive exercise through a longer window, six months, in order to master the challenges and reap the benefits of the enhanced exercise experience. Additionally, this study design began to tease apart the impact the of component parts of exergaming (e.g., physical exercise only vs. mental exercise only), as well as explore possible neurobiological mechanisms and neuroimaging markers that tentatively shed light and nudge future research regarding the ways in which the body and mind might interact for neuroprotection or amelioration of cognitive decline. A particular strength of this study is the use of alternate forms and additional serial testing (via single bout and 3M evaluation) that preceded the final 6-month evaluation such that practice or learning effects should have largely "washed out" or likely plateaued by that point (Beglinger et al., 2005), thus greater confidence can be placed in the results as representing a genuine effect.

A significant limitation of this study is the difficulty participants experienced in engaging a new behavioral approach to preventing or curbing cognitive decline. Attrition far exceeded our expectations based on past pilots and standard rates noted in the literature. The fact that this study focused on persons with sMCI, who face more than the usual challenges in starting a new exercise regimen, was likely a major contributing factor. Additionally, the requirement set out initially by grant reviewers and medical center IRBs that persons with MCI be considered a vulnerable population and must exercise in a limited environment with professional oversight (i.e., physical therapy clinics) proved daunting as participants were unwilling or unable to arrange transport 3–7×/wk to engage in regular exercise. Obtaining approval to make the equipment more accessible within retirement communities and neighborhood

[13]As noted above, both ACC and PFC were analyzed in order to replicate prior research which reported each ROI correlated with outcomes (e.g., exercise dose or cognition), but because of the overlap of these ROIs only one is shown here for clarity.

wellness centers did help somewhat, but nevertheless, retention remained a significant issue. The resultant small sample does diminish statistical power, although despite this, effects were sizeable enough to detect. Additionally, a small sample limits our ability to ask nuanced questions of the dataset which the study design would have facilitated if a larger sample had been obtained. For example, it was an a priori goal to compare known subtypes of MCI (i.e., amnestic vs. not) to see what, if any, impact subtype of MCI might have had on participants' abilities to learn and engage the more challenging exer-score videogame. This will have to wait for a future trial with a larger sample, perhaps by recruiting, as was necessary herein, those yet undiagnosed, but going beyond a screening tool, a future study could prospectively build in the mechanisms for a complete clinical workup of MCI as well. Nevertheless, much was learned regarding the needs of MCI patients and families in the conduct of such a trial, and will enhance future trial designs and interventions (see below). It will remain challenging however, to balance ideals about statistical power with the reality and importance of continuing to conduct research with clinical samples.

Future research is needed to address limitations of this study and improve retention and adherence to these types of behavioral interventions which have promising findings despite the variety of hindrances. For example, to try to address the challenges of enrolling and retaining MCI participants, our lab has been developing a more strategic and tailored in-home approach to facilitate adoption of this type of long-term behavioral intervention. We have developed a portable, adaptive, tablet-based neuro-exergame[14], *Memory Lane™*, specifically designed to target executive function by way of integrating specific mental challenges presented via a relatively simple, in-home interactive Physical and Cognitive Exercise System (iPACES™[15]). While still only available for research purposes, the design had limited bulkiness of equipment and used budget components such that a large clinical trial will remain feasible (for example, an under-table pedaler paired with a budget tablet). Preliminary results from single bout use of our prototype iPACES™ have been promising (Anderson-Hanley et al., 2017), and we hope these various studies will encourage others to identify, design, and implement novel behavioral interventions to combat and ameliorate cognitive decline. Indeed there are a number of other open protocols currently recruiting to innovative behavioral interventions (Legault et al., 2011; Lee et al., 2016); for example, the Aerobic Exercise and Cognitive Training Trial (ACT) out of the University of Minnesota is enrolling patients with MCI to better understand the benefit of combined physical and mental activities (NCT03313895), and the Multidomain Alzheimer Prevention Trial (MAPT) combines physical and cognitive exercise, while also layering a nutritional component that may be able to further maximize any cognitive benefit derived (Vellas et al., 2014). Some research teams have been pushing the envelope on the possibilities given advancing technologies and have even explored web-connected exergaming to facilitate participation (Bamidis et al., 2011; Konstantinidis et al., 2017). The availability of such innovative interventions through data-yielding clinical trials is heartening to many individuals and families already facing the challenges of cognitive decline.

Given the encroaching dementia epidemic, it behooves researchers and society at large to continue to press for innovative and effective solutions that aim to maximize cognitive benefits. In this way we can hope to make meaningful contributions to the important cause of slowing or preventing the onset of cognitive decline. It is likely that a multi-factorial approach will yield the greatest impact, but there is much work to be done to clarify which components and intensities (e.g., of physical and mental exercise, nutritional and/or social supports, etc.), to meld and leverage for the best and most meaningful impact on brain health so as to ensure sustained cognitive functions in later life. Furthermore, it seems likely that there is a great deal to learn about factors that predict response to any intervention, including physical and mental exercise. It may be that certain genetic factors, such as ApoE status may moderate the body's ability to spark a given neurobiological cascade and thus reap the benefits of a given intervention such as interactive physical and cognitive exercise (Raichlen and Alexander, 2014). The more we learn about these underlying mechanisms and the nuanced effects exposed by analyzing larger samples, the more effective we can be in designing and tailoring interventions (Morrison-Bogorad et al., 2007; Lieberman, 2009; Larson, 2010; Read and Shortell, 2011; Gerling and Mandryk, 2014; Barha et al., 2016) to do the most good for the greatest number of people as fast as we can, especially now that so many are faced with sliding into the long suffering.

AUTHOR NOTES

Thank you to:

- Our participants and site administrators from: Albany Medical Center, Stratton VA Medical Center, Sunnyview Rehabilitation Hospital, Beverwyck, CDPHP Wellness Center, Coburg Village, Glen Eddy, Hawthorne Ridge, Jewish Community Center of Niskayuna, Kimgsway Community, Prestwick Chase, Schaffer Heights, and the YMCA of Saratoga Springs.

- Research assistants: Chris Avanessian, Joel Gideon, Julie Warren, and the NY6 2016 Summer Research Team: Elizabeth

[14]Neuro-exergaming (Anderson-Hanley et al., 2016, 2017), is an adaptation of existing terms and used herein to indicate the integration of neurogaming with exergaming for the express purpose of benefiting brain health and fostering improved cognitive function

[15]iPACES™ 2013-present, patent pending No. 62/140,991; BSK Ref. No.: 416P1700A

Altman, Zachariah Arnold, Amelia Denney, Casey Terzian, Jennifer Vu, and Emily West.

- Colleagues who provided advice and assistance at various stages of this project: Drs. Adam Brickman, Amanda Damjanovic, Michael Hogan, Michael McCann, and Jeffrey Woods.
- Dr. Gaetano Pastena and the clinical team at Community Care Niskayuna and Latham who assisted in collection of 3T MRI imaging.
- Ross Stensrud of Interactive Fitness Holdings for technical assistance with data retrieval from the Expresso bike platforms utilized in this study.

Earlier versions of these results were presented at the annual meetings of: the Society for Neuroscience Chapter, the International Neuropsychological Society, and the American Academy for Clinical Neuropsychology.

AUTHOR CONTRIBUTIONS

CA-H, NB, MM, VY, DH wrote pieces of the manuscript; CA-H, NB, EZ, RG, MD contributed to study design, implementation and interpretation; BC contributed to biomarker data analysis and interpretation; KM contributed to exosome study design, data analysis and interpretation; DH contributed to MRI data analysis and interpretation; PA contributed to study design, exercise science factors, implementation and interpretation; AK contributed to study design, interpretation.

REFERENCES

Ahlskog, J. E., Geda, Y. E., Graff-Radford, N. R., and Petersen, R. C. (2011). Physical exercise as a preventive or disease-modifying treatment of dementia and brain aging. *Mayo Clin. Proc.* 86, 876–884. doi: 10.4065/mcp.2011.0252

Alzheimer's Association (2014). Alzheimer's association report: Alzheimer's disease facts and figures. *Alzheimer's Demen.* 10, 47–92. Available online at: https://www.cdc.gov/aging/pdf/2013-healthy-brain-initiative.pdf

Alzheimer's Association and Centers for Disease Control and Prevention (2013). *The Healthy Brain Initiative: The Public Health Road Map for State and National Partnerships, 2013–2018*: Chicago, IL: Alzheimer's Association.

Al-Yahya, E., Dawes, H., Smith, L., Dennis, A., Howells, K., and Cockburn, J. (2011). Cognitive motor interference while walking: a systematic review and meta-analysis. *Neurosci. Biobehav. Rev.* 35, 715–728. doi: 10.1016/j.neubiorev.2010.08.008

Anderson-Hanley, C., Barcelos, B., Maloney, M., Michel, M., Striegnitz, S., and Saulnier, T. (2016). "Neuropsychological effects of an Interactive Physical & Cognitive Exercise System (iPACES) for older adults: pilot comparison of in-home neuro-exergame versus neuro-game," in *Presentation at the Annual Meeting of the International Neuropsychological Society* (Boston, MA).

Anderson-Hanley, C., Arciero, P. J., Barcelos, N., Nimon, J., Rocha, T., Thurin, M., et al. (2014). Executive function and self-regulated exergaming adherence among older adults. *Front. Hum. Neurosci.* 8:989. doi: 10.3389/fnhum.2014.00989

Anderson-Hanley, C., Arciero, P. J., Brickman, A., Nimon, J., Okuma, N., Westen, S., et al. (2012). Exergaming improves older adult cognition: a cluster randomized clinical trial. *Am. J. Prev. Med.* 42, 109–119. doi: 10.1016/j.amepre.2011.10.016

Anderson-Hanley, C., Maloney, M., Barcelos, N., Striegnitz, K., and Kramer, A. F. (2017). Neuropsychological benefits of neuro-exergaming for older adults: a pilot study of an interactive physical and cognitive exercise system (iPACES^{TM}). *J. Aging Phys. Activity* 25, 73–83. doi: 10.1123/japa.2015-0261

Angevaren, M., Aufdemkampe, G., Verhaar, H. J., Aleman, A., and Vanhees, L. (2008). Physical activity and enhanced fitness to improve cognitive function in older people without known cognitive impairment. *Cochrane Database Syst. Rev.* 3:CD005381. doi: 10.1002/14651858.CD005381.pub3

Anguera, J. A., Boccanfuso, J., Rintoul, J. L., Al-Hashimi, O., Faraji, F., and Gazzaley, A. (2013). Video game training enhances cognitive control in older adults. *Nature* 501, 97–101. doi: 10.1038/nature12486

Bahar-Fuchs, A., Clare, L., and Woods, B. (2013). Cognitive training and cognitive rehabilitation for persons with mild to moderate dementia of the Alzheimer's or vascular type: a review. *Alzheimer's Res. Ther.* 5:35. doi: 10.1186/alzrt189

Baker, L. D., Frank, L. L., Foster-Schubert, K., Green, P. S., Wilkinson, C. W., McTiernan, A., et al. (2010). Effects of aerobic exercise on mild cognitive impairment: a controlled trial. *Arch. Neurol.* 67, 71–79. doi: 10.1001/archneurol.2009.307

Bamidis, P. D., Fissler, P., Papageorgiou, S. G., Zilidou, V., Konstantinidis, E. I., Billis, A. S., et al. (2015). Gains in cognition through combined cognitive and physical training: the role of training dosage and severity of neurocognitive disorder. *Front. Aging Neurosci.* 7:152. doi: 10.3389/fnagi.2015.00152

Bamidis, P. D., Konstantinidis, E. I., Billis, A., Frantzidis, C., Tsolaki, M., Hlauschek, W., et al. (2011). "A Web services-based exergaming platform for senior citizens: the Long Lasting Memories project approach to e-health care," in *Conference Proceedings:... Annual International Conference Of The IEEE Engineering In Medicine And Biology Society. IEEE Engineering In Medicine And Biology Society. Annual Conference, 20112505-2509* (Boston, MA).

Bamidis, P. D., Vivas, A. B., Styliadis, C., Frantzidis, C., Klados, M., Schlee, W., et al. (2014). A review of physical and cognitive interventions in aging. *Neurosci. Biobehav. Rev.* 44, 206–220. doi: 10.1016/j.neubiorev.2014.03.019

Barcelos, N., Shah, N., Cohen, K., Hogan, M. J., Mulkerrin, E., Arciero, P. J., et al. (2015). Aerobic and cognitive exercise (ACE) pilot study for older adults: executive function improves with cognitive challenge while exergaming. *J. Int. Neuropsychol. Soc.* 21, 768–779. doi: 10.1017/S1355617715001083

Barha, C. K., Galea, L. A., Nagamatsu, L. S., Erickson, K. I., and Liu-Ambrose, T. (2016). Personalising exercise recommendations for brain health: considerations and future directions. *Brit. J. Sports Med.* 51, 636–639. doi: 10.1136/bjsports-2016-096710

Barnes, D. E., Santos-Modesitt, W., Poelke, G., Kramer, A. F., Castro, C., Middleton, L. E., et al. (2013). The mental activity and exercise (MAX) trial. A randomized controlled trial to enhance cognitive function in older adults. *JAMA* 173, 797–804. doi: 10.1001/jamainternmed.2013.189

Barry, G., Galna, B., and Rochester, L. (2014). The role of exergaming in Parkinson's disease rehabilitation: a systematic review of the evidence. *J. Neuroeng. Rehabil.* 11:33. doi: 10.1186/1743-0003-11-33

Batistela, M. S., Josviak, N. D., Sulzbach, C. D., and de Souza, R. R. (2017). An overview of circulating cell-free microRNAs as putative biomarkers in Alzheimer's and Parkinson's Diseases. *Int. J. Neurosci.* 127, 547–558. doi: 10.1080/00207454.2016.1209754

Beglinger, L. J., Gaydos, B., Tangphao-Daniels, O., Duff, K., Kareken, D. A., Crawford, J., et al. (2005). Practice effects and the use of alternate forms in serial neuropsychological testing. *Arch. Clin. Neuropsychol.* 20, 517–529. doi: 10.1016/j.acn.2004.12.003

Bellar, D., Glickman, E. L., Juvancic-Heltzel, J., and Gunstad, J. (2011). Serum insulin like growth factor-1 is associated with working memory, executive function, and selective attention in a sample of healthy, fit older adults. *Neuroscience* 178, 133–137. doi: 10.1016/j.neuroscience.2010.12.023

Bertoldi, K., Cechinel, L. R., Schallenberger, B., Corssac, G. B., Davies, S., Guerreiro, I. K., et al. (2017). Circulating extracellular vesicles in the aging process: impact of aerobic exercise. *Mol. Cell. Biochem.* 440, 115–125. doi: 10.1007/s11010-017-3160-4

Bherer, L. (2015). Cognitive plasticity in older adults: effects of cognitive training and physical exercise. *Ann. N. Y. Acad. Sci.* 1337, 1–6. doi: 10.1111/nyas.12682

Black, J. E., Isaacs, K. R., Anderson, B. J., Alcantara, A. A., and Greenough, W. T. (1990). Learning causes synaptogenesis, whereas motor activity causes angiogenesis, in cerebellar cortex of adult rats. *Proc. Natl. Acad. Sci. U.S.A.* 87, 5568–5572. doi: 10.1073/pnas.87.14.5568

Boot, W. R., and Kramer, A. F. (2014). The brain games conundrum: does cognitive training really sharpen the mind? *Cerebrum* 2014, 1–15.

Boyke, J., Driemeyer, J., Gaser, C., Büchel, C., and May, A. (2008). Training-induced brain structure changes in the elderly. *J. Neurosci.* 28, 7031–7035. doi: 10.1523/JNEUROSCI.0742-08.2008

Brookmeyer, R., Gray, S., and Kawas, C. (1998). Projections of Alzheimer's disease in the United States and the public health impact of delaying disease onset. *Amer. J. Public Health* 88, 1337–1342. doi: 10.2105/AJPH.88.9.1337

Brown, B. M., Peiffer, J. J., and Martins, R. N. (2013). Multiple effects of physical activity on molecular and cognitive signs of brain aging: can exercise slow neurodegeneration and delay Alzheimer's disease? *Mol. Psychiatry* 18, 864–874. doi: 10.1038/mp.2012.162

Burdette, J. H., Laurienti, P. J., Espeland, M. A., Morgan, A., Telesford, Q., Vechlekar, C. D., et al. (2010). Using network science to evaluate exercise-associated brain changes in older adults. *Front. Aging Neurosci.* 2:23. doi: 10.3389/fnagi.2010.00023

Burzynska, A. Z., Jiao, Y., Knecht, A. M., Fanning, J., Awick, E. A., Chen, T., et al. (2017). White matter integrity declined over 6-months, but dance intervention improved integrity of the fornix of older adults. *Front. Aging Neurosci.* 9:59. doi: 10.3389/fnagi.2017.00059

Ceccarelli, A., Rocca, M. A., Pagani, E., Falini, A., Comi, G., and Filippi, M. (2009). Cognitive learning is associated with gray matter changes in healthy human individuals: a tensor-based morphometry study. *Neuroimage* 48, 585–589. doi: 10.1016/j.neuroimage.2009.07.009

Chao, Y., Scherer, Y., and Montgomery, C. (2014). Effects of using nintendo wii exergames in older adults: a review of the literature. *J. Aging Health* 27, 379–402. doi: 10.1177/0898264314551171

Chapman, S. B., Aslan, S., Spence, J. S., DeFina, L. F., Keebler, M. W., Didehbani, N., et al. (2013). Shorter term aerobic exercise improves brain, cognition, and cardiovascular fitness in aging. *Front. Aging Neurosci.* 5:75. doi: 10.3389/fnagi.2013.00075

Chapman, S. B., Aslan, S., Spence, J. S., Keebler, M. W., DeFina, L. F., Didehbani, N., et al. (2016). Distinct brain and behavioral benefits from cognitive vs. physical training: a randomized trial in aging adults. *Front. Hum. Neurosci.* 10:338. doi: 10.3389/fnhum.2016.00338

Chodzko-Zajko, W. J., Proctor, D. N., Fiatarone Singh, M. A., Minson, C. T., Nigg, C. R., Salem, G. J., et al. (2009). American College of sports medicine position stand. exercise and physical activity for older adults. *Med. Sci. Sports Exerc.* 41, 1510–1530. doi: 10.1249/MSS.0b013e3181a0c95c

Churchill, J. D., Galvez, R., Colcombe, S., Swain, R. A., Kramer, A. F., and Greenough, W. T. (2002). Exercise, experience and the aging brain. *Neurobiol. Aging* 23, 941–955. doi: 10.1016/S0197-4580(02)00028-3

Coelho, F. G., Andrade, L. P., Pedroso, R. V., Santos-Galduroz, R. F., Gobbi, S., Costa, J. L., et al. (2013b). Multimodal exercise intervention improves frontal cognitive functions and gait in Alzheimer's disease: a controlled trial. *Geriatr. Gerontol. Int.* 13, 198–203. doi: 10.1111/j.1447-0594.2012.00887.x

Coelho, F. G., Gobbi, S., Andreatto, C. A. A., Corazza, D. I., Pedroso, R. V., and Santos-Galduróz, R. F. (2013a). Physical exercise modulates peripheral levels of brain-derived neurotrophic factor (BDNF): a systematic review of experimental studies in the elderly. *Arch. Gerontol. Geriatr.* 56, 10–15. doi: 10.1016/j.archger.2012.06.003

Colcombe, S. J., Erickson, K. I., Scalf, P. E., Kim, J. S., Prakash, R., McAuley, E., et al. (2006). Aerobic exercise training increases brain volume in aging humans. *J. Gerontol.* 61, 1166–1170. doi: 10.1093/gerona/61.11.1166

Colcombe, S., and Kramer, A. F. (2003). Fitness effects on the cognitive function of older adults: a meta-analytic study. *Psychol. Sci.* 14, 125–130. doi: 10.1111/1467-9280.t01-1-01430

Colcombe, S. J., Kramer, A. F., Erickson, K. I., Scalf, P., McAuley, E., Cohen, N. J., et al. (2004). Cardiovascular fitness, cortical plasticity, and aging. *Proc. Natl. Acad. Sci. U.S.A.* 101, 3316–3321. doi: 10.1073/pnas.0400266101

Cotman, C. W., Berchtold, N. C., and Christie, L.-A. (2007). Exercise builds brain health: key roles of growth factor cascades and inflammation. *Trends Neurosci.* 30, 464–472. doi: 10.1016/j.tins.2007.06.011

Curlik, D., and Shors, T. (2013). Training your brain: do mental and physical (MAP) training enhance cognition through the process of neurogenesis in the hippocampus? *Neuropharmacology* 64, 506–514. doi: 10.1016/j.neuropharm.2012.07.027

D'Elia, L. G., Satz, P., Uchiyama, C. L., and White, T. (1996). *Color Trails Test Manual.* Odessa, FL: Psychological Assessment Resources.

Desikan, R. S., Ségonne, F., Fischl, B., Quinn, B. T., Dickerson, B. C., Blacker, D., et al. (2006). An automated labeling system for subdividing the human cerebral cortex on MRI scans into gyral based regions of interest. *Neuroimage* 31, 968–980. doi: 10.1016/j.neuroimage.2006.01.021

Desjardins-Crépeau, L., Berryman, N., Fraser, S. A., Vu, T. T. M., Kergoat, M.-J., Li, K. Z., et al. (2016). Effects of combined physical and cognitive training on fitness and neuropsychological outcomes in healthy older adults. *Clin. Interv. Aging* 11:1287. doi: 10.2147/CIA.S115711

Destrieux, C., Fischl, B., Dale, A., and Halgren, E. (2010). Automatic parcellation of human cortical gyri and sulci using standard anatomical nomenclature. *Neuroimage* 53, 1–15. doi: 10.1016/j.neuroimage.2010.06.010

Dhami, P., Moreno, S., and DeSouza, J. X. (2015). New framework for rehabilitation—Fusion of cognitive and physical rehabilitation: the hope for dancing. *Front. Psychol.* 5:1478. doi: 10.3389/fpsyg.2014.01478

Diamond, A. (2013). Executive functions. *Annu. Rev. Psychol.* 64, 135–168. doi: 10.1146/annurev-psych-113011-143750

Dimitrova, J., Hogan, M., Khader, P., O'Hora, D., Kilmartin, L., Walsh, J. C., et al. (2016). Comparing the effects of an acute bout of physical exercise with an acute bout of interactive mental and physical exercise on electrophysiology and executive functioning in younger and older adults. *Aging Clin. Exp. Res.* 29, 959–967. doi: 10.1007/s40520-016-0683-6

Dinoff, A., Herrmann, N., Swardfager, W., Liu, C. S., Sherman, C., Chan, S., et al. (2016). The effect of exercise training on resting concentrations of peripheral brain-derived neurotrophic factor (BDNF): a meta-analysis. *PLoS ONE* 11:e0163037. doi: 10.1371/journal.pone.0163037

Domenech, P., and Koechlin, E. (2015). Executive control and decision-making in the prefrontal cortex. *Curr. Opin. Behav. Sci.* 1, 101–106. doi: 10.1016/j.cobeha.2014.10.007

Edelmann, E., Lessmann, V., and Brigadski, T. (2014). Pre- and postsynaptic twists in BDNF secretion and action in synaptic plasticity. *Neuropharmacology* 76, 610–627. doi: 10.1016/j.neuropharm.2013.05.043

Eggenberger, P., Schumacher, V., Angst, M., Theill, N., and de Bruin, E. D. (2015). Does multicomponent physical exercise with simultaneous cognitive training boost cognitive performance in older adults? A 6-month randomized controlled trial with a 1-year follow-up. *Clin. Interv. Aging* 10, 1335–1349. doi: 10.2147/CIA.S87732

Eggenberger, P., Wolf, M., Schumann, M., and de Bruin, E. D. (2016). Exergame and balance training modulate prefrontal brain activity during walking and enhance executive function in older adults. *Front. Aging Neurosci.* 8:66. doi: 10.3389/fnagi.2016.00066

Ehlers, D. K., Daugherty, A. M., Burzynska, A. Z., Fanning, J., Awick, E. A., Chaddock-Heyman, L., et al. (2017). Regional brain volumes moderate, but do not mediate, the effects of group-based exercise training on reductions in loneliness in older adults. *Front. Aging Neurosci.* 9:110. doi: 10.3389/fnagi.2017.00110

Erickson, K. I., Hillman, C., and Kramer, A. F. (2015). Physical activity, brain, and cognition. *Curr. Opin. Behav. Sci.* 4, 27–32. doi: 10.1016/j.cobeha.2015.01.005

Erickson, K. I., Miller, D. L., and Roecklein, K. A. (2012). The aging hippocampus: interactions between exercise, depression, and BDNF. *Neuroscientist* 18, 82–97. doi: 10.1177/1073858410397054

Erickson, K. I., Voss, M. W., Prakash, R. S., Basak, C., Szabo, A., Chaddock, L., et al. (2011). Exercise training increases size of hippocampus and improves memory. *Proc. Natl. Acad. Sci. U.S.A.* 108, 3017–3022. doi: 10.1073/pnas.1015950108

Etnier, J. L., and Chang, Y. K. (2009). The effect of physical activity on executive function: a brief commentary on definitions, measurement issues, and the current state of the literature. *J. Sport Exerc. Psychol.* 31, 469–483. doi: 10.1123/jsep.31.4.469

Ettenhofer, M. L., Hambrick, D. Z., and Abeles, N. (2006). Reliability and stability of executive functioning in older adults. *Neuropsychology* 20, 607–613. doi: 10.1037/0894-4105.20.5.607

Fabel, K., Wolf, S., Ehninger, D., Babu, H., Galicia, P., and Kempermann, G. (2009). Additive effects of physical exercise and environmental enrichment on adult hippocampal neurogenesis in mice. *Front. Neurosci.* 3:50. doi: 10.3389/neuro.22.002.2009

Fabre, C., Chamari, K., Mucci, P., Masse-Biron, J., and Prefaut, C. (2002). Improvement of cognitive function by mental and/or individualized aerobic training in healthy elderly subjects. *Int. J. Sports Med.* 23, 415–421. doi: 10.1055/s-2002-33735

Faul, F., Erdfelder, E., Lang, A.-G., and Buchner, A. (2007). G*Power 3: a flexible statistical power analysis program for the social, behavioral, and biomedical sciences. *Behav. Res. Methods* 39, 175–191. doi: 10.3758/BF03193146

Fiatarone, S. M. A., Gates, N., Saigal, N., Wilson, G. C., Meiklejohn, J., Brodaty, H., et al. (2014). The Study of Mental and Resistance Training (SMART) study-resistance training and/or cognitive training in mild cognitive impairment: a randomized, double-blind, double-sham controlled trial. *J. Am. Med. Dir. Assoc.* 15, 873–880. doi: 10.1016/j.jamda.2014.09.010

Fischl, B., Salat, D. H., Busa, E., Albert, M., Dieterich, M., Haselgrove, C., et al. (2002). Whole brain segmentation: automated labeling of neuroanatomical structures in the human brain. *Neuron* 33, 341–355. doi: 10.1016/S0896-6273(02)00569-X

Fissler, P., Kuster, O., Schlee, W., and Kolassa, I.-T. (2013). Novelty interventions to enhance broad cognitive abilities and prevent dementia: synergistic approaches for the facilitation of positive plastic change. *Progress. Brain Res.* 207, 403–434. doi: 10.1016/B978-0-444-63327-9.00017-5

Flöel, A., Ruscheweyh, R., Krüger, K., Willemer, C., Winter, B., Völker, K., et al. (2010). Physical activity and memory functions: are neurotrophins and cerebral gray matter volume the missing link? *Neuroimage* 49, 2756–2763. doi: 10.1016/j.neuroimage.2009.10.043

Forbes, D., Forbes, S. C., Blake, C. M., Thiessen, E. J., and Forbes, S. (2015). Exercise programs for people with dementia. *Cochrane Database Syst. Rev.* CD006489. doi: 10.1002/14651858.CD006489.pub4

Forte, R., Boreham, C. G., Leite, J. C., De Vito, G., Brennan, L., Gibney, E. R., et al. (2013). Enhancing cognitive functioning in the elderly: multicomponent vs resistance training. *Clin. Interv. Aging* 8, 9–27. doi: 10.2147/CIA.S36514

Foster, P. P. (2013). How does dancing promote brain reconditioning in the elderly? *Front. Aging Neurosci.* 5:4. doi: 10.3389/fnagi.2013.00004

Frantzidis, C. A., Ladas, A. I., Vivas, A. B., Tsolaki, M., and Bamidis, P. D. (2014). Cognitive and physical training for the elderly: evaluating outcome efficacy by means of neurophysiological synchronization. *Int. J. Psychophysiol.* 93, 1–11. doi: 10.1016/j.ijpsycho.2014.01.007

Freitas, S., Simões, M. R., Marôco, J., Alves, L., and Santana, I. (2012). Construct validity of the Montreal Cognitive Assessment (MoCA). *J. Int. Neuropsychol. Soc.* 18, 242–250. doi: 10.1017/S1355617711001573

Gage, F. H. (2002). Neurogenesis in the adult brain. *J. Neurosci.* 22, 612–613. doi: 10.1523/JNEUROSCI.22-03-00612.2002

Gallo, A., and Alevizos, I. (2013). Isolation of circulating microRNA in saliva. *Methods Mol. Biol.* 1024, 183–190. doi: 10.1007/978-1-62703-453-1_14

Galvan, V., and Bredesen, D. E. (2007). Neurogenesis in the adult brain: implications for Alzheimer's disease. *CNS Neurol. Disord. Drug Targets* 6, 303–310.

Gates, N. (2013). The effect of exercise training on cognitive function in older adults with mild cognitive impairment: a meta-analysis of randomized controlled trials. *Amer. J. Geriatr. Psychiatry* 21, 1086–1098. doi: 10.1016/j.jagp.2013.02.018

Geda, Y. E., Roberts, R. O., Knopman, D. S., Christianson, T. J., Pankratz, V. S., Ivnik, R. J., et al. (2010). Physical exercise, aging, and mild cognitive impairment. *Arch. Neurol.* 67, 80–86. doi: 10.1001/archneurol.2009.297

Geerlings, M. I., Sigurdsson, S., Eiriksdottir, G., Garcia, M. E., Harris, T. B., Gudnason, V., et al. (2015). Salivary cortisol, brain volumes, and cognition in community-dwelling elderly without dementia. *Neurology* 85, 976–983. doi: 10.1212/WNL.0000000000001931

Gerling, K., and Mandryk, R. (2014). Custom-designed motion-based games for older adults: a review of literature in human-computer interaction. *Gerontechnology* 12, 68–80. doi: 10.4017/gt.2013.12.2.001.00

González-Palau, F., Franco, M., Bamidis, P., Losada, R., Parra, E., Papageorgiou, S. G., et al. (2014). The effects of a computer-based cognitive and physical training program in a healthy and mildly cognitive impaired aging sample. *Aging Ment. Health* 18, 838–846. doi: 10.1080/13607863.2014.899972

Gordon, B. A., Rykhlevskaia, E. I., Brumback, C. R., Lee, Y., Elavsky, S., Konopack, J. F., et al. (2008). Neuroanatomical correlates of aging, cardiopulmonary fitness level, and education. *Psychophysiology* 45, 825–838. doi: 10.1111/j.1469-8986.2008.00676.x

Grandes, G., Sanchez, A., Sanchez-Pinilla, R. O., Torcal, J., Montoya, I., Lizarraga, K., et al. (2009). Effectiveness of physical activity advice and prescription by physicians in routine primary care: a cluster randomized trial. *Arch. Intern. Med.* 169, 694–701. doi: 10.1001/archinternmed.2009.23

Grandjean, J., D'Ostilio, K., Phillips, C., Balteau, E., Degueldre, C., Luxen, A., et al. (2012). Modulation of brain activity during a Stroop inhibitory task by the kind of cognitive control required. *PLoS ONE* 7:e41513. doi: 10.1371/journal.pone.0041513

Greenough, W. T., Cohen, N. J., and Juraska, J. M. (1999). New neurons in old brains: learning to survive? *Nat. Neurosci.* 2, 203–205. doi: 10.1038/6300

Hannay, J. H., and Lezak, M. D. (2004). "The neuropsychological examination: interpretation," in *Neuropsychological Assessment, 4th Edn.* eds M. D. Lezak, D. B. Howieson, and D. W. Loring (New York, NY: Oxford University Press), 133–156.

Harrison, J., Minassian, S. L., Jenkins, L., Black, R. S., Koller, M., and Grundman, M. (2007). A neuropsychological test battery for use in Alzheimer disease clinical trials. *Arch. Neurol.* 64, 1323–1329. doi: 10.1001/archneur.64.9.1323

Hayes, S. M., Hayes, J. P., Cadden, M., and Verfaellie, M. (2013). A review of cardiorespiratory fitness-related neuroplasticity in the aging brain. *Front. Aging Neurosci.* 5:31. doi: 10.3389/fnagi.2013.00031

Hess, N. C. L., Dieberg, G., McFarlane, J. R., and Smart, N. A. (2014). The effect of exercise intervention on cognitive performance in persons at risk for, or with, dementia: a systematic review and meta-analysis. *Healthy Aging Res.* 3:3. doi: 10.12715/har.2014.3.3

Heyn, P., Abreu, B. C., and Ottenbacher, K. J. (2004). The effects of exercise training on elderly persons with cognitive impairment and dementia: a meta-analysis. *Arch. Phys. Med. Rehabil.* 85, 1694–1704. doi: 10.1016/j.apmr.2004.03.019

Hillman, C., Erickson, K., and Kramer, A. (2008). Be smart, exercise your heart: exercise effects on brain and cognition. *Nat. Rev. Neurosci.* 9, 58–65. doi: 10.1038/nrn2298

Hiyamizu, M., Morioka, S., Shomoto, K., and Shimada, T. (2012). Effects of dual task balance training on dual task performance in elderly people: a randomized controlled trial. *Clin. Rehabil.* 26, 58–67. doi: 10.1177/0269215510394222

Hosseini, S. H., Bruno, J. L., Baker, J. M., Gundran, A., Harbott, L. K., Gerdes, J. C., et al. (2017). Neural, physiological, and behavioral correlates of visuomotor cognitive load. *Sci. Rep.* 7:8866. doi: 10.1038/s41598-017-07897-z

Hotting, K., and Roder, B. (2013). Effects of physical exercise on neuroplasticity and cognition. *Neurosci. Biobehav. Rev.* 37, 2243–2257. doi: 10.1016/j.neubiorev.2013.04.005

Houx, P. J., Shepherd, J., Blauw, G.-J., Murphy, M. B., Ford, I., Bollen, E. L., et al. (2002). Testing cognitive function in elderly populations: The PROSPER study. *J. Neurol. Neurosurg. Psychiatr.* 73, 385–389. doi: 10.1136/jnnp.73.4.385

Huang, E. J., and Reichardt, L. F. (2001). Neurotrophins: roles in neuronal development and function. *Annu. Rev. Neurosci.* 24, 677–736. doi: 10.1146/annurev.neuro.24.1.677

Huntley, J. D., Gould, R. L., Liu, K., Smith, M., and Howard, R. J. (2015). Do cognitive interventions improve general cognition in dementia? A meta-analysis and meta-regression. *BMJ Open* 5:e005247. doi: 10.1136/bmjopen-2014-005247

Jak, A. J., Bondi, M. W., Delano-Wood, L., Wierenga, C., Corey-Bloom, J., Salmon, D. P., et al. (2009). Quantification of five neuropsychological approaches to defining mild cognitive impairment. *Am. J. Geriatr. Psychiatry* 17, 368–375. doi: 10.1097/JGP.0b013e31819431d5

Jak, A. J., Preis, S. R., Beiser, A. S., Seshadri, S., Wolf, P. A., Bondi, M. W., et al. (2016). Neuropsychological criteria for mild cognitive impairment and dementia risk in the Framingham Heart Study. *J. Int. Neuropsychol. Soc.* 22, 937–943. doi: 10.1017/S1355617716000199

Jessberger, S., and Gage, F. H. (2014). Adult neurogenesis: bridging the gap between mice and humans. *Trends Cell Biol.* 24, 558–563. doi: 10.1016/j.tcb.2014.07.003

Jonasson, L. S., Nyberg, L., Kramer, A. F., Lundquist, A., Riklund, K., and Boraxbekk, C. J. (2017). Aerobic exercise intervention, cognitive performance, and brain structure: Results from the Physical Influences on Brain in Aging (PHIBRA) Study. *Front. Aging Neurosci.* 8:336. doi: 10.3389/fnagi.2016.00336

Julayanont, P., Brousseau, M., Chertkow, H., Phillips, N., and Nasreddine, Z. S. (2014). Montreal Cognitive Assessment Memory Index Score (MoCA-MIS) as a predictor of conversion from mild cognitive impairment to Alzheimer's disease. *J. Am. Geriatr. Soc.* 62, 679–684. doi: 10.1111/jgs.12742

Karlawish, J. (2008). Measuring decision-making capacity in cognitively impaired individuals. *Neurosignals* 16, 91–98. doi: 10.1159/000109763

Karr, J. E., Areshenkoff, C. N., Rast, P., and Garcia-Barrera, M. A. (2014). An empirical comparison of the therapeutic benefits of physical exercise and cognitive training on the executive functions of older adults: a meta-analysis of controlled trials. *Neuropsychology* 28, 829–845. doi: 10.1037/neu0000101

Karssemeijer, E. A., Aaronson, J. A., Bossers, W. J., Smits, T., Olde Rikkert, M. M., and Kessels, R. C. (2017). Positive effects of combined cognitive and physical exercise training on cognitive function in older adults with mild cognitive impairment or dementia: a meta-analysis. *Ageing Res. Rev.* 40, 75–83. doi: 10.1016/j.arr.2017.09.003

Kattenstroth, J., Kalisch, T., Holt, S., Tegenthoff, M., and Dinse, H. R. (2013). Six months of dance intervention enhances postural, sensorimotor, and cognitive performance in elderly without affecting cardio-respiratory functions. *Front. Aging Neurosci.* 5:5. doi: 10.3389/fnagi.2013.00005

Kleemeyer, M. M., Polk, T. A., Schaefer, S., Bodammer, N. C., Brechtel, L., and Lindenberger, U. (2017). Exercise-induced fitness changes correlate with changes in neural specificity in older adults. *Front. Hum. Neurosci.* 11:123. doi: 10.3389/fnhum.2017.00123

Klusmann, V., Evers, A., Schwarzer, R., Schlattmann, P., Reischies, F. M., Heuser, I., et al. (2010). Complex mental and physical activity in older women and cognitive performance: a 6-month randomized controlled trial. *J. Gerontol.* 65, 680–688. doi: 10.1093/gerona/glq053

Knaepen, K., Goekint, M., Heyman, E. M., and Meeusen, R. (2010). Neuroplasticity - exercise-induced response of peripheral brain-derived neurotrophic factor: a systematic review of experimental studies in human subjects. *Sports Med.* 40, 765–801. doi: 10.2165/11534530-000000000-00000

Konstantinidis, E. I., Bamparopoulos, G., and Bamidis, P. D. (2017). Moving real exergaming engines on the web: the webfitforall case study in an active and healthy ageing living lab environment. *IEEE J. Biomed. Health Inform.* 21, 859–866. doi: 10.1109/JBHI.2016.2559787

Kraft, E. (2012). Cognitive function, physical activity, and aging: possible biological links and implications for multimodal interventions. *Aging Neuropsychol. C* 19, 248–263. doi: 10.1080/13825585.2011.645010

Kramer, A. F., Hahn, S., Cohen, N. J., Banich, M. T., McAuley, E., Harrison, C. R., et al. (1999). Ageing, fitness and neurocognitive function. *Nature* 400, 418–419. doi: 10.1038/22682

Kramer, A., and Erickson, K. (2007). Capitalizing on cortical plasticity: Influence of physical activity on cognition and brain function. *Trends Cogn. Sci.* 11, 342–348. doi: 10.1016/j.tics.2007.06.009

Kramer, A., Wickens, C., and Donchin, E. (1985). Processing of stimulus properties: evidence for dual-task integrality. *J. Exp. Psychol.* 11, 393–408. doi: 10.1037/0096-1523.11.4.393

Kumar, S., and Reddy, P. H. (2016). Are circulating microRNAs peripheral biomarkers for Alzheimer's disease? *Biochim. Biophys. Acta* 1862, 1617–1627. doi: 10.1016/j.bbadis.2016.06.001

Lam, M., Eng, G. K., Rapisarda, A., Subramanium, M., Kraus, M., Keefe, R. E., et al. (2013). Formulation of the age–education index: measuring age and education effects in neuropsychological performance. *Psychol. Assess.* 25, 61–70. doi: 10.1037/a0030548

Lansbergen, M. M., Kenemans, J. L., and van Engeland, H. (2007). Stroop interference and attention-deficit/hyperactivity disorder: a review and meta-analysis. *Neuropsychology* 21, 251–262. doi: 10.1037/0894-4105.21.2.251

Lara, J., Cooper, R., Nissan, J., Ginty, A. T., Khaw, K.-T., Deary, I. J., et al. (2015). A proposed panel of biomarkers of healthy ageing. *BMC Med.* 13:222. doi: 10.1186/s12916-015-0470-9

Larson, E. (2010). Prospects for delaying the rising tide of worldwide, late-life dementias. *Int. Psychogeriatr.* 22, 1196–1202. doi: 10.1017/S1041610210001080

Lauenroth, A., Ioannidis, A. E., and Teichmann, B. (2016). Influence of combined physical and cognitive training on cognition: a systematic review. *BMC Geriatr.* 16:141. doi: 10.1186/s12877-016-0315-1

Law, L. L., Barnett, F., Yau, M. K., and Gray, M. A. (2014). Effects of combined cognitive and exercise interventions on cognition in older adults with and without cognitive impairment: a systematic review. *Ageing Res. Rev.* 15, 61–75. doi: 10.1016/j.arr.2014.02.008

Leckie, R. L., Oberlin, L. E., Voss, M. W., Prakash, R. S., Szabo-Reed, A., Chaddock-Heyman, L., et al. (2014). BDNF mediates improvements in executive function following a 1-year exercise intervention. *Front. Hum. Neurosci.* 8:985. doi: 10.3389/fnhum.2014.00985

Lee, Y. Y., Wu, C. Y., Teng, C. H., Hsu, W. C., Chang, K. C., and Chen, P. (2016). Evolving methods to combine cognitive and physical training for individuals with mild cognitive impairment: study protocol for a randomized controlled study. *Trials* 17:526. doi: 10.1186/s13063-016-1650-4

Legault, C., Jennings, J. M., Katula, J. A., Dagenbach, D., Gaussoin, S. A., Sink, K. M., et al. (2011). Designing clinical trials for assessing the effects of cognitive training and physical activity interventions on cognitive outcomes: The Seniors Health and Activity Research Program Pilot (SHARP-P) study, a randomized controlled trial. *BMC Geriatr.* 11:27. doi: 10.1186/1471-2318-11-27

Leßmann, V., and Brigadski, T. (2009). Mechanisms, locations, and kinetics of synaptic BDNF secretion: an update. *Neurosci. Res.* 65, 11–22. doi: 10.1016/j.neures.2009.06.004

Li, M., Huang, M., Li, S., Tao, J., Zheng, G., and Chen, L. (2017). The effects of aerobic exercise on the structure and function of DMN-related brain regions: a systematic review. *Int. J. Neurosci.* 127, 634–649. doi: 10.1080/00207454.2016.1212855

Li, S., Yan, Y., Jiao, Y., Gao, Z., Xia, Y., Kong, L., et al. (2016). Neuroprotective effect of osthole on neuron synapses in an alzheimer's disease cell model via upregulation of MicroRNA-9. *J. Mol. Neurosci.* 60, 71–81. doi: 10.1007/s12031-016-0793-9

Lieberman, D. A. (2009). "Designing serious games for learning and health in informal and formal settings," in *Serious Games: Mechanisms and Effects*, eds U. Ritterfeld, M. Cody, and P. Vorderer (New York, NY: Routledge), 117–130.

Lipardo, D. S., Aseron, A. C., Kwan, M. M., and Tsang, W. W. (2017). Effect of exercise and cognitive training on falls and fall-related factors in older adults with mild cognitive impairment: a systematic review. *Arch. Phys. Med. Rehabil.* 98, 2079–2096. doi: 10.1016/j.apmr.2017.04.021

Lommatzsch, M., Zingler, D., Schuhbaeck, K., Schloetcke, K., Zingler, C., Schuff-Werner, P., et al. (2005). The impact of age, weight and gender on BDNF levels in human platelets and plasma. *Neurobiol. Aging* 26, 115–123. doi: 10.1016/j.neurobiolaging.2004.03.002

Lorens-Martín, M., Torres-Alemán, I., and Trejo, J. L. (2009). Reviews: mechanisms mediating brain plasticity: IGF-1 and adult hippocampal neurogenesis. *Neuroscientist* 15, 134–148. doi: 10.1177/1073858408331371

Maass, A., Duzel, S., Brigads, T., Goerke, M., Becke, A., Sobieray, U., et al. (2016). Relationships of peripheral IGF-1, VEGF and BDNF levels to exercise-related changes in memory, hippocampal perfusion and volumes in older adults. *Neuroimage* 131, 142–154. doi: 10.1016/j.neuroimage.2015.10.084

Maillot, P., Perrot, A., and Hartley, A. (2012). Effects of interactive physical-activity video- game training on physical and cognitive function in older adults. *Psychol. Aging* 3, 589–600. doi: 10.1037/a0026268

Mandel, A., Ozdener, H., and Utermohlen, V. (2011). Brain-derived neurotrophic factor in human saliva: ELISA optimization and biological correlates. *J. Immunoassay Immunochem.* 32, 18–30. doi: 10.1080/15321819.2011.538625

Marquez, D. X., Wilson, R., Aguiñaga, S., Vásquez, P., Fogg, L., Yang, Z., et al. (2017). Regular latin dancing and health education may improve cognition of late middle-aged and older latinos. *J. Aging Phys. Act.* 25, 482–489. doi: 10.1123/japa.2016-0049

Marshall, G. A., Rentz, D. M., Frey, M. T., Locascio, J. J., Johnson, K. A., and Sperling, R. A. (2011). Executive function and instrumental activities of daily living in mild cognitive impairment and Alzheimer's disease. *Alzheimer's Dementia* 7, 300–308. doi: 10.1016/j.jalz.2010.04.005

Martin, M., Clare, L., Altgassen, A. M., Cameron, M. H., and Zehnder, F. (2011). Cognition-based interventions for healthy older people and people with mild cognitive impairment. *Cochrane Database Syst. Rev.* 1:CD006220. doi: 10.1002/14651858.CD006220.pub2

McAuley, E., Mullen, S. P., Szabo, A. N., White, S. M., Wojcicki, T. R., Mailey, E. L., et al. (2011). Self-regulatory processes and exercise adherence in older adults: Executive function and self-efficacy effects. *Am. J. Prev. Med.* 41, 284–290. doi: 10.1016/j.amepre.2011.04.014

Mills, K. L., and Tamnes, C. K. (2014). Methods and considerations for longitudinal structural brain imaging analysis across development. *Dev. Cogn. Neurosci.* 9, 172–190. doi: 10.1016/j.dcn.2014.04.004

Monteiro-Junior, R. S., de Tarso Maciel-Pinheiro, P., da Matta Mello Portugal, E., da Silva Figueiredo, L. F., Terra, R., Carneiro, L. F., et al. (2017). Effect of exercise on inflammatory profile of older persons: systematic review and meta-analyses. *J. Phys. Act. Health* 15, 64–71. doi: 10.1123/jpah.2016-0735

Morrison-Bogorad, M., Cahan, V., and Wagster, M. (2007). Brain health interventions: the need for further research. *Alzheimers Dem.* 3, S80–S85. doi: 10.1016/j.jalz.2007.01.015

Muijden, J. V., Band, G. P. H., and Hommel, B. (2012). Online games training aging brains: limited transfer to cognitive control functions. *Front. Hum. Neurosci.* 6: 221. doi: 10.3389/fnhum.2012.00221

Müller, P., Rehfeld, K., Schmicker, M., Hökelmann, A., Dordevic, M., Lessmann, V., et al. (2017). Evolution of neuroplasticity in response to physical activity in old age: the case for dancing. *Front. Aging Neurosci.* 9:56. doi: 10.3389/fnagi.2017.00056

Nasreddine, Z. S., Phillips, N. A., Bédirian, V., Charbonneau, S., Whitehead, V., Collin, I., et al. (2005). The montreal cognitive assessment, MoCA: a brief screening tool for mild cognitive impairment. *J. Am. Geriatr. Soc.* 53, 695–699. doi: 10.1111/j.1532-5415.2005.53221.x

National Alzheimer's Project Act (2011). *National Alzheimer's Project Act of 2011. Public Law. No. 111-375.*

Nishiguchi, S., Yamada, M., Tanigawa, T., Sekiyama, K., Kawagoe, T., Suzuki, M., et al. (2015). A 12-week physical and cognitive exercise program can improve cognitive function and neural efficiency in community-dwelling older adults: a randomized controlled trial. *J. Am. Geriatr. Soc.* 63, 1355–1363. doi: 10.1111/jgs.13481

Ogawa, E. F., You, T., and Leveille, S. G. (2016). Potential benefits of exergaming for cognition and dual-task function in older adults: a systematic review. *J. Aging Phys. Activ.* 24:332336. doi: 10.1123/japa.2014-0267

Olson, A. K., Eadie, B. D., Ernst, C., and Christie, B. R. (2006). Environmental enrichment and voluntary exercise massively increase neurogenesis in the adult hippocampus via dissociable pathways. *Hippocampus* 16, 250–260. doi: 10.1002/hipo.20157

Oswald, W. D., Gunzelmann, T., Rupprecht, R., and Hagen, B. (2006). Differential effects of single versus combined cognitive and physical training with older adults: the SimA study in a 5- year perspective. *Eur. J. Aging* 3, 179–192. doi: 10.1007/s10433-006-0035-z

Owen, A., Hampshire, A., Grahn, J. A., Stenton, R., Dajani, S., Burns, A. S., et al. (2010). Putting brain training to the test. *Nature* 465, 775–778. doi: 10.1038/nature09042

Park, H., and Poo, M. (2013). Neurotrophin regulation of neural circuit development and function. *Nat. Rev. Neurosci.* 14, 7–23. doi: 10.1038/nrn3379

Párrizas, M., Brugnara, L., Esteban, Y., González-Franquesa, A., Canivell, S., Murillo, S., et al. (2015). Circulating miR-192 and miR-193b are markers of prediabetes and are modulated by an exercise intervention. *J. Clin. Endocrinol. Metab.* 100, E407–E415. doi: 10.1210/jc.2014-2574

Payne, B. R., Jackson, J. J., Noh, S. R., and Stine-Morrow, E. L. (2011). In the zone: Flow state and cognition in older adults. *Psychol. Aging* 26, 738–743. doi: 10.1037/a0022359

Pereira, F. S., Yassuda, M. S., Oliveira, A. M., and Forlenza, O. V. (2008). Executive dysfunction correlates with impaired functional status in older adults with varying degrees of cognitive impairment. *Int. Psychogeriatr.* 20, 1104–1115. doi: 10.1017/S1041610208007631

Pfaffl, M. W., Horgan, G. W., and Dempfle, L. (2002). Relative expression software tool (REST (c)) for group-wise comparison and statistical analysis of relative expression results in real-time PCR. *Nucleic Acids Res.* 30:e36. doi: 10.1093/nar/30.9.e36

Phillips, C., Baktir, M. A., Das, D., Lin, B., and Salehi, A. (2015). The link between physical activity and cognitive dysfunction in Alzheimer disease. *Phys. Ther.* 95, 1046–1060. doi: 10.2522/ptj.20140212

Phillips, C., Baktir, M. A., Srivatsan, M., and Salehi, A. (2014). Neuroprotective effects of physical activity on the brain: a closer look at trophic factor signaling. *Front. Cell. Neurosci.* 8:170. doi: 10.3389/fncel.2014.00170

Podhorna, J., Krahnke, T., Shear, M., and Harrison, J. E. (2016). Alzheimer's Disease Assessment Scale-Cognitive subscale variants in mild cognitive impairment and mild Alzheimer's disease: change over time and the effect of enrichment strategies. *Alzheimer's Res. Ther.* 8:8. doi: 10.1186/s13195-016-0170-5

Podsiadlo, D., and Richardson, S. (1991). The timed "Up & Go": a test of basic functional mobility for frail elderly persons. *J. Am. Geriatr. Soc.* 39, 142–148. doi: 10.1111/j.1532-5415.1991.tb01616.x

Pusic, K. M., Pusic, A. D., and Kraig, R. P. (2016). Environmental enrichment stimulates immune cell secretion of exosomes that promote CNS myelination and may regulate inflammation. *Cell. Mol. Neurobiol.* 36, 313–325. doi: 10.1007/s10571-015-0269-4

Rahe, J., Becker, J., Fink, G. R., Kessler, J., Kukolja, J., Rahn, A., et al. (2015). Cognitive training with and without additional physical activity in healthy older adults: cognitive effects, neurobiological mechanisms, and prediction of training success. *Front. Aging Neurosci.* 7:187. doi: 10.3389/fnagi.2015.00187

Raichlen, D. A., and Alexander, G. E. (2014). Exercise, APOE genotype, and the evolution of the human lifespan. *Trends Neurosci.* 37, 247–255. doi: 10.1016/j.tins.2014.03.001

Read, J. L., and Shortell, S. M. (2011). Interactive games to promote behavior change in prevention and treatment. *JAMA* 305, 1704–1705. doi: 10.1001/jama.2011.408

Redick, T. S., Shipstead, Z., Harrison, T. L., Hicks, K. L., Fried, D. E., Hambrick, D. Z., et al. (2013). No evidence of intelligence improvement after working memory training: a randomized, placebo-controlled study. *J. Exp. Psychol. Gen.* 142, 359–379. doi: 10.1037/a0029082

Rehfeld, K., Müller, P., Aye, N., Schmicker, M., Dordevic, M., Kaufmann, J., et al. (2017). Dancing or fitness sport? The effects of two training programs on hippocampal plasticity and balance abilities in healthy seniors. *Front. Hum. Neurosci.* 11:305. doi: 10.3389/fnhum.2017.00305

Reuter, M., Schmansky, N. J., Rosas, H. D., and Fischl, B. (2012). Within-subject template estimation for unbiased longitudinal image analysis. *Neuroimage* 62, 1402–1418. doi: 10.1016/j.neuroimage.2012.02.084

Riancho, J., Vázquez-Higuera, J. L., Pozueta, A., Lage, C., Kazimierczak, M., Bravo, M., et al. (2017). MicroRNA profile in patients with Alzheimer's disease: analysis of miR-9-5p and miR-598 in raw and exosome enriched cerebrospinal fluid samples. *J. Alzheimer's Dis.* 57, 483–491. doi: 10.3233/JAD-161179

Roberts, R., and Knopman, D. S. (2013). Classification and epidemiology of MCI. *Clin. Geriatr. Med.* 29, 753–772. doi: 10.1016/j.cger.2013.07.003

Ruigrok, A. V., Salimi-Khorshidi, G., Lai, M., Baron-Cohen, S., Lombardo, M. V., Tait, R. J., et al. (2014). A meta-analysis of sex differences in human brain structure. *Neurosci. Biobehav. Rev.* 39, 34–50. doi: 10.1016/j.neubiorev.2013.12.004

Ruijter, J. M., Thygesen, H. H., Schoneveld, O. J., Das, A T., Berkhout, B., and Lamers, W. H. (2006). Factor correction as a tool to eliminate between-session variation in replicate experiments: application to molecular biology and retrovirology. *Retrovirology* 3:2. doi: 10.1186/1742-4690-3-2

Ruijter, J. M., Ramakers, C., Hoogaars, W. M., Karlen, Y., Bakker, O., van den Hoff, M. J., et al. (2009). Amplification efficiency: linking baseline and bias in the analysis of quantitative PCR data. *Nucleic Acids Res.* 37:e45. doi: 10.1093/nar/gkp045

Russell, A. P., Lamon, S., Boon, H., Wada, S., Güller, I., Brown, E. L., et al. (2013). Regulation of miRNAs in human skeletal muscle following acute endurance exercise and short-term endurance training. *J. Physiol.* 591, 4637–4653. doi: 10.1113/jphysiol.2013.255695

Sano, M., Ernesto, C., Thomas, R. G., Klauber, M. R., Schafer, K., Grundman, M., et al. (1997). A controlled trial of selegiline, alpha-tocopherol, or both as treatment for Alzheimer's disease. The Alzheimer's Disease Cooperative Study. *N. Engl. J. Med.* 336, 1216–1222. doi: 10.1056/NEJM199704243361704

Satoh, M., Ogawa, J., Tokita, T., Nakaguchi, N., Nakao, K., Kida, H., et al. (2014). The effects of physical exercise with music on cognitive function of elderly people: Mihama-Kiho Project. *PLoS ONE* 9:e95230. doi: 10.1371/journal.pone.0095230

Schaefer, S., and Schumacher, V. (2011). The interplay between cognitive and motor functioning in healthy older adults: findings from dual-task studies and suggestions for intervention. *Gerontology* 57, 239–246. doi: 10.1159/000322197

Schoene, D., Lord, S. R., Delbaere, K., Severino, C., Davies, T. A., and Smith, S. T. (2013). A randomized controlled pilot study of home-based step training in older people using videogame technology. *PLoS ONE* 8:e57734. doi: 10.1371/journal.pone.0057734

Schoene, D., Valenzuela, T., Lord, S. R., and de Bruin, E. D. (2014). The effect of interactive cognitive-motor training in reducing fall risk in older people: a systematic review. *BMC Geriatr.* 14:107. doi: 10.1186/1471-2318-14-107

Schoene, D., Valenzuela, T., Toson, B., Delbaere, K., Severino, C., Garcia, J., et al. (2015). Interactive cognitive-motor step training improves cognitive risk factors of falling in older adults - a randomized controlled trial. *PLoS ONE* 10:e0145161. doi: 10.1371/journal.pone.0145161

Sexton, C. E., Betts, J. F., Demnitz, N., Dawes, H., Ebmeier, K. P., and Johansen-Berg, H. (2016). A systematic review of MRI studies examining the relationship between physical fitness and activity and the white matter of the ageing brain. *Neuroimage* 131, 81–90. doi: 10.1016/j.neuroimage.2015.09.071

Shah, T., Verdile, G., Sohrabi, H., Campbell, A., Putland, E., Cheetham, C., and et al. (2014). A combination of physical activity and computerized brain training improves verbal memory and increases cerebral glucose metabolism in the elderly. *Transl. Psychiatry* 4:e487. doi: 10.1038/tp.2014.122

Shatil, E. (2013). Does combined cognitive training and physical activity training enhance cognitive abilities more than either alone? A four-condition randomized controlled trial among healthy older adults. *Front. Aging Neurosci.* 5:8. doi: 10.3389/fnagi.2013.00008

Simons, D. J., Boot, W. R., Charness, N., Gathercole, S. E., Chabris, C. F., Hambrick, D. Z., et al. (2016). Do 'brain-training' programs work? *Psychol. Sci. Public Interest* 17, 103–186. doi: 10.1177/1529100616661983

Smith, P. J., Blumenthal, J. A., Hoffman, B. M., Cooper, H., Strauman, T. A., et al. (2010). Aerobic exercise and neurocognitive performance: a meta-analytic review of randomized control trials. *Psychosom. Med.* 72, 239–252. doi: 10.1097/PSY.0b013e3181d14633

Snyder, A., Anderson-Hanley, C., and Arciero, P. J. (2012). Virtual and live social facilitation while exergaming: competitiveness moderates effort. *J. Sport Exerc. Psychol.* 34, 252–259. doi: 10.1123/jsep.34.2.252

Stanmore, E., Stubbs, B., Vancampfort, D., de Bruin, E. D., and Firth, J. (2017). The effect of active video games on cognitive functioning in clinical and non-clinical populations: a meta-analysis of randomized controlled trials. *Neurosci. Biobehav. Rev.* 78, 34–43. doi: 10.1016/j.neubiorev.2017.04.011

Strauss, E., Sherman, E. M. S., and Spreen, O. (2006). *A Compendium of Neuropsychological Tests, 3rd Edn.* New York, NY: Oxford University Press.

Studenski, S., Carlson, M. C., Fillit, H., Greenough, W. T., Kramer, A., and Rebok, G. W. (2006). From bedside to bench: does mental and physical activity promote cognitive vitality in late life? *Sci. Aging Knowledge Environ.* 10:pe21. doi: 10.1126/sageke.2006.10.pe21

Styliadis, C., Kartsidis, P., Paraskevopoulos, E., Ioannides, A. A., and Bamidis, P. D. (2015). Neuroplastic effects of combined computerized physical and cognitive training in elderly individuals at risk for dementia: an eLORETA controlled study on resting states. *Neural Plast.* 2015, 172–192. doi: 10.1155/2015/172192

Suo, C., Singh, M. F., Gates, N., Wen, W., Sachdev, P., Brodaty, H., et al. (2016). Therapeutically relevant structural and functional mechanisms triggered by physical and cognitive exercise. *Mol. Psychiatry* 21, 1633–1642. doi: 10.1038/mp.2016.19

Suzuki, T., Shimada, H., Makizako, H., Doi, T., Yoshida, D., Tsutsumimoto, K., et al. (2012). Effects of multicomponent exercise on cognitive function in older adults with amnestic mild cognitive impairment: a randomized controlled trial. *BMC Neurol.* 12:128. doi: 10.1186/1471-2377-12-128

Szuhany, K. L., Bugatti, M., and Otto, M. W. (2014). A meta-analytic review of the effects of exercise on brain-derived neurotrophic factor. *J. Psychiatr. Res.* 60, 56–64. doi: 10.1016/j.jpsychires.2014.10.003

Teixeira, C. L., Rezende, T. J., Weiler, M., Nogueira, M. H., Campos, B. M., Pegoraro, L. F., et al. (2016). Relation between aerobic fitness and brain structures in amnestic mild cognitive impairment elderly. *Age* 38:51. doi: 10.1007/s11357-016-9912-3

ten Brinke, L. F., Bolandzadeh, N., Nagamatsu, L. S., Hsu, C. L., Davis, J. C., Miran-Khan, K., et al. (2015). Aerobic exercise increases hippocampal volume in older women with probable mild cognitive impairment: a 6-month randomised controlled trial. *Br. J. Sports Med.* 49, 248–254. doi: 10.1136/bjsports-2013-093184

Terry, P. C., Lane, A. M., and Fogarty, G. J. (2003). Construct validity of the Profile of Mood States-Adolescents for use with adults. *Psychol. Sport Exerc.* 4, 125–139. doi: 10.1016/S1469-0292(01)00035-8

Theill, N., Schumacher, V., Adelsberger, R., Martin, M., and Jäncke, L. (2013). Effects of simultaneously performed cognitive and physical training in older adults. *BMC Neurosci.* 14:103. doi: 10.1186/1471-2202-14-103

Thery, C., Amigorena, S., Raposo, G., and Clayton, A. (2006). Isolation and characterization of exosomes from cell culture supernatants and biological fluids. *Curr. Protoc. Cell. Biol.* Chapter 3:Unit 3 22. doi: 10.1002/0471143030.cb0322s30

Thielen, J., Kärgel, C., Müller, B. W., Rasche, I., Genius, J., Bus, B., et al. (2016). Aerobic activity in the healthy elderly is associated with larger plasticity in memory related brain structures and lower systemic inflammation. *Front. Aging Neurosci.* 8:319. doi: 10.3389/fnagi.2016.00319

Thomas, A. G., Dennis, A., Bandettini, P. A., and Johansen-Berg, H. (2012). The effects of aerobic activity on brain structure. *Front. Psychol.* 3:86. doi: 10.3389/fpsyg.2012.00086

Toril, P., Reales, J. M., and Ballesteros, S. (2014). Video game training enhances cognition of older adults: a meta-analytic study. *Psychol. Aging* 29, 706–716. doi: 10.1037/a0037507

Trachtenberg, J. T., Chen, B. E., Knott, G. W., Feng, G., Sanes, J. R., Welker, E., et al. (2002). Longterm *in vivo* imaging of experience-dependent synaptic plasticity in adult cortex. *Nature* 420, 788–794. doi: 10.1038/nature01273

Train the Brain Consortium (2017). Randomized trial on the effects of a combined physical/cognitive training in aged MCI subjects: the Train the Brain study. *Sci. Rep.* 7:39471. doi: 10.1038/srep39471

Tsai, S., Chen, P., Calkins, M. J., Wu, S., and Kuo, Y. (2016). Exercise counteracts aging-related memory impairment: a potential role for the astrocytic metabolic shuttle. *Front. Aging Neurosci.* 8:57. doi: 10.3389/fnagi.2016.00057

Van der Elst, W., Van Boxtel, M. J., Van Breukelen, G. P., and Jolles, J. (2006). The stroop color-word test: influence of age, sex, and education; and normative data for a large sample across the adult age range. *Assessment* 13, 62–79. doi: 10.1177/1073191105283427

van Praag, H. (2008). Neurogenesis and exercise: past and future directions. *Neuromol. Med.* 10, 128–140. doi: 10.1007/s12017-008-8028-z

Van Praag, H., Shubert, T., Zhao, C., and Gage, F. H. (2005). Exercise enhances learning and hippocampal neurogenesis in aged mice. *J. Neurosci.* 25, 8680–8685. doi: 10.1523/JNEUROSCI.1731-05.2005

Van Schaik, P., Blake, J., Pernet, F., Spears, I., and Fencott, C. (2008). Virtual augmented exercise gaming for older adults. *CyberPsychol. Behav.* 11, 103–106. doi: 10.1089/cpb.2007.9925

Vaughan, S., Wallis, M., Polit, D., Steele, M., Shum, D., and Morris, N. (2014). The effects of multimodal exercise on cognitive and physical functioning and brain-derived neurotrophic factor in older women: a randomised controlled trial. *Age Ageing* 43, 623–629. doi: 10.1093/ageing/afu010

Vellas, B., Carrie, I., Gillette-Guyonnet, S., Touchon, J., Dantoine, T., Dartigues, J. F., et al. (2014). MAPT Study: a multidomain approach for preventing Alzheimer's disease: design and baseline data. *J. Prevent. Alzheimer's Dis.* 1, 13–22.

Veterans Administration Medical Center (VAMC). (2007). *Impaired Decision Making Capacity Screening Assessment Form. Unpublished document.* Syracuse, NY: VAMC. Available online at: https://www.visn2.va.gov/VISN2/research/syr/docs/IDMC_Assesment_Form.doc

Vickers, A. J. (2005). Parametric versus non-parametric statistics in the analysis of randomized trials with non-normally distributed data. *BMC Med. Res. Methodol.* 5:35. doi: 10.1186/1471-2288-5-35

Vidoni, E. D., Johnson, D. K., Morris, J. K., Van Sciver, A., Greer, C. S., Billinger, S. A., et al. (2015). Dose-response of aerobic exercise on cognition: a community-based, pilot randomized controlled trial. *PLoS ONE* 10:e0131647. doi: 10.1371/journal.pone.0131647

Vijayakumar, N., Whittle, S., Yücel, M., Dennison, M., Simmons, J., and Allen, N. B. (2014). Thinning of the lateral prefrontal cortex during adolescence predicts emotion regulation in females. *Soc. Cogn. Affect. Neurosci.* 9, 1845–1854. doi: 10.1093/scan/nst183

Vital, T. M., Stein, A. M., de Melo Coelho, F. G., Arantes, F. J., Teodorov, E., and Santos-Galduróz, R. F. (2014). Physical exercise and vascular endothelial growth factor (VEGF) in elderly: a systematic review. *Arch. Gerontol. Geriatr.* 59, 234–239. doi: 10.1016/j.archger.2014.04.011

Voss, M. W., Prakash, R. S., Erickson, K. I., Basak, C., Chaddock, L., Kim, J. S., et al. (2010). Plasticity of brain networks in a randomized intervention trial of exercise training in older adults. *Front. Aging Neurosci.* 2:32. doi: 10.3389/fnagi.2010.00032

Voss, M., Vivar, C., Kramer, A. F., and van Praag, H. (2013). Bridging animal and human models of exercise-induced brain plasticity. *Trends Cogn. Sci.* 17, 525–544. doi: 10.1016/j.tics.2013.08.001

Wang, C., Yu, J., Wang, H., Tan, C., Meng, X., and Tan, L. (2014). Non-pharmacological interventions for patients with mild cognitive impairment: a meta-analysis of randomized controlled trials of cognition-based and exercise interventions. *J. Alzheimer's Dis.* 42, 663–678. doi: 10.3233/JAD-140660

Wang, P., Liu, H., Zhu, X., Meng, T., Li, H., and Zuo, X. (2016). Action video game training for healthy adults: a meta-analytic study. *Front. Psychol.* 7:907. doi: 10.3389/fpsyg.2016.00907

Wang, X., and Goh, D. H. (2017). Video game acceptance: a meta-analysis of the extended technology acceptance model. *Cyberpsychol. Behav. Soc. Netw.* 20, 662–671. doi: 10.1089/cyber.2017.0086

Wecker, N. S., Kramer, J. H., Wisniewski, A., Delis, D. C., and Kaplan, E. (2000). Age effects on executive ability. *Neuropsychology* 14, 409–414. doi: 10.1037/0894-4105.14.3.409

Weinstein, A. M., Voss, M. W., Prakash, R. S., Chaddock, L., Szabo, A., White, S. M., et al. (2012). The association between aerobic fitness and executive function is mediated by prefrontal cortex volume. *Brain Behav. Immun.* 26, 811–819. doi: 10.1016/j.bbi.2011.11.008

Willis, S. L., Tennstedt, S. L., Marsiske, M., Ball, K., Elias, J., Koepke, K. M., et al. (2006). Long-term effects of cognitive training on everyday functional outcomes in older adults. *JAMA* 296, 2805–2814. doi: 10.1001/jama.296.23.2805

Witwer, K. W., Buzás, E. I., Bemis, L. T., Bora, A., Lässer, C., Lötvall, J., et al. (2013). Standardization of sample collection, isolation and analysis methods in extracellular vesicle research. *J. Extracell. Vesicles* 2. doi: 10.3402/jev.v2i0.20360

Wong, C. N., Chaddock-Heyman, L., Voss, M. W., Burzynska, A. Z., Basak, C., Erickson, K. I., et al. (2015). Brain activation during dual-task processing is associated with cardiorespiratory fitness and performance in older adults. *Front. Aging Neurosci.* 7:154. doi: 10.3389/fnagi.2015.00154

Yokoyama, H., Okazaki, K., Imai, D., Yamashina, Y., Takeda, R., Naghavi, N., et al. (2015). The effect of cognitive-motor dual-task training on cognitive function and plasma amyloid beta peptide 42/40 ratio in healthy elderly persons: a randomized controlled trial. *BMC Geriatr.* 15:60. doi: 10.1186/s12877-015-0058-4

Young, J., Angevaren, M., Rusted, J., and Tabet, N. (2015). Aerobic exercise to improve cognitive function in older people without known cognitive impairment. *Cochrane Database Syst. Rev.* CD005381. doi: 10.1002/14651858.CD005381.pub4

Zatorre, R. J., Douglas Fields, R., and Johansen-Berg, H. (2012). Plasticity in gray and white: Neuroimaging changes in brain structure during learning. *Nat. Neurosci.* 15, 528–536. doi: 10.1038/nn.3045

Zhang, R., Zhang, Q., Niu, J., Lu, K., Xie, B., Cui, D., et al. (2014). Screening of microRNAs associated with Alzheimer's disease using oxidative stress cell model and different strains of senescence accelerated mice. *J. Neurol. Sci.* 338, 57–64. doi: 10.1016/j.jns.2013.12.017

Zheng, G., Xia, R., Zhou, W., Tao, J., and Chen, L. (2016). Aerobic exercise ameliorates cognitive function in older adults with mild cognitive impairment: a systematic review and meta-analysis of randomised controlled trials. *Brit. J. Sports Med.* doi: 10.1136/bjsports-2015-095699. [Epub ahead of print].

Zhu, X., Yin, S., Lang, M., He, R., and Li, J. (2016). The more the better? A meta-analysis on effects of combined cognitive and physical intervention on cognition in healthy older adults. *Ageing Res. Rev.* 31, 67–79. doi: 10.1016/j.arr.2016.07.003

Zilidou, V. I., Konstantinidis, E. I., Romanopoulou, E. D., Karagianni, M., Kartsidis, P., and Bamidis, P. D. (2016). "Investigating the effectiveness of physical training through exergames: focus on balance and aerobic protocols," in *International Conference on, Technology and Innovation in Sports, Health and Wellbeing (TISHW)* (Vila Real: IEEE), 1–6.

Zokaei, N., MacKellar, C., Cepukaityte, G., Patai, E. Z., and Nobre, A. C. (2016). Cognitive training in the elderly: bottlenecks and new avenues. *J. Cogn. Neurosci.* 29, 1473–1482. doi: 10.1162/jocn_a_01080

14

Resting State Default Mode Network Connectivity, Dual Task Performance, Gait Speed and Postural Sway in Older Adults with Mild Cognitive Impairment

Rachel A. Crockett, Chun Liang Hsu, John R. Best and Teresa Liu-Ambrose*

Aging, Mobility, and Cognitive Neuroscience Laboratory, Department of Physical Therapy, Djavad Mowafaghian Centre for Brain Health, University of British Columbia, Vancouver, BC, Canada

***Correspondence:**
Teresa Liu-Ambrose
teresa.ambrose@ubc.ca

Aging is associated with an increased risk of falling. In particular, older adults with mild cognitive impairment (MCI) are more vulnerable to falling compared with their healthy counterparts. Major contributors to this increased falls risk include a decline in dual task performance, gait speed, and postural sway. Recent evidence highlights the potential influence of the default mode network (DMN), the frontoparietal network (FPN), and the supplementary motor area (SMA) on dual task performance, gait speed, and postural sway. The DMN is active during rest and deactivates during task-oriented processes, to maintain attention and stay on task. The FPN and SMA are involved in top-down attentional control, motor planning, and motor execution. The DMN shows less deactivation during task in older adults with MCI. This lack of deactivation is theorized to increase competition for resources between the DMN and task-related brain regions (e.g., the FPN and SMA), increasing distraction from the task and reducing task performance. However, no study has yet investigated the relationship between the between-network connectivity of the DMN with these regions and dual task walking, gait speed or postural sway. We hypothesized that greater functional connectivity both within the DMN and between DMN–FPN and DMN–SMA, will be associated with poorer performance during dual task walking, slower gait speed, and greater postural sway in older adults with MCI. Forty older adults with MCI were measured on a dual task-walking paradigm, gait speed over a 4-m walk, and postural sway using a sway-meter. Greater within-DMN connectivity was significantly correlated with poorer dual task performance. Furthermore, greater inter-network connectivity between the DMN and SMA was significantly correlated with slower gait speed and greater postural sway on the eyes open floor sway task. Thus, greater resting state DMN functional connectivity may be an underlying neural mechanism for reduced dual task ability, slower gait speed, and greater postural sway, resulting in the increased risk of mobility disability and falling in older adults with MCI.

Keywords: functional connectivity, default mode network, dual task, gait speed, postural sway, mild cognitive impairment

INTRODUCTION

Walking has long been considered an automated skill required for daily functioning and independent living. In reality, walking requires the complex neural coordination of visual, proprioceptive, and vestibular sensory incoming information (Beurskens and Bock, 2012). Furthermore, walking in everyday life is not performed as a single task since environmental demands require the ability to perform additional cognitive tasks at the same time (i.e., dual task), such as walking while talking (Yuan et al., 2015). Thus, walking depends on higher-order cognitive processes, known as executive functions (Yogev et al., 2008). Research consistently demonstrates that executive functions are important for successful dual task performance (Coppin et al., 2006).

The risk for developing impaired mobility (e.g., slow walking) increases with age (Verghese et al., 2009; Seidler et al., 2010). Falls are a significant consequence of impaired mobility (Fuller, 2000) with the majority of falls occurring during dual task conditions, such as walking while performing a secondary task (Tideiksaar, 1996). Thus, it is hypothesized that falls may not be a result of balance deficits in isolation, but the inability to effectively allocate attention to postural stability in dual task situations (Lajoie et al., 1996). This hypothesis is supported by observations such as older adults who stop walking while engaged in conversation (i.e., less able to dual task) are more likely to fall than those who continue walking (Lundin-Olsson et al., 1997). Recent evidence also highlights the importance of maintaining dual task ability in older adults beyond falls risk; Montero-Odasso et al. (2017) demonstrated that reduced dual task gait performance among older adults with mild cognitive impairment (MCI) was associated with progression to dementia.

MCI is considered the prodromal stage for dementia and is characterized by global brain atrophy and cognitive decline beyond normal aging but that does not impact daily living (Feldman and Jacova, 2005). Older adults with MCI are also found to have a greater decline in physical functioning (Aggarwal et al., 2006) and poorer performance under dual task conditions (Nascimbeni et al., 2015). Consequently, those with MCI are five times as likely to fall compared to cognitively intact older adults (Tinetti et al., 1988). Despite this, knowledge regarding the underlying neural correlates associated with dual task and gait performance in MCI is lacking. A better understanding of the neural basis for impaired dual task and mobility in this population can inform future strategies to prevent the progression of MCI and subsequently reduce the risk of mobility disability and falling.

Current evidence suggests that both the cognitive and motor impairments associated with MCI have a common neurobiological basis (Silbert et al., 2008; Callisaya et al., 2013). Of relevance, aging is characterized by disruptions in the functional connectivity of neural networks that support both cognitive and motor functions. Recent evidence highlights the potential involvement of the default mode network (DMN) and the frontoparietal network (FPN). The DMN is involved in autobiographical memory, memory consolidation, and self-referential thought (Andrews-Hanna et al., 2007; Buckner et al., 2008). It is active during rest and deactivates during task-oriented processes, to maintain attention and stay on task (Raichle et al., 2001). However, the DMN shows less deactivation on task for older adults and those with MCI (Lustig et al., 2003; Mevel et al., 2011). Although findings are inconsistent, it is thought this lack of deactivation may be due to greater resting state DMN functional connectivity (Mevel et al., 2011). It is suggested that as the posterior components of the network are among the first brain regions to be affected by both age and MCI-related atrophy (Buckner et al., 2005; Choo et al., 2010), compensation occurs as connections between the DMN and frontal regions increase (Davis et al., 2008), leading to a net increase in resting state functional connectivity and a lack of deactivation on task. This lack of deactivation while on task is theorized to increase distraction and reduce cognitive performance (Gardini et al., 2014). With age, walking becomes more dependent on executive functioning (Coppin et al., 2006). Therefore a decline in cognitive performance is subsequently hypothesized to also have a detrimental impact on walking in older adults and those with MCI.

The FPN is involved in top-down attentional control and allocation of available neural resources to important cognitive processes (Corbetta, 1998; Scolari et al., 2015), as well as in motor planning and motor execution (Ptak et al., 2017). It has also been associated with dual task walking performance. Compared to normal walking, performance on a walking while talking task was associated with greater functional connectivity between the prefrontal and supplementary motor areas (SMA) of the FPN and sensorimotor network, respectively (Yuan et al., 2015).

Much like the FPN, the SMA is a key structure for the execution and control of voluntary movement, motor planning (Roland et al., 1980; Eccles, 1982), and for maintaining attention on a motor task (Johansen-Berg and Matthews, 2000). Unlike some of the deeper brain structures, functional activation of the SMA can be assessed while walking using imaging techniques such as near infrared spectroscopy. Research using this technique, has found that an increase in activation of the SMA was associated with declines in gait performance under dual task conditions (Lu et al., 2015). Thus, the SMA may play an important role in the maintenance of gait performance during dual task walking.

Research focusing on the relationship between the DMN and the task-related networks responsible for motor functioning is lacking. However, one study did find that greater functional connectivity between the DMN and FPN was associated with reduced performance on a finger-tapping task in older fallers, indicative of an inability to focus attention on the task (Hsu et al., 2014). It is theorized that in older adults, this greater connectivity between the DMN and task-related networks at rest may suggest the DMN is remaining active on task, competing for resources with the task-related networks, and subsequently causing a decline in performance. This competition for resources is likely exacerbated under dual task conditions (Tombu and Jolicœur, 2003) and is hypothesized to underlie the relationship between cognitive and motor functioning decline, leading to an increased risk of falls and mobility disability in older adults and those with MCI. However, to our knowledge, no research has yet investigated the effect of the functional between-network connectivity of the DMN in relation to dual task walking paradigms.

In addition to reduced dual task performance, slower gait speed and increased postural sway are considered major factors contributing to an increased risk of falls. Older adults with MCI were found to have significantly slower gait speed (Eggermont et al., 2010) and greater postural sway (Liu-Ambrose et al., 2008) compared to healthy older adults. Both the SMA and components of the FPN have been associated with having a functional role in controlling gait speed (Harada et al., 2009; Yuan et al., 2015) and maintaining postural stability (Mihara et al., 2008). Therefore, maladaptive connectivity between these regions and the DMN may also negatively impact gait speed and postural stability, further contributing to an increased risk of falling. No research has yet investigated this potential relationship.

Consequently, the primary objective of this study was to investigate the relationship between the functional connectivity within the DMN and the between-network connectivity of the DMN with both the FPN and SMA (i.e., DMN–FPN and DMN–SMA) during a dual task walking paradigm in older adults with MCI. In addition, the secondary objective was to explore the association of within-network and between-network connectivity with gait speed and postural sway.

We hypothesized that greater functional connectivity within the DMN, between DMN–FPN, as well as between the DMN–SMA will be associated with poorer dual task walking performance, slower gait speed and greater postural sway. The rationale and hypotheses for this study are highlighted in **Figure 1**.

MATERIALS AND METHODS

Participants

Forty community dwelling older adults with MCI are included in this cross-sectional study. MCI was defined as: (1) a Montreal Cognitive Assessment (MoCA) score <26/30; (2) have subjective memory complaints (SMC); (3) no significant functional impairment, as determined by a score $\geq$6/8 on the Lawton and Brody Instrumental Activities of Daily Living Scale; and (4) no dementia.

Participants were recruited from metropolitan Vancouver and interested individuals were telephone screened to confirm general eligibility according to the inclusion and exclusion criteria. We included those who: (1) were aged $\geq$60 years; (2) scored $\leq$26/30 on the MoCA (Nasreddine et al., 2005); (3) had SMC, defined as the self-reported feeling of memory worsening with an onset within the last 5 years, as determined by interview (Gifford et al., 2014); (4) preserved general cognition as indicated by a Mini-Mental State Examination (Folstein et al., 1975) score $\geq$24/30; (5) score $\geq$6/8 on the Lawton and Brody (Lawton and Brody, 1969) Instrumental Activities of Daily Living Scale; (6) were right hand dominant as measured by the Edinburgh Handedness Inventory (Oldfield, 1971); (7) were living independently in their own homes; (8) had visual acuity of at least 20/40, with or without corrective lenses; and (9) provided informed consent. We excluded those who: (1) had a formal diagnosis

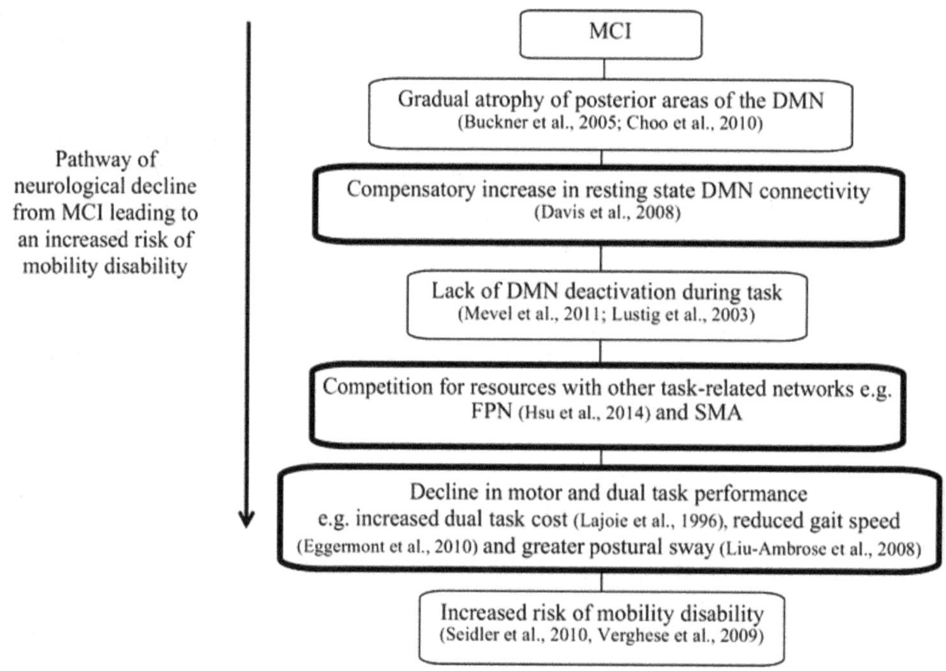

FIGURE 1 | The pathway of neurological decline leading to increased risk of mobility disability in patients with mild cognitive impairment (MCI). The boxes highlighted in black indicate the hypothesized components of this theory that this study aims to investigate.

of neurodegenerative disease, stroke, dementia (of any type), or psychiatric condition; (2) had clinically significant peripheral neuropathy or severe musculoskeletal or joint disease; (3) were taking psychotropic medication; (4) had a history indicative of carotid sinus sensitivity; (5) were living in a nursing home, extended care facility, or assisted-care facility; or (6) were ineligible for magnetic resonance imaging (MRI) scanning. All participants provided written consent and ethics approval was acquired from the Vancouver Coastal Research Health Institute and University of British Columbia's Clinical Research Ethics Board.

Descriptive Variables

Age was quantified in years and education level was assessed by self-report. Standing height was measured as stretch stature to the 0.1 cm per standard protocol. Weight was measured twice to the 0.1 kg on a calibrated digital scale. As previously stated, the MoCA was used as a classification tool for MCI. The MoCA is a 30-point test that covers multiple cognitive domains (Nasreddine et al., 2005). The MoCA has been found to have good internal consistency and test–retest reliability and was able to correctly identify 90% of a large sample of MCI individuals from two different clinics (Nasreddine et al., 2005).

Dual Task

Participants were also asked to perform a dual task involving a cognitive task while walking. Better performance on dual task measures is associated with better task switching, working memory, and divided attention (Schaefer and Schumacher, 2010). The cognitive task was the serial subtracting sevens task whereby the participant is required to start subtracting sevens aloud from a randomly given number. The walking task was performed on a GAITRite mat (McDonough et al., 2001), which was used to record the time between the first step onto the mat and the last step off of the mat for each task. Participants were instructed to begin walking 1 m before they reached the mat and finish once they made it to 1 m past the end of the mat to control for acceleration and deceleration effects. The participants were first asked to walk three times at a self-selected pace across the mat to give a mean walking time. They then performed the subtracting sevens task standing still (off of the mat) for 30 s. For the dual task component they were asked to walk at a self-selected pace and begin the serial subtraction once on the mat. This was repeated three times to get a mean dual task time. Dual task cost was then calculated by subtracting the mean walking only time from the dual task time, divided by the walking only time [(dual task − walking time)/walking time]. A lower dual task cost score indicated better dual task performance.

Usual Gait Speed

Participants walked at their usual pace along a 4-m path. To avoid acceleration and deceleration effects, participants started walking 1 m before reaching the 4-m path and completed their walk 1 m beyond it.

Usual gait speed (m/s) was calculated from the mean of two trials. The test–retest reliability of usual gait speed in our laboratory is 0.95 (ICC; Liu-Ambrose et al., 2006).

Postural Sway

Balance was assessed using the eyes open floor and foam sway component of the Physiological Profile Assessment© 18 (Prince of Wales Medical Research Institute, Randwick, Sydney, NSW, Australia; Lord et al., 2003). Participants were asked to stand with their feet hip width apart and look straight ahead for 30 s, first on the hard floor and secondly on a 3-inch high-density foam cushion. The task was stopped if the participant grabbed for support. A pen attached to a rod and connected to a band around the participants' waist was set to lie parallel to the ground and rest on a large paper grid (sway-meter). Sway was calculated as the largest distance covered across the grid.

Functional Magnetic Resonance Imaging Acquisition

The MRI scans were conducted at the University of British Columbia (UBC) Hospital in Vancouver at the UBC MRI research center. A 3.0-Tesla Intera Achieva MRI Scanner with an 8-channel SENSE neurovascular coil was used. During the scanning procedure, the participants were told to rest with their eyes open, remaining completely still and thinking of nothing in particular for the duration of the session.

The scanning session consisted of an initial resting-state scan with 360 dynamic images of 36 slices (3 mm thick) with a repetition time (TR) of 2000 ms, an echo time (TE) of 30 ms, a flip angle (FA) of 90°, a field of view (FoV) of 240 mm and an acquisition matrix of 80 × 80. High-resolution anatomical T1 images were also acquired with 170 slices (1 mm thick), TR of 7.7 ms, TE of 3.6 ms, FA of 8°, FoV of 256 mm, and an acquisition matrix of 256 × 200.

fMRI Pre-processing

FSL (FMRIB's Software Library), MATLAB (Matrix Laboratory), and toolboxes from Statistical Parametric Mapping (SPM) were used to carry out image processing. The Optimized Brain Extraction Tool (optiBET) (Lutkenhoff et al., 2014) was used to remove any excess unwanted structures in high resolution T1 images, e.g., skull, eyes, etc. The rigid body motion correction was done using MCFLIRT with the absolute and relative mean displacement extracted and included as covariates in the statistical analysis. The Multivariate Exploratory Linear Optimized Decomposition into Independent Components (MELODIC) further removed any additional artifacts. FSL Motion Outliers was used to determine any data points that were corrupted with a large amount of motion. A confound matrix was used to remove the effects of these time points on any subsequent analyses. The Gaussian kernel of full-width-half-maximum (FWHM) 6 mm was used for spatial smoothing and temporal filtering was applied to create a signal between $0.008 < f < 0.08$ Hz, which is the optimal range for analyzing resting-state functional connectivity data.

The functional MRI data was registered to the corresponding high resolution T1 anatomical image for each participant, which was then registered to standardized 152 T1 Montreal

Neurological Institute (MNI) space. Regression of the cerebral spinal fluid, white matter and global brain signal was used to remove noise from any physiological or non-physiological sources. Finally, to account for the delay of hemodynamic response, the first four volumes of data were discarded.

Functional Connectivity Analysis

The main focus of the functional connectivity analysis was to investigate the connectivity firstly within the DMN and secondly the inter-network connectivity between the DMN and the FPN and SMA independently. Previous studies guided the region of interest (ROI) selection for the analysis of the DMN, FPN, and SMA (Voss et al., 2010; Hsu et al., 2014). The ROIs within each network and their respective MNI space coordinates can be seen in **Table 1**. In order to analyze the overall interconnectivity between brain networks, the average of all the pairwise ROI–ROI correlations for each network was calculated. Preprocessed time-series data were extracted for each ROI with 14 mm diameter spherical ROIs drawn around their respective MNI coordinates in standard space. The time-series data for each ROI were then cross-correlated with every brain voxel to create functional connectivity maps of each neural network. Ordinary least-squares regression using FSL's flameo (Beckman et al., 2003) was used to calculate group-level between subject results. The statistical map thresholding was set at $Z = 2.33$, with a cluster correction of $p < 0.05$.

Data Analysis

Statistical analysis was conducted using the IBM SPSS Statistic 19 for Windows (SPSS Inc., Chicago, IL, United States). Descriptive data are reported for variables of interest. Alpha was set at $p \leq 0.05$ for all analyses.

Partial correlations, adjusted for age and MoCA, were performed to investigate the association between: (1) dual task performance and DMN functional connectivity; and (2) measures of gait speed and postural sway and DMN functional connectivity

Additional partial correlational analyses were also conducted to determine whether functional between-network connectivity between the DMN–FPN and DMN–SMA were correlated with dual task performance, gait speed, and postural sway.

RESULTS

Participants

A total of 40 participants were included in this study (see **Table 2**). However, five participants did not complete the dual task measure leaving 35 participants for analysis.

Based on visual inspection of the data there appeared to be a few outliers in the dual task cost results. Upon further analysis of all of the behavioral measures, two extreme outliers (mean ± 3 SD) were found in the dual task cost results. However, the removal of these outliers did not affect the results and as such, all data were included in the final analyses.

Partial Correlations: Dual Task Performance, Gait Speed, Postural Sway, and DMN Functional Connectivity

Partial correlation analyses showed a significant association between mean DMN functional connectivity and dual task cost ($r = 0.427$; $p = 0.013$), such that greater DMN connectivity was associated with poorer dual task performance. No other significant correlations were found ($p \geq 0.05$). The resting state connectivity map for the DMN can be seen in **Figure 2**.

TABLE 1 | Region of interests (ROIs) with MNI coordinates for each network.

Network	ROI	X	Y	Z
DMN	PCC	8	−56	30
	FMC	−2	54	−12
	BMTG	58	−10	−18
		−52	−14	−20
	BPHG	24	−26	−20
		−26	−24	−20
	LMFG	−30	20	50
	BLOC	54	−62	32
		−44	−72	30
FPN	RIPS	25	−62	53
	BVV	36	−62	0
		−44	−60	−6
	RSMG	32	−38	38
	BLSOC	26	−64	54
		−26	−60	52
	BFEF	28	−4	58
		−26	−8	54
SMN	SMA	−5	−1	52

DMN, default mode network; PCC, posterior cingulate cortex; FMC, frontal medial cortex; BMTG, bilateral middle temporal gyrus; BPHG, bilateral parahippocampal gyrus; LMFG, left middle frontal gyrus; BLOC, bilateral occipital cortex; FPN, frontoparietal network; RIPS, right inferior parietal sulcus; BVV, bilateral ventral visual; RSMG, right supramarginal gyrus; BLSOC, bilateral superior occipital cortex; BFEF, bilateral frontal eye field; SMN, sensorimotor network; SMA, supplementary motor area.

TABLE 2 | Participant characteristics.

Variables		Mean (SD) or *n*
N		40
Female		21
Age (years)		76.75 (5.8)
Weight (kg)		74.16 (14.4)
MMSE (max 30)		27.50 (1.3)
MoCA (max 30)		22.30 (2.7)
Dual task cost	Single task time (s)	4.96 (1.4)
	Dual task time (s)	6.40 (2.7)
	Dual task cost	0.20 (0.2)
Gait speed (m/s)		1.17 (0.2)
Eyes open postural sway	Floor sway (mm)	64.48 (25.6)
	Foam sway (mm)	182.12 (87.4)

MMSE, Mini-Mental Status Examination; MoCA, Montreal Cognitive Assessment.

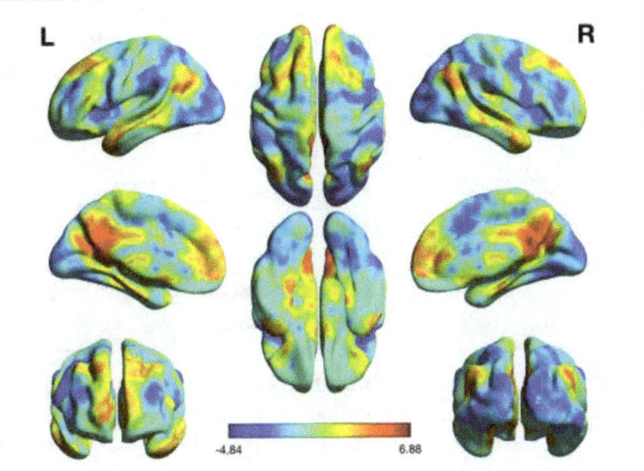

FIGURE 2 | Resting state functional connectivity of the default mode network.

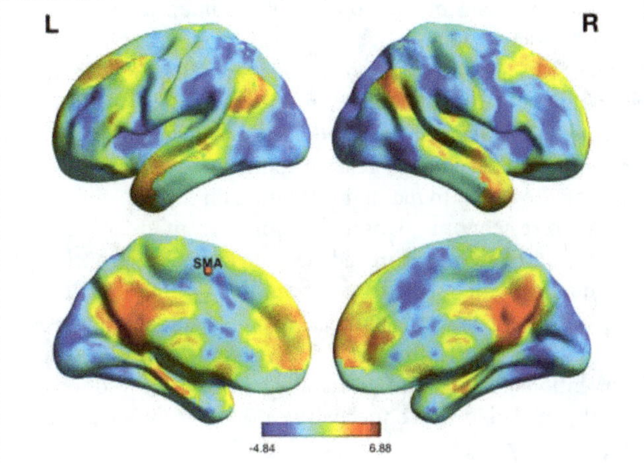

FIGURE 3 | Resting state functional connectivity between the default mode network and supplementary motor area.

Partial Correlations: Dual Task Performance, Gait Speed, Postural Sway, and Functional Between-network Connectivity between the DMN–FPN and DMN–SMA

Mean resting state between-network DMN–SMA functional connectivity was significantly correlated with gait speed ($r = -0.440$; $p = 0.01$) as well as postural sway under the eyes open floor condition ($r = 0.365$; $p = 0.037$). Thus, greater between-network DMN–SMA functional connectivity was associated with slower gait speed and greater postural sway under the eyes open floor condition. Results of the partial correlation analyses are reported in **Table 3**. The resting state between network connectivity map for the DMN and SMA can be seen in **Figure 3**.

DISCUSSION

We found that greater resting state DMN functional connectivity was significantly associated with greater dual task cost among community-dwelling older adults with MCI. It was previously discussed that greater DMN connectivity at rest is indicative of a lack of deactivation on task in older adults with MCI (Lustig et al., 2003; Mevel et al., 2011), which would subsequently result in a decrease in task performance. The association between greater DMN connectivity and reduced dual task performance found in this study is therefore likely evidence for a lack of deactivation of the DMN on task.

TABLE 3 | Partial correlation results.

	Dual task cost	Gait speed	EO floor sway	EO foam sway
DMN	0.427*	−0.125	0.075	−0.162
DMN–FPN	0.140	−0.108	−0.190	0.18
DMN–SMA	0.012	−0.440*	0.365*	0.36

*Adjusted for age and MoCA; *p < 0.05. EO, eyes open.*

One possible explanation for greater dual task cost being associated with greater DMN connectivity is provided by the capacity sharing theory. This theory states that because attentional resources are limited, when a person is required to perform two attention-demanding tasks simultaneously, the performance of at least one of these tasks will deteriorate (Tombu and Jolicœur, 2003). Therefore, if the greater DMN connectivity at rest were evidence of a lack of deactivation on task, this would suggest that the DMN is providing additional competition for resources, reducing those available for task-related functioning and subsequently reducing performance on the task. In addition to competing for resources generally, the DMN would be using these resources to fuel a functional process responsible for increasing distraction from the task, further amplifying its negative impact on task performance.

Walking in everyday life is not performed as a single task. Hence, the dual task walking measure has been associated with replicating the demands of the environment whilst walking (Tideiksaar, 1996). Findings from the current study indicate that patients with MCI are unable to meet the cognitive demands required to maintain walking performance in everyday life due to a lack of resources available and reduced ability to maintain attention on the task. It is plausible that an increase in distraction whilst attempting dual task walking may contribute to the increase in falls risk seen in older adults with MCI.

In addition, we also found that the functional connectivity between the DMN and SMA was significantly associated with slower gait speed and increased postural sway. Given that the DMN would normally deactivate on task (Raichle et al., 2001), intact resting state DMN–SMA connectivity would usually be an indication that during task performance, when the SMA is active, the DMN is deactivated. In this case, greater connectivity between these brain regions at rest is negatively correlated with gait speed and thus suggests there is interference between these networks on task; most plausibly that the DMN is influencing the SMA by remaining active on task.

The SMA has been shown to play an active role in motor planning (Roland et al., 1980), and in maintaining attention on a motor task (Johansen-Berg and Matthews, 2000). Through the DMN remaining active, increasing competition for resources and reducing the ability to maintain attention on the task, the SMA is unable to create motor plans with as much accuracy or efficiency. This would likely result in reduced quality of gait control and subsequently, gait speed. In addition, this decline in gait speed will further contribute to an increased risk of falls (Verghese et al., 2009; Espy et al., 2010). It would be useful to establish whether interventions targeted at increasing gait speed are also found to alter this maladaptive connectivity in order to provide support for this theory.

The SMA has also been implicated in postural control. Findings from Viallet et al. (1992) lead to the suggestion that the SMA was responsible for selecting the relevant circuits of phasic postural adjustments in order to maintain posture. Consequently, if an increase in DMN activity on task were to add competition for resources to the SMA, it is likely that there would be a decrease in the ability to select the correct postural adjustments to maintain balance, leading to the increased sway evident in this study.

It is important to note that greater connectivity between the DMN and SMA only correlated with performance on the floor sway task and not performance on the foam sway task. It is thought this is because the foam sway task may require more overt attention. Whereas, the participants may be less inclined to intentionally focus on the floor sway task because they are not so obviously unstable. This may be better explained by the capacity model of attention, which states that when a task is less cognitively demanding, more resources remain available to be allocated to task-irrelevant networks (Kahneman, 1973). In this case, the additional resources are allocated to the DMN. It may therefore be that when performing the foam sway task, participants were able to overcome the DMN interference by actively allocating more resources to the task-related regions than when performing the floor sway task. However, this can only be considered a speculative explanation as participants were not asked about how much attention they paid to the task and task-related neuronal activity could not be measured. This theory is also contradictory to the capacity sharing theory that has been used to explain the findings in relation to dual task performance, known to be a cognitively demanding task. Investigating the effect of the DMN–SMA connectivity over progressively more challenging postural tasks would be beneficial to determine which theory is most likely to explain these results.

There was no relationship found between connectivity of the DMN and FPN at rest and any of the behavioral measures. Due to the lack of previous literature in this area it is not completely clear why this may be. One of the studies that did find increased connectivity between the DMN and FPN during the performing of a motor task, found the increase in connectivity was specific to older adults classified as fallers rather than non-fallers (Hsu et al., 2014). Consequently, it may be that the FPN is more resistant to the influence of the DMN until a later stage in mobility decline. Further research is required to investigate the effect of the DMN on the FPN across several stages of falls risk, ideally comparing healthy older adults to those with MCI and those classified as fallers in order to establish at what stage connectivity between the DMN and FPN may become detrimental, if at all.

This study only compared resting state brain network connectivity with behavioral measures and did not investigate brain activity on task. Due to the limitations of functional MRI (fMRI) scanning (i.e., sensitivity to movement artifacts), and the lack of MRI-safe apparatus it was not possible for us to assess activity of the DMN and associated networks while performing motor tasks such as walking. Thus, caution must be taken when interpreting these results, as they are only correlational. To support our findings, future studies should aim to investigate the functional connectivity both within and between these networks whilst simultaneously performing a motor task. It is also important to acknowledge that there may be other underlying factors that could account for these results. For example, this study did not investigate the impact of potential sex differences or the underlying structural integrity of these networks, which may have provided an alternative explanation of the findings. Consequently, future studies should aim to identify any sex differences and compare both the structural and functional associations between these networks and mobility factors in order to better understand the underlying neurobiological factors contributing to increased falls risk. In addition, our study consisted of community-dwelling older adults with MCI exclusively and we did not have ethical clearance to collect any data pertaining to the race or ethnicity of our participants, as this was not related to our hypotheses. Thus, we acknowledge that this may make the generalizability of our findings ambiguous. Furthermore, some evidence highlights the potential influence of the cerebellum on the networks discussed in this study (Habas et al., 2009). Although this was not one of the main focuses of the current study, it may be beneficial to additionally investigate the role of the cerebellum in relation to these networks in future research. Due to the exploratory nature of this study and the small sample size, no adjustments were made to the significance value in order to control for multiple comparisons. It is acknowledged that this increases the likelihood of a type I error and future studies with larger sample sizes are needed to confirm our current findings. Finally, walking was performed indoors on a GAITRite mat and a verbal subtraction task was used for the dual task, consistent with other studies using a dual task walking paradigm (Beurskens and Bock, 2012). However, it would be useful to determine the specific effects of other cognitive and motor tasks whilst walking over varying terrains as well, as this is likely to be more representative of real-world scenarios.

Our results show that increased resting state DMN connectivity is associated with a decrease in dual task performance, slower gait speed and increased postural sway in older adults with MCI; either via greater within network connectivity or between-network connectivity with the SMA. This supports the theory proposed initially in **Figure 1**. To our knowledge, this is the first study to investigate the role of the DMN on dual task performance and motor functioning in people with MCI. These findings can be used to determine if interventions targeted to improve gait, cognition, and/or dual tasking specifically, can reduce the maladaptive effects of greater DMN connectivity in older adults vulnerable to an increased risk of mobility disability.

AUTHOR CONTRIBUTIONS

RC, TL-A, and CLH were involved in designing and performing the study. All authors contributed to the data analysis. RC, TL-A, and CLH were involved in the interpretation of results. RC wrote the first draft of the manuscript. TL-A, JB, and CLH wrote portions of the manuscript and critically reviewed the manuscript. All authors have read and approved the manuscript.

FUNDING

Funding was provided by an Alzheimer Society Research Program Grant No. F13-05246 to TL-A.

REFERENCES

Aggarwal, N. T., Wilson, R. S., Beck, T. L., Bienias, J. L., and Bennett, D. A. (2006). Motor dysfunction in mild cognitive impairment and the risk of incident Alzheimer disease. *Arch. Neurol.* 63, 1763–1769. doi: 10.1001/archneur.63.12.1763

Andrews-Hanna, J. R., Snyder, A. Z., Vincent, J. L., Lustig, C., Head, D., Raichle, M. E., et al. (2007). Disruption of large-scale brain systems in advanced aging. *Neuron* 56, 924–935. doi: 10.1016/j.neuron.2007.10.038

Beckman, C. F., Jenkinson, M., and Smith, S. M. (2003). General multilevel linear modeling for group analysis in FMRI. *Neuroimage* 20, 1052–1063. doi: 10.1016/S1053-8119(03)00435-X

Beurskens, R., and Bock, O. (2012). Age-related deficits of dual-task walking: a review. *Neural Plast.* 2012:131608. doi: 10.1155/2012/131608

Buckner, R. L., Andrews-Hanna, J. R., and Schacter, D. L. (2008). The brain's default network: anatomy, function, and relevance to disease. *Ann. N. Y. Acad. Sci.* 1124, 1–38. doi: 10.1196/annals.1440.011

Buckner, R. L., Snyder, A. Z., Shannon, B. J., LaRossa, G., Sachs, R., Fotenos, A. F., et al. (2005). Molecular, structural, and functional characterization of Alzheimer's disease: evidence for a relationship between default activity, amyloid, and memory. *J. Neurosci.* 25, 7709–7717. doi: 10.1523/JNEUROSCI.2177-05.2005

Callisaya, M. L., Beare, R., Phan, T. G., Blizzard, L., Thrift, A. G., Chen, J., et al. (2013). Brain structural change and gait decline: a longitudinal population-based study. *J. Am. Geriatr. Soc.* 61, 1074–1079. doi: 10.1111/jgs.12331

Choo, I. L., Lee, D. Y., Oh, J. S., Lee, J. S., Lee, D. S., Song, I. C., et al. (2010). Posterior cingulate cortex atrophy and regional cingulum disruption in mild cognitive impairment and Alzheimer's disease. *Neurobiol. Aging* 31, 772–779. doi: 10.1016/j.neurobiolaging.2008.06.015

Coppin, A. K., Shumway-Cook, A., Saczynski, J. S., Patel, K. V., Ble, A., Ferrucci, L., et al. (2006). Association of executive function and performance of dual-task physical tests among older adults: analyses from the InChianti study. *Age Ageing* 35, 619–624. doi: 10.1093/ageing/afl107

Corbetta, M. (1998). Frontoparietal cortical networks for directing attention and the eye to visual locations: identical, independent, or overlapping neural systems? *Proc. Natl. Acad. Sci. U.S.A.* 95, 831–838. doi: 10.1073/pnas.95.3.831

Davis, S. W., Dennis, N. A., Daselarr, S. M., Fleck, M. S., and Cabeza, R. (2008). Que PASA? The posterior-anterior shift in aging. *Cereb. Cortex* 18, 1201–1209. doi: 10.1093/cercor/bhm155

Eccles, J. C. (1982). The initiation of voluntary movements by the supplementary motor area. *Arch. Psychiatr. Nervenkr.* 231, 423–441. doi: 10.1007/BF00342722

Eggermont, L. H., Gavett, B. E., Volkers, K. M., Blankevoort, C. G., Scherder, E. J., Jefferson, A. L., et al. (2010). Lower-extremity function in cognitively healthy aging, mild cognitive impairment, and Alzheimer's disease. *Arch. Phys. Med. Rehabil.* 91, 584–588. doi: 10.1016/j.apmr.2009.11.020

Espy, D. D., Yang, F., Bhatt, T., and Pai, Y. C. (2010). Independent influence of gait speed and step length on stability and fall risk. *Gait Posture* 32, 378–382. doi: 10.1016/j.gaitpost.2010.06.013

Feldman, H. H., and Jacova, C. (2005). Mild cognitive impairment. *Am. J. Geriatr. Psychiatry* 13, 645–655. doi: 10.1176/appi.ajgp.13.8.645

Folstein, M. F., Folstein, S. E., and McHugh, P. R. (1975). "Mini-mental state". A practical method for grading the cognitive state of patients for the clinician. *J. Psychiatr. Res.* 12, 189–198. doi: 10.1016/0022-3956(75)90026-6

Fuller, G. F. (2000). Falls in the elderly. *Am. Fam. Physician* 61, 2159–2168.

Gardini, S., Venneri, A., Sambataro, F., Cuetos, F., Fasano, F., Marchi, M., et al. (2014). Default mode network in mild cognitive impairment: a maladaptive compensatory mechanism associated with poor semantic memory performance. *J. Alzheimers Dis.* 45, 457–470. doi: 10.3233/JAD-142547

Gifford, K. A., Liu, D., Lu, Z., Tripodis, Y., Cantwell, N. G., Palmisano, J., et al. (2014). The source of cognitive complaints predicts diagnostic conversion differentially among nondemented older adults. *Alzheimers Dement.* 10, 319–327. doi: 10.1016/j.jalz.2013.02.007

Habas, C., Kamdar, N., Nguyen, D., Keller, K., Beckmann, C. F., Menon, V., et al. (2009). Distinct cerebellar contributions to intrinsic connectivity networks. *J. Neurosci.* 29, 8586–8594. doi: 10.1523/JNEUROSCI.1868-09.2009

Harada, T., Miyai, I., Suzuki, M., and Kubota, K. (2009). Gait capacity affects cortical activation patterns related to speed control in the elderly. *Exp. Brain Res.* 3, 445–454. doi: 10.1007/s00221-008-1643-y

Hsu, C. L., Voss, M. W., Handy, T. C., Davis, J. C., Nagamatsu, L. S., Chan, C., et al. (2014). Disruptions in brain networks of older fallers are associated with subsequent cognitive decline: a 12-month prospective exploratory study. *PLOS ONE* 9:e93673. doi: 10.1371/journal.pone.0093673

Johansen-Berg, H., and Matthews, P. M. (2000). Attention to movement modulates activity in sensori-motor areas, including primary motor cortex. *Exp. Brain Res.* 142, 13–24. doi: 10.1007/s00221-001-0905-8

Kahneman, D. (1973). *Attention and Effort.* Englewood Cliffs, NJ: Prentice Hall Inc.

Lajoie, Y., Teasdale, N., Bard, C., and Fleury, M. (1996). Upright standing and gait: Are there changes in attentional requirements related to normal aging? *Exp. Aging Res.* 22, 185–198. doi: 10.1080/03610739608254006

Lawton, M. P., and Brody, E. M. (1969). Assessment of older people: self-maintaining and instrumental activities of daily living. *Gerontologist* 9, 179–186. doi: 10.1093/geront/9.3_Part_1.179

Liu-Ambrose, T., Khan, K. M., Donaldson, M. G., Eng, J. J., Lord, S. R., and McKay, H. A. (2006). Falls-related self-efficacy is independently associated with balance and mobility in older women with low bone mass. *J. Gerontol. A Biol. Sci. Med. Sci.* 61, 832–838. doi: 10.1093/gerona/61.8.832

Liu-Ambrose, T. Y., Ashe, M. C., Graf, P., Beattie, B. L., and Khan, K. M. (2008). Increased risk of falling in older community-dwelling women with mild cognitive impairment. *Phys. Ther.* 88, 1482–1491. doi: 10.2522/ptj.20080117

Lord, S. R., Menz, B. H., and Tiedemann, A. (2003). A physiological profile approach to falls risk assessment and prevention. *Phys. Ther.* 83, 237–252.

Lu, C. F., Liu, Y. C., Yang, Y. R., Wu, Y. T., and Wang, R. Y. (2015). Maintaining gait performance by cortical activation during dual-task interference: a functional near-infrared spectroscopy study. *PLOS ONE* 10:e0129390. doi: 10.1371/journal.pone.0129390

Lundin-Olsson, L., Nyberg, L., and Gustafson, Y. (1997). "Stops walking when talking" as a predictor of falls in elderly people. *Lancet* 349:617. doi: 10.1016/S0140-6736(97)24009-2

Lustig, C., Snyder, A. Z., Bhakta, M., O'Brien, K. C., McAvoy, M., Raichle, M. E., et al. (2003). Functional deactivations: change with age and dementia of the

Alzheimer type. *Proc. Natl. Acad. Sci. U.S.A.* 100, 14504–14509. doi: 10.1073/pnas.2235925100

Lutkenhoff, E. S., Rosenberg, M., Chiang, J., Zhang, K., Pickard, J. D., Owen, A. M., et al. (2014). Optimized brain extraction for pathological brains (optiBET). *PLOS ONE* 9:e115551. doi: 10.1371/journal.pone.0115551

McDonough, A. L., Batavia, M., Chen, F. C., Kwon, S., and Ziai, J. (2001). The validity and reliability of the GAITRite system's measurements: a preliminary evaluation. *Arch. Phys. Med. Rehabil.* 82, 419–425. doi: 10.1053/apmr.2001.19778

Mevel, K., Chételat, G., Eustache, F., and Desgranges, B. (2011). The default mode network in healthy aging and Alzheimer's disease. *Int. J. Alzheimers Dis.* 2011:535816. doi: 10.4061/2011/535816

Mihara, M., Miyai, I., Hatakenaka, M., Kubota, K., and Sakoda, S. (2008). Role of the prefrontal cortex in human balance control. *Neuroimage* 43, 329–336. doi: 10.1016/j.neuroimage.2008.07.029

Montero-Odasso, M. M., Sarquis-Adamson, Y., Speechley, M., Borrie, M. J., Hachinski, V. C., Wells, J., et al. (2017). Association of dual-task gait with incident dementia in mild cognitive impairment: results from the gait and brain study. *JAMA Neurol.* 74, 857–865. doi: 10.1001/jamaneurol.2017.0643

Nascimbeni, A., Caruso, S., Salatino, A., Carenza, M., Rigano, M., Raviolo, A., et al. (2015). Dual task-related gait changes in patients with mild cognitive impairment. *Funct. Neurol.* 30, 59–65.

Nasreddine, Z. S., Phillips, N. A., Bedirian, V., Charbonneau, S., Whitehead, V., Collin, I., et al. (2005). The Montreal Cognitive Assessment, MoCA: a brief screening tool for mild cognitive impairment. *J. Am. Geriatr. Soc.* 53, 695–699. doi: 10.1111/j.1532-5415.2005.53221.x

Oldfield, R. C. (1971). The assessment and analysis of handedness: the Edinburgh inventory. *Neuropsychologia* 9, 97–113. doi: 10.1016/0028-3932(71)90067-4

Ptak, R., Schnider, A., and Fellrath, J. (2017). The dorsal frontoparietal network: a core system for emulated action. *Trends Cogn. Sci.* 21, 589–599. doi: 10.1016/j.tics.2017.05.002

Raichle, M. E., MacLeod, A. M., Snyder, A. Z., Powers, W. J., Gusnard, D. A., and Shulman, G. L. (2001). A default mode of brain function. *Proc. Natl. Acad. Sci. U.S.A.* 98, 676–682. doi: 10.1073/pnas.98.2.676

Roland, P. E., Larsen, B., Lassen, N. A., and Skinhoj, E. (1980). Supplementary motor area and other cortical areas in organization of voluntary movements in man. *J. Neurophysiol.* 43, 118–136.

Schaefer, S., and Schumacher, V. (2010). The interplay between cognitive and motor functioning in healthy older adults: findings from dual-task studies and suggestions for intervention. *Gerontology* 57, 239–246. doi: 10.1159/000322197

Scolari, M., Seidl-Rathkopf, K., and Kastner, S. (2015). Functions of the human frontoparietal attention network: evidence from neuroimaging. *Curr. Opin. Behav. Sci.* 1, 32–39. doi: 10.1016/j.cobeha.2014.08.003

Seidler, R. D., Bernard, J. A., Burutolu, T. B., Fling, B. W., Gordon, M. T., Gwin, J. T., et al. (2010). Motor control and aging: links to age-related brain structural, functional, and biochemical effects. *Neurosci. Biobehav. Rev.* 34, 721–733. doi: 10.1016/j.neubiorev.2009.10.005

Silbert, L. C., Nelson, C., Howieson, D. B., Moore, M. M., and Kaye, J. A. (2008). Impact of white matter hyperintensity volume progression on rate of cognitive and motor decline. *Neurology* 71, 108–113. doi: 10.1212/01.wnl.0000316799.86917.37

Tideiksaar, R. (1996). Preventing falls: how to identify risk factors, reduce complications. *Geriatrics* 51, 49–50.

Tinetti, M. E., Speechley, M., and Ginter, S. F. (1988). Risk factors for falls among elderly persons living in the community. *N. Engl. J. Med.* 319, 1701–1707. doi: 10.1056/NEJM198812293192604

Tombu, M., and Jolicœur, P. (2003). A central capacity sharing model of dual-task performance. *J. Exp. Psychol. Hum. Percept. Perform.* 29, 3–18. doi: 10.1037/0096-1523.29.1.3

Verghese, J., Holtzer, R., Lipton, R. B., and Wang, C. (2009). Quantitative gait markers and incident fall risk in older adults. *J. Gerontol. A Biol. Sci. Med. Sci.* 64A, 896–901. doi: 10.1093/Gerona/glp033

Viallet, F., Massion, J., Massarino, R., and Khalil, R. (1992). Coordination between posture and movement in a bimanual load lifting task: putative role of a medial frontal region including the supplementary motor area. *Exp. Brain Res.* 88, 674–684. doi: 10.1007/BF00228197

Voss, M. W., Prakash, R. S., Erickson, K. I., Basak, C., Chaddock, L., Kim, J. S., et al. (2010). Plasticity of brain networks in a randomized intervention trial of exercise training in older adults. *Front. Aging Neurosci.* 2:32. doi: 10.3389/fnagi.2010.00032

Yogev, G., Hausdorff, J. M., and Giladi, N. (2008). The role of executive function and attention in gait. *Mov. Disord.* 23, 329–472. doi: 10.1002/mds.21720

Yuan, J., Blumen, H. M., Verghese, J., and Holtzer, R. (2015). Functional connectivity associated with gait velocity during walking and walking-while-talking in aging: a resting-state fMRI study. *Hum. Brain Mapp.* 36, 1484–1493. doi: 10.1002/hbm.22717

15

Open- and Closed-Skill Exercise Interventions Produce Different Neurocognitive Effects on Executive Functions in the Elderly: A 6-Month Randomized, Controlled Trial

Chia-Liang Tsai[1]**, *Chien-Yu Pan*[2], *Fu-Chen Chen*[2] *and Yu-Ting Tseng*[1,3]

[1] *Institute of Physical Education, Health and Leisure Studies, National Cheng Kung University, Tainan, Taiwan,* [2] *Department of Physical Education, National Kaohsiung Normal University, Kaohsiung, Taiwan,* [3] *School of Kinesiology, University of Minnesota, Minneapolis, MN, United States*

Correspondence:
Chia-Liang Tsai
andytsai@mail.ncku.edu.tw

This study aimed to explore the effects of open- and closed-skill exercise interventions on the neurocognitive performance of executive functions in the elderly. Sixty-four healthy elderly males were randomly assigned to either a closed-skill (bike riding or brisk walking/jogging, $n = 22$), open-skill (table tennis, $n = 21$), or control ($n = 21$) group. Various neuropsychological [e.g., accuracy rates (AR) and reaction time (RT)] and electrophysiological [e.g., event-related potential (ERP) P3 component] measures were assessed during a variant of the task-switching paradigm, as well as an N-back task at baseline and after either a 6-month exercise intervention or control period. The results showed that, when performing the task-switching paradigm, the two exercise groups relative to control group showed significantly faster RTs in the switch trials after the exercise intervention. However, the RT facilitation in the non-switch and switch trials post-exercise relative to pre-exercise only emerged in the open-skill group. In terms of the N-back task, the two exercise groups significantly increased ARs in the 1-back condition after the exercise intervention, and the beneficial AR effect on the 2-back condition only emerged in the closed-skill group. In addition, the two exercise groups exhibited significantly larger P3 amplitudes on the frontal-to-parietal cortex areas after the exercise intervention relative to the baseline when performing the two cognitive tasks. These neurocognitive results still remained unchanged even when the confounding factors (e.g., cardiorespiratory fitness, social participation, and BMI) were controlled for. The present study concluded that, although 6-month open- and closed-skill exercise interventions facilitate overall electrophysiological effects (i.e., increased ERP P3 amplitudes) on the frontal-to-parietal cortices in the elderly, the two exercise modes produced different levels of neuropsychologically beneficial effects on RTs of the task-switching paradigm (i.e., lessened RTs) and ARs of the N-back task (i.e., enhanced ARs). The distinctive neurocognitive changes induced by open- and closed-skill exercise have implications for task switching and working memory in elderly individuals, especially with such cognitive functioning impairments.

Keywords: cognition, behavior, event-related potential, exercise modes, elderly

INTRODUCTION

Life expectancy has been increasing in developed countries, resulting in a rapid growth in the elderly population. Since aging is the main risk factor for neurodegenerative diseases (e.g., Alzheimer's disease), which affect a substantial and growing part of the global population (Rodríguez-Arellano et al., 2016), one important issue is how to counteract such neurocognitive declines in order to reduce the medical costs associated with geriatric care. Although a decrease in certain cognitive functions is an unavoidable part of normal aging, the degree to which this occurs varies within the healthy older population. Among an array of cognitive functions, the executive-control processes and brain areas that support them have been shown to undergo large age-related performance declines (West, 1996; Colcombe and Kramer, 2003; Anderson and McConnell, 2007), as seen in capacities such as working memory (Wingfield et al., 1988), visuospatial attention (Greenwood et al., 1993), and task switching (Friedman et al., 2008).

The vast majority of related studies have proposed that physical fitness and exercise are factors that strongly promote healthy cognitive aging (Lee et al., 2012; Kimura et al., 2013; Tsai et al., 2015). Improvements in physical fitness via exercise training are thus reflected in enhancements of a number of cognitive functions, such as processing speed, visuospatial function, and control processes (e.g., inhibition, planning, scheduling, and working memory) in older adults, with the largest effect sizes being on tests thought to depend more on the executive function (e.g., task switching, inhibitory control, and working memory; Diamond, 2013) (Hall et al., 2001; Voelcker-Rehage et al., 2010; Guiney and Machado, 2013; Tsai et al., 2015). However, a broad range of physical exercise types is possible, and different kinds of exercise seem to have specific effects on neurocognitive performance, due to the differences in the secretion of some biomarkers (e.g., brain-derived neurotrophic factor, insulin-like growth factor-1, and homocysteine) in the neurochemical system (Neeper et al., 1995; Liu-Ambrose et al., 2010; Cassilhas et al., 2012; Tsai et al., 2014b,c), and the differences in brain tissue volumes and activation patterns induced by different types of exercise (Luft et al., 2008; Park et al., 2008; Liu-Ambrose et al., 2010; Erickson et al., 2011; Tsai and Wang, 2015; Tsai et al., 2016). These earlier works seem to support the view that different types of physical exercise could affect the brain in different ways.

Different forms of physical exercise with different cognitive executive process loads and different motor-coordination skills have been reported to be strongly associated with improved neurocognitive performances (Voelcker-Rehage et al., 2011; Tsai et al., 2016). Therefore, the present study divided exercise into two main modes, open- and closed-skill (Di Russo et al., 2010; Dai et al., 2013; Tsai and Wang, 2015), since the former (e.g., table tennis and badminton) requires rich cognitive and executive loadings and different sets of motor-coordination skills to adapt to a unpredictable/changing environment and various opponents (van Praag et al., 2000; Artola et al., 2006; Di Russo et al., 2010), while the later (e.g., running and biking) is performed according to the individual's own pace in a stable and predictable environment (Di Russo et al., 2010). From the perspective of motor-coordination skill, Voelcker-Rehage et al. (2011) found that older adults experienced beneficial effects on executive control (assessed using the Flanker task) and perceptual speed (assessed using the Visual Search task) due to cardiorespiratory and coordination training. However, the two exercise modes produced different effects on speed and accuracy, with coordination training leading to improved accuracy rates (ARs) on executive control and perceptual speed, but cardiorespiratory training only leading to better ARs on executive control. In terms of reaction time (RT), only the perceptual speed task was significantly improved by coordination training. In addition, cardiorespiratory training increased activation of the sensorimotor network in the elderly, while coordination training elevated activation of the visual–spatial network (Voelcker-Rehage et al., 2011). In contrast, Hötting et al. (2012) found that, although significant increases in episodic memory learning scores were found for both the cycling and stretching/coordination groups as compared with the sedentary control group, cycling training had greater effects on the episodic memory recognition scores than the stretching/coordination training. They also found that the latter was particularly effective in improving selective attention as compared with the cycling training. This suggests a specific relation between particular types of exercise and cognitive functions, with the increase in memory functions being linked to an increase in cardiovascular fitness, whereas the increase in attention is more pronounced after stretching/coordination training. The two exercise modes (i.e., open- and closed-skills) thus seem to be capable of producing different effects on the various cognitive domains (Voss et al., 2010) and neural processes (Tsai and Wang, 2015; Tsai et al., 2016).

Although recent studies have explored the effects of open- and closed-skill exercise on neuropsychological performance in disabled athletes (Di Russo et al., 2010) and the young adults (Wang et al., 2013a,b), and neurocognitive (neuropsychological and electrophysiological) performances in the elderly (Dai et al., 2013; Tsai and Wang, 2015; Tsai et al., 2016), the findings in the rather limited research literature remain somewhat ambiguous. More importantly, even though previous cross-sectional studies have demonstrated that regular participation in open- and closed-skill exercise has distinct benefits for neurocognitive performances (e.g., specific cost, RT, P3 amplitudes, and strength of inhibitory control) in the elderly when performing the task switching paradigm (Dai et al., 2013; Tsai and Wang, 2015) and visuospatial attention task (Tsai et al., 2016), the elderly subjects who showed more of the benefits of open-skill exercise on neurocognitive performance might have had some inherently better aspects of their executive control functions (e.g., visuospatial attention and task switching) as compared to their counterparts participating in the closed-skill exercise mode, and this may have induced them to adopt this kind of exercise (Snowden et al., 2011). Therefore, these cross-sectional studies cannot establish causality between exercise and cognitive aging, which is nonetheless required for more accurate and effective public health recommendations (Snowden et al., 2011; Miller et al., 2012), as well as to better explain the beneficial effects of the two exercise modes.

Two cognitive tasks, the task-switch paradigm and N-back task, were adopted in the current study to investigate the impacts of the various exercise-mode mechanisms responsible for specific kinds of executive-control functioning, since earlier works found that open- and closed-skill exercise could have different neurocognitive effects on different cognitive tasks executive functions (Di Russo et al., 2010; Dai et al., 2013; Tsai and Wang, 2015; Tsai et al., 2016), and, crucially, open-skill exercise (e.g., table tennis) affects more of the prefrontal cortex areas responsible for attention, task-switching and inhibition, while closed-skill exercise (e.g., jogging) works more on the hippocampus, which is important for memory (e.g., long-term memory and working memory; Axmacher et al., 2010; Burrel, 2015). Moreover, there are previous reports of age- and physical-activity-related impacts on the neuropsychological (e.g., AR and RT) and electrophysiological [e.g., event-related potential (ERP) P3 component] outcomes of the task-switching paradigm (Hillman et al., 2006; Friedman et al., 2008; Adrover-Roig and Barceló, 2010; Guiney and Machado, 2013) and N-back task (Voelcker-Rehage et al., 2010; Guiney and Machado, 2013; Saliasi et al., 2013) among elderly subjects.

ERP recordings made during the cognitive task performance permitted on-line measures of cognitive processes on the order of milliseconds, which cannot be obtained by neuropsychological performance alone (Tsai et al., 2014b). Given that the P3 activity has nonspecific qualities that are often associated with indexing stimulus evaluations and the intensity of the concomitant executive function processes (e.g., task-set updating processes and reconfiguration, updating working memory, integrating information into existing networks) (Kok, 2001; Kieffaber and Hetrick, 2005; Nicholson et al., 2005; Polich, 2007), the ERP component was used to illustrate the effects of the different exercise-mode interventions on executive cognitive functions in the elderly in the present study. With regard to the electrophysiological index, the P3 activity induced by the task-switch paradigm represents the set of processes subsumed under the construct of the task-set reconfiguration (Kieffaber and Hetrick, 2005; Nicholson et al., 2005). ERP P3 represents the memory-related neural processing that is involved in categorizing incoming information and updating the context of the working memory (e.g., encoding, rehearsal, recognition, and retrieval) (Duncan-Johnson and Donchin, 1977; Donchin and Coles, 1988; Rugg, 1995).

To date there is a lack of intervention research on the impact of open- and closed-skill exercise modes on various forms of executive function (e.g., task switching and working memory) involved in cognitive aging in older adults. The main goal of this study was thus to clarify the distinctive effects of a 6-month open- and closed-skill exercise intervention on the neuropsychological (e.g., AR and RT) and electrophysiological (e.g., ERP P3 latency and amplitude) performances in older adults with a sedentary life-style when performing the task-switching paradigm and N-back task, with rigorous controls on the confounding factors in neurocognitive performance [e.g., cardiorespiratory fitness, social participation, and body mass index (BMI), since these parameters could be changed to different extents after exercise] (Messier and Gagnon, 2009; Miller et al., 2012). The elderly subjects with regular open-skill exercise participation in the literature general show better switch-related neurocognitive performances than those with only closed-skill experience (Dai et al., 2013; Tsai and Wang, 2015), and short-term closed-skill exercise intervention (e.g., resistance exercise) cannot improve task-switching performance (Kimura et al., 2010), while closed-skill exercise training with the goal of enhancing cardiorespiratory fitness can facilitate white matter integrity, increase the size of the hippocampus, and improve memory performance in the elderly (Erickson et al., 2011; Ruscheweyh et al., 2011; Voss et al., 2013; Maass et al., 2016) and have more benefits on memory functions than stretching/coordination training (Hötting et al., 2012). As such, we hypothesized the following: (1) that a 6-month open-skill exercise intervention (e.g., table tennis) in contrast to a closed-exercise one (e.g., bike riding or brisk walking/jogging) would have more benefits for neurocognitive performance with regard to task-switching in the elderly; and (2) that closed-skill exercise would have more beneficial effects on the cognitive functioning involving the memory domains.

MATERIALS AND METHODS

Participants

Sixty-four community-dwelling men were recruited with the use of an informative flyer and underwent screening by a standardized telephone interview, with subjects being eligible for inclusion in this study if they (1) were aged 60–80 years old and a non-smoker; (2) were living independently in their own home with a sedentary life-style; and (3) did not have a current medical condition for which exercise is contraindicated. The participants consisted solely of men because neurocognitive and endocrinological responses to exercise could be gender-dependent (Baker et al., 2010). They then underwent a routine laboratory testing and medical examination, including blood pressure and heart rate measurements, electrocardiography, a standardized neurological and psychiatric examination, and a structured interview on previous medical history to ascertain whether they were free of a history of neurological disorders, brain injury, depressive symptoms [scores above 13 on the Beck Depression Inventory, 2nd edition (BDI-II)], and cognitive impairment [scores below 26 on the Mini Mental State Examination (MMSE)] (Ruscheweyh et al., 2011). The Edinburgh Handedness Inventory assessed all participants as right-handed (Oldfield, 1971). Written informed consent, as approved by the Institutional Ethics Committees in the organization within which the study was performed, was obtained from all the participants.

Procedures

The Consolidated Standards of Reporting Trials (CONSORT) flowchart outlining the number of participants from first contact to study completion is shown in **Figure 1**. The original cohort consisted of 79 participants. After the assessment of a physician specializing in geriatric care, two subjects were excluded due to a history of heart disease, five due to neurological disorders, musculoskeletal problems, or psychiatric illness (e.g., scores

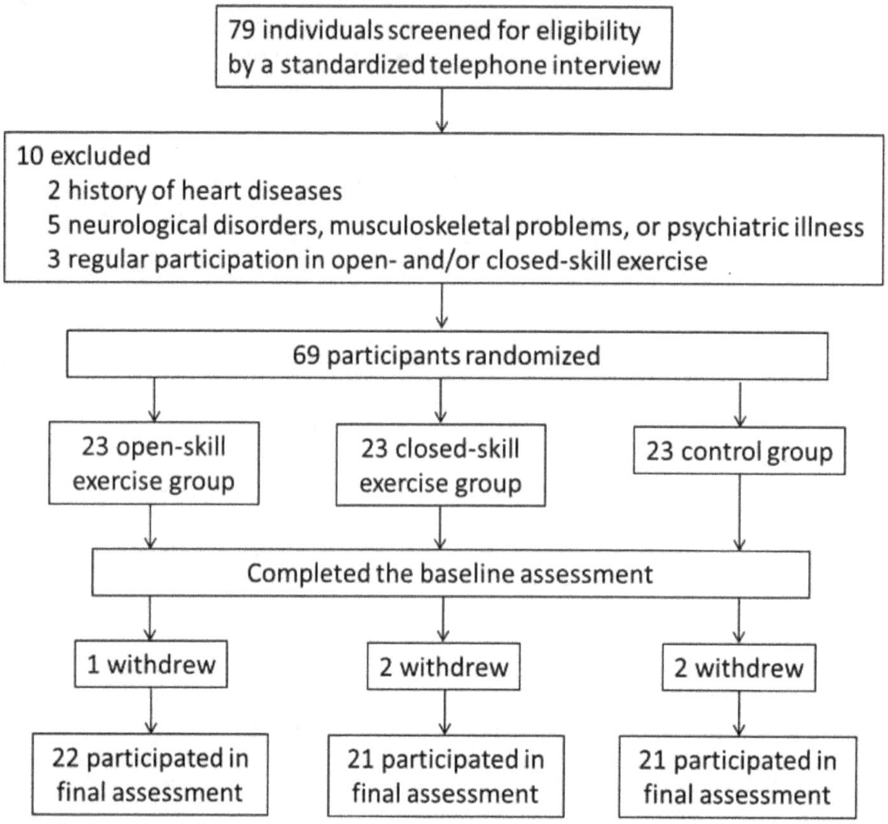

FIGURE 1 | The CONSORT (Consolidated Standards of Reporting Trials) flowchart.

above 13 on the BDI-II or below 26 on the MMSE), and three due to regular participation in open- and/or closed-skill exercise in the previous 3 months. The remaining 69 participants were randomly assigned to either an open-skill, closed-skill, or active control group by drawing an envelope with the treatment assignment enclosed after matching for age.

Before the exercise intervention, the participants visited the cognitive neurophysiology laboratory on two separate occasions. During the first session, each participant completed an informed consent form, the basic information form (e.g., a medical history and demographic questionnaire), and a handedness inventory. Two certified fitness instructors then completed all assessments of senior functional physical fitness for each participant. On a separate day within 1 week of the completion of the baseline evaluation, the participants performed two cognitive tasks (i.e., a task-switching paradigm and an N-back task) in a counter balanced order with concomitant electrophysiological recording (i.e., event-related potentials, ERPs).

Before the final exercise interventions were completed, one participant in the open-skill group, two in the closed-skill group, and two in the active control group, terminated their participation, leaving 64 participants in the final sample (open-skill, $n = 22$; closed-skill, $n = 21$; active control, $n = 21$). The three groups did not significantly differ at baseline in any of the demographic characteristics, including years of formal education, body mass index, systolic and diastolic pressure, social participation, MMSE, BDI-II, and senior functional physical fitness (see **Table 1**). Within 1 week after completing a 24-week exercise intervention, the participants completed the same questionnaires and senior functional physical fitness assessment, and received the same neurocognitive measurements, as in the pre-exercise procedure. Compliance with the prescribed training protocol remained high throughout the study period (90 ± 2%).

Training Protocol

Open-Skill Exercise Condition

The participants in the open-skill group were trained individually and regularly in a series of 40-min sessions that took place three times per week for 24 weeks, with the following structure: a warm-up, the main part of table tennis training, playing games of table tennis with the coach, and cooling down at the end. The training intervention was carried out in a sequence of increasing complexity. The table tennis training program was intended to improve the participants' general skills, and had seven main components over the whole training session: (a) footwork (e.g., ready position, one-, two-, and cross-step), (b) serving (including how to give sidespin, backspin, topspin, no-spin, and so on), (c) forehand and backhand driving, (d) forehand bouncing, backhand bouncing, and alternate bouncing, (e) smashing, (f) continuously hitting back a ball that was randomly delivered by

TABLE 1 | Demographic characteristics of the open-skill exercise, closed-skill and control groups before and after the exercise intervention.

	Open-skill ($n = 22$)			Closed-skill ($n = 21$)			Control ($n = 21$)		
	Pre-exercise	**Post-exercise**	***p***	**Pre-exercise**	**Post-exercise**	***p***	**Pre-exercise**	**Post-exercise**	***p***
Age (years)	66.88 ± 4.74		–	66.15 ± 4.90		–	65.70 ± 3.54		–
Education (years)	12.50 ± 4.09		–	12.62 ± 2.97		–	10.62 ± 3.20		–
Height (cm)	162.90 ± 6.71	162.88 ± 6.74	0.329	159.70 ± 7.24	159.57 ± 7.12	0.186	161.20 ± 7.94	160.68 ± 8.54	0.329
Weight (kg)	62.65 ± 9.11	62.71 ± 8.99	0.329	60.98 ± 9.11	58.86 ± 9.55	0.005	62.04 ± 10.57	61.95 ± 10.47	0.329
BMI (kg/m^2)	23.65 ± 3.64	23.68 ± 3.61	0.329	23.79 ± 3.65	23.04 ± 2.99	0.007	23.83 ± 3.29	23.94 ± 3.20	0.458
Systolic pressure (mmHg)	128.68 ± 22.95	125.82 ± 18.02	0.076	129.29 ± 21.79	124.57 ± 20.99	0.125	132.05 ± 25.12	129.33 ± 24.59	0.313
Diastolic pressure (mmHg)	75.86 ± 11.62	74.14 ± 9.13	0.296	78.62 ± 11.65	74.76 ± 10.76	0.151	79.48 ± 10.58	77.67 ± 12.07	0.347
Social participation	10.23 ± 2.07	10.73 ± 1.91	0.031*	9.57 ± 2.40	9.90 ± 2.28	0.090	9.95 ± 2.04	9.62 ± 1.99	0.090
Memory depth	18.50 ± 5.57	19.45 ± 5.41	0.404	17.10 ± 7.15	20.14 ± 4.60	0.059	18.24 ± 3.89	18.67 ± 4.46	0.410
MMSE	28.73 ± 1.28	28.05 ± 2.73	0.252	27.48 ± 3.03	28.95 ± 1.40	0.082	27.67 ± 1.80	28.19 ± 1.43	0.299
BDI-II	3.68 ± 3.72	3.09 ± 3.05	0.221	5.04 ± 4.14	4.71 ± 8.16	0.877	3.38 ± 3.38	2.47 ± 3.03	0.092
FITNESS									
Grip (kg)	28.90 ± 6.75	29.13 ± 6.74	0.834	26.98 ± 10.03	24.65 ± 9.50	0.368	27.81 ± 7.62	26.84 ± 6.82	0.338
Arm Curl (number)	18.09 ± 4.60	21.82 ± 3.40	<0.001*	17.24 ± 3.22	17.29 ± 2.57	0.942	17.47 ± 4.32	16.95 ± 3.69	0.451
Chair Stand (sec)	15.18 ± 3.80	19.41 ± 5.90	0.001*	18.08 ± 6.35	17.95 ± 4.04	0.932	15.80 ± 4.98	16.10 ± 2.96	0.757
8-Foot Up-and-Go (sec)	6.03 ± 1.38	5.53 ± 1.03	0.012*	6.97 ± 3.73	5.54 ± 1.04	0.086	6.32 ± 1.09	6.35 ± 1.05	0.859
Back Scratch (cm)	−3.23 ± 11.98	−2.11 ± 9.66	0.315	−1.43 ± 11.14	−1.55 ± 9.37	0.924	−0.64 ± 7.31	0.43 ± 9.58	0.383
Chair Sit-and-Reach (cm)	19.85 ± 5.27	20.40 ± 3.06	0.532	17.09 ± 2.02	17.04 ± 2.16	0.782	18.58 ± 2.38	19.33 ± 2.84	0.181
VO_{2max} (mL/kg/min)	25.63 ± 9.66	30.32 ± 12.03	0.071	26.83 ± 5.44	31.01 ± 4.25	0.001*	24.11 ± 6.61	23.79 ± 6.71	0.735

*BMI, body mass index; MMSE, Mini Mental State Examination; BDI-II, Beck Depression Inventory, 2nd edition; VO_{2max}, maximal oxygen uptake. *$p < 0.05$.*

the ball-projection machine from fixed or random directions, and (g) comprehensive practice. Training for each skill began with a simple movement and then progressed to more complex variations. The assessor for the neurocognitive tests and the exercise leader/coach were blinded to group membership. A more detailed training manual is available on request from the authors.

Closed-Skill Exercise Condition

Participants in the closed-skill group attended three supervised exercise sessions per week for 24 consecutive weeks on a bicycle ergometer or a motor-driven treadmill (Medtrack ST55, Quinton Instrument Company, United States), with exercise intensity corresponding to 50–60% of the individual target heart rate reserve (HRR) during the first 2 weeks and 70–75% of the HRR for the remainder of the program. Each aerobic exercise session involved a 5-min warm-up period, followed by 30 min of continuous bike riding or brisk walking/jogging at an intensity that would maintain the heart rate within the assigned training range, and 5 min of cool-down. A Polar HR monitor (RX800CX, Finland) was used to monitor each participant's heart rate during the exercise.

Control Condition

Participants in the active control group attended a balance and stretching program led by a trained exercise leader three times a week for 24 weeks. Every class included a 5-min warm-up period, static stretching and balance training, and a 5-min cool-down period. Different stretching and balancing techniques used various equipment, such as balance boards and fitness balls, to maintain the participants' interest.

Physical Fitness Assessment

The Senior Functional Physical Fitness (SFPF) test (Rikli and Jones, 2012) is a battery of tests that was used to assess the participants' physical fitness in the current study. The participants first undertook 10 min' warm-up before the test and then completed the component tests in the designated order. Five items in the SFPF test were measured, as follows: (1) the Arm Curl test, which assesses arm muscle (specifically of the biceps) strength endurance, with the score being the number of repetitions in 30 s using the elbow of the dominant hand to flex and extend with a weight (men: 8 lb; women: 5 lb) through the complete range of motion; (2) the Chair Stand test, which measures lower body strength, based on the number of repetitions in 30 s using a full standing position from a chair and then returning to a fully seated position; (3) the 8-Foot Up-and-Go test, which evaluates agility and dynamic balance, using the number of seconds needed to get up from a seated position from a chair, walk eight feet, and return to a fully seated position on the chair; (4) the Back Scratch test, which assess upper body (shoulder) flexibility based on the number of centimeters being short of touching (minus score) or overlapping (plus score) between the third fingertip of each hand; (5) the Chair Sit-and-Reach test, which assesses the flexibility of the lower extremities, with the score being the distance in centimeters between the fingertips and toes; the number of centimeters short of reaching the toes (minus score) or reached beyond the toes (plus score).

With regard to cardiorespiratory fitness, the Rockport Fitness Walking Test was used to estimate VO_{2max} (Kline et al., 1987), in which the participants were required to walk one mile as quickly as possible, during which their heart rate was continuously recorded using a Polar HR monitor.

Cognitive Tasks

Task-Switching Paradigm

The task switching paradigm employed in the present study has been shown to effectively assess the variations among elderly subjects who regularly participate in open- and closed-skill types of exercise (Tsai and Wang, 2015). The stimulus used in this test was a white digit (1–9, excluding 5) shown focally in the center of the screen against a black background. The same digit was not repeated in successive trials, and the digits were put into eight task blocks (blocks 1–2 and 7–8: homogeneous tasks; blocks 3–6: heterogeneous tasks), with a short rest period in the middle of each. The homogenous (i.e., non-switch) blocks each included 56 trials. Within each homogenous block, the participants only responded if the focal digit was greater or less than 5 (e.g., blocks 1 and 7), or if it was odd or even (e.g., blocks 2 and 8). The heterogeneous (i.e., task-switching) blocks contained 224 trials, each with 20 switches. With the heterogeneous blocks, the participants started with one task (e.g., even/odd) and then switched to the other (e.g., more/less than 5), as signaled by a simultaneously presented rectangle drawn around the digit, after at least seven or no more than 13 intervening trials. The participants were asked to press one of two buttons on a small response box that they held in the right hand as quickly and accurately as possible. The digit was shown on the screen until the participants pressed the response button, and the following trial began 500ms after the RT response. The prompts "more less" or "even odd" appeared simultaneously with and below the digit during all trials, dependent on which was appropriate to the task. The homogenous and heterogeneous blocks were counterbalanced across participants. All the participants were given instructions about the tasks, and both single-task and task-switch trials were practiced before the formal test until they understood the whole procedure.

N-back Task

A continuous stream of white letters (stimuli) with pseudo-random sequences of vowels and consonants was presented with 10% gray noise, embedded in a 50% random noise gray rectangular background patch, on a computer screen. Targets were defined according to the N-back design. Participants pressed a button with the index finger of their right hands as soon as a target appeared, and no motor response was needed for non-target trials. Stimuli were presented for a duration of 500 ms, followed by a 3 s inter-trial-interval during which a dot helped participants maintain fixation. The cognitive task consisted of three different working-memory-load conditions: (1) a simple detection (control) condition with sequential letters or background patches without any letters being presented, during which the participants responded when the background patches without letters appeared (memory-free condition); (2) the 1-back condition, with the target being any letter identical to the one immediately preceding it (moderately demanding); (3) the 2-back condition, with the target being any letter that was identical to the one presented two trials back (highly demanding). Before the formal test, the participants were given the task instructions and initially practiced a brief version of the task, consisting of two blocks of 45 trials each (one block of moderately demanding and one of highly demanding trials). Following this practice, the participants completed nine blocks of trials with 120 trials in each (three blocks per condition). Nine blocks were tested following the sequence: blocks 1, and 8–9: the control condition, blocks 2, and 6–7: the 1-back condition, and blocks 3–5: the 2-back condition. No feedback was provided during this period.

ERPs Recording and Analysis

Continuous electroencephalographic (EEG) signals were acquired from 18 electrodes (F7, F3, Fz, F4, F8, C3, Cz, C4, T5, T3, T4, T6, P3, Pz, P4, O1, Oz, and O2) placed using a 10/20 extended Quik-Cap system (Compumedics Neuroscan, Inc., El Paso, TX). Horizontal and vertical electrooculogram (EOG) activity for eye movements was monitored bipolarly with ocular electrodes placed on the supero-lateral right canthus and infero-lateral to the left eye. A ground electrode was placed on the mid-forehead on the Quik-Cap. References were placed at vertex by default, but were subsequently re-referenced off-line to averaged mastoids. The values of interelectrode impedance were kept at 5 KΩ for all electrodes. The raw EEG signal was recorded with an A/D rate of 500 Hz/channel, a band-pass filter of 0.1–50 Hz, and a 60-Hz notch filter using an on-line amplifier. These data were written continuously to hard disk for off-line analysis using Neuroscan Scan 4.3 analysis software (Compumedics Neuroscan, Inc., El Paso, USA).

Trials with a response error or EEG artifacts (e.g., VEOG, HEOG, and electromyogram) exceeding peak-to-peak deflections over 100 μV were discarded before averaging. ERPs were extracted off-line and averaged in epochs starting 200 ms prior to stimulus activity onset, and lasting for 1,000 ms of post-stimulus activity. Since the ERP P3 component is widely examined among studies that independently and simultaneously investigate the externalizing spectrum and executive functioning (Baskin-Sommers et al., 2014), it was the focus of the current work. The effects of the two cognitive tasks on the P3 component in the elderly were clearly visible in the frontal-parietal regions of the scalp in the current study (see also Kieffaber and Hetrick, 2005; Friedman et al., 2008; Baskin-Sommers et al., 2014). Three electrodes (Fz, Cz, Pz) were thus analyzed in the present work (Themanson et al., 2006; Tusch et al., 2016). P3 mean amplitudes were calculated for the time-window between 300 and 600 ms post stimulus.

Data Processing and Statistical Analyses

One-way analysis of variance (ANOVA) was used to examine the homogeneity of the demographic backgrounds of the participants at the baseline in the open-skill, closed-skill, and control groups. A two-tailed paired t-test was used to analyze the differences within the three groups at baseline and at 24 weeks.

Different trials/conditions in the two cognitive tasks were subjected to neuropsychological (i.e., AR and RT) and electrophysiological (i.e., P3 amplitude) statistical analyses. Only the RT and ERP data corresponding to correct answers were averaged according to the task trial/condition. With regard to the task-switching paradigm, two switch costs were determined by the RTs performance: (1) general-switch cost, which was obtained by subtracting the mean RT between homogeneous trials during homogeneous blocks and non-switch trials during heterogeneous blocks; (2) specific-switch cost, which was calculated by subtracting the mean RT between non-switch trials and switch trials during heterogeneous blocks.

Task Switching Paradigm

With regard to the neuropsychological performance, the AR and RT were separately submitted to a 3 (*Group*: open-skill vs. closed-skill vs. control) × 2 (*Time*: pre-exercise vs. post-exercise) × 3 [*Trial*: homogeneous (during homogeneous blocks) vs. non-switch vs. switch (during heterogeneous blocks)] mixed repeated measures analysis of variance (RM–ANOVA). In terms of the electrophysiological performance, the P3 latency and amplitude from ERP recordings were submitted to a 3 (*Group*: open-skill vs. closed-skill vs. control) × 2 (*Time*: pre-exercise vs. post-exercise) × 3 (*Trial*: homogeneous vs. non-switch vs. switch) × 3 (*Electrode*: Fz vs. Cz vs. Pz) RM–ANOVA.

N-back Task

With regard to the neuropsychological performance, the AR and RT were separately submitted to a 3 (*Group*: open-skill vs. closed-skill vs. control) × 2 (*Time*: pre-exercise vs. post-exercise) × 3 (*Condition*: 0-back vs. 1-back vs. 2-back) RM–ANOVA. In terms of the electrophysiological performance, the P3 latency and amplitude from ERP recordings were submitted to a 3 (*Group*: open-skill vs. closed-skill vs. control) × 2 (*Time*: pre-exercise vs. post-exercise) × 3 (*Condition*: 0-back vs. 1-back vs. 2-back) × 3 (*Electrode*: Fz vs. Cz vs. Pz) RM–ANOVA.

Bonferroni *post-hoc* analyses were performed when there was a significant difference. Simple main effects were determined following observation of any significant interaction effects. Because cardiorespiratory fitness, social participation, and BMI are confounding factors on cognitive performance (Messier and Gagnon, 2009; Miller et al., 2012), the neuropsychological and electrophysiological performances of the three groups after the exercise intervention were assessed separately using an analysis of covariance (ANCOVA) to examine the effects on the neurocognitive performance in relation to different types of intervention, with the three post-exercise factors as a covariate. The Greenhouse–Geisser (G–G) correction adjusted the significance levels of the F ratios whenever RM–ANOVA detected a major violation of the sphericity assumption. Partial Eta squared (η_p^2) was used to calculate effect sizes for significant main effects and interactions, with the following criteria used to determine the magnitude of mean effect size: 0.01–0.059 indicated a small effect size; 0.06–0.139, a medium effect size; and >0.14, a large effect size. A p-value less than 0.05 for the differences between the mean values is considered statistically significant.

RESULTS

Demographic Characteristics

Table 1 presents an overview of the pre- and post-exercise characteristics of the participants. At baseline there were no significant differences (all $ps > 0.05$) at the group level with regard to age, height, weight, BMI, systolic and diastolic pressure in the three groups (i.e., open-skill, closed-skill, and control). Other confounding factors (e.g., the years of education, social participation, memory depth, global cognitive function, depression, and cardiorespiratory fitness) in relation to cognition and the tests of functional fitness also did not achieve significant difference in the three groups (all $ps > 0.05$) across the three groups at baseline. Paired t-tests showed that after the exercise intervention the open-skill group had significantly improved scores for the social participation, arm curl, chair stand, and 8-foot up-and-go items, and approached significance for the level of cardiorespiratory fitness (VO_{2max}); and the results for the closed-skill group showed that the values of weight and BMI decreased significantly, the level of cardiorespiratory fitness was significantly enhanced, and the performance of memory depth approached significance.

Accuracy Rate (AR)

Task-Switching Paradigm

As shown in **Figure 2**, RM–ANOVA performed on the ARs only highlighted the main effects of *Time* [$F_{(1, 61)} = 10.36$, $p = 0.002$, $\eta_p^2 = 0.15$] and *Trial* [$F_{(2, 122)} = 35.57$, $p < 0.001$, $\eta_p^2 = 0.37$], with a higher AR post- (90.96%) than pre-exercise (88.53%) and with the following trial gradient across the three groups: homogeneous (93.52%) > non-switch (88.96%) > switch (86.75%).

N-back Task

RM–ANOVA performed on the ARs for the N-back task revealed the main effects of *Time* [$F_{(1, 61)} = 20.45$, $p < 0.001$, $\eta_p^2 = 0.25$] and *Condition* [$F_{(2, 122)} = 129.89$, $p < 0.001$, $\eta_p^2 = 0.68$], with a higher AR for post- (90.61%) than pre-exercise (88.43%), and with the following condition gradient: 0-back (98.01%) > 1-back (90.17%) > 2-back (80.37%). The interactions between *Time* × *Group* [$F_{(2, 61)} = 4.74$, $p = 0.012$, $\eta_p^2 = 0.14$], *Time* × *Condition* [$F_{(2, 122)} = 10.51$, $p < 0.001$, $\eta_p^2 = 0.15$], and *Time* × *Group* × *Condition* [$F_{(4, 122)} = 2.61$, $p = 0.012$, $\eta_p^2 = 0.39$] were also significant. *Post-hoc* analysis for the *Time* × *Group* × *Condition* interaction showed that (1) there were no significant differences at any condition among the three groups at baseline and after the exercise intervention (all $ps > 0.05$); and (2) when post- compared to pre-exercise, the open- [$F_{(1, 21)} = 4.44$, $p = 0.047$] and closed-skill [$F_{(1, 20)} = 21.45$, $p < 0.001$] groups exhibited significantly higher ARs in the 1-back condition, and only the closed-skill [$F_{(1, 20)} = 36.59$, $p < 0.001$] group exhibited a significantly higher AR in the 2-back condition. In addition, the significant post- and pre-exercise differences in ARs among the three groups only emerged in the 2-back condition, with a greater improvement after the exercise intervention for the closed-skill group than the open-skill and control groups (closed-skill vs. open-skill: $p = 0.002$; closed-skill vs. control: $p =$

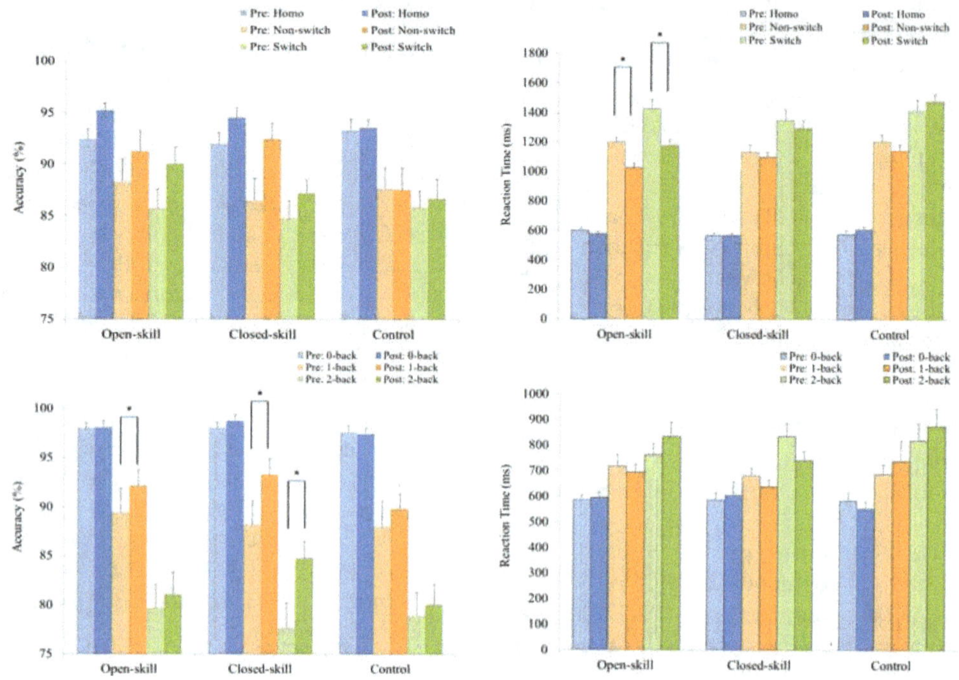

FIGURE 2 | Grand mean accuracy rate (the left side) and reaction time (the right side) performance (mean ± SE) of the open-skill, closed-skill, and control groups during the task-switching (**upper**) and N-back (**lower**) tasks before and after the exercise intervention. *Significantly different ($p < 0.05$).

0.001). Even when the post-exercise cardiorespiratory fitness, social participation, and BMI were controlled for, the results of ANCOVA on the ARs in the 2-back condition still indicated a significant difference in the three groups [$F_{(2, 58)} = 9.90$, $p < 0.001$], with *post-hoc* analysis indicating that closed-skill group performed significantly better than the open-skill (closed-skill vs. open-skill: $p < 0.001$) and control (closed-skill vs. control: $p < 0.001$) groups after the exercise intervention.

Reaction Time (RT)

Task-Switching Paradigm

As illustrated in **Figure 2**, RM–ANOVA conducted on mean RTs revealed the main effects of *Time* [$F_{(1, 61)} = 10.22$, $p = 0.002$, $\eta_p^2 = 0.14$] and *Trial* [$F_{(2, 122)} = 490.16$, $p < 0.001$, $\eta_p^2 = 0.89$], suggesting that RTs were faster post- (999.2 ms) rather than pre-exercise (1,056.1 ms), and that RTs followed the trial gradient: homogeneous (587.4 ms) < non-switch (1,136.6 ms) < switch (1,358.9 ms). The interactions of *Time* × *Group* [$F_{(2, 61)} = 7.34$, $p = 0.001$, $\eta_p^2 = 0.19$], *Time* × *Condition* [$F_{(2, 122)} = 5.55$, $p = 0.005$, $\eta_p^2 = 0.08$], and *Time* × *Condition* × *Group* [$F_{(4, 122)} = 3.69$, $p = 0.007$, $\eta_p^2 = 0.11$] were also significant. *Post-hoc* analysis for the *Time* × *Condition* × *Group* interaction showed that (1) the open- and closed-skill groups showed significantly faster responses than the control group in the switch trials after the exercise intervention [$F_{(2, 61)} = 10.31$, $p < 0.001$; open-skill vs. control: $p < 0.001$; closed-skill vs. control: $p = 0.027$], and (2) when post- compared to pre-exercise, the open-skill group responded faster in the non-switch [$F_{(1, 21)} = 24.80$, $p < 0.001$] and switch [$F_{(1, 21)} = 27.15$, $p < 0.001$] trials. Even when the post-exercise cardiorespiratory fitness, social participation, and BMI were controlled for, the results of ANCOVA on the RTs in switch trials still indicated a significant difference in the three groups [$F_{(2, 58)} = 7.70$, $p = 0.001$], with *post-hoc* analysis indicating that the two exercise groups showed significantly faster responses than the control group (open-skill vs. control: $p < 0.001$; closed-skill vs. control: $p = 0.027$) after the exercise intervention.

In terms of RT switch costs, RM-ANOVA for the general-switch cost revealed the main effect of *Time* [$F_{(1, 61)} = 15.01$, $p < 0.001$, $\eta_p^2 = 0.20$], indicating that the general-switch cost was smaller post- (501.9 ms) rather than pre-exercise (596.5 ms) across the three groups. RM-ANOVA for the specific-switch cost revealed that the interaction of *Time* × *Group* [$F_{(2, 61)} = 3.35$, $p = 0.042$, $\eta_p^2 = 0.10$] was significant. *Post-hoc* analysis showed that only the value of the specific-switch cost approached significance [$F_{(1, 21)} = 4.33$, $p = 0.050$] post-exercise (149.2 ± 163.0 ms) relative to pre-exercise (227.5 ± 208.1 ms) in the open-skill group.

N-back Task

RM–ANOVA conducted on mean RTs for the N-back task only revealed a main effect of *Condition* [$F_{(2, 92)} = 210.94$, $p < 0.001$, $\eta_p^2 = 0.82$], with the following gradient: 0-back (586.8 ms) < 1-back (693.5 ms) < 2-back (812.4 ms).

P3 Latency

Task-Switching Paradigm

As shown in **Figures 3, 5**, no significant difference was observed with regard to any main effect or interaction in the P3 latency. These results indicate that the P3 latencies did not show obvious changes between three groups when performing the

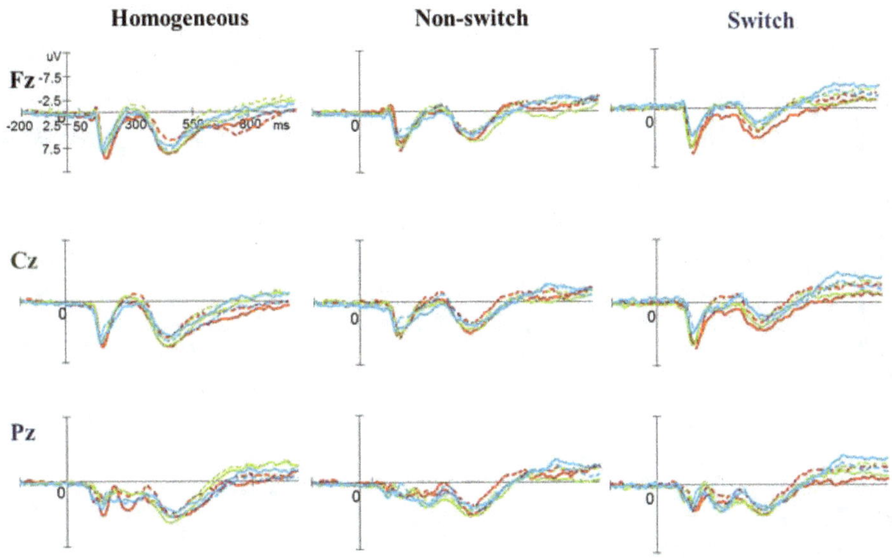

FIGURE 3 | Grand average event-related potential waveforms of three electrodes (Fz, Cz, and Pz) for three conditions (homogeneous, non-switch, and switch) for the P3 component in the task-switching paradigm at baseline (dashed line) and after exercise intervention (solid line) in the open-skill (red), closed-skill (green), and control groups (blue).

task-switching paradigm throughout the exercise intervention stage.

N-back Task

No significant difference was observed with regard to any main effect or interaction in the P3 latency. These results indicate that the P3 latencies did not show obvious changes when performing the N-back task between three groups throughout the exercise intervention stage.

P3 Amplitude

Task-Switching Paradigm

As shown in **Figures 3**, **5**, RM–ANOVA performed on the P3 amplitudes of the task-switching paradigm showed main effects of *Time* [$F_{(1, 61)} = 30.30$, $p < 0.001$, $\eta_p{}^2 = 0.33$], *Condition* [$F_{(2, 122)} = 39.35$, $p < 0.001$, $\eta_p^2 = 0.39$] and *Electrode* [$F_{(2, 122)} = 15.99$, $p < 0.001$, $\eta_p^2 = 0.21$], with the *post-hoc* analyses indicating that the P3 amplitudes were larger post- (4.89 μV) rather than pre-exercise (3.82 μV); the P3 amplitudes in the three conditions had the following gradient: homogeneous (5.85 μV) > non-switching (3.99 μV) > switching (3.22 μV); and significantly greater amplitudes at the Fz (4.73 μV) and Cz (4.57 μV) electrodes were found as compared to the Pz (3.77 μV) electrode. The interactions of *Time* × *Group* [$F_{(2, 61)} = 11.47$, $p < 0.001$, $\eta_p{}^2 = 0.27$] and *Condition* × *Electrode* [$F_{(4, 244)} = 13.96$, $p < 0.001$, $\eta_p{}^2 = 0.19$] were also significant. *Post-hoc* analysis for the *Time* × *Group* interaction showed that (1) there were no significant differences among the three groups at baseline [$F_{(2, 61)} = 0.04$; $p = 0.961$]; (2) there were significant differences among the three groups after the exercise intervention [$F_{(2, 61)} = 6.37$; $p = 0.003$], with *post-hoc* analysis showing that both open- (5.79 μV) and closed-skill (5.38 μV) groups showed significantly larger P3 amplitudes as compared to the control group (3.50 μV) after the intervention (open-skill vs. control: $p = 0.004$; closed-skill vs. control: $p = 0.025$); and (3) both the open- and closed-skill groups exhibited significantly larger P3 amplitudes [open-skill: $F_{(1, 21)} = 32.99$, $p < 0.001$; closed-skill: $F_{(1, 20)} = 23.34$, $p < 0.001$] across all three conditions and electrodes after the intervention relative to baseline. Even when the post-exercise cardiorespiratory fitness, social participation, and BMI were controlled for, the results of ANCOVA on the averaged P3 amplitudes in the three conditions and three electrodes still indicated significant post-exercise group differences [$F_{(2, 58)} = 8.07$, $p = 0.001$], with *post-hoc* analysis indicating that the two exercise groups showed significantly larger P3 amplitudes than the control group (open-skill vs. control: $p < 0.001$; closed-skill vs. control: $p = 0.003$) after the intervention.

N-back Task

As illustrated in **Figures 4**, **6**, RM–ANOVA performed on the P3 amplitudes of the N-back task showed the main effects of *Time* [$F_{(1, 61)} = 13.42$, $p = 0.001$, $\eta_p{}^2 = 0.18$] and *Condition* [$F_{(2, 122)} = 9.85$, $p < 0.001$, $\eta_p{}^2 = 0.14$], with the *post-hoc* analyses indicating the P3 amplitudes were larger post- (3.57 μV) rather than pre-exercise (2.27 μV); and significantly greater amplitudes at the 0-back (3.31 μV) and 1-back (3.27 μV) conditions were found as compared to the 2-back (2.19 μV) condition. The interaction of *Time* × *Group* [$F_{(2, 61)} = 3.89$, $p = 0.026$, $\eta_p{}^2 = 0.11$] was also significant, with *post-hoc* analysis indicating that (1) there were no significant differences among the three groups at baseline [$F_{(2, 61)} = 0.02$; $p = 0.985$]; (2) there were significant differences among the three groups after the exercise intervention [$F_{(2, 61)} = 6.09$; $p = 0.004$], with *post-hoc* analysis showing that both open- (4.02 μV) and closed-skill (4.52 μV) groups showed significantly

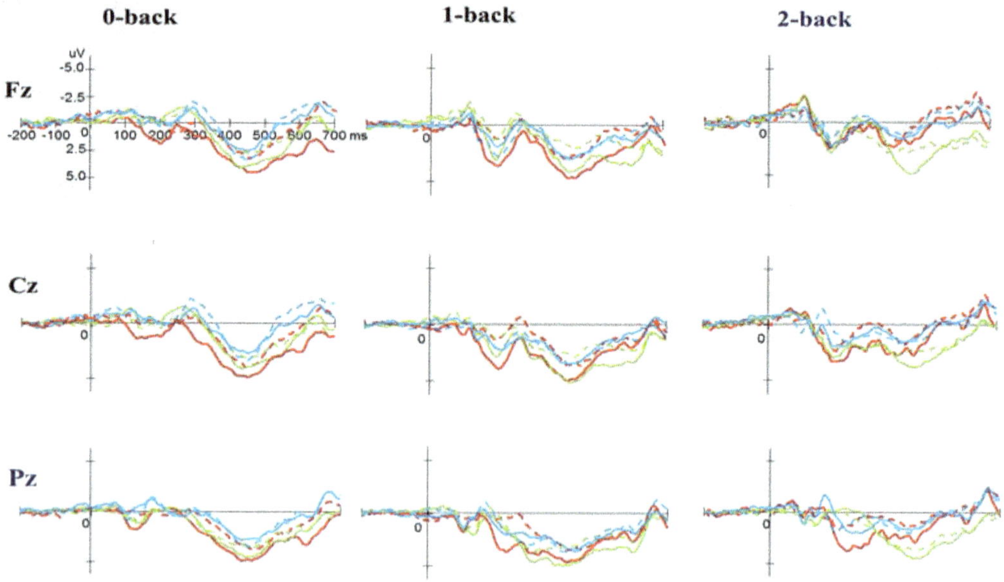

FIGURE 4 | Grand average event-related potential waveforms of three electrodes (Fz, Cz, and Pz) for three conditions (0-, 1-, and 2-back) for the P3 component in the N-back task at baseline (dashed line) and after exercise intervention (solid line) in the open-skill (red), closed-skill (green), and control groups (blue).

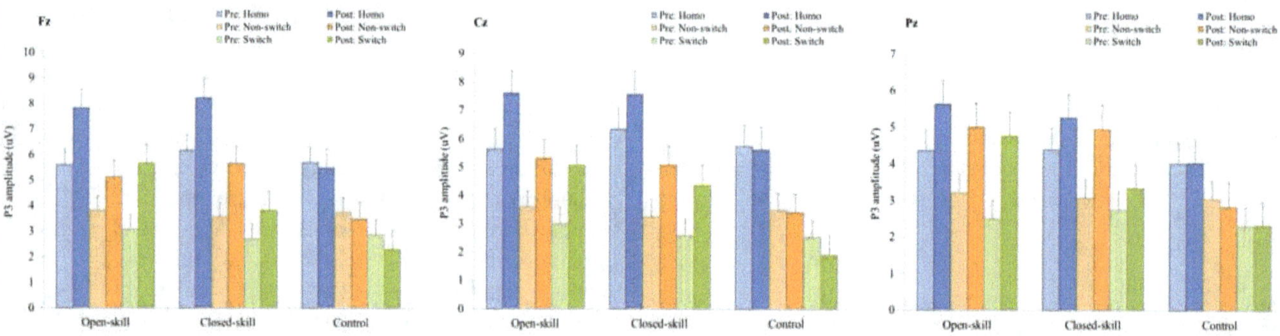

FIGURE 5 | P3 amplitudes (mean ± SE) of three electrodes (Fz, Cz, and Pz) for three conditions (homogeneous, non-switch, and switch) during the task-switching paradigm in the open-skill, closed-skill, and control groups before and after the exercise intervention.

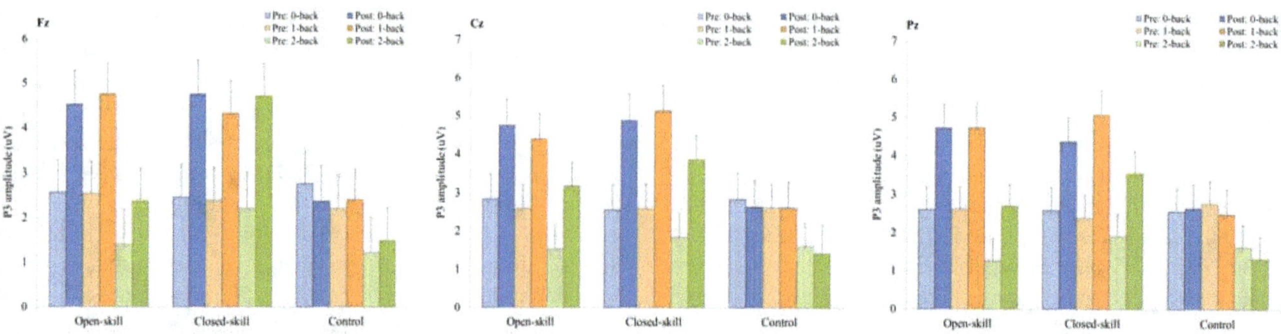

FIGURE 6 | P3 amplitudes (mean ± SE) of three electrodes (Fz, Cz, and Pz) for three conditions (0-, 1-, and 2-back) during the N-back task in the open-skill, closed-skill, and control groups before and after the exercise intervention.

larger P3 amplitudes as compared to the control group (2.17 μV) after the intervention (open-skill vs. control: $p = 0.032$; closed-skill vs. control: $p = 0.005$); and (3) both the open- and closed-skill groups exhibited significantly larger P3 amplitudes [open-skill: $F_{(1, 21)} = 7.59$, $p = 0.012$; closed-skill: $F_{(1, 20)} = 16.83$, $p = 0.001$] across all three conditions and electrodes after the intervention relative to baseline. Even when the post-exercise cardiorespiratory fitness, social participation, and BMI were controlled for, the results of ANCOVA on the averaged P3 amplitudes in the three conditions and three electrodes still indicated significant post-exercise group differences [$F_{(2, 58)} = 5.56$, $p = 0.006$], with *post-hoc* analysis indicating that the two exercise group showed significantly larger P3 amplitudes than the control group (open-skill vs. control: $p = 0.016$; closed-skill vs. control: $p = 0.002$).

DISCUSSION

Main Findings

The present study aimed to explore the effects of 6-month open- (e.g., table tennis) and closed-skill (e.g., bike riding or brisk walking/jogging) exercise interventions on neurocognitive performance in the elderly when performing the task-switching paradigm and N-back task. The findings showed that, with regard to the neuropsychological performance, after participation in the two types of exercise the elderly participants did not increase their ARs in the task-switching paradigm, but showed significantly faster responses than the control group in the switch trials of the heterogeneous condition after the exercise intervention. In addition, compared to the baseline, regular participation in open-skill exercise for 6 months could effectively enhance RTs in the elderly when performing the non-switch and switch trials of the heterogeneous condition, and the specific-switch cost approached significance post- relative to pre-exercise in the open-skill group. In terms of the N-back task, although performing the open- and closed-skill exercise for 6 months did not improve RTs in the elderly when performing such a cognitive task, the ARs in the 1-back condition were significantly enhanced after the exercise intervention in both exercise groups, and the beneficial effects on the 2-back condition only emerged in the closed-skill group. In terms of electrophysiological performance, both open- and closed-skill groups exhibited significantly larger P3 amplitudes across conditions and electrodes after the exercise intervention relative to baseline when performing not only the task-switching paradigm, but also the N-back task. These post-exercise neurocognitive benefits still remained even when the confounding factors (e.g., cardiorespiratory fitness, social participation, and BMI) were controlled for.

Neuropsychological Performances

In the present study, the older adults participating in the open-skill types of exercise (e.g., table tennis) not only had to follow the rules of the game, but also switch strategies and select relevant sensory information when encountering the various skill levels of the other players within a constantly changing environment (Di Russo et al., 2010). In addition, they needed to continually adapt or switch to more suitable movements/responses to initiate appropriate actions or inhibit inappropriate ones based on the opponent's actions. The capabilities of motoric and cognitive switching are thus facilitated during this type of exercise. Indeed, with regard to neuropsychological performance in the task-switching paradigm, although no differences in ARs were found among the three groups after the exercise intervention in the present study, only the open-skill group showed faster responses in the non-switch and switch trials of the heterogeneous condition and a lower specific-switch cost after participation in 6-month table tennis exercise training. This result is in line with the previous findings of cross-sectional research (Tsai and Wang, 2015). Since task switching involves stimulus perception and identification, attentional reallocation, task-set updating, response conflict detection, and monitoring processing (Friedman et al., 2008), the elderly subjects participating in the open-skill exercise modes could show greater cognitive flexibility at switching from one task to another. However, both the open and closed-skill groups showed significantly faster responses when compared to the control group in the switch trials of the heterogeneous condition after the exercise intervention, partly supporting the findings of earlier studies which showed that, relative to the control group, the older adults who regularly participated in physical exercise or regular participation in open- or closed-skill exercise displayed a generalized reduction in the time efficiency of the central processing of cognitive functions when performing a task switching paradigm (Hillman et al., 2006; Themanson et al., 2006; Dai et al., 2013; Tsai and Wang, 2015). In addition, it is worth pointing out that, after engaging in 6-month open- or closed-skill exercise, no improvement in the general-switch cost was found in the older adults in the present study, suggesting that the two exercise modes could not facilitate the process of selecting between and coordinating the two competing tasks (Friedman et al., 2008).

Although the older adults participating in the closed-skill types of exercise (e.g., bike riding and jogging) in the present study stayed in a predictable and stable environment to perform the related exercise at their own pace (Di Russo et al., 2010), and thus they had a lower cognitive load than seen with the open-skill exercise, their cardiorespiratory fitness was significantly enhanced. This was because, compared to the open-skill exercise, repeatedly performing similar movements coupled with continuously higher HR maintenance could much more effectively improve cardiorespiratory fitness. Previous studies have demonstrated that physical exercise interventions aimed at increasing cardiorespiratory fitness are associated with improvements in the neuropsychological (e.g., response accuracy) and electrophysiological (e.g., P3 and CNV components) performances of working memory in preadolescent children (Pesce et al., 2009; Kamijo et al., 2011; Tsai et al., 2014a) and the elderly (Voss et al., 2013). The potential mechanisms could be that such an exercise mode can increase cerebral blood flow (Seifert and Secher, 2011), cerebral structure (Colcombe et al., 2003), and brain-derived neutrophic factors (Seifert et al., 2010), and regulate hippocampal neurogenesis and synaptic plasticity (Erickson et al., 2009). Given that previous studies have linked cardiorespiratory fitness to enhanced memory in the elderly (Kramer et al., 2001; Voss et al., 2013), and aerobic exercise is associated with increased hippocampal size and function (Erickson et al., 2011), it is not surprising that the closed-skill group in the present study participating in the exercise type that had the greatest impact on cardiorespiratory fitness showed improved ARs on the N-back task involving moderate and high working-memory demands, which require continual processing and updating (Bopp and Verhaeghen, 2005), although there were still no significantly different ARs among the three groups post-exercise. Nevertheless, it should be noted that the open-skill group also exhibited significantly higher ARs on the N-back task involving a moderate working-memory demand (i.e., the 1-back condition) after the exercise intervention, suggesting that the potentially neuropsychological benefit derived from the open-skill exercise on the working memory should not be negated in the elderly. One possible explanation for this is that the effect of improved cardiorespiratory fitness approached significance in the elderly participating in the table tennis intervention in the present study. The results on the relation between the N-back task and exercise modes in the present study were partly in line with Hötting et al.'s (2012) findings that cycling training improved learning and recognition scores in an episodic memory test in middle-aged adults, while stretching/coordination training only improved the learning score, and such beneficial effects could be attributed in an increase in cardiovascular fitness. However, it is worth noting that, when the cofounding factors (also including cardiorespiratory fitness) were controlled for in the present study, the beneficial effect on the AR in the 2-back condition still remained for the closed-skill group relative to the open-skill and control groups. Therefore, the potential mechanisms of the effects (e.g., the increases in the hippocampal size/function and the cerebral blood flow) of the closed-skill exercise on the working memory in the elderly are worth exploring in the future (Erickson et al., 2011).

Electrophysiological Indices

P3 latencies did not show obvious changes after 6-month exercise intervention in the two exercise groups, suggesting that the perceptual/central processing could not be facilitated by the open- and closed-skill exercise in the elderly when performing the two cognitive tasks. In line with a previous study reporting a larger P3 amplitude for the active rather than for the sedentary elderly when performing the task switching paradigm (Hillman et al., 2006), the older adults participating in the 6-month open- and closed-skill exercises programs in the present study could effectively increase their P3 amplitudes and so have larger P3 amplitudes across all conditions relative to the control group, suggesting that the two physical exercise modes could facilitate the attentional set that makes it possible to better evaluate the stimulus in either of the two tasks. However, the open- and closed-skill groups exhibited similar benefits on the neural processes at work in processing the current task-switching paradigm. These results are somewhat inconsistent with those of a previous cross-sectional study (Tsai and Wang, 2015), in which the older adults regularly participating in open-skill exercise (e.g., table tennis and badminton) showed a significantly larger P3 amplitude in the switch condition when performing the task-switching paradigm compared to their counterparts participating in closed-skill exercise. The lack of consistency in these results may be attributable to the inherently better task-switching capacity that may encourage some older adults to choose an open-skill exercise mode (Snowden et al., 2011; Tsai and Wang, 2015). The current 6-month exercise intervention study seems to clarify that both open- and closed-skill exercise modes could produce similar electrophysiological benefits across all conditions when older adults perform the task-switching paradigm. However, even though lower P3-and-RT correlation was found in the older individuals (Pfefferbaum et al., 1980), the distinctive effects of open-skill exercise on neuropsychological performance (i.e., better exercise-training-induced effects on specific-switch cost and RTs in the heterogeneous conditions) in the elderly, as mentioned above, cannot be ignored.

Similarly, relative to the open-skill exercise, although a closed-skilled exercise intervention could have more neuropsychological benefits (i.e., significantly increasing ARs under the high load condition) on the elderly when performing the N-back task, the effects of greater P3 amplitudes were comparable in the two exercise groups in the present study. This suggests that not only closed- but also open-skill exercise could facilitate the memory-related neural processing which is involved in categorizing incoming information and updating the context of the working memory (e.g., encoding, rehearsal, recognition, and retrieval), due to the greater efficiency by which cognitive resources are allocated (Duncan-Johnson and Donchin, 1977; Donchin and Coles, 1988; Rugg, 1995). Although there were no significant between-group AR differences post-exercise among the three groups, the increase in exercise-induced P3 amplitudes observed in the two exercise groups after the 6-month interventions, as compared with the figures seen before training, could reveal that they allocated more resources for target classification and evaluation, which might result in higher ARs in the working memory task since larger overall P3 amplitudes during the N-back could be associated with better task performance in older adults (Tusch et al., 2016). However, the P3 amplitude could be influenced by a greater latency jitter of P3 in the high than in the low memory condition (Kok, 2001), and regular exercise could change P3 latency in the older adults (see review, Hillman et al., 2003), the potential response jitter thus needs to be clarified in further investigations, since different conditions in the two cognitive tasks are involved in different cognitive loads in the present study.

It is worth noting that there was no significant interaction of *Time* × *Group*× *Electrode* in the present study, suggesting that 6-month open- and closed-skill exercise interventions induced similar electrophysiological effects (i.e., increased P3 amplitudes) from the frontal to parietal cortices. However, previous studies have suggested that different physical exercises could affect the brain in different ways (Erickson et al., 2011; Voelcker-Rehage et al., 2011; Burrel, 2015). For example, Erickson et al. (2011) found that 1-year of aerobic exercise training could effectively increase the size of the anterior hippocampus in the elderly, but not the caudate nucleus and thalamus volumes, accompanied by improved memory function. Moreover, such effects were not shown in the individuals performing a stretching and toning program. Voelcker-Rehage et al.'s (2011) longitudinal research reported that although the older adults participating in cardiorespiratory training aimed at enhancing cardiorespiratory fitness or coordination training to increase fine- and gross-motor body coordination could improve their executive functioning and perceptual speed, although with different effects on speed and accuracy, the two types of exercise had different impacts on neural activity, with an increased activation of the sensorimotor network and less prefrontal activation in the cardiovascular-training group, and increased activation in the visual-spatial network (e.g., right inferior frontal gyrus, superior parietal cortex, thalamus, and caudate body) in the coordination-training group. In addition, animal studies showed that regular cardiovascular training in rats did not increase the number of synapses, but could increase the density of capillaries (Black et al., 1990) and shorten the diffusion distance from the blood vessels in the molecular layer of the paramedian lobule (Isaacs et al., 1992). In contrast, regular complex motor-skill training in the rats did not increase the density of capillaries, but could substantially increase the number of synapses per Purkinje neuron and blood vessels, thus maintaining the diffusion distance (Isaacs et al., 1992). These findings from both human and animal studies suggest that different types of exercise intervention (e.g., open- vs. closed-skill) could produce distinct training effects on the brain tissues and neural activations. However, in the present study the effects of exercise interventions on neural activity in the frontal-to-parietal cortices seem to be comprehensively covered. In fact, in terms of aging, cognition, and brain function, the phenomenon of dedifferentiation, which characterizes a simple marker of cognitive decline, is often found in the elderly. That is, the regions of the brain that are recruited to perform a variety of cognitive tasks are less specific among older rather than younger adults (Cabeza, 2001), possibly due to additional cortical areas being recruited to compensate for losses in neural efficiency in the former. Therefore, while increased prefrontal activation to compensate for processing impairment, particularly in posterior areas, is a consequence of age-related structural and functional declines in various brain regions (Greenwood, 2007), the findings of the present study suggest that both open- and closed-skill exercise modes could not only facilitate anterior cortical processing efficiency, but also compensate for neural processing impairment in the posterior cortical areas due to cognitive aging. In addition, whether the improvement in cognitive function that results from the open- and closed-skill exercise would produce more distinctive effects in different age groups is one area for future works to address. It is likely that longitudinal assessments of the effects of open- and closed exercise interventions on electrophysiological performance in young adults would help clarify the benefits of different types of exercise with regard to cognitive functions.

Colcombe and Kramer's (2003) meta-analytic study suggested that aerobic fitness training increases cognitive performance by 0.5 SD on average, regardless of the exercise training method and types of cognitive task, especially in the executive-control processes. Therefore, although the distinct benefits of open- and closed-skill exercises on both working memory and task switching performance were found in the present research, cardiorespiratory fitness could play an important role and have a beneficial influence on these two types of cognitive functions in older adults (Netz et al., 2011; Voelcker-Rehage et al., 2011; Wang et al., 2016). Additionally, in light of evidence that depression, education, social stimulation, and BMI could also mediate the exercise-cognition association in the elderly (Miller et al., 2012; Ronan et al., 2016; Tomioka et al., 2016), adequate controls to take into account the confounding factors that participants in the intervention groups are impacted by, in addition to physical exercise, need to be considered. Indeed, in the present study the two groups showed different levels of improvements in cardiorespiratory fitness, social participation, and BMI after participation in either open- or closed-skilled exercise. However, when including these improved confounding factors as covariates in the analysis of the improved neurocognitive performance after the exercise intervention, the difference among the three groups remained significant, showing that both types of exercise modes do indeed lead to improved neurocognitive performance.

Strengths and Weaknesses

Although a number of confounding factors which could mediate the exercise-cognition association were rigorously controlled for in the current study, some potential limitations of this work need to be addressed. First, since changes in the brain and neurocognitive performance are not always proportional to each other, a decrease in brain size and plasticity that results in cognitive changes is associated with normal aging (Peters, 2006). Further MRI/fMRI studies to explore the changes in the sizes/densities of the brain tissues and in patterns of brain activation would be helpful to understand the complex relationship between different exercise modes and neurocognitive performance, and to determine the exact mechanism of cognitive enhancement in the elderly. Second, some exercise items that do not aim to increase cardiorespiratory fitness are also included in the category of closed-skill exercise, such as resistance exercise and yoga. It would thus be informative in the future to compare the neurocognitive performances of elderly adults on different cognitive tasks using these closed-skill exercise items, in order to more clearly explain the effects of the closed-skill exercise intervention on executive functioning, especially in the memory domains, in this population. Lastly, the ERP recordings in the present study were referred to a linked mastoid reference, and this is not an ideal zero reference, and thus the task-related effect could have been impacted by this, and a potential bias produced (Yao, 2001). However, the adopted reference did not change the topography map of the P300 components (Yang et al., 2017), and the P3 amplitudes decreased significantly with increasing cognitive loads (Kok, 2001) in the present study. These findings suggest that the electrophysiological findings from such a reference site are still reliable. However, further EEG-fMRI studies aiming to explore the effects of exercise interventions might consider applying the Reference Electrode Standardization Technique (REST) (Yao, 2001; Yao et al., 2005) as the reference method for ERP data (Yang et al., 2017).

CONCLUSIONS

Extending earlier cross-sectional studies on aging that relied on volunteer participants, which could inevitably include some selection bias with an overrepresentation of individuals with inherently higher executive functioning, the present study of a 6-month exercise intervention confirmed recent cross-sectional results showing that open- and closed-skill exercise modes relate differently to various forms of executive functioning (e.g., task switching and working memory) in relation to cognitive aging in older adults. However, the current findings more clearly revealed that both open- and closed-skill exercise could effectively enhance overall brain cortical activity. These beneficial effects of the two exercise interventions on the neuropsychological and electrophysiological performances in the elderly remained unchanged after statistical adjustment for improved cardiorespiratory fitness, social participation, and BMI. Although exercise is a simple and healthy lifestyle factor that has been proposed to be protective against neurocognitive declines during aging, possibly even retarding or reversing age-associated degeneration in the brain, different exercise modes seem to have different effects on various forms of executive function in the elderly.

AUTHOR CONTRIBUTIONS

CT designed the study, wrote the protocol, and the first draft of the manuscript. CP analyzed the data. FC and YT helped collect data.

ACKNOWLEDGMENTS

This research was supported by a grant from the Ministry of Science and Technology in Taiwan (MOST 102-2628-H-006-003-MY3). The authors are also grateful to the participants who gave their precious time to facilitate the work reported here.

REFERENCES

Adrover-Roig, D., and Barceló, F. (2010). Individual differences in aging and cognitive control modulate the neural indexes of context updating and maintenance during task switching. *Cortex* 46, 434–450. doi: 10.1016/j.cortex.2009.09.012

Anderson, L. A., and McConnell, S. R. (2007). Cognitive health: an emerging public health issue. *Alzheimers Dement.* 3, S70–S73. doi: 10.1016/j.jalz.2007.01.018

Artola, A., von Frijtag, J. C., Fermont, P. C., Gispen, W. H., Schrama, L. H., Kamal, A., et al. (2006). Long-lasting modulation of the induction of LTD and LTP in rat hippocampal CA1 by behavioural stress and environmental enrichment. *Eur. J. Neurosci.* 23, 261–272. doi: 10.1111/j.1460-9568.2005.04552.x

Axmacher, N., Henseler, M. M., Jensen, O., Weinreich, I., Elger, C. E., and Fell, J. (2010). Cross-frequency coupling supports multi-item working memory in the human hippocampus. *Proc. Natl. Acad. Sci. U.S.A.* 107, 3228–3233. doi: 10.1073/pnas.0911531107

Baker, L. D., Frank, L. L., Foster-Schubert, K., Green, P. S., Wilkinson, C. W., McTiernan, A., et al. (2010). Effects of aerobic exercise on mild cognitive impairment: a controlled trial. *Arch. Neurol.* 67, 71–79. doi: 10.1001/archneurol.2009.307

Baskin-Sommers, A. R., Krusemark, E. A., Curtin, J. J., Lee, C., Vujnovich, A., and Newman, J. P. (2014). The impact of cognitive control, incentives, and working memory load on the P3 responses of externalizing prisoners. *Biol. Psychol.* 96, 86–93. doi: 10.1016/j.biopsycho.2013.12.005

Black, J. E., Isaacs, K. R., Anderson, B. J., Alcantara, A. A., and Greenough, W. T. (1990). Learning causes synaptogenesis, whereas motor activity causes angiogenesis, in cerebellar cortex of adult rats. *Proc. Natl. Acad. Sci. U.S.A.* 87, 5568–5572. doi: 10.1073/pnas.87.14.5568

Bopp, K. L., and Verhaeghen, P. (2005). Aging and verbal memory span: a meta-analysis. *J. Gerontol. B. Psychol. Sci. Soc. Sci.* 60, 223–233. doi: 10.1093/geronb/60.5.P223

Burrel, T. (2015). Circuit train your brain. *New Scientist* 227, 32–37. doi: 10.1016/S0262-4079(15)31032-0

Cabeza, R. (2001). "Functional neuroimaging of cognitive aging," in *Handbook of Functional Neuroimaging of Cognition*, eds R. Cabeza and A. Kingstone (Cambridge, MA: MIT Press), 331–377.

Cassilhas, R. C., Lee, K. S., Fernandes, J., Oliveira, M. G., Tufik, S., Meeusen, R., et al. (2012). Spatial memory is improved by aerobic and resistance exercise through divergent molecular mechanisms. *Neuroscience* 202, 309–317. doi: 10.1016/j.neuroscience.2011.11.029

Colcombe, S. J., Erickson, K. I., Raz, N., Webb, A. G., Cohen, N. J., McAuley, E., et al. (2003). Aerobic fitness reduces brain tissue loss in aging humans. *J. Gerontol. A Biol. Sci. Med.* Sci. 58, 176–180. doi: 10.1093/gerona/58.2.M176

Colcombe, S., and Kramer, A. F. (2003). Fitness effects on the cognitive function of older adults: a meta-analytic study. *Psychol. Sci.* 14, 125–130. doi: 10.1111/1467-9280.t01-1-01430

Dai, C. T., Chang, Y. K., Huang, C. J., and Hung, T. M. (2013). Exercise mode and executive function in older adults: an ERP study of task-switching. *Brain Cogn.* 83, 153–162. doi: 10.1016/j.bandc.2013.07.007

Diamond, A. (2013). Executive functions. *Annu. Rev. Psychol.* 64, 135–168. doi: 10.1146/annurev-psych-113011-143750

Di Russo, F., Bultrini, A., Brunelli, S., Delussu, A. S., Polidori, L., Taddei, F., et al. (2010). Benefits of sports participation for executive function in disabled athletes. *J. Neurotrauma* 27, 2309–2319. doi: 10.1089/neu.2010.1501

Donchin, E., and Coles, M. G. H. (1988). Is the P300 component a manifestation of context updating? *Behav. Brain Sci.* 11, 357–374. doi: 10.1017/S0140525X00058027

Duncan-Johnson, C. C., and Donchin, E. (1977). On quantifying surprise: the variation of event-related potentials with subjective probability. *Psychophysiology* 14, 456–467. doi: 10.1111/j.1469-8986.1977.tb01312.x

Erickson, K. I., Prakash, R. S., Voss, M. W., Chaddock, L., Hu, L., Morris, K. S., et al. (2009). Aerobic fitness is associated with hippocampal volume in elderly humans. *Hippocampus* 19, 1030–1039. doi: 10.1002/hipo.20547

Erickson, K. I., Voss, M. W., Prakash, R. S., Basak, C., Szabo, A., Chaddock, L., et al. (2011). Exercise training increases size of hippocampus and improves memory. *Proc. Natl. Acad. Sci. U.S.A.* 108, 3017–3022. doi: 10.1073/pnas.1015950108

Friedman, D., Nessler, D., Johnson, R. Jr., Ritter, W., and Bersick, M. (2008). Age-related changes in executive function: an event-related potential (ERP) investigation of task-switching. *Neuropsychol. Dev. Cogn. B Aging Neuropsychol. Cogn.* 15, 95–128. doi: 10.1080/13825580701533769

Greenwood, P. M. (2007). Functional plasticity in cognitive aging: review and hypothesis. *Neuropsychology* 21, 657–673. doi: 10.1037/0894-4105.21.6.657

Greenwood, P. M., Parasuraman, R., and Haxby, J. V. (1993). Changes in visuospatial attention over the adult lifespan. *Neuropsychologia* 31, 471–485. doi: 10.1016/0028-3932(93)90061-4

Guiney, H., and Machado, L. (2013). Benefits of regular aerobic exercise for executive functioning in healthy populations. *Psychon Bull Rev.* 20, 73–86. doi: 10.3758/s13423-012-0345-4

Hall, C. D., Smith, A. L., and Keele, S. W. (2001). The impact of aerobic activity on cognitive function in older adults: a new synthesis based on the concept of executive control. *Eur. J. Cogn. Psychol.* 13, 279–300. doi: 10.1080/09541440126012

Hillman, C. H., Erickson, K. I., and Kramer, A. F. (2003). Be smart, exercise your heart: exercise effects on brain and cognition. *Nat. Rev. Neurosci.* 9, 58–65. doi: 10.1038/nrn2298

Hillman, C. H., Kramer, A. F., Belopolsky, A. V., and Smith, D. P. (2006). A cross-sectional examination of age and physical activity on performance and event-related brain potentials in a task switching paradigm. *Int. J. Psychophysiol.* 59, 30–39. doi: 10.1016/j.ijpsycho.2005.04.009

Hötting, K., Reich, B., Holzschneider, K., Kauschke, K., Schmidt, T., Reer, R., et al. (2012). Differential cognitive effects of cycling versus stretching/coordination training in middle-aged adults. *Health Psychol.* 31, 145–155. doi: 10.1037/a0025371

Isaacs, K. R., Anderson, B. J., Alcantara, A. A., Black, J. E., and Greenough, W. T. (1992). Exercise and the brain: angionesis in the adult rat cerebellum after vigorous physical activity and motor skill learning. *J. Cereb. Blood Flow Metab.* 12, 110–119. doi: 10.1038/jcbfm.1992.14

Kamijo, K., Pontifex, M. B., O'Leary, K. C., Scudder, M. R., Wu, C. T., Castelli, D. M., et al. (2011). The effects of an afterschool physical activity program on working memory in preadolescent children. *Dev. Sci.* 14, 1046–1058. doi: 10.1111/j.1467-7687.2011.01054.x

Kieffaber, P. D., and Hetrick, W. P. (2005). Event-related potential correlates of task switching and switch costs. *Psychophysiology* 42, 56–71. doi: 10.1111/j.1469-8986.2005.00262.x

Kimura, K., Obuchi, S., Arai, T., Naqasawa, H., Shiba, Y., Watanabe, S., et al. (2010). The influence of short-term strength training on health-related quality of life and executive cognitive function. *J. Physiol. Anthropol.* 29, 95–101. doi: 10.2114/jpa2.29.95

Kimura, K., Yasunaga, A., and Wang, L. Q. (2013). Correlation between moderate daily physical activity and neurocognitive variability in healthy elderly people. *Arch. Gerontol. Geriatr.* 56, 109–117. doi: 10.1016/j.archger.2012.10.004

Kline, G. M., Porcari, J. P., Hintermeister, R., Freedson, P. S., Ward, A., McCarron, R. F., et al. (1987). Estimation of VO_{2max} from a one-mile track walk, gender, age, and body weight. *Med. Sci. Sports Exerc.* 19, 253–259. doi: 10.1249/00005768-198706000-00012

Kok, A. (2001). On the utility of P3 amplitude as a measure of processing capacity. *Psychophysiology* 38, 557–577. doi: 10.1017/S0048577201990559

Kramer, A. K., Hahn, S., McAuley, E., Cohen, N. J., Banich, M. T., Harrison, C., et al. (2001). "Exercise, aging and cognition: healthy body, healthy mind ?," in *Human Factors Interventions for the Health Care of Older Adults*, eds W. Rogers and A. D. Fisk (Hillsdale, NJ: Erlbaum), 92–120.

Lee, I. M., Shiroma, E. J., Lobelo, F., Puska, P., Blair, S. N., Katzmarzyk, P. T.;, et al. (2012). Effect of physical inactivity on major non-communicable diseases worldwide: an analysis of burden of disease and life expectancy. *Lancet* 380, 219–229. doi: 10.1016/S0140-6736(12)61031-9

Liu-Ambrose, T., Nagamatsu, L. S., Graf, P., Beattie, B. L., Ashe, M. C., and Handy, T. C. (2010). Resistance training and executive functions: a 12-month randomized controlled trial. *Arch. Intern. Med.* 170, 170–178. doi: 10.1001/archinternmed.2009.494

Luft, A. R., Macko, R. F., Forrester, L. W., Villagra, F., Ivey, F., Sorkin, J. D., et al. (2008). Treadmill exercise activates subcortical neural networks and improves walking after stroke: a randomized controlled trial. *Stroke* 39, 3341–3350. doi: 10.1161/STROKEAHA.108.527531

Maass, A., Düzel, S., Brigadski, T., Goerke, M., Becke, A., Sobieray, U., et al. (2016). Relationships of peripheral IGF-1, VEGF and BDNF levels to exercise-related changes in memory, hippocampal perfusion and volumes in older adults. *Neuroimage* 131, 142–154. doi: 10.1016/j.neuroimage.2015.10.084

Messier, C., and Gagnon, M. (2009). Cognitive decline associated with dementia and type 2 diabetes: the interplay of risk factors. *Diabetologia* 52, 2471–2474. doi: 10.1007/s00125-009-1533-2

Miller, D. I., Taler, V., Davidson, P. S., and Messier, C. (2012). Measuring the impact of exercise on cognitive aging: methodological issues. *Neurobiol. Aging* 33, 622.e29–622.e43. doi: 10.1016/j.neurobiolaging.2011.02.020

Neeper, S. A., Gomez-Pinilla, F., Choi, J., and Cotman, C. (1995). Exercise and brain neurotrophins. *Nature* 373:109.

Netz,. Y., Dwolatzky, T., Zinker, Y., Argov, E., and Agmon, R. (2011). Aerobic fitness and multidomain cognitive function in advanced age. *Int. Psychogeriatr.* 23, 114–124. doi: 10.1017/S1041610210000797

Nicholson, R., Karayanidis, F., Poboka, D., Heathcote, A., and Michie, P. T. (2005). Electrophysiological correlates of anticipatory task-switching processes. *Psychophysiology* 42, 540–554. doi: 10.1111/j.1469-8986.2005.00350.x

Oldfield, R. C. (1971). The assessment and analysis of handedness: the Edinburgh inventory. *Neuropsychologia* 9, 97–113. doi: 10.1016/0028-3932(71)90067-4

Park, J. W., Kwon, Y. H., Lee, M. Y., Bai, D., Nam, K. S., Cho, Y. W., et al. (2008). Brain activation pattern according to exercise complexity: a functional MRI study. *NeuroRehabilitation* 23, 283–288.

Pesce, C., Crova, C., Cereatti, L., Casella, R., and Bellucci, M. (2009). Physical activity and mental performance in preadolescents: effects of acute exercise on free-recall memory. *Ment. Health Phys. Act.* 2, 16–22. doi: 10.1016/j.mhpa.2009.02.001

Peters, R. (2006). Ageing and the brain. *Postgrad. Med. J.* 82, 84–88. doi: 10.1136/pgmj.2005.036665

Pfefferbaum, A., Ford, J. M., Roth, W. T., and Kopell, B. S. (1980). Age differences in P3-reaction time associations. *Electroencephalogr. Clin. Neurophysiol.* 49, 257–265. doi: 10.1016/0013-4694(80)90220-5

Polich, J. (2007). Updating P300: an integrative theory of P3a and P3b. *Clin. Neurophysiol.* 118, 2128–2148. doi: 10.1016/j.clinph.2007.04.019

Rikli, R. E., and Jones, C. J. (2012). *Senior Fitness Test Manual, 2nd Edn.* Champaign, IL: Human Kinetics.

Rodríguez-Arellano, J. J., Parpura, V., Zorec, R., and Verkhratsky, A. (2016). Astrocytes in physiological aging and Alzheimer's disease. *Neuroscience* 323, 170–182. doi: 10.1016/j.neuroscience.2015.01.007

Ronan, L., Alexander-Bloch, A. F., Wagstyl, K., Farooqi, S., Brayne, C., Tyler, L. K., et al. (2016). Obesity associated with increased brain age from midlife. *Neurobiol. Aging* 47, 63–70. doi: 10.1016/j.neurobiolaging.2016.07.010

Rugg, M. D. (1995). "ERP studies of memory," in *Electrophysiology of Mind. Event-related Potentials and Cognition*, eds M. D. Rugg and M. G. H. Coles (Oxford: Oxford University Press), 132–170.

Ruscheweyh, R., Willemer, C., Krüger, K., Duning, T., Warnecke, T., Sommer, J., et al. (2011). Physical activity and memory functions: an interventional study. *Neurobiol. Aging* 32, 1304–1319. doi: 10.1016/j.neurobiolaging.2009.08.001

Saliasi, E., Geerligs, L., Lorist, M. M., and Maurits, N. M. (2013). The relationship between P3 amplitude and working memory performance differs in young and older adults. *PLoS ONE* 8:e63701. doi: 10.1371/journal.pone.0063701

Seifert, T., Brassard, P., Wissenberg, M., Rasmussen, P., Nordby, P., Stallknecht, B., et al. (2010). Endurance training enhances BDNF release from the human brain. *Am. J. Physiol. Regul. Integr. Comp. Physiol.* 298, R372–R377. doi: 10.1152/ajpregu.00525.2009

Seifert, T., and Secher, N. H. (2011). Sympathetic influence on cerebral blood flow and metabolism during exercise in humans. *Prog. Neurobiol.* 95, 406–426. doi: 10.1016/j.pneurobio.2011.09.008

Snowden, M., Steinman, L., Mochan, K., Grodstein, F., Prohaska, T. R., Thurman, D. J., et al. (2011). Effect of exercise on cognitive performance in community-dwelling older adults: Review of intervention trials and recommendations for public health practice and research. *J. Am. Geriatr. Soc.* 59, 704–716. doi: 10.1111/j.1532-5415.2011.03323.x

Themanson, J. R., Hillman, C. H., and Curtin, J. J. (2006). Age and physical activity influences on action monitoring during task switching. *Neurobiol. Aging* 27, 1335–1345. doi: 10.1016/j.neurobiolaging.2005.07.002

Tomioka, K., Kurumatani, N., and Hosoi, H. (2016). Social participation and cognitive decline among community-dwelling older adults: a community-based longitudinal study. *J. Gerontol. B Psychol. Sci. Soc. Sci.* doi: 10.1093/geronb/gbw059. [Epub ahead of print].

Tsai, C. L., Chang, Y. K., Chen, F. C., Hung, T. M., Pan, C. Y., and Wang, C. H. (2014a). Effects of cardiorespiratory fitness enhancement on deficits in visuospatial working memory in children with developmental coordination disorder: a cognitive electrophysiological study. *Arch. Clin. Neuropsychol.* 29, 173–185. doi: 10.1093/arclin/act081

Tsai, C. L., Chen, F. C., Pan, C. Y., Wang, C. H., Huang, T. H., and Chen, T. C. (2014b). Impact of acute aerobic exercise and cardiorespiratory fitness on visuospatial attention performance and serum BDNF level. *Psychoneuroendocrinology* 41, 121–131. doi: 10.1016/j.psyneuen.2013.12.014

Tsai, C. L., Wang, C. H., Chen, F. C., Pan, C. Y., Huang, S. Y., and Tseng, Y. T. (2016). The effects of different exercise types on visuospatial attention in the elderly. *Psychol. Sport Exer.* 26, 130–138. doi: 10.1016/j.psychsport.2016.06.013

Tsai, C. L., Wang, C. H., Pan, C. Y., and Chen, F. C. (2015). The effect of long-term resistance exercise on the relationship between neurocognitive performance and GH, IGF-1, and homocysteine levels in the elderly. *Front. Behav. Neurosci.* 9:23. doi: 10.3389/fnbeh.2015.00023

Tsai, C. L., Wang, C. H., Pan, C. Y., Chen, F. C., Huang, T. H., and Chou, F. Y. (2014c). Executive function and endocrinological responses to acute resistance exercise. *Front. Behav. Neurosci.* 8:262. doi: 10.3389/fnbeh.2014.00262

Tsai, C. L., and Wang, W. L. (2015). Exercise-mode-related changes in task-switching performance in the elderly. *Front. Behav. Neurosci.* 9:56. doi: 10.3389/fnbeh.2015.00056

Tusch, E. S., Alperin, B. R., Ryan, E., Holcomb, P. J., Mohammed, A. H., and Daffner, K. R. (2016). Changes in neural activity underlying working memory after computerized cognitive training in older adults. *Front. Aging Neurosci.* 8:255. doi: 10.3389/fnagi.2016.00255

van Praag, H., Kempermann, G., and Gage, F. H. (2000). Neural consequences of environmental enrichment. *Nat. Rev. Neurosci.* 1, 191–198. doi: 10.1038/35044558

Voelcker-Rehage, C., Godde, B., and Staudinger, U. M. (2010). Physical and motor fitness are both related to cognition in old age. *Eur. J. Neurosci.* 31, 167–176. doi: 10.1111/j.1460-9568.2009.07014.x

Voelcker-Rehage, C., Godde, B., and Staudinger, U. M. (2011). Cardiovascular and coordination training differentially improve cognitive performance and neural processing in older adults. *Front. Hum. Neurosci.* 5:26. doi: 10.3389/fnhum.2011.00026

Voss, M. W., Heo, S., Prakash, R. S., Erickson, K. I., Alves, H., Chaddock, L., et al. (2013). The influence of aerobic fitness on cerebral white matter integrity and cognitive function in older adults: Results of a one-year exercise intervention. *Hum. Brain Mapp.* 34, 2972–2985. doi: 10.1002/hbm.22119

Voss, M. W., Kramer, A. F., Basak, C., Prakash, R. S., and Robers, B. (2010). Are expert athletes 'expert' in the cognitive laboratory? A meta-analytic review of cognition and sport expertise. *Appl. Cogn. Psychol.* 24, 812–826. doi: 10.1002/acp.1588

Wang, C. H., Chang, C. C., Liang, Y. M., Chiu, W. S., Tseng, P., Hung, D. L., et al. (2013a). Open vs. closed sports and the modulation of inhibitory control. *PLoS ONE* 8:e55773. doi: 10.1371/journal.pone.0055773

Wang, C. H., Chang, C. C., Liang, Y. M., Shih, C. M., Muggleton, N. G., and Juan, C. H. (2013b). Temporal preparation in athletes: a comparison of tennis players and swimmers with sedentary controls. *J. Mot. Behav.* 45, 55–63. doi: 10.1080/00222895.2012.740522

Wang, C. H., Shih, C. M., and Tsai, C. L. (2016). The relation between aerobic fitness and cognitive performance: is it mediated by brain potentials? *J. Psychophysiol.* 30, 102–113. doi: 10.1027/0269-8803/a000159

West, R. (1996). An application of prefrontal cortex function theory to cognitive aging. *Psychol. Bull.* 120, 272–292. doi: 10.1037/0033-2909.120.2.272

Wingfield, A., Stine, E. A., Lahar, C. J., and Aberdeen, J. S. (1988). Does the capacity of working memory change with age? *Exp. Aging Res.* 14, 103–107. doi: 10.1080/03610738808259731

Yang, P., Fan, C., Wang, M., and Li, L. (2017). A comparative study of average, linked mastoid, and REST references for ERP components acquired during fMRI. *Front. Neurosci.* 11:247. doi: 10.3389/fnins.2017.00247

Yao, D. (2001). A method to standardize a reference of scalp EEG recordings to a point at infinity. *Physiol. Meas.* 22, 693–711. doi: 10.1088/0967-3334/22/4/305

Yao, D., Wang, L., Oostenveld, R., Nielsen, K. D., Arendt-Nielsen, L., and Chen, A. (2005). A comparative study of different references for EEG spectral mapping: the issue of the neutral reference and the use of the infinity reference. *Physiol. Meas.* 26, 173–184. doi: 10.1088/0967-3334/26/3/003

16

Inhibitory Control, Task/Rule Switching and Cognitive Planning in Vascular Dementia: Are there any Differences from Vascular Aging?

Krystallia Pantsiou[1], *Ourania Sfakianaki*[1], *Vasileios Papaliagkas*[2*], *Dimitra Savvoulidou*[1], *Vassiliki Costa*[3], *Georgia Papantoniou*[4] *and Despina Moraitou*[1*]

[1] Lab of Psychology, Department of Experimental and Cognitive Psychology, School of Psychology, Aristotle University of Thessaloniki, Thessaloniki, Greece, [2] Laboratory of Clinical Neurophysiology, Aristotle University of Thessaloniki, Thessaloniki, Greece, [3] 1st Neurology Department, AHEPA Hospital, Aristotle University of Thessaloniki, Thessaloniki, Greece, [4] Department of Early Childhood Education, School of Education, University of Ioannina, Ioannina, Greece

***Correspondence:**
Vasileios Papaliagkas
vpapal@auth.gr
Despina Moraitou
demorait@psy.auth.gr

Recent studies have shown that patients diagnosed with Vascular Dementia (VaD) exhibit deficits in executive functions. According to "vascular hypothesis of cognitive aging," community-dwelling older adults having risk factors for vascular disease development (RVD) may suffer from cognitive decline of the same type. The aim of the study was to assess the level of specific executive functions (EF) that have been revealed as most affected by vascular abnormalities, in older adults with incipient VaD and RVD. Subsequently specific ways of EF measuring could be suggested for more accurate diagnosis of early stage VaD. The study compared three adult groups (N = 60): (a) patients diagnosed with incipient VaD, according to DSM-5 criteria (n = 20); (b) community-dwelling older adults presenting cardiovascular risk factors (RVD; n = 20); (c) healthy young adult controls (n = 20). Three types of executive functions were examined: inhibitory control, cognitive flexibility as rule/task switching, and planning. The following D-KEFS subtests were administered for their evaluation: The 'Color-Word Interference Test,' the 'Verbal Fluency Test,' and the 'Tower Test.' Mixed-measures ANOVA, MANOVA, and one-way ANOVA as well as Scheffe *post hoc* test were applied to the data of the scores in each condition of each test. The results showed that VaD patients had significantly lower performance in test conditions requiring switching and planning, compared to RVD group and young controls. The specific deficits of VaD patients, compared to older adults presenting RVD according to multiple-group path analyses were: more uncorrected errors in inhibition, the use of semantic knowledge primarily instead of switching ability to switch between semantic categories, as well as a lower level of movement precision in planning.

Keywords: cold executive functions, D-KEFS subtests, early stage vascular dementia, periventricular white matter hyperintensities, vascular hypothesis of cognitive aging

INTRODUCTION

Recent epidemiological studies showed that Vascular Dementia (VaD) is the second most common type of dementia in Western countries after Alzheimer's disease (AD). Specifically, it affects approximately 5.6% of people older than 60 years old (O'Brien and Thomas, 2015). A meta-analysis of the prevalence of VaD showed that 26% of dementia cases met the NINDS-AIREN criteria for VaD, with a rate for people over 65 years between 0.6 and 2.1% (Kalaria et al., 2008;

Rodriguez et al., 2008; Rizzi et al., 2014; Elahi and Miller, 2017). Many studies suggest that the rates of VaD increase with advancing age, a finding which is related to both genders (O'Brien and Thomas, 2015).

The term 'VaD' is used to describe a group of dementias associated with vascular brain lesions, which can cause ischemic lesions including large vessel disease (e.g., CVAs and large-vessel atherosclerosis) or small vessel disease (e.g., lacunar -very small-infarcts in the deeper white matter of the brain). The use of the term is also linked to the description of dementias associated with extensive intracerebral hemorrhages or to more focal ischemic strokes (cerebral infarctions) impairing the efficient blood supply in cortical and/or subcortical brain regions, as well as to abnormalities in hemodynamic status (Reilly et al., 2010; Korczyn et al., 2012). The presence of vascular lesions in the brain has not always been associated with cognitive decline. There are cases where large ischemic lesions are not associated with cognitive deficits whereas small vascular lesions are likely to lead to cognitive decline and loss of functionality (O'Brien and Thomas, 2015). Vascular lesions have also been observed during 'normal aging' but they do not always cause dementia phenomena.

Hence, many researchers are concerned about the suitability of the term 'VaD' for the description of the aforementioned group of dementias and have suggested to replace it with the term 'Vascular Cognitive Impairment (VCI),' which refers to cognitive deficits induced by various cerebrovascular lesions (Hachinski and Bowler, 1993; Román et al., 2004; Erkinjuntti, 2007; Dichgans and Leys, 2017). The main reason for the suggestion of this replacement is that the 'traditional' criteria for defining VaD were based on, and affected by the criteria established for AD. Hence, memory loss and impairment of everyday functioning were considered diagnostic criteria for VaD whilst none of them was necessarily the case in early VaD (Bowler, 2007). Therefore, VaD could only be identified in late stages. This underestimation of VaD incidence led to the development of the new concept of VCI, the criteria of which can be applied to diagnose VaD in early stage, and subsequently to lead to timely treatment (Bowler, 2007). Similarly, DSM-5 (American Psychiatric Association, 2013) uses the term 'Vascular Neurocognitive Disorder (VNCD).'

The VNCD is distinguished into probable or possible. Probable VNCD is diagnosed if one of the following is present: (a) clinical criteria supported by neuroimaging evidence which confirms the cerebrovascular disease; (b) cognitive deficits that are temporally related to one or more documented cerebrovascular events; and (c) an evidence of both clinical and genetic cerebrovascular disease. Diagnosis of possible VNCD occurs when although clinical criteria are met there is no available evidence from neuroimaging and no establishment of the temporal relationship of neurocognitive disorder with one or more cerebrovascular events.

Executive Functions in Vascular Dementia

Cognitive profiles of dementias, and especially of VaD, have been best understood due to the findings of recent neuropsychological research (Lindeboom and Weinstein, 2004; Traykov et al., 2005; Jacova et al., 2007; Nelson, 2007; Epelbaum et al., 2011; Hoffman, 2013). In this context, dysexecutive impairments have been revealed as an early feature of VaD in its various types. 'Executive Functions (EF)' (or otherwise 'Cognitive control') is an umbrella term for higher-order cognitive processes, which are supported by frontal regions and their distributed networks. They are considered as higher-order abilities because they coordinate other, cognitive, affective, and motor abilities during the execution of complex tasks (Lippa and Davis, 2010; Moreira et al., 2017). At a theoretical level, they have been divided into cold or cool EF and hot EF (Lippa and Davis, 2010; Moreira et al., 2017). Cold or cool EF include 'pure cognitive' or logical, goal-directed abilities such as planning, inhibition, flexibility/switching, and working memory updating. Hot EF abilities are activated when affect (e.g., motivation, emotion-regulation, metacognitive feelings etc.) is involved. Nevertheless, this distinction might not be straightforward and it has been suggested that the two types of EF are rather interdependent (Lippa and Davis, 2010; Moreira et al., 2017). Cognitive psychology and clinical neuropsychology approach EF -mainly but not only in terms of measurement- in different ways. The latter has tried to develop all-inclusive tasks/tests/scales to measure EF, in terms of the various EF abilities that should be recruited to perform in a measure. On the other hand, cognitive psychology 'supports' the development of 'clear' measures of EF. In other words, it stipulates that each task should be designed to measure a primary EF as well as component functions that contribute to performance on this task (Lippa and Davis, 2010; Moreira et al., 2017).

With regards to VaD, cold EF abilities have been extensively studied, as compared to hot EF abilities, and they are revealed, along with processing speed, to be among the first cognitive abilities that decline. Regarding memory functioning, some studies showed that in VaD patients a decline is noticed in the ability to organize the information that is going to be recalled. According to them this decline is attributed to the relationship between this specific ability and EF. The aforementioned conclusion results from the findings of a study (Di Cesare et al., 2012) in which a group of VCI participants, who were outpatients with a positive history of chronic cerebral vascular disorder, were compared with healthy younger and older adults, by means of a serial learning task of concrete frequent words. Similar conclusions were obtained from another study (Levy and Chelune, 2007) in which, groups of participants diagnosed with different dementia types, including VaD, were compared with the use of a battery of tests which are consisted of learning tasks, a verbal memory test, tasks measuring attention and executive functions as well as instruments measuring affect and emotions. In a recent longitudinal study, Livner et al. (2009) investigated two aspects of episodic memory, retrospective (free and cued recall task) and prospective (task developed for the purpose of the study), in people with AD and VaD as multi-infarct or strategic dementia. Based on the findings, they concluded that deficits in prospective memory in VaD are directly related to frontal – subcortical regions. Lamar et al. (2007) studied the relationship between leukoaraiosis in patients diagnosed with AD, VaD (probable/possible), and mixed AD/VaD, and alterations in working memory capacity measured via a modified Digit Span Backward paradigm. Their results suggest that high degrees of leukoaraiosis in people with working memory deficits are connected, to some extent, to their inability to inhibit over-learned and automatic procedural memories.

In the same vein, it seems that language skills remain intact during the various stages of VaD (even in the most progressive stages) in contrast with verbal fluency. In specific, studies which compared groups of participants diagnosed with different dementia types, including VaD, as well as groups of cognitively impaired, non-demented (CIND and vascular CIND) participants, showed that people with VaD had low scores in phonemic fluency, (Duff Canning et al., 2004) a finding which was mainly attributed to dysfunction of frontal lobes (but see Jones et al., 2006). In the same vein, during the first phase of a longitudinal study (Bagnoli et al., 2012) participants with preclinical AD and preclinical VaD as multi-infarct or strategic dementia, were examined in category and letter fluency with the use of a task of early and late word generation 3 years before the dementia diagnosis. It was found that the two groups had the same performance in letter fluency. However, preclinical VaD group outperformed their preclinical AD counterparts in category fluency which is considered to be more dependent on the medial-temporal lobe.

Visuospatial skills have been assessed by the Clock Drawing Test (CDT). Mild visuospatial deficits are observed in patients with VaD. Such deficits are depicted not only in construction abilities but also in executive control function (Graham et al., 2004; Lee et al., 2009). In particular, studies in which the CDT was used to assess the visuospatial skills of patients with subcortical VaD, confirmed spatial and planning deficits in these patients. A possible interpretation of this finding associates the observed deficits with frontal-subcortical circuit dysfunction (Graham et al., 2004). Lee et al. (2009) who studied the characteristics of CDT errors in different types of dementia, including subcortical VaD, concluded that errors in VaD are mainly associated with impairments of planning functions.

Hence, most studies show that there is a relationship between VaD in its various types and deficits in executive functions (Moorhouse et al., 2010; De Witte et al., 2011). Moreover, two review studies (Gunning-Dixon and Raz, 2000; Oosterman et al., 2004) on cognition in cerebral small vessel disease (CSVD; it refers to pathological processes that affect small arteries, capillaries, and small veins in the brain), which is considered the most common cause of subcortical vascular pathology and corresponding cognitive impairment, resulted in findings supporting executive dysfunction in CSVD. However, one of them (Oosterman et al., 2004) showed that there is indeed a significant relationship between white matter lesions and executive functions but only with regards to timed tests.

Moreover, a recent review study (Vasquez and Zakzanis, 2015) aiming at examining the cognitive profile of vascular CIND, showed that, when persons with vascular CIND are compared to persons with non-vascular CIND, they demonstrate impairments in executive functions and processing speed. However, their comparison with healthy controls suggests performance decrements across a broad range of cognitive domains., Phonemic fluency, Stroop interference, Wisconsin Card Sorting Test in various versions, Trail Making Test B and B-A (switching), and Clock Drawing are the tools mostly used in the aforementioned studies (Vasquez and Zakzanis, 2015) to measure executive functions in VaD and VCI.

Nevertheless, today, diagnosis of small vessel disease, at least at the clinical level, includes executive dysfunction manifested not only by impaired capacity to use complex information and formulate plans, but also by incapability to exercise self-control (Wallin et al., 2018). In this context, new batteries, such as the 'Executive Interview 25,' the 'Frontal Assessment Battery,' the 'INECO Frontal Screening,' and the 'Frontier Executive Screen' have been developed to measure executive functions (Moreira et al., 2017). However, more research is needed, mainly at the psychometrics level in order their usefulness to be established comparatively to traditional tasks measuring the same abilities, as well as to tests of general intelligence. Moreover, future studies would be appropriate to show the usefulness of the aforementioned tools for each neurodegenerative condition (Moreira et al., 2017; Wallin et al., 2018).

Hence, the latest diagnostic criteria for VaD (American Psychiatric Association, 2013) include the presence of cognitive impairments in frontal - executive functions (Rockwood, 2002; Desmond, 2004). Deficits in executive functions are mainly associated with subcortical regions (e.g., thalamus, caudate) and their connection with frontal–subcortical circuits (Desmond, 2004; Royall et al., 2004; Moorhouse et al., 2010; Meguro et al., 2013). Greater deficits in these functions are more frequently observed in people with severe white matter lesions (Gunning-Dixon and Raz, 2003; Buckner, 2004; Nakamizo et al., 2013).

In this vein, the present study aimed at developing a small and reliable tool to differentiate diagnosis of VaD from cognitive aging due to vascular risk factors. This tool will be comprised by a battery of tests measuring specific executive functions that have been revealed as the most vulnerable dimensions of cognition in VaD.

Vascular Aging in Community Dwelling Older Adults

The theoretical approach of the 'vascular hypothesis of cognitive aging' (Spiro and Brady, 2008) posits that risk factors for the emergence of vascular disease, affect primarily cognitive functions that are supported by the frontal brain regions (van den Berg et al., 2009; Jellinger, 2013; Kling et al., 2013). A disruption to fronto-subcortical network seems to be one of the main factors that contribute to decline in executive functions. The network might be damaged by white matter lesions, microbleeds affecting connecting pathways of the network, as well as lacunes or microbleeds at subcortical structures of the network (van den Berg et al., 2009; Jellinger, 2013; Kling et al., 2013).

At the conceptual level, the 'vascular hypothesis' (Spiro and Brady, 2011) posits that age is only a descriptive variable of cognitive declines that occur as people age. This theoretical perspective suggests health rather than age as a candidate explanatory process. The term 'health' includes 'disease' as the opposite end of a continuum starting with 'health.'

Older adults usually have health issues, such as elevations in various risk factors for disease, higher prevalence of disease, including subclinical situations, pure control of disease, widespread or even wrong use of medication etc. Taking all these into account, the 'vascular hypothesis' posits that instead of focusing on diagnostic categories, such as 'dementia,' and introducing new ones, such as 'Mild Cognitive Impairment (MCI),' 'Subjective Cognitive Impairment (SCI)' etc., in order to move faster on diagnosis, it might be more useful to consider cognitive aging itself as a long pathophysiological process of 'brain at risk' (Hachinski, 2007; Spiro and Brady, 2011). Recent findings indicating that even 'healthy' older adults can demonstrate a degree of vascular abnormality, suggest that there is indeed a continuum of vascular degeneration in aging, which can result in different degrees of cognitive decline, ranging from trivial to clinically relevant changes (Hachinski, 2007; Spiro and Brady, 2011).

Hypertension is one of the most important risk factors for vascular dysfunction (Moss and Jonak, 2007; Knecht et al., 2009; Sharifi et al., 2011; Areosa Sastre et al., 2017). Several studies suggest that hypertension causes pathological changes in the brain before the presence of acute events (e.g., stroke). Cognitive functions that are more affected by hypertension seem to be attention and executive functions (switching mainly) (Knecht et al., 2009; Sharifi et al., 2011; Areosa Sastre et al., 2017). In the same context, the effect of diabetes mellitus on vascular function and cognitive abilities (Yen et al., 2010; Blom et al., 2013; Hugenschmidt et al., 2013; Spauwen et al., 2013; Zhang et al., 2014) has also been demonstrated by relevant research as an additional risk factor. High levels of cholesterol, homocysteine, and ethanol (Schreurs, 2010; Ehrlich and Humpel, 2012; Niu et al., 2013; Galper et al., 2015) are included to additional physiological risk factors for cerebral vascular disorders.

Given that community dwelling older adults, without a diagnosis of dementia or MCI, usually present risk factors for developing vascular disease, it was considered useful to compare this group with patients diagnosed with incipient VaD, since the existence of risk factors could be a prodromal stage to the development of VaD.

The Purpose and the Hypotheses of the Study

The aim of the study was to assess the level of some executive functions that have been revealed as the most affected by vascular abnormalities, (van den Berg et al., 2009; Moorhouse et al., 2010; De Witte et al., 2011; Jellinger, 2013; Kling et al., 2013) in patients with incipient VaD and community dwelling older adults presenting vascular risk factors, in order to suggest specific ways of measuring the executive functions for a more accurate diagnosis of VaD at the neuropsychological level. Since we could hardly find any healthy older adults, presenting no vascular risk factors to participate in the healthy controls' group of the study, and as our aim was to reveal and estimate the extent of the potential declines in executive functions due to vascular risk factors and VaD, we decided to include a group of healthy young adults in the sample of the study. We considered it useful to assess young adults' performance as an 'index' of the best possible performance in the tests, since it is well-established in the literature of lifespan development that fluid intelligence, including cognitive control, is at the highest possible level in this age-group (Salthouse, 2010; Spiro and Brady, 2011).

The hypotheses of the study were formulated as follows:

> Hypothesis 1: we hypothesized that older adults diagnosed with incipient VaD would show a lower performance in *inhibition* tasks, compared to community dwelling older adults who are at risk of developing vascular disease. Both older adult groups were expected to have a lower performance in the same tasks compared to a healthy young adult group.
>
> Hypothesis 2: Similarly, it was expected that patients with incipient VaD would show a lower performance in tasks requiring a *combination of inhibition and switching abilities* mainly, compared to older adults with risk factors for vascular disease. Both older adult groups were expected to have a lower performance in the same tasks compared to healthy young adult group.
>
> Hypothesis 3: *Planning* is a complex process which integrates into the theoretical framework of cognitive control: in fact, it represents, among others, *the combined use of inhibition, switching, and updating processes.* Thus, it was expected that older adults with a diagnosis of incipient VaD would show a lower performance in planning tasks, compared to community dwelling older adults who are at risk of developing vascular disease. Both older adult groups were expected to have a lower performance in the same tasks compared to healthy young adult group.

MATERIALS AND METHODS

Participants

The sample comprised a total of 60 adults (29 males, 31 females). Their age ranged from 20 to 85 years (M = 57.73, SD = 25.26). There were three groups: (a) healthy young adult controls (n = 20, 6 men and 14 women, age range: 20–25 years, M = 22.75, SD = 1.58); (b) community dwelling older adults who are at risk of developing vascular disease (RVD, n = 20, 13 men and 7 women, age range: 71–85 years, M = 75.85, SD = 4.47); (c) older adults with a diagnosis of incipient VaD. The diagnosis of VaD was made according to the criteria of probable VNCD (DSM-5, American Psychiatric Association, 2013; VaD, n = 20, 10 men and 10 women, age range: 68–83 years, M = 74.60, SD = 5.17).

The two groups of older adults did not differ significantly in age [$t(38) = 0.81, p > 0.05$] and gender [$t(38) = 0.94, p > 0.05$]. Female gender was overrepresented compared to male gender in the young adult group. The participants' educational level varied; 23 participants (38.3%) had a low educational level (LEL: 0–9 years of education), 13 (21.7%) had a medium one (MEL: 10–12 years education), and 24 (40%) were highly educated (HEL: 13 or more years of education). The groups of older adults did not differ in educational level [$\chi^2(2,40) = 0.120, p > 0.05$]. In the VaD group, 11 participants had a LEL, 7 had a MEL, and 2 had a HEL. In the RVD group, 12 participants had a LEL, 6 had a MEL, and 2 had a HEL. All participants of the young adult group had a high educational level.

Young adults and older adults with risk factors came from the general population. History of psychosis and existence of addiction were exclusion criteria for the whole sample. Hypertension, hypercholesterolemia, and diabetes were also exclusion criteria for young adults. These criteria were selected because the authors wanted to ensure the absence of factors that could possibly provoke vascular disorders in this group. Moreover, none of the young participants was taking medication.

On the contrary, the inclusion criterion for older adults with risk factors (RVD) was a self-report of a diagnosis of hypertension, hypercholesterolemia and/or diabetes (one or more of the above), while a self-reported diagnosis of a growth-related cognitive disorder (any type of dementia or MCI) constituted an exclusion criterion for this group.

Older adults diagnosed with incipient VaD were recruited from the inpatient unit of Memory disorders and AD of the 1st Neurology Department of the Aristotle University of Thessaloniki which is located in the AHEPA Hospital. For the diagnosis of VaD (as probable VNCD), patients underwent clinical examination, laboratory tests (blood tests, biochemical tests, thyroid tests, B12, folic acid, etc.) and neuroimaging (CT/MRI). The inclusion criteria were the following: (a) clinical evidence that was consistent with a vascular etiology [(1) temporal relationship between the presence of cognitive deficits and the onset of one or more strokes, (2) evidence of early decline in cognitive abilities, such as complex attention and frontal-executive functions], (b) a cerebrovascular disease which could be indicated by medical history, physical examination, and/or neuroimaging examination, (c) cognitive deficits that could not be explained by another organic or brain disease, and (d) a degree of cognitive decline that did not prevent the daily functioning of the person.

In particular, the diagnosis of VaD was given after clinical and neuropsychological examination. Clinical examination consisted of neurological examination, biochemical and neuroimaging tests (MRI/CT/SPECT). Neuropsychological examination included the Mini Mental State Examination (MMSE), (Folstein et al., 1975; Fountoulakis et al., 2000) the Sort Cognitive Performance Test (SKT), (Lehfield and Erzigkeit, 1997) the Clinical Dementia Rating scale (CDR), (Berg, 1988) the Ishihara Tests for Color-Blindness, (Ishihara, 1992), and the Hamilton Depression Rating Scale (HDRS) (Hamilton, 1960). Based on these examinations, the neurologist was able to diagnose VaD.

The participants in this study were selected among the patients diagnosed with incipient VaD, by one of the authors (Prof. Vassiliki Costa). They were patients diagnosed with specific lesions in the brain. The majority of them had been diagnosed with multi-infarct dementia (bilateral thromboembolic events), some others with leukoaraiosis and decrease in brain volume. It is important to note that none of the participants had been diagnosed with severe hemorrhagic or ischemic stroke in the past, however, as it was found in the MRI, some of them suffered small ischemic attacks. The functional level of all participants was not affected in specific domains as clothing, dressing, feeding and use of toilet. 75% of the VaD patients reported that they had hypertension, 35% hypercholesterolemia, and 30% diabetes and for these reasons they were taking medication. The Geriatric Depression Scale - 15 (GDS-15) (Sheikh and Yesavage, 1986; Fountoulakis et al., 1999) was used to examine the incidence of depressive symptoms. No scores indicative of depressive symptomatology were observed in the overall rating of the GDS-15 (score ≤ 5). In MMSE (Folstein et al., 1975; Fountoulakis et al., 2000) a wider band of scores (25–30) as compared to RVD group was observed. However, these values do not indicate the presence of cognitive impairment related to dementia (see **Table 1**).

In the RVD group, 75% reported having hypertension, 30% high cholesterol, and 40% reported a diagnosis of diabetes, and therefore they were taking medication. None of the participants in this group showed scores indicating depressive symptomatology in the GDS-15 (score ≤ 5). Another exclusion criterion used in this group was the performance in the MMSE, as scores under 24 are indicative of the presence of dementia symptoms. The scores of the participants ranged from 28/30 to 30/30.

TABLE 1 | Individual – demographic - clinical information for each sample group of the study.

Sample Groups	YA[1]	RVD	VaD
	(*n* = 20)	(*n* = 20)	(*n* = 20)
Age (in years): M *(SD)*	22.75 *(1.58)*	75.85 *(4.47)*	74.60 *(5.17)*
Gender: male/female *(n)*	6/14	13/7	10/10
Educational level: low/middle/high *(n)*	0/0/20	12/6/2*	11/7/2*
Geriatric Depression Scale – 15: M *(SD)*	–	1.95 *(1.43)*	1.50 *(1.31)*
Mini Mental State Examination: M *(SD)*	–	28.90 *(0.71)***	27.00 *(1.48)***
Hypertension (%)	–	75% (self-reported)	75%
Hypercholesterolemia (%)	–	30% (self-reported)	35%
Diabetes (%)	–	40% (self-reported)	30%

[1] *VaD, older adults diagnosed with Vascular Dementia according to the criteria of probable Vascular Neurocognitive Disorder; RVD, community dwelling older adults having risk factors for vascular disease development; YA, young adults.* $^*\chi^2(2,40) = 0.120$, $p > 0.05$. $^{**}p < 0.05$.

The mean GDS-15 score of the RVD group (M = 1.95, SD = 1.43) did not differ [$t(38) = 1.03, p > 0.05$] from the mean GDS-15 score of the VaD group (M = 1.50, SD = 1.31). On the contrary, there was a significant difference [$t(27.4) = 5.14, p < 0.05$] in the mean scores of MMSE between RVD (M = 28.9, SD = 0.718) and VaD group (M = 27.0, SD = 1.48). The first group had a higher performance.

Tools

Based on the literature suggesting early impairments of cold EF abilities, such as inhibition and planning, in VaD and VCI, and adopting a cognitive perspective for measuring EF, we chose to assess cold EF abilities, namely inhibition, cognitive flexibility/switching, and planning with the use of specific tests of the Delis-Kaplan Executive Function System (D-KEFS) (Delis et al., 2001). The D-KEFS includes tests that are administered to determine whether poor performance is due to specific impairment in EF, or impairment in lower-order cognitive abilities. Contrast measure scores, completion time, correct answers, and error analyses provided by the D-KEFS tests are factors which enable the assessment of an individual's executive functioning (Delis et al., 2001; Homack et al., 2005)

Delis-Kaplan Executive Function System: Color – Word Interference Test, Standard Form – D-KEFS C-WIT, SF (Delis et al., 2001)

This test is based on Stroop's experiment (1935) and measures the ability to inhibit a dominant and automatic verbal response. The participants have to inhibit an overlearned verbal response (e.g., reading the printed words) to generate a contradictory response (e.g., naming the color of the word). The test comprises four conditions: (a) naming the three basic colors (green, red and blue), (b) reading words written in black that are naming colors, (c) naming the dissonant ink colors in which the words are printed (inhibition), and (d) switching between naming the color of the words and reading the words (inhibition/switching). There is a time limit for each condition, i.e., 90 s in the first two conditions and 180 s for the following two. The examiner interrupts the test when the participant cannot complete the task within the given time.

There are two training sessions in each condition to ensure that participants have understood the task. In the first condition, the participant has to name the colors of squares (green, red, and blue). In the second condition, he/she has to read black-colored words naming the above three colors. The third condition comprises of color words written in incompatible color from the one they name. The participant has to name the color of the word instead of reading the word. Finally, in the fourth condition the participant has to (1) name the color of the word and (2) read the framed word instead of naming its color. The instructions for these tasks are displayed at the top left side of the stimulus booklet that is given to the participant. The test follows some discontinue rules as well. That is, the examiner administers the third condition only if the participant succeeds in finishing the first two ones the examiner is entitled to interrupt the administration of the test in case that participants have difficulty in the training sessions or if participants perform three consecutive uncorrected errors. Given that the contrast scores in this test have been found to display poor reliability, (Homack et al., 2005) it was decided that in this study, the examiner would record the time until the completion of the task with the restriction that there should not be an overrun of the time limit. The examiner had also to record the total of wrong answers in the form of corrected and uncorrected errors in each condition.

Plenty of clinical studies examined the validity of D-KEFS – C-WIT and showed that people with frontal lobe epilepsy, cardiovascular disorder, chronic kidney failure, AD, and Huntington's disease have a low performance in the third and fourth condition (Kramer et al., 2002; Delis et al., 2004).

Delis-Kaplan Executive Function System: Verbal Fluency Test, Standard Form – D-KEFS VF, SF (Delis et al., 2001)

This test assesses crystallized intelligence and executive functions. It is comprised of three testing conditions: (a) phonemic fluency, (b) semantic (category) fluency, and (c) category switching. In the first condition, the participant has to say as many words starting with the letters F, A, and S as he/she can within 60 s. The rules of this condition are as follows: (1) Names of persons or locations are excluded of the words to be stated by the participants, (2) Numbers do not count as words, and (3) Derivatives of the words already stated by the participants are not credited with additional points. In the second condition, the participant is asked to generate as many words that belong to a designated semantic category (animals and men names) as he/she can within 60 s. Finally, in the third condition the participants are asked to generate as many fruit and furniture names as they can, switching between these two semantic categories within 60 s.

The score of phonemic fluency condition consists of the total sum of the correct answers for each letter. The ranking scale is from 0 to 1, each correct word is credited with 1 point and the wrong ones (words that do not fall within the rules or word repetitions) with 0. The score of the second condition consists of the total sum of the correct answers in each category. The ranking scale is the same as in the first condition, namely 1 point for each correct word and 0 points for irrelevant or repeated words. Lastly, the third condition score is derived from the total sum of correct words in each category (3a) and the total sum of correct switches between the semantic categories (3b). Correct answers are marked with 1 point while wrong ones with 0 points.

D-KEFS VF factor analysis revealed a three-factor solution. The first factor was labeled "conceptual flexibility," the second one "monitoring," and the third one "inhibition" (Latzman and Markon, 2010; Fine and Delis, 2011). The results showed that the first condition (phonemic fluency) of the D-KEFS VF had modest loadings on inhibition factor (0.35) in the 20–49 age range and a higher loading (0.61) in the 50–89 age range. The second condition (semantic fluency) had modest loadings on monitoring factor (0.39) in the 20–49 age range and higher loadings on inhibition factor (0.60) in the 50–89 age range. Lastly, the third condition (category switching) had an extremely high loading on monitoring factor (0.97) in both age ranges.

The test also assesses crystallized intelligence, the ability to use learned knowledge and experience. In other words, it is associated with the accumulated knowledge that is derived from the individual's vocabulary depth and from the world knowledge.

Delis-Kaplan Executive Function System: Tower Test, Standard Form – D-KEFS – TT, SF (Delis et al., 2001)

In this test, participants have to make towers along three vertical pegs using five disks. Each participant has to solve the issue of the task using a specific minimum number of moves. The test consists of a wooden board with three vertical pegs, five wooden disks that vary in size and color (shades of blue), a timer, a recording and a stimulus booklet. The test comprises nine problems of increasing difficulty. Each problem has a specific time for completion, 30 s for the first three problems, 60 s for the fourth, 120 s for the fifth and sixth, 180 s for the seventh, and 240 s for the eighth and ninth problem. There are two rules in this test which are given both orally and in writing. The first rule is that only one disk can be moved at a time, and the second one is that no disk must be placed on top of a smaller disk. In each problem the examiner slides the disks onto the pegs, in a specific order, and shows the participant a picture of the tower he has to do (the final position of the disks). In the first problem, the participant has to use two disks the number of which is increased during the administration of the test. If the participant fails to solve the problem, the examiner shows him/her the solution. This aid only applies to the first and second problems. The examiner records the completion time of the first move (optionally), the total number of moves, the whole of rules violation (optionally), the completion time of the problem, and whether the problem was solved (yes or no). If the participant exceeds the time provided, the examiner interrupts the resolution of the problem and scores it with 0. The examiner interrupts the administration of the test in case that participants perform three consecutive failures (i.e., exceeded the given time, making an incorrect version of the tower, using fewer moves than the those origianally predefined).

The scores of D-KEFS TT used in this study are the following: (a) the total number of administered problems, (b) the total number of violations of the rules, (c) the total achievement score which is derived from the sum of the total of correct solutions (the scoring is based on the number of moves). The range of raw scores extends from 0 (zero problems solved) to 30 (all problems solved within the given time and with the minimum number of moves). In the present study, (d) the precision of movements was also measured, which results from the ratio of the total number of movements to the total number of the minimum predefined movements for each administered problem. This measurement assesses the state of planning awareness and the ability to learn heuristic strategies when solving problems.

D-KEFS TT is a tool which assesses complex executive functioning. Factor analysis (Latzman and Markon, 2010) showed positive loadings on spatial planning, learning rules, inhibition, and the ability to define and maintain cognitive sets. The validity of the tool has been studied by various studies in people with brain damage. A recent study showed that people with cardiovascular disease had achieved a lower overall score compared to control group (Jefferson et al., 2006; Fine and Delis, 2011).

Procedure

The above tools were merged to create a battery. Two different versions of this battery, as far as the order of administration is concerned, were designed to avoid order effects. The battery tests were individually administrated and the length of the test administration was almost an hour. The examination took place in a quiet and comfortable environment.

Young adults and older adults presenting risk factors for developing vascular disease were recruited from the community by the first author (Krystallia Pantsiou) via convenience sampling. They were examined at a place of their own choice. Patients diagnosed with incipient VaD, were recruited from the inpatient unit of Memory disorders and AD, of the AHEPA hospital, and they were examined by the same author in an office of the unit.

Ethics Statement

The authors assert that all procedures contributing to this work comply with the ethical standards of the relevant national and institutional committees on human experimentation and with the Helsinki Declaration of 1975, as revised in 2008. All participants participated voluntarily in the study. They were informed about the procedure and the aim of the study, and subsequently they provided their written consent for participation. The Ethics Committee of the School of Psychology of the Aristotle University of Thessaloniki, after reviewing the research protocol, confirmed that all ethical guidelines for research on human subjects were followed (011/16-06-2017).

Statistical Analysis

The data analysis was conducted in SPSS version 21 (IBM Corp, 2012). The analyses carried out were (a) mixed-measures ANOVA, (b) repeated measures ANOVA, (c) multivariate analysis of variance (MANOVA), (d) one-way ANOVA. The aim of these analyses was to compare the performance between the three groups as well as the performance of each group in each condition of a test. Levene's test was used to assess the equality of variances, Box's Test for the assessment of the equivalence of covariance matrices, and Mauchly's test of sphericity for the assessment of within-subject factor. Authors used Greenhouse-Geisser for thecorrection of sphericity violations. Partial eta-squared (η^2) was used for the estimation of the effect size. Scheffe test (plus Bonferroni correction) was adopted for *post hoc* comparisons: even if there are issues related to test's conservatism, given the exploratory 'nature' of this study, we considered Scheffe procedure as the best choice due to the following reasons: it tests all possible comparisons, it is robust in relation to non-normality, and it provides maximum protection against type I error, which was our main concern in this study (Armstrong and Hilton, 2006).

In the next step, data analysis was conducted in EQS version 6.1 (Bentler, 2005). Specifically, structural equation modeling (SEM) on covariance matrices was used. The 'Robust maximum likelihood estimation' procedure was performed due to small sample size and data kurtosis. The specific SEM technique applied to the data was path analysis. This technique was used to examine the directional relations between the constructs – observed variables which emerged from the measurements of each test (Kline, 2005). Lagrange Multiplier and Wald test (Brown, 2006) were conducted to investigate the elements of the model that didn't fit the data well. In specific, a series of multiple-group path analysis were conducted to examine and compare the relations between the variables in the three groups, in order to reveal potential differences in the way participants of each grouprecruit executive functions when needed. Regarding the confirmation of a path model, a significance level of Goodness of Fit Index χ^2 that is $p > .05$ is indicative of a good fit of the model to the data. In this study, authors calculated the Satorra-Bentler χ^2 index (Bentler, 2005) due to the statistical analysis they chose to perform (Robust procedure). In addition, when the value of Root Mean Square Error of Approximation (RMSEA) is <0.05, it is also an indication of the good fit of the model to the data. RMSEA values ranging from 0.06 to 0.08 indicate a reasonable and therefore acceptable approximation error. RMSEA value is relatively "expanded" in cases of small sample size ($n < 100$) and that is reflected in confidence interval range (90% CI). This means that RMSEA should be considered as a model fit index, however, with caution (Bollen, 1990). Comparative Fit Index (CFI) examines whether the data fit a hypothesized measurement model compared to the basic model. Values greater than 0.90 indicate adequate fit of the model to the data, whereas values close to 1.00 indicate a good fit.

RESULTS

Color – Word Interference Test, Standard Form: Inhibition and Switching

Initially, means and standard deviations (SD) of test scores in all C-WIT conditions were calculated for all groups. Subsequently, a series of analyses of variance (ANOVA) was applied in order to examine the 'quantitative' differences between the three groups in the variables under examination for the first three C-WIT conditions. Finally, a Multiple-Group Path Analysis was performed for the third C-WIT condition in order to examine the main differences between the three groups, in cases of the application of the executive function of inhibition.

Total Corrected and Non-corrected Errors

A 3 × 3 mixed design ANOVA (three groups of participants × three conditions of C-WIT) showed a significant main effect of the participant group, $F(2,57) = 15.84, p < 0.0001$, $\eta^2 = 0.35$, condition, $F(1.07,61.04) = 53.21$, $p < 0.0001$, $\eta^2 = 0.48$, as well as a significant group – condition interaction, $F(2.14,61.04) = 21.21, p < 0.0001, \eta^2 = 0.42$.

With regards to the significant main effect of the participant group, Scheffe's method of multiple comparisons showed that more statistically significant errors were made by the VaD group compared to the RVD group, $p = 0.01$, and to young adult group, $p < 0.0001$. The difference between the last two groups was non-significant, $p = 0.057$. A series of repeated measures ANOVA applied to the data in each group, showed that the group of young adults did not show statistically significant differences in the total number of errors in all three C-WIT conditions, $F(1.23,23.49) = 2.13$, $p = 0.07$. On the other hand, the group of adults with RVD showed differences in the errors in all three conditions, $F(1.22,23.28) = 11.78$, $p = 0.001$, with the highest number of errors (corrected and not corrected) being observed in the third condition, followed by the first and the second conditions. The VaD group showed significant differences in the total number of errors, $F(1.00,19.17) = 39.55$, $p < 0.0001$, with a greater number of errors being observed in the third C-WIT condition compared to the second condition (see **Table 2A**).

TABLE 2A | D-KEFS Color – Word Interference Test, Standard Form: comparisons of the three sample groups in total scores as well as of each group performance in the first three conditions.

	Type of score	Group type		
		VaD[1]	RVD	YA
	Total *n* of errors (*M* and *SD*)	2.71 (0.30)*	1.36 (0.30)*	0.31 (0.30)*
	Task completion time (*M* and *SD*)	73.46 (3.45)*	60.26 (3.45)*	33.75 (3.45)*
Group type	**Type of score**	**Condition type**		
		(1) Naming the colors	**(2) Reading words in black**	**(3) Naming the dissonant ink colors (Inhibition)**
VaD	Total *n* of errors (*M* and *SD*)	0.10 (0.45)*	0.00 (0.00)*	8.05 (5.71)*
	Task completion time (*M* and *SD*)	47.65 (2.28)*	34.25 (1.58)*	138.50 (9.47)*
RVD	Total *n* of errors (*M* and *SD*)	1.05 (1.19)*	0.10 (0.45)*	2.95 (3.20)*
	Task completion time (*M* and *SD*)	47.15 (3.18)*	40.25 (4.66)*	93.40 (7.95)*
YA	Total *n* of errors (*M* and *SD*)	0.25 (0.55)	0.10 (0.31)	0.60 (0.88)
	Task completion time (*M* and *SD*)	30.35 (1.24)*	22.45 (0.89)*	48.45 (2.06)*

[1] *VaD, older adults diagnosed with Vascular Dementia according to the criteria of probable Vascular Neurocognitive Disorder; RVD, community dwelling older adults having risk factors for vascular disease development; YA, young adults. *p < 0.017 (after Bonferroni correction).*

Task Completion Time

A 3 × 3 mixed design ANOVA was applied with the participant group (young adults, RVD, VaD) as a between-group variable and the C-WIT condition (first three conditions) as a within-group variable. The results of the analysis showed that there is a main group effect, $F(2,57) = 34.25$, $p < 0.0001$, $\eta^2 = 0.54$, a main condition effect, $F(1.01,62.94) = 212.84$, $p < 0.0001$, $\eta^2 = 0.78$, as well as a significant group – condition interaction, $F(2.20,62.94) = 32.04, p < 0.0001, \eta^2 = 0.52$.

With regard to the main group effect, Scheffe's multiple comparison showed that the VaD group had a significantly longer task completion time compared to young adults, $p < 0.0001$. The VaD group also differed from the young adult group, $p < 0.0001$.

For further analysis of the main condition effect, repeated measures ANOVA was applied to the data of each group. For the group of young adults, $F(1.28,24.47) = 145.63$, $p < 0.0001$, significant differences were observed in the completion time between the three conditions. Similar results were observed for both the RVD group, $F(1.22,23.17) = 55.06, p < 0.0001$, as well as for the VaD patients, $F(1.03,19.70) = 109.28$, $p < 0.0001$. However, despite the fact that the prototype of differences observed is almost similar among all groups, the young adult group spent much less time to complete the 3rd condition, compared to older adults with RVD and VaD (see **Table 2A**).

Multiple-Group Path Analysis Models for the 3rd C-WIT Condition (Inhibition)

This analysis investigated the directed relations between the total number of errors (corrected and non-corrected), the total number of corrected errors, the total number of uncorrected errors and the completion time of the third condition in all three groups of participants. The results showed that different path models were confirmed for each group, Satorra-Bentler χ^2 (3, $N = 60$) = 2.20, $p = 0.53$, CFI = 1.00, RMSEA = 0.00 (90% CI: 0.00 –0.19). In specific, regarding the group of young adults, no relations were observed between the measurements. However, the model for RVD adults appears to be interesting. In this case, it was found that the number of uncorrected errors is positively associated with the completion time (i.e., associated with increased time), while the number of corrected errors has a compensatory function, as associated with reduced completion time. Furthermore, a different model was confirmed for VaD adults, since the total number of uncorrected errors is positively associated with both the total number of errors and the completion time of the condition (see **Figure 1**).

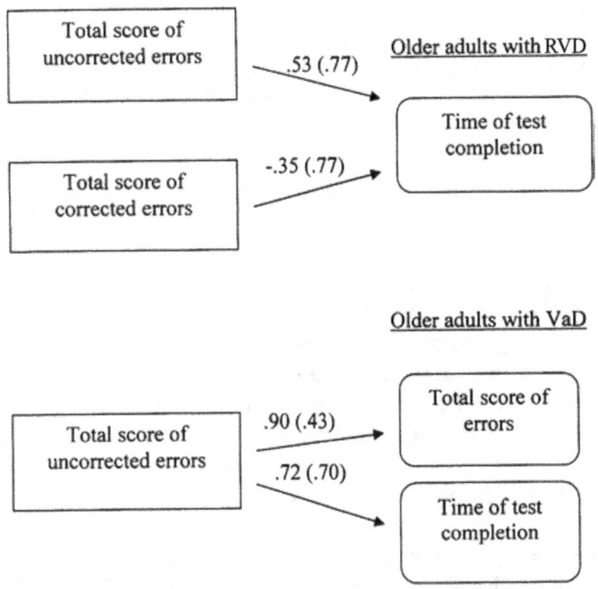

FIGURE 1 | Multiple-group path model displaying differences in inhibitory control (3rd condition of Color – Word Interference Test) between older adults at risk of developing vascular disease (RVD) and Vascular Dementia (VaD) patients. All relationships are statistically significant for $p < 0.05$. Measurement error is given in parenthesis.

Findings Regarding the Score in the 4th C-WIT Condition (Inhibition and Switching)

In this condition, only 8 participants from the group of VaD adults completed the test. Following the instructions, the fourth condition was not administered, because participants experienced great difficulty in the practice lines of this condition. For this reason it was not included in the aforementioned analyses. Regarding the group of RVD adults, although only one participant could not complete the fourth condition, the differences from young adults in both the number of errors and the completion time of the condition were statistically significant: Errors: $F(1,38) = 21.71, p < 0.0001$. Completion time: $F(1,38) = 51.51, p < 0.0001$ (see **Table 2B**).

Verbal Fluency Test: Inhibition and Switching

Means and SD were calculated for VFT conditions for all groups. Then, a series of analyses of variance was applied in order to examine the differences between the three groups on the relevant variables. Finally, based on Pearson correlations between variables and taking into account the sample size, a multiple-group path analysis was applied to the data of the second and third condition of VFT.

TABLE 2B | D-KEFS Color – Word Interference Test, Standard Form: comparisons of the sample groups in the fourth condition: Switching between naming the color of the words and reading the words.

Type of score	Group type		
	VaD[1]	RVD	YA
Total *n* of errors (*M* and *SD*)	–	5.42 (4.11)***	1.00 (1.00)***
Task completion time (*M* and *SD*)	–	121.47 (40.27)***	54.25 (11.33)***

[1] *VaD, older adults diagnosed with Vascular Dementia according to the criteria of probable Vascular Neurocognitive Disorder; RVD, community dwelling older adults having risk factors for vascular disease development; YA, young adults.* ***$p < 0.001$.

Total Correct Answers-Words

Initially, a 3 × 3 mixed design ANOVA was performed with the participant group (young adults, RVD, VaD) as a between-groups factor and the condition of VFT (three conditions) as a within-subjects factor. A significant main effect of the participant group was found, $F(2,57) = 78.20$, $p < 0.0001$, $\eta^2 = 0.73$, as well as a main effect of the condition type, $F(2,114) = 288.35$, $p < 0.0001$, $\eta^2 = 0.83$, and a significant group – condition interaction, $F(2,114) = 11.95$, $p < 0.0001$, $\eta^2 = 0.29$.

Subsequently, analysis of variance was applied with the participant group as the independent variable and performance in each of the three conditions as the dependent variables: According to Pillai's trace, the group effect was found to be significant, $V = 0.78$, $F(2,57) = 12.03$, $p < 0.0001$, $\eta^2 = 0.39$. In particular, the group effect on the total number of correct responses in the phonemic fluency condition (1), $F(2,57) = 42.95$, $p < 0.0001$, $\eta^2 = 0.60$, in the semantic fluency condition (2), $F(2,57) = 56.13$, $p < 0.0001$, $\eta^2 = 0.66$, and in the semantic fluency condition under switching rules (3a), $F(2,57) = 24.74$, $p < 0.0001$, $\eta^2 = 0.46$, was statistically significant. Scheffe's *post hoc* comparison showed that young adults produced more words in the first condition, as compared to RVD and VaD groups, $p < .0001$. No significant differences were observed between the two older adult groups, $p = 0.48$. Similar results were observed in the second condition: young adults had a higher performance compared to RVD and VaD groups, $p < 0.0001$, whereas the difference between the two older adult groups was not significant, $p = 0.13$. It was found that in the condition '3a' VaD adults produced a reduced number of words, compared to RVD, $p = 0.016$, and young adult groups, $p < 0.0001$. A significant difference was also observed between the last two groups, $p < 0.0001$ (see **Table 3**).

For a further analysis of the main condition effect repeated measures ANOVA was used to compare the data of each group. Young adults showed a statistically significant difference in the responses produced in all three conditions, $F(2,38) = 138.90$, $p < 0.0001$. In particular, they produced a greater number of correct words in the first and second condition, compared to the third, $p < 0.0001$. Similar results were observed for the RVD group, $F(1.48,28.17) = 50.57$, $p < 0.0001$, and also for the VaD group, $F(2,38) = 150.52$, $p < 0.0001$ (see **Table 3**).

Total Repetitions and Total Errors in the Three Conditions of VFT

A univariate analysis of variance showed that the three groups did not differ significantly in the total number of repetitions they did, $F(2,57) = 1.86$, $p = 0.16$, as well as in the total number of their errors, $F(2,57) = 1.76$, $p = 0.18$.

Total Number of Switches in the Third Condition (Semantic Fluency Under Rules of Switching) of VFT (Condition '3b')

A univariate analysis of variance was performed, that showed a significant effect of the participant group on the total number of correct switches, $F(2,57) = 13.09$, $p < 0.0001$, $\eta^2 = 0.31$. Scheffe's multiple comparison showed that young adults achieved a significantly higher number of switches, compared to RVD and VaD groups, $p = 0.006$ and $p < 0.0001$, respectively (**Table 3**). However, there was no significant difference between the two groups of older adults, $p = 0.27$.

Multiple-Group Path Analysis Models for VFT

A multiple-group path analysis was used to examine the directed relations between semantic fluency (2nd condition), the words produced in the condition of semantic fluency with switching (condition '3a') and the total number of switches (condition '3b'). It must be noted that the error in measuring word production under switching condition was set to be equal in the two older adult groups. The data from young adults were not used in the analyses, because the aforementioned variable-scores were not significantly inter-correlated. The results for the two older adult groups, Satorra-Bentler χ^2 (1, N = 40) = 0.70, $p = 0.39$, CFI = 1.00, RMSEA = 0.00 (90% CI: 0.00 −0.39), showed that for the RVD group it was confirmed a model in which the number of switches (condition '3b') is positively associated with the production of words in the condition '3a'. On the other hand, a different model was confirmed for VaD adults. In this case, semantic fluency (2nd condition) appeared to be positively associated with the word production under switching rules (3a condition) (**Figure 2**).

Tower test: planning

Means and SDs were calculated for all measurements in all TT conditions for all groups. Subsequently, a series of analyses of variance was applied in order to examine the differences between the three groups of the sample on the variables under

TABLE 3 | D-KEFS: Verbal Fluency Test: Standard Form: comparisons of the three sample groups as well as of each group performance in the three conditions.

Condition type	Type of score	Group type		
		VaD[1]	RVD	YA
(1) Phonemic fluency	Total *n* of correct words (*M* and *SD*)	25.05 (4.33)*	28.45 (10.76)*	45.80 (6.18)*
(2) Semantic fluency	Total *n* of correct words (*M* and *SD*)	22.95 (5.28)*	27.10 (5.53)*	43.00 (7.82)*
(3a) Semantic fluency with switching	Total *n* of correct words (*M* and *SD*)	8.45 (0.80)***	11.80 (0.70)***	16.55 (0.93)***
(3b) Semantic fluency with switching	Total *n* of switches (*M* and *SD*)	8.85 (0.83)*	10.80 (0.83)*	14.80 (0.83)*

*[1] VaD, older adults diagnosed with Vascular Dementia according to the criteria of probable Vascular Neurocognitive Disorder; RVD, community dwelling older adults having risk factors for vascular disease development; YA = young adults. *p < 0.017; ***p < 0.001.*

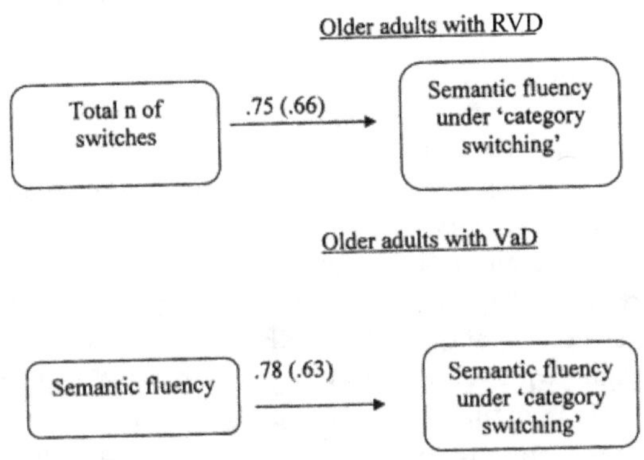

FIGURE 2 | Multiple-group path model displaying differences in cognitive flexibility (Verbal Fluency Test: condition 3) between older adults at risk of developing vascular disease (RVD) and Vascular Dementia (VaD) patients. All relationships are statistically significant for $p < 0.05$. Measurement error is given in parenthesis.

TABLE 4 | D-KEFS: Tower Test: comparisons of the three sample groups in four scores.

Type of score	Group type		
	VaD[1]	**RVD**	**YA**
Total *n* of problems (*M* and *SD*)	7.00 (0.23)*	8.25 (0.23)*	8.95 (0.23)*
Total *n* of rule violations (*M* and *SD*)	8.85 (0.85)*	4.80 (0.85)*	1.80 (0.85)*
Precision of movements (*M* and *SD*)	0.83 (0.15)*	1.65 (0.15)*	1.85 (.15)*
Total achievement score (*M* and *SD*)	8.90 (0.74)*	12.20 (0.74)*	17.40 (.74)*

*[1] VaD, older adults diagnosed with Vascular Dementia according to the criteria of probable Vascular Neurocognitive Disorder; RVD, community dwelling older adults having risk factors for vascular disease development; YA, young adults. *p < 0.013 (after Bonferroni correction).*

examination, namely the total number of problems given, the total number of violations, the precision of movements and the total achievement score. Based on the calculated Pearson correlations between variables of TT and taking into account the small sample size, a multiple-group path analysis was applied to the data of TT.

In more detail, analysis of variance was applied with the participants' group as the independent variable and the four performance variables as dependent ones: the main effect of group was found to be significant, $V = 0.85$, $F(2,57) = 10.33$, $p < 0.0001$, $\eta^2 = 0.42$. In particular, the group effect was significant on (a) the total number of problems given, $F(2,57) = 17.47$, $p < 0.0001$, $\eta^2 = 0.38$, (b) the total number of rule violations, $F(2,57) = 17.09$, $p < 0.0001$, $\eta^2 = 0.37$, (c) the precision of movements, $F(2,57) = 11.79$, $p < 0.0001$, $\eta^2 = 0.29$, and (d) the total achievement score, $F(2,57) = 33.45$, $p < 0.0001$, $\eta^2 = 0.54$.

Scheffe's multiple comparison showed that VaD patients were given less problems (because of their inability to achieve the task or to resolve it correctly) compared to young adults and RVD group, $p < 0.0001$ and 0.001, respectively. Similar findings were found for the total number of violations, where significant differences were observed among all three groups, with the group of VaD patients showing the higher number of rule violations, $p < 0.0001$ and 0.004, respectively. A reduced precision of movements was observed in the VaD group compared to the other two groups, $p < 0.0001$ and 0.002, respectively. Finally, regarding the total achievement score, significant differences were observed among the three groups, with young adults to show higher score compared to RVD and VaD groups, $p < 0.0001$. The difference between the two older adult groups was also found to be significant, $p = 0.008$ (see **Table 4**).

Multiple-Group Path Analysis Models for TT

A multiple-group path analysis was applied to TT data to examine the directed relations between the total number of the problems given, the precision of movement and the total score achieved in all groups, for TT data. The results showed that different models were confirmed for each group, Satorra-Bentler $\chi^2(1, N = 60) = 0.90$, $p = 0.34$, CFI = 1.00 and RMSEA = 0.00 (90%CI: 0.00 −0.33). Regarding young adults, there was no relationship between measurements. For the RVD group, the confirmed model showed that only the total number of problems given was positively associated with the total score achieved. Regarding the VaD group, the confirmed model showed that both the total number of given problems and the precision of movements were positively linked to the total score

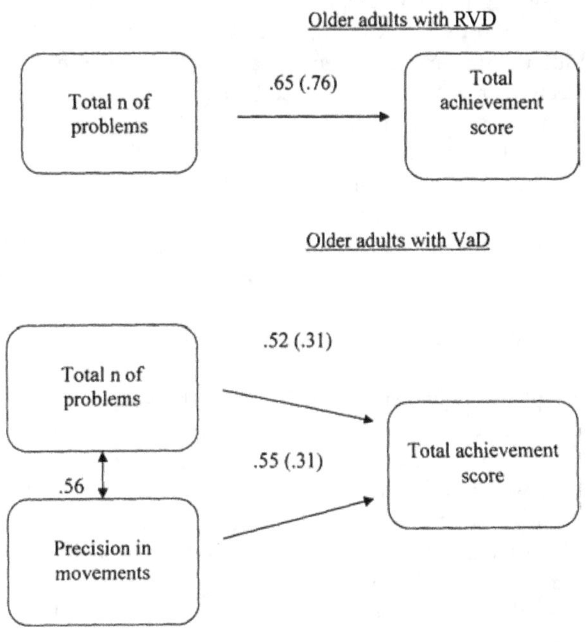

FIGURE 3 | Multiple-groups path model displaying differences in cognitive planning (Tower Test) between older adults at risk of developing vascular disease (RVD) and Vascular Dementia (VaD) patients. All relationships are statistically significant for $p < 0.05$. Measurement error is given in parenthesis.

achieved. There was also a significant correlation between the precision of movements and the number of problems given (see **Figure 3**).

DISCUSSION

Cognitive Control in Vascular Dementia: Inhibition

Based on the extant literature supporting EF deficit in VaD, (Moorhouse et al., 2010; De Witte et al., 2011; Vasquez and Zakzanis, 2015; Moreira et al., 2017) the aim of this study was to go a step further in terms of examining whether older patients with incipient VaD would show a low performance in cold EF tasks mainly requiring the application of three types of executive functions, namely inhibition, switching (or set-shifting), and planning. The investigation of discrete EF abilities, in which older adults diagnosed with incipient VaD and community dwelling older adults with risk factors for vascular disease development (RVD) could show a pattern of 'clear' differences, was considered a subject with great interest, which would enable the development of a short and reliable diagnostic tool for early stage VaD.

'Inhibitory control' is the process of altering one's learned behavioral responses in a way that makes it easier to achieve a particular goal. In this vein, an inhibitory control task measures one's ability to overcome their habitual or dominant response to a stimulus in order to implement a different response. In this study, inhibition was examined with the D-KEFS Color - Word Interference Test (Delis et al., 2001) which is based on selective information processing in the presence of disruptive stimuli.

According to the findings, the number, and mainly the type of errors (mostly uncorrected) in D-KEFS – C-WIT inhibition condition (3rd) might be an indicator of the differentiation between incipient VaD patients and community dwelling older adults presenting risk factors for vascular disease development. Theoretically, it has been argued that the ability to correct errors requires control and adjustment of behavior and is related to metacognitive skills which are impaired in old age (Delis et al., 2001). Thus the inability of VaD patients to correct their wrong responses may reflect a deficit in their metacognitive control system. Based on the findings, the first signs of such a deficit may be evident in community dwelling older adults with RVD, as compared to healthy young controls. However, it seems that at this phase individuals maintain their inhibitory control at a relatively adequate level, since they can correct a part of their errors, displaying metacognitive control to some extent, and perform well in tasks requiring inhibition.

With regards to the completion time, the findings indicated that in the inhibition condition, VaD patients took more time to complete the task, compared to young adults. According to Delis et al. (2001) persons who demonstrate a relatively good performance in naming and reading (1st and 2nd conditions), but have an increased response time and mainly make uncorrected errors in the inhibition condition, tend to be characterized by severe deficits in inhibitory control. Given the aforementioned findings, this pattern of performance is fully confirmed for VaD patients. In addition, first signs of deficit in inhibitory control, in terms of response time, /become visible in older adults with RVD when they are compared to young adults.

Taking into account the significantly increased overall response time and the total error score of VaD patients, in the D-KEFS – C-WIT compared to the other two groups, it can be suggested that *the Hypothesis 1 was partially confirmed* at least in the case of examining inhibitory control via a Stroop-type task: older adults diagnosed with incipient VaD have generally shown lower performance in the D-KEFS – C-WIT compared to older adults with RVD and young adults, while there are some indications of inhibitory control deficit in RVD group compared to young adults. In verification of these findings, Kramer et al. (2002) suggest that subcortical ischemic vascular disease is associated with impaired inhibition even in individuals without a diagnosis of dementia. It is noteworthy that in previous studies a significant contribution of the frontal and subcortical regions has been found in the ability to inhibit, (Lenartowicz et al., 2010) and especially of the anterior cingulate cortex, (Alvarez and Emory, 2006) and frontal gyrus (Leung et al., 2000).

A recent systematic review and meta-analysis study (Sudo et al., 2017) suggested a specific inhibitory control deficit in small vessel cognitive impairment (SVCI), based on the findings of a series of studies that used the Stroop test. The results of this review showed significant differences between SVCI patients and healthy controls in the number of errors as well as in the completion time of the 3rd condition of the Stroop test. The suggested interpretation for this deficit is that it is potentially due to vulnerability to interlobar disconnection on account of periventricular white matter abnormalities (Banich et al., 2000). Neurophysiological studies have indicated that periventricular white matter receives blood supply from terminal vessels of long perforating arteries in areas where branches of large cerebral vessels are encountered. However, most such arteries are very tortuous and this makes their areas vulnerable to hypoperfusion due to arteriosclerosis (Banich et al., 2000). In the same vein, another study (Dunet et al., 2016) which examined the relationship of cognitive impairment with functional connectivity between the basal ganglia and cingulate cortex in vascular parkinsonism, showed that inhibitory control and errors in the Stroop test are related to increased caudate nucleus functional connectivity with the perigenual anterior cingulate cortex, and decreased caudate nucleus functional connectivity with the posterior cingulate cortex at resting-state, respectively. White matter lesions, indicative of small vessel disease, were found to partially contribute in this pattern.

The D-KEFS VF was also used in this study to examine inhibitory control (see Materials and Methods). The findings showed that it is not able to differentiate VaD patients and older adults with RVD. A possible reason for this may be that D-KEFS VF doesn't require the same level of inhibitory control as the D-KEFS C-WIT, while both older adult groups can function relatively well at the level required by D-KEFS VF. In any case, this finding is important, considering the widespread use of the verbal fluency task in neuropsychological examination as well as the findings of previous studies which showed a relationship of VaD and deficits in phonemic fluency (Duff Canning et al., 2004;

Jones et al., 2006). However, the aforementioned meta-analysis and a series of studies on VCI did not replicate this relationship (Banich et al., 2000). Methodological reasons (e.g., different stage of VCI) may be responsible for this inconsistency.

Cognitive Control in Vascular Dementia: Inhibition *plus* Switching

'Task or rule switching' represents a kind of cognitive flexibility that involves the ability to shift attention between one task/rule and another. This ability allows a person to adapt efficiently to different environmental situations. In this study, switching was examined via the administration of the D-KEFS C-WIT (condition 4) and the D-KEFS VF (condition 3). Despite the fact that the two tests examine the same EF abilities, namely switching in conjunction with inhibitory control, it was considered that different results could be found due to the different lower-order cognitive abilities required to perform in each test.

In relation to the 4th condition of the D-KEFS C-WIT, the findings showed that community dwelling older adults with RVD presented a lower performance compared to young adults. The conclusion drawn is that the ability to control a situation declines when task requirements increase and this is particularly obvious in older adults. This finding seems to corroborate those of previous studies suggesting significant age-related effects on the combined application of inhibition and switching (Bryan and Luszcz, 2000; Plumet et al., 2005; Adornetti, 2016; Lam et al., 2017).

Nevertheless, in the present study, many VaD patients failed to complete the 4th condition. This is indicative of the increased difficulty of the patients with the specific neuropathology compared to community dwelling older adults, when they are asked to recruit two executive functions in combination, one of which had to be an expression of cognitive flexibility. Hence, it appears that failure to complete 'inhibition plus switching' condition of the D-KEFS C-WIT recommends a performance standard which can work as a 'clear indicator' of the differentiation between VaD patients and older adults with RVD.

However, with regard to the differentiation between the last group and young adults, confounding variables such as age-related factors and education should be taken into account, (Bryan and Luszcz, 2000; Plumet et al., 2005) in addition to potential early signs of neurodegeneration.

According to the findings, older adults with VaD and with RVD differentiated in the 3rd condition of the D-KEFS VF. Delis et al. (2001) claim that normal performance in phonological fluency (1st) and semantic fluency (2nd) conditions of the D-KEFS VF together with low performance in the semantic fluency under switching (3rd) condition indicate deficits in cognitive flexibility and not in verbal fluency. Based on the findings, it appears that such deficits are so severe in incipient VaD patients that they rely on their semantic knowledge to complete this condition without practically employing switching ability. Inversely, increased performance under switching recruitment (number of words generated) of older adults with RVD reflects that there is no such severe decline in set-shifting ability in this group, compared to VaD patients. On the other hand, the higher performance of young adults in the same condition compared to older adults with RVD, may indicate a progressive decline in cognitive flexibility along with age as well as its corresponding health deterioration (Bryan and Luszcz, 2000; Gunning-Dixon and Raz, 2003; Plumet et al., 2005; Spiro and Brady, 2008; Adornetti, 2016; Lam et al., 2017).

Several studies argue that there is an increase in interference and a decline in switching in people with severe white matter lesions (Lam et al., 2017). According to the findings of the same systematic review and meta-analysis study, (Sudo et al., 2017) which examined inhibitory control measured by the Stroop test, the decline of cognitive flexibility, as measured by the Trail Making Test – B in small vessel disease, also represents a specific EF deficit that might be attributed to the increased vulnerability to interlobar disconnection due to periventricular white matter hyperintensities.

Furthermore, Tsutsumimoto et al. (2015) used in their study the Trail Making Test to measure switching in MCI patients. According to their findings (gross) gray matter volume was both significantly and negatively associated with this EF ability. In the same light, another study in which gray matter correlates (regions of interest) of set-shifting in neurocognitive disorders was examined with the use of three D-KEFS tests [Design Fluency (non-verbal analog to Verbal Fluency), Trail Making, and Color-Word Interference] (Delis et al., 2001) and voxel-based morphometry, suggests that the switching performance correlated with focal regions in prefrontal and posterior parietal cortices. Interestingly, bilateral prefrontal cortex and the right posterior parietal lobe were identified as common sites for switching across all tasks. This finding is important as different types of tasks that measure set-shifting appear to have different underlying neuroanatomy to some extent (Kramer et al., 2007; Pa et al., 2010). Hence, VaD patients might experience lesions at least in the common areas that support switching, even from the initial stage of the disease.

In conclusion, the findings of this study showed that the level of switching ability can differentiate VaD even in the very first stage (Hypothesis 2). In fact, it appears that cognitive flexibility deficits are more severe and more obvious in incipient VaD compared to inhibitory control decline. Thus, the neuropsychological tests that are used to diagnose early stage VaD should include more than one conditions examining set-shifting.

Cognitive Control in Vascular Dementia: Planning

'Cognitive planning' encompasses the neuropsychological processes involved in the formulation, evaluation and selection of a sequence of thoughts and actions in order a desired goal to be achieved. It is considered a complex EF ability in terms of involving functions such as the 'updating' component of working memory, inhibitory control, and task/rule switching (Jefferson et al., 2006).

In this study, young adults and the two older adult groups showed a significant difference between them in two of the four examined variables (total achievement score and total rule violations). Community dwelling older adults with RVD were significantly worse than young adults in the aforementioned variables but they had almost the same level of precision in movements and solved the same number of Tower Test problems as young adults: this pattern of performance could be indicative of a progressive decline in planning along with age that starts with rule violations which indicate deficits in production and preservation (Miyake et al., 2000; Homack et al., 2005; Lee et al., 2009; Moreira et al., 2017). A step further, incipient VaD patients showed lower performance than the other two groups in all variables measured: this finding reflects a more generalized deficit of planning ability in VaD. Therefore, D-KEFS – TT appears to be a very promising tool for differentiating incipient VaD from vascular cognitive impairment in aging (Hypothesis 3).

Moreover, different patterns of variable associations were revealed in older adults with RVD and VaD patients: the more problems solved the higher the total score in the first older adult group. However, the performance of VaD patients was additionally affected by the precision in movements. According to Delis et al. (2001) a close-to-zero ratio in the precision in movements in combination with a low total achievement score indicate one's inability to find correct problem-solving strategies as well as impairments in careful planning ability. VaD patients systematically presented this behavioral pattern. Furthermore, they failed to solve more complex problems, while the administration had to be interrupted whenever high-level planning was required.

The findings of the present study corroborate the results of previous research aimed at examining cognitive changes associated with moderate to severe white matter hyperintensities and less than 5 lacunes (Sudo et al., 2013, 2015). These studies indicated that a series of 'impure' EF tasks that assess complex EF abilities, such as planning, appear to be able to distinguish patients from healthy adults in the earliest pathological neuroimaging of cerebrovascular disease. Functional neuroimaging studies suggested that complex EF employ areas of an extensive neural network including prefrontal, parietal, medial and superior temporal cortices as well as subcortical structures. Leukoaraiosis as well as the onset of excessive white matter hyperintensities may lead to disconnection of those areas (Sudo et al., 2013, 2015).

With regards to Tower Test, in specific, fMRI studies indicated the involvement of the dorsolateral PFC (dlPFC) and anterior cingulate cortex (ACC) in the TT performance (Moreira et al., 2017). According to Foster et al. (2014) selective pyramidal cell atrophy in the dlPFC might partially explain the lower performance in TT. Aberrant functional connectivity between medial prefrontal cortex and ACC might also underlie the impaired complex EF ability (Zhou et al., 2016).

In conclusion, the present study shows that the D-KEFS – TT is an important tool for differentiating between incipient VaD and vascular aging of community dwelling older adults (Hypothesis 3).

Nevertheless, given that all EF tools used in this study are timed tests, processing speed could also be considered a function that is seriously affected in VaD. This is well-established in the extant literature and the main reason for this impairment is periventricular white matter hyperintensities (Gunning-Dixon and Raz, 2000; Oosterman et al., 2004; Vasquez and Zakzanis, 2015; Moreira et al., 2017; Sudo et al., 2017). Finally, it should be taken into account that the D-KEFS tests which were used in the present study measure cold EF mainly supported by dlPFC. However, it has been claimed that damage, at least in some central locations of the dlPFC, lead to defects in general intelligence (g) and not exclusively in EF (Barbey et al., 2013; Keifer and Tranel, 2013).

TABLE 5 | Differences in inhibitory control, task/rule switching, and cognitive planning as indicators for differentiation between Vascular Dementia and vascular aging.

Vascular Dementia Vs. Vascular Aging
Color – Word Interference Test
• more errors
Color – Word Interference Test: inhibition (3rd condition)
• uncorrected errors → increased time to complete the condition vs. two types of errors → differential effects on response time
Color – Word Interference Test: inhibition *plus* switching (4th condition)
• failure to complete the condition vs. success to complete the condition
Verbal Fluency Test: inhibition *plus* switching (3rd condition)
• fewer words generated
• semantic fluency (2nd condition) → generating words (3a condition) *Vs.* n of correct switches (3b condition) → generating words (3a condition)
Tower test: planning
• greater number of violations
• fewer problems administered
• lower-level precision in movements
• lower total achievement score
• precision in movements and total n of problems administered → total achievement score *Vs.* total n of problems → total achievement score

CONCLUSION

At the theoretical level, the present study showed that deficits in complex or/and combined cold EF are more prominent in incipient VaD patients, compared to basic abilities of cognitive control. Specifically, the findings indicated that cognitive planning and cognitive flexibility are considerably affected by VaD progression even in the very first stages. On the contrary, inhibitory control does not seem to be a very useful indicator for the differential diagnosis of incipient VaD. At the applied level, this means that specific timed tests for the examination of planning and set-shifting should be 'in a prominent position' in the neuropsychological batteries administered for VaD evaluation. In this direction, the present study suggests some very specific indicators that can be used to differentiate incipient VaD from vascular aging experienced by community dwelling older adults (see **Table 5**), based on the findings which derived from a detailed examination of three EF abilities, that is planning, cognitive flexibility, and inhibitory control.

However, this study can be only considered preliminary and replication is deemed necessary to ensure the reliability and validity of the findings.

Limitations and Future Research

A number of limitations of the study have to be pointed out. First, the size of the sample was small due to the difficulty in recruiting participants diagnosed with incipient VaD as well as healthy controls of the same age, gender, and educational level. The administration of a broader battery of tools developed to measure specific EF abilities, not only cold but also hot EF, on a larger sample, may demonstrate more reliable and valid findings regarding executive functioning in vascular aging and incipient VaD. Moreover, it was also difficult to recruit a reliable number of patients with a diagnosis of a specific type of VaD. This is an important limitation, as different deficits have been reported on cognitive tests in specific types of VaD. As regards vascular aging, community dwelling older adult participants in the study reported that they have been diagnosed with specific risk factors. Hence, there was no objective examination and other risk factors for the development of vascular disease (e.g., diet, obesity) were not taken into account. The design of the study was cross-sectional and did not allow to 'capture' the trajectory of the change in vascular health during the lifespan. The cooperation of different scientific fields in a longitudinal study would enable a detailed observation of any changes occurring in the human brain, the way they are reflected on cognitive functions, and the time when the pathology starts. Other dementia groups should also be added to the sample, in order to differentiate VaD from other dementia types at the executive functioning level at an early stage of the disease. Moreover, more ecologically valid instruments or real life situations should be used to measure specific EF in the future.

AUTHOR CONTRIBUTIONS

KP designed the study under the supervision of DM, examined all participants, and participated in the statistical processing of the data and the writing of the manuscript. OS and VP participated in the writing of the manuscript. DS corrected the writing style of the manuscript. VC provided all patients diagnosed with VaD by her Clinic as well as all participants with vascular risk factors. GP participated in the statistical processing of the data and provided the main neuropsychological instrument of the study. DM brought the general supervision in all phases of the study which is a part of a broader research project of the same as principal investigator.

REFERENCES

Adornetti, I. (2016). On the phylogenesis of executive functions and their connection with language evolution. *Front. Psychol.* 7:1426. doi: 10.3389/fpsyg.2016.01426

Alvarez, J. A., and Emory, E. (2006). Executive function and the frontal lobes: a meta-analytic review. *Neuropsychol. Rev.* 16, 17–42. doi: 10.1007/s11065-006-9002-x

American Psychiatric Association (2013). *Diagnostic and Statistical Manual of Mental Disorders*, 5th Edn. Arlington, VA: American Psychiatric Publishing. doi: 10.1176/appi.books.9780890425596

Areosa Sastre, A., Vernooij, R. W., González-Colaço Harmand, M., and Martínez, G. (2017). Effect of the treatment of type 2 diabetes mellitus on the development of cognitive impairment and dementia. *Cochrane Database Syst. Rev.* 6:CD003804.

Armstrong, R. A., and Hilton, A. (2006). Post hoc ANOVA tests. *Microbiologist* 6, 34–36.

Bagnoli, S., Failli, Y., Piaceri, I., Rinnoci, V., Bessi, V., Tedde, A., et al. (2012). Suitability of neuropsychological tests in patients with vascular dementia (VaD). *J. Neurol. Sci.* 322, 41–45. doi: 10.1016/j.jns.2012.05.045

Banich, M. T., Milham, M. P., Atchley, R., Cohen, N. J., Webb, A., Wszalek, T., et al. (2000). fMRI studies of stroop tasks reveal unique roles of anterior and posterior brain systems in attentional selection. *J. Cogn. Neurosci.* 12, 988–1000. doi: 10.1162/08989290051137521

Barbey, A. K., Colom, R., and Grafman, J. (2013). Dorsolateral prefrontal contributions to human intelligence. *Neuropsychologia* 51, 1361–1369. doi: 10.1016/j.neuropsychologia.2012.05.017

Bentler, P. M. (2005). *EQS 6.1. U.S.A.* Encino, CA: Multivariate Software, Inc.

Berg, L. (1988). Clinical dementia rating (CDR). *Psychopharmacol. Bull.* 24, 637–639.

Blom, K., Emmelot-Vonk, M. H., and Koek, H. L. (2013). The influence of vascular risk factors on cognitive decline in patients with dementia: a systematic review. *Maturitas* 76, 113–117. doi: 10.1016/j.maturitas.2013.06.011

Bollen, K. A. (1990). Overall fit in covariance structure models: two types of sample size effects. *Psychol. Bull.* 107:256. doi: 10.1037/0033-2909.107.2.256

Bowler, J. V. (2007). Modern concept of vascular cognitive impairment. *Br. Med. Bull.* 83, 291–305. doi: 10.1093/bmb/ldm021

Brown, T. A. (2006). *Confirmatory Factor analysis for Applied Research.* New York, NY: The Guilford Press.

Bryan, J., and Luszcz, M. A. (2000). Measurement of executive function: considerations for detecting adult age differences. *J. Clin. Exp. Neuropsychol.* 22, 40–55. doi: 10.1076/1380-3395(200002)22:1;1-8;FT040

Buckner, R. L. (2004). Memory and executive function in aging and AD: multiple factors that cause decline and reserve factors that compensate. *Neuron* 44, 195–208. doi: 10.1016/j.neuron.2004.09.006

De Witte, L., Brouns, R., Kavadias, D., Engelborghs, S., De Deyn, P. P., and Mariën, P. (2011). Cognitive, affective and behavioural disturbances following vascular thalamic lesions: a review. *Cortex* 47, 273–319. doi: 10.1016/j.cortex.2010.09.002

Delis, D. C., Kaplan, E., and Kramer, J. H. (2001). *Delis-Kaplan Executive Function System.* San Antonio, TX: Psychological Corporation.

Delis, D. C., Kramer, J. H., Kaplan, E., and Holdnack, J. (2004). Reliability and validity of the Delis-Kaplan executive function system: an update. *J. Int. Neuropsychol. Soc.* 10, 301–303. doi: 10.1017/S1355617704102191

Desmond, D. W. (2004). The neuropsychology of vascular cognitive impairment: is there a specific cognitive deficit? *J. Neurol. Sci.* 226, 3–7. doi: 10.1016/j.jns.2004.09.002

Di Cesare, F., D' Ilario, D., and Fioravanti, M. (2012). Differential characteristics of the aging process and the vascular cognitive impairment in the organization of memory retrieval. *J. Neurol. Sci.* 322, 148–151. doi: 10.1016/j.jns.2012.07.042

Dichgans, M., and Leys, D. (2017). Vascular cognitive impairment. *Circ. Res.* 120, 573–591. doi: 10.1161/CIRCRESAHA.116.308426

Duff Canning, S. J., Leach, L., Stuss, D. T., Ngo, L., and Black, S. E. (2004). Diagnostic utility of abbreviated fluency measures in Alzheimer's disease and vascular dementia. *Neurology* 62, 556–562. doi: 10.1212/WNL.62.4.556

Dunet, V., Deverdun, J., Charroud, C., Le Bars, E., Molino, F., Menjot de Champfleur, S., et al. (2016). Cognitive impairment and basal ganglia functional connectivity in vascular parkinsonism. *AJNR Am. J. Neuroradiol.* 2010, 2310–2316. doi: 10.3174/ajnr.A4889

Ehrlich, D., and Humpel, C. (2012). Chronic vascular risk factors (cholesterol, homocysteine, ethanol) impair spatial memory, decline cholinergic neurons and induce blood-brain barrier leakage in rats in vivo. *J. Neurol. Sci.* 322, 92–95. doi: 10.1016/j.jns.2012.07.002

Elahi, F. M., and Miller, B. L. (2017). A clinicopathological approach to the diagnosis of dementia. *Nat. Rev. Neurol.* 13, 457–476. doi: 10.1038/nrneurol.2017.96

Epelbaum, S., Benisty, S., Reyes, S., O' Sullivan, M., Jouvent, E., Düring, M., et al. (2011). Verbal memory impairment in subcortical ischemic vascular disease: a descriptive analysis in CADASIL. *Neurobiol. Aging* 32, 2172–2182. doi: 10.1016/j.neurobiolaging.2009.12.018

Erkinjuntti, T. (2007). Cerebrovascular disease, vascular cognitive impairment and dementia. *Psychiatry* 7, 15–19. doi: 10.1016/j.mppsy.2007.11.002

Fine, E. M., and Delis, D. C. (2011). "Delis–kaplan executive functioning system," in *Encyclopedia of Clinical Neuropsychology*, eds J. S. Kreutzer, J. DeLuca, and B. Caplan (New York, NY: Springer).

Folstein, M. F., Folstein, S. E., and McHugh, P. R. (1975). Mini-mental state". A practical method for grading the cognitive state of patients for the clinician. *J. Psychiatr. Res.* 12, 189–198. doi: 10.1016/0022-3956(75)90026-6

Foster, V., Oakley, A. E., Slade, J. Y., Hall, R., Polvikoski, T. M., Burke, M., et al. (2014). Pyramidal neurons of the prefrontal cortex in poststroke, vascular and other ageing-related dementias. *Brain* 137, 2509–2521. doi: 10.1093/brain/awu172

Fountoulakis, K. N., Tsolaki, M., Chantzi, H., and Kazis, A. (2000). Mini mental state examination (MMSE): a validation study in Greece. *Am. J. Alzheimers Dis. Other Demen.* 15, 342–345. doi: 10.1177/153331750001500604

Fountoulakis, K. N., Tsolaki, M., Iacovides, A., Yesavage, J., O'Hara, R., Kazis, A., et al. (1999). The validation of the short form of the Geriatric Depression Scale (GDS) in Greece. *Aging* 11, 367–372.

Galper, B. Z., Wang, Y. C., and Einstein, A. J. (2015). Strategies for primary prevention of coronary heart disease based on risk stratification by the ACC/AHA lipid guidelines, ATP III guidelines, coronary calcium scoring, and C-reactive protein, and a global treat-all strategy: a comparative–effectiveness modeling study. *PLoS One* 10:e0138092. doi: 10.1371/journal.pone.0138092

Graham, N. L., Emery, T., and Hodges, J. R. (2004). Distinctive cognitive profiles in Alzheimer's disease and subcortical vascular dementia. *J. Neurol. Neurosur. Psychiatry* 75, 61–71.

Gunning-Dixon, F. M., and Raz, N. (2000). The cognitive correlates of white matter abnormalities in normal aging: a quantitative review. *Neuropsychology* 14, 224–232. doi: 10.1037/0894-4105.14.2.224

Gunning-Dixon, F. M., and Raz, N. (2003). Neuroanatomical correlates of selected executive functions in middle-aged and older adults: a prospective MRI study. *Neuropsychologia* 41, 1929–1941. doi: 10.1016/S0028-3932(03)00129-5

Hachinski, V. (2007). The 2005 Thomas Willis Lecture: stroke and vascular cognitive impairment: a transdisciplinary, translational and transactional approach. *Strok* 38, 1396–1403. doi: 10.1161/01.STR.0000260101.08944.e9

Hachinski, V. C., and Bowler, J. V. (1993). Vascular dementia. *Neurology* 43, 2159–2160. doi: 10.1212/WNL.43.10.2159-a

Hamilton, M. (1960). A rating scale for depression. *J. Neurol. Neurosurg. Psychiatry* 23, 56–62. doi: 10.1136/jnnp.23.1.56

Hoffman, M. (2013). Frontal network syndrome testing: clinical tests and positron emission tomography brain imaging help distinguishing the 3 most common dementia subtypes. *Am. J. Alzheimers Dis. Other Demen.* 28, 477–484. doi: 10.1177/1533317513488920

Homack, S., Lee, D., and Riccio, C. A. (2005). Test review: delis–Kaplan executive function system. *J. Clin. Exp. Neuropsychol.* 27, 599–609. doi: 10.1080/13803390490918444

Hugenschmidt, C. E., Hsu, F.-C., Hayasaka, S., Carr, J. J., Freedman, B. I., Nyenhuis, D. L., et al. (2013). The influence of subclinical cardiovascular disease and related risk factors on cognition in type 2 diabetes mellitus: the DHS-Mind study. *J. Diabetes Complications* 27, 422–428. doi: 10.1016/j.jdiacomp.2013.04.004

IBM Corp (2012). *IBM SPSS Statistics for Windows, Version 21.0*. Armonk, NY: IBM Corp.

Ishihara, S. (1992). *Ishihara's Tests for Colour-Blindness, 24 Plates Ed.* Tokyo: Kanehara and Co.

Jacova, C., Kertesz, A., Blair, M., Fisk, J. D., and Feldman, H. H. (2007). Neuropsychological testing and assessment for dementia. *Alzheimers Dement.* 3, 299–377. doi: 10.1016/j.jalz.2007.07.011

Jefferson, A. L., Paul, R. H., Ozonoff, A., and Cohen, R. A. (2006). Evaluating elements of executive functioning as predictors of instrumental activities of daily living (IADLs). *Arch. Clin. Neuropsychol.* 21, 311–320. doi: 10.1016/j.acn.2006.03.007

Jellinger, K. A. (2013). Pathology and pathogenesis of vascular cognitive impairment – a critical update. *Front. Aging Neurosci.* 5:17. doi: 10.3389/fnagi.2013.00017

Jones, S., Laukka, E. J., and Bäckman, L. (2006). Differential verbal fluency deficits in the preclinical stages of Alzheimer's disease and vascular dementia. *Cortex* 42, 347–355. doi: 10.1016/S0010-9452(08)70361-7

Kalaria, R. N., Maestre, G. E., Arizaga, R., Friedland, R. P., Galasko, D., Hall, K., et al. (2008). Alzheimer's disease and vascular dementia in developing countries: prevalence, management, and risk factors. *Lancet Neurol.* 7, 812–826. doi: 10.1016/S1474-4422(08)70169-8

Keifer, E., and Tranel, D. (2013). A neuropsychological investigation of the Delis-Kaplan executive function system. *J. Clin. Exp. Neuropsychol.* 35, 1048–1059. doi: 10.1080/13803395.2013.854319

Kline, R. (2005). *Principles and Practice of Structural Equation Modeling*, 2nd Edn. New York, NY: The Guilford Press.

Kling, M. A., Trojanowski, J. Q., Wolk, D. A., Lee, V. M. Y., and Arnold, S. E. (2013). Vascular disease and dementias: paradigm shifts to drive in new directions. *Alzheimers Dement.* 9, 76–92. doi: 10.1016/j.jalz.2012.02.007

Knecht, S., Wersching, H., Lohmann, H., Berger, K., and Ringelstein, E. B. (2009). How much does hypertension affect cognition? Explained variance in cross-sectional analysis of non-demented community-dwelling individuals in the SEARCH study. *J. Neurol. Sci.* 283, 149–152. doi: 10.1016/j.jns.2009.02.362

Korczyn, A. D., Vakhapova, V., and Grinberg, L. T. (2012). Vascular dementia. *J. Neurol. Sci.* 322, 2–10. doi: 10.1016/j.jns.2012.03.027

Kramer, J. H., Quitania, L., Dean, D., Neuhaus, J., Rosen, H. J., Halabi, C., et al. (2007). Magnetic resonance imaging correlates of set shifting. *J. Int. Neuropsychol. Soc.* 13, 386–392. doi: 10.1017/S1355617707070567

Kramer, J. H., Reed, B. R., Mungas, D., Weiner, M. W., and Chui, H. C. (2002). Executive dysfunction in subcortical ischemic vascular disease. *J. Neurol. Neurosurg. Psychiatry* 72, 217–220. doi: 10.1136/jnnp.72.2.217

Lam, C. L. M., Yiend, J., and Lee, T. M. C. (2017). Imaging and neuropsychological correlates of white matter lesions in different subtypes of Mild Cognitive Impairment: a systematic review. *NeuroRehabilitation* 41, 189–204. doi: 10.3233/NRE-171471

Lamar, M., Price, C. C., Libon, D. J., Penney, D. L., Kaplan, E., Grossman, M., et al. (2007). Alterations in working memory as a function of leukoaraiosis in dementia. *Neuropsychologia* 45, 245–254. doi: 10.1016/j.neuropsychologia.2006.07.009

Latzman, R. D., and Markon, K. E. (2010). The factor structure and age-related factorial invariance of the Delis-Kaplan Executive Function System (D-KEFS). *Assessment* 17, 172–184. doi: 10.1177/1073191109356254

Lee, A. Y., Kim, J. S., Choi, B. H., and Sohn, E. H. (2009). Characteristics of clock drawing test (CDT) errors by the dementia type: quantitative and qualitative analyses. *Arch. Gerontol. Geriatr.* 48, 58–60. doi: 10.1016/j.archger.2007.10.003

Lehfield, H., and Erzigkeit, H. (1997). The SKT – A short cognitive performance test for assessing deficits of memory and attention. *Int. Psychogeriatr.* 9(Suppl. 1), 115–121. doi: 10.1017/S104161029700478X

Lenartowicz, A., Kalar, D. J., Congdon, E., and Poldrack, R. A. (2010). Towards an ontology of cognitive control. *Top. Cogn. Sci.* 2, 678–692. doi: 10.1111/j.1756-8765.2010.01100.x

Leung, H., Skudlarski, P., Gatenby, J. C., Peterson, B. S., and Gore, J. C. (2000). An event-related functional MRI study of the Stroop color word interference task. *Cereb. Cortex* 10, 552–560. doi: 10.1093/cercor/10.6.552

Levy, J. A., and Chelune, G. J. (2007). Cognitive - behavioral profiles of neurodegenerative dementias: beyond Alzheimer's disease. *J. Geriatr. Psychiatry Neurol.* 20, 227–238. doi: 10.1177/0891988707308806

Lindeboom, J., and Weinstein, H. (2004). Neuropsychology of cognitive ageing, minimal cognitive impairment, Alzheimer's disease, and vascular cognitive impairment. *Eur. J. Pharmacol.* 490, 86–86. doi: 10.1016/j.ejphar.2004.02.046

Lippa, S. M., and Davis, R. N. (2010). Inhibition/switching is not necessarily harder than inhibition: an analysis of the D-KEFS color-word interference test. *Arch. Clin. Neuropsychol.* 25, 146–152. doi: 10.1093/arclin/acq001

Livner, A, Laukka, E. J., Karlsson, S., and Bäckman, L. (2009). Prospective and retrospective memory in Alzheimer's disease and vascular dementia: similar patterns of impairment. *J. Neurol. Sci.* 283, 235–239. doi: 10.1016/j.jns.2009.02.377

Meguro, K., Akanuma, K., Ouchi, Y., Meguro, M., Nakamura, K., and Yamaguchi, S. (2013). Vascular dementia with left thalamic infarction:

neuropsychological and behavioral implications suggested by involvement of the thalamic nucleus and the remote effect on cerebral cortex. the Osaki-Tajiri project. *Psychiatry Res. Neuroimaging* 213, 56–62. doi: 10.1016/j.pscychresns. 2012.12.004

Miyake, A, Friedman, N. P., Emerson, M. J., Witzki, A. H., and Howerter, A. (2000). The unity and diversity of executive functions and their contributions to complex "frontal lobe" tasks: a latent variable analysis. *Cogn. Psychol.* 41, 49–100. doi: 10.1006/cogp.1999.0734

Moorhouse, P., Song, X., Kenneth, R., Black, S., Kertesz, A., Gauthier, S., et al. (2010). Executive dysfunction in vascular cognitive impairment in the consortium to investigate vascular impairment of cognition study. *J. Neurol. Sci.* 288, 142–146. doi: 10.1016/j.jns.2009.09.017

Moreira, H. S., Costa, A. S., Castro, S. L., Lima, C. F., and Vicente, S. G. (2017). Assessing executive dysfunction in neurodegenerative disorders: a critical review of brief neuropsychological tools. *Front. Aging Neurosci.* 9:369. doi: 10.3389/fnagi.2017.00369

Moss, M. B., and Jonak, E. (2007). Cerebrovascular disease and dementia: a primate model of hypertension and cognition. *Alzheimers Dement.* 3, S6–S15. doi: 10. 1016/j.jalz.2007.01.002

Nakamizo, A, Kikkawa, Y, Hiwatashi, A, Matsushima, T, and Sasaki, T (2013). Executive function and diffusion in frontal white matter of adults with moyamoya disease. *J. Stroke Cerebrovasc. Dis.* 23, 457–461. doi: 10.1016/j. jstrokecerebrovasdis.2013.03.022

Nelson, N. W. (2007). Differential diagnosis of Alzheimer's dementia and vascular dementia. *Dis. Mon.* 53, 148–151. doi: 10.1016/j.disamonth.2007.04.004

Niu, M.-J., Yin, F.-Z., Liu, L.-X., Fang, Y., Xuan, X.-M., and Wu, C.-F. (2013). Non-high-density lipoprotein cholesterol and other risk factors of mild cognitive impairment among Chinese type 2 diabetic patients. *J. Diabetes Complications* 27, 443–446. doi: 10.1016/j.jdiacomp.2013.06.001

O'Brien, J. T., and Thomas, A. (2015). Vascular dementia. *Lancet* 386, 1698–1706. doi: 10.1016/S0140-6736(15)00463-8

Oosterman, J. M., Sergeant, J. A., Weinstein, H. C., and Scherder, E. J. A. (2004). Timed executive functions and white matter in aging with and without cardiovascular risk factors. *Rev. Neurosci.* 15, 439–462. doi: 10.1515/ REVNEURO.2004.15.6.439

Pa, J., Possin, K. L., Wilson, S. M., Quitania, L. C., Kramer, J. H., Boxer, A. L., et al. (2010). Gray matter correlates of set-shifting among neurodegenerative disease, mild cognitive impairment, and healthy older adults. *J. Int. Neuropsychol. Soc.* 16, 640–650. doi: 10.1017/S1355617710000408

Plumet, J., Gaonac'h, D., and Gil, R. (2005). Neuropsychological assessment of executive functions in women: the effects of age and education. *Neuropsychology* 19, 566–577. doi: 10.1037/0894-4105.19.5.566

Reilly, J., Rodriguez, A., Lamy, M., and Neils-Strunjas, J. (2010). Cognition, language, and clinical pathological features of non-Alzheimers Dementias: an overview. *J. Commun. Disord.* 43, 438–452. doi: 10.1016/j.jcomdis.2010.04.011

Rizzi, L., Rosset, I., and Roriz-Cruz, M. (2014). Global epidemiology of dementia: Alzheimer's and vascular types. *Biomed Res. Int.* 2014:908915. doi: 10.1155/ 2014/908915

Rockwood, K. (2002). Vascular cognitive impairment and vascular dementia. *J. Neurol. Sci.* 203–204, 23–27. doi: 10.1016/S0022-510X(02)00255-1

Rodriguez, J. J. L., Ferri, C. P., Acosta, D., Guerra, M., Huang, Y., Jacob, K. S., et al. (2008). Prevalence of dementia in Latin America, India, and China: a population-based cross-sectional survey. *Lancet* 372, 464–474. doi: 10.1016/ S0140-6736(08)61002-8

Román, G. C., Sachdev, P., Royall, D. K., Roger, A., Bullock, R. A., Orgogozo, J.-M., et al. (2004). Vascular cognitive disorder: a new diagnostic category updating vascular cognitive impairment and vascular dementia. *J. Neurol. Sci.* 226, 81–87. doi: 10.1016/j.jns.2004.09.016

Royall, D. R., Palmer, R., Chido, L. K., and Polk, M. J. (2004). Declining executive control in normal aging predicts change in functional status: the freedom house study. *J. Am. Geriatr. Soc.* 52, 346–352. doi: 10.1111/j.1532-5415.2004.52104.x

Salthouse, T. A. (2010). Selective review of cognitive aging. *J. Int. Neuropsychol. Soc.* 16, 754–760. doi: 10.1017/S1355617710000706

Schreurs, B. G. (2010). The effects of cholesterol on learning and memory. *Neurosci. Biobehav. Rev.* 34, 1366–1379. doi: 10.1016/j.neubiorev.2010.04.010

Sharifi, F., Hedayat, M., Fakhrzadeh, H., Mahmoudi, M. J., Ghaderpanahi, M., Mirarefin, M., et al. (2011). Hypertension and cognitive impairment: Kahrizak elderly study. *Int. J. Gerontol.* 5, 212–216. doi: 10.1016/j.ijge.2011.12.001

Sheikh, J. I., and Yesavage, J. A. (1986). "Geriatric Depression Scale (GDS). Recent evidence and development of a shorter version," in *Clinical Gerontology: A Guide to Assessment and Intervention*, ed. T. L. Brink (New York, NY: The Haworth Press, Inc), 165–173.

Spauwen, P. J., Kohler, S., Verhey, F. R., Stehouwer, C. D., and van Boxtel, M. P. (2013). Effects of type 2 diabetes on 12-year cognitive change: results from the Maastricht aging study. *Diabetes Care* 36, 1554–1561. doi: 10.2337/dc12-0746

Spiro, A., and Brady, C. (2008). "Integrating health into cognitive aging research and theory," in *Handbook of Cognitive Aging: Interdisciplinary Perspectives*, eds S. Hofer and D. Alwin (Thousand Oaks, CA: Sage), 260–283. doi: 10.4135/ 9781412976589.n16

Spiro, A. III, and Brady, C. B. (2011). Integrating health into cognitive aging: toward a preventive cognitive neuroscience of aging. *J. Gerontol. Ser. B Psychol. Sci. Soc. Sci.* 66B, i17–i25. doi: 10.1093/geronb/gbr018

Sudo, F. K., Alves, G. S., Tiel, C., Ericeira-Valente, L., Moreira, D. M., Laks, J., et al. (2015). Neuroimaging criteria and cognitive performance in vascular mild cognitive impairment A systematic review. *Dement. Neuropsychol.* 9, 394–404. doi: 10.1590/1980-57642015DN94000394

Sudo, F. K., Amado, P., Alves, G. S., Laks, J., and Engelhardt, E. (2017). A continuum of executive function deficits in early subcortical vascular cognitive impairment: a systematic review and meta-analysis. *Dement. Neuropsychol.* 11, 371–380. doi: 10.1590/1980-57642016dn11-040006

Sudo, F. K., Eduardo, C., Alves, O., Alves, G. S., Ericeira-valente, L., Tiel, C., et al. (2013). White matter hyperintensities, executive function and global cognitive performance in vascular mild cognitive impairment. *Arq. Neuropsiquiatr.* 71, 431–436. doi: 10.1590/0004-282X20130057

Traykov, L., Baudic, S., Raoux, N., Latour, F., Rieu, D., Smagghe, A., et al. (2005). Patterns of memory impairment and perseverative behavior discriminate early Alzheimer's disease from subcortical vascular dementia. *J. Neurol. Sci.* 229-230, 75–79. doi: 10.1016/j.jns.2004.11.006

Tsutsumimoto, K., Makizako, H., Shimada, H., Doi, T., and Suzuki, T. (2015). Set-shifting ability is associated with gray matter volume in older people with mild cognitive impairment. *Dement. Geriatr. Cogn. Disord. Extra* 5, 395–403. doi: 10.1159/000438721

van den Berg, E., Kloppenborg, R. P., Kessels, R. P., Kappelle, L. J., and Biessels, G. J. (2009). Type 2 diabetes mellitus, hypertension, dyslipidemia and obesity: a systematic comparison of their impact on cognition. *Biochim. Biophys. Acta* 1792, 470–481. doi: 10.1016/j.bbadis.2008.09.004

Vasquez, B. P., and Zakzanis, K. K. (2015). The neuropsychological profile of vascular cognitive impairment not demented: a meta-analysis. *J. Neuropsychol.* 9, 109–136. doi: 10.1111/jnp.12039

Wallin, A., Román, G. C., Esiri, M., et al. (2018). Update on vascular cognitive impairment associated with subcortical small-vessel disease. *J. Alzheimers Dis.* 62, 1417–1441. doi: 10.3233/JAD-170803

Yen, C.-H., Yeh, C.-J., Wang, C.-C., Liao, W.-C., Chen, S.-C., Chen, C.-C., et al. (2010). Determinants of cognitive impairment over time among the elderly in Taiwan: results of the national longitudinal study. *Arch. Gerontol. Geriatr.* 50, S53–S57. doi: 10.1016/S0167-4943(10)70014-5

Zhang, Y., Zhang, X., Zhang, J., Liu, C., Yuan, O., Yin, X., et al. (2014). Gray matter volume abnormalities in type 2 diabetes mellitus with and without mild cognitive impairment. *Neurosci. Lett.* 562, 1–6. doi: 10.1016/j.neulet.2014. 01.006

Zhou, X., Hu, X., Zhang, C., Wang, H., Zhu, X., Xu, L., et al. (2016). Aberrant functional connectivity and structural atrophy in subcortical vascular cognitive impairment: relationship with cognitive impairments. *Front. Aging Neurosci.* 8:14. doi: 10.3389/fnagi.2016.00014

17

MEG Beamformer-Based Reconstructions of Functional Networks in Mild Cognitive Impairment

Maria E. López[1,2†], Marjolein M. A. Engels[3†], Elisabeth C. W. van Straaten[4,5], Ricardo Bajo[6], María L. Delgado[7,8], Philip Scheltens[3], Arjan Hillebrand[4], Cornelis J. Stam[4] and Fernando Maestú[2,6,8]*

[1] Laboratory of Neuropsychology, Universitat de les Illes Balears, Palma de Mallorca, Spain, [2] Networking Research Center on Bioengineering, Biomaterials and Nanomedicine, Madrid, Spain, [3] Alzheimer Center and Department of Neurology, Neuroscience Campus Amsterdam, VU University Medical Center, Amsterdam, Netherlands, [4] Department of Clinical Neurophysiology and MEG Center, Neuroscience Campus Amsterdam, VU University Medical Center, Amsterdam, Netherlands, [5] Nutricia Advanced Medical Nutrition, Nutricia Research, Utrecht, Netherlands, [6] Laboratory of Cognitive and Computational Neuroscience, Center for Biomedical Technology, Complutense University of Madrid and Technical University of Madrid, Madrid, Spain, [7] Seniors Center of the District of Chamartín, Madrid, Spain, [8] Department of Basic Psychology II, Complutense University of Madrid, Madrid, Spain

***Correspondence:**
Maria E. López
meugenia.lopez@uib.es

† These authors have contributed equally to this work.

Subjects with mild cognitive impairment (MCI) have an increased risk of developing Alzheimer's disease (AD), and their functional brain networks are presumably already altered. To test this hypothesis, we compared magnetoencephalography (MEG) eyes-closed resting-state recordings from 29 MCI subjects and 29 healthy elderly subjects in the present exploratory study. Functional connectivity in different frequency bands was assessed with the phase lag index (PLI) in source space. Normalized weighted clustering coefficient (normalized Cw) and path length (normalized Lw), as well as network measures derived from the minimum spanning tree [MST; i.e., betweenness centrality (BC) and node degree], were calculated. First, we found altered PLI values in the lower and upper alpha bands in MCI patients compared to controls. Thereafter, we explored network differences in these frequency bands. Normalized Cw and Lw did not differ between the groups, whereas BC and node degree of the MST differed, although these differences did not survive correction for multiple testing using the False Discovery Rate (FDR). As an exploratory study, we may conclude that: (1) the increases and decreases observed in PLI values in lower and upper alpha bands in MCI patients may be interpreted as a dual pattern of disconnection and aberrant functioning; (2) network measures are in line with connectivity findings, indicating a lower efficiency of the brain networks in MCI patients; (3) the MST centrality measures are more sensitive to detect subtle differences in the functional brain networks in MCI than traditional graph theoretical metrics.

Keywords: mild cognitive impairment, magnetoencephalography, phase lag index, brain networks, minimum spanning tree

INTRODUCTION

Mild Cognitive Impairment

Mild cognitive impairment (MCI) is an intermediate state between normal aging and dementia. Patients suffering from MCI have an increased risk of developing dementia, in particular Alzheimer's disease (AD; Shah et al., 2000; Farias et al., 2005). Those MCI subjects with positive biomarkers for AD (i.e., amyloid deposition and neural injury markers such as accumulations of intracellular tau or medial temporal lobe atrophy [MTA]) are regarded to be at the symptomatic pre-dementia phase of AD, and are often referred to as "MCI due to AD" (Albert et al., 2011). The pathological processes that these biomarkers indicate are well described in AD (Braak and Braak, 1991) and are known to produce synaptic disruptions. AD has been described as a "disconnection syndrome," not only at the cellular level, but also at the macroscale, since the connections in the brain networks also seem to be disrupted (Blennow et al., 1996; Selkoe, 2002; Delbeuck et al., 2003; Arendt, 2009; Takahashi et al., 2010). In fact, structural and functional changes have been described in MCI subjects, suggesting that this disconnection of brain networks already begins during the MCI-stage of AD (Pijnenburg et al., 2004; Koenig et al., 2005; Buldú et al., 2011; Wang et al., 2013).

Functional Connectivity

One of the main concepts used to understand how the different brain areas interact is functional connectivity (Friston, 1994), which reflects the statistical interdependencies between two-time series of physiological activity. Several resting-state electroencephalography (EEG) and magnetoencephalography (MEG) studies have found decreases in functional connectivity, especially in higher frequency bands (i.e., alpha and beta bands), in MCI patients compared to healthy controls (Moretti et al., 2008; Gómez et al., 2009; López et al., 2014b; Cuesta et al., 2015). This change in synchronization pattern is quite similar to that described for AD patients (Stam and van Dijk, 2002; Jeong, 2004; Stam et al., 2006), although increased connectivity has also been described for AD involving posterior brain regions (Stam et al., 2006; Alonso et al., 2011). Reductions in functional connectivity in MCI have also been observed between regions of the default mode network (DMN), with a parallel disruption of the anatomical connections (Garcés et al., 2014; Pineda-Pardo et al., 2014). However, some resting-state studies comparing different MCI groups have also detected a specific hypersynchronization pattern in high frequency bands (alpha and beta) in those MCI subjects who finally developed AD (López et al., 2014a), or those who presented abnormal concentration of phospho-tau (p-tau) protein in the cerebrospinal fluid (CSF; Canuet et al., 2015). In a recent multicenter study, this profile of hypersynchronization was used to obtain a high percentage of correct classification of MCI and healthy controls (Maestú et al., 2015).

Brain Networks

Based on the estimated functional connectivity between time series, a weighted network can be reconstructed using graph theory (Bullmore and Sporns, 2009). For this purpose, brain systems are described as sets of nodes (i.e., brain regions or sensors) and links (i.e., functional connections between nodes). The topology of these networks can then be characterized, for example, providing information about the local integration of the network (e.g., the "clustering coefficient") as well as the global integration (e.g., the "path length"; see Rubinov and Sporns, 2010 for a review). A small-world network has a high local connectedness (quantified by a large clustering coefficient) and a high global integration (quantified by a short path length) and has been regarded as a network with an optimal topology for the transfer of information. AD patients exhibit brain networks that appear to have a sub-optimal topology in which the networks have shifted toward a more random configuration. This was mainly characterized by a loss of small-worldness (see Tijms et al., 2013 for a review), supporting the hypothesis of the disconnection syndrome. However, Tijms et al. (2013) also show that the results differ drastically between studies. Only few studies, using different approaches and modalities, have explored the network topology in MCI, reporting a disturbed balance between local and global integration [functional Magnetic Resonance imaging (fMRI); Wang et al., 2013; MEG; Buldú et al., 2011; Pineda-Pardo et al., 2014]. Methodological difficulties make the comparison between networks of different sizes and different edge densities challenging, if not impossible (Lee et al., 2006; van Wijk et al., 2010; Stam, 2014; Tewarie et al., 2015). This might lead to contradicting results that could be due to differences in modalities (Tijms et al., 2013), but also due to methodological biases (van Wijk et al., 2010). One solution is to reconstruct the minimum spanning tree (MST; Stam, 2014). The MST is a sub-graph of the complete network, which forms a backbone of the original graph. It is uniquely defined whilst avoiding the arbitrary choices of traditional approaches, therefore solving the limitations of previous graph studies (van Wijk et al., 2010; Tewarie et al., 2015). Despite its advantages and application in other neurological disorders (Ortega et al., 2008; Fraschini et al., 2014; Olde Dubbelink et al., 2014; Otte et al., 2015; Tewarie et al., 2015), there is only one fMRI study and one EEG study that has used the MST in comparing healthy elders and AD patients (Çiftçi, 2011; Engels et al., 2015), and none that studied the MST in patients with MCI.

For this reason, we performed an MEG study with MCIs and healthy controls with the aim to characterize how the functional network organization in the MCI stage differs from that of controls. To this end, we estimated MEG resting-state functional connectivity between cortical regions and characterized the topology of the reconstructed MST. We expected to find subtle differences in functional connectivity between MCI patients and controls while the graph theoretical measures will show a clear disrupted topological pattern in MCI. We expected that the novel MST measures give more insight in the network changes of MCI than the traditional network measures (normalized Cw and normalized Lw).

MATERIALS AND METHODS

Subjects

Magnetoencephalography recordings were obtained from 58 subjects (29 MCI patients and 29 healthy elderly subjects). The MCI group was recruited from the Hospital Universitario San Carlos (Madrid), and the control group from the Seniors Center of the District of Chamartin (Madrid). All subjects were right handed (Oldfield, 1971) and native Spanish speakers.

All participants were screened by means of standardized diagnostic instruments and also received an exhaustive neuropsychological assessment. To evaluate their global and cognitive functional status there were used: the Spanish version of the Mini-Mental State Examination (MMSE; Lobo et al., 1979), the Global Deterioration Scale (GDS; Reisberg et al., 1982), the Functional Assessment Questionnaire (FAQ; Pfeffer et al., 1982), the Geriatric Depression Scale-Short Form (GDS-SF; Yesavage et al., 1982), the Hachinski Ischemic Score (Rosen et al., 1980), the questionnaire for Instrumental Activities of Daily Living (Lawton and Brody, 1969), and the Functional Assessment Staging (FAST; Auer and Reisberg, 1997).

Additionally, all subjects underwent an extensive neuropsychological assessment to explore their cognitive functioning by using the following tests: direct and inverse digit span test (DDS and IDS, Wechsler Memory Scale III, WMS-III; Wechsler, 1997), immediate and delayed recall (IR and DR, WMS-III; Wechsler, 1997), phonemic and semantic fluency (PhF and SF, controlled oral word association test; Benton and Hamsher, 1989), ideomotor praxis of Barcelona test (IP; Peña-Casanova, 1990), Visual Object and Space Perception Test (VOSP; Warrington and James, 1991), Boston Naming Test (BNT; Kaplan et al., 1983), and Trail-Making Test (TMT), parts A and B (TMT-A and TMT-B; Reitan, 1958).

The MCI diagnosis was established according to the National Institute on Aging- Alzheimer Association (NIA-AA) criteria (Albert et al., 2011), which includes: (i) self- or informant-reported cognitive complaints; (ii) objective evidence of impairment in one or more cognitive domains; (iii) preserved independence in functional abilities; and (iv) not demented (McKhann et al., 2011). Besides meeting the clinical criteria, MCI participants had signs of neuronal injury (hippocampal volume measured by magnetic resonance imaging (MRI). So, they might be considered as "MCI due to AD" with an intermediate likelihood (Albert et al., 2011).

None of the participants had a history of psychiatric or neurological disorders (other than MCI). General inclusion criteria were: an age between 65 and 80, a modified Hachinski score $\leq$ 4, a short-form Geriatric Depression Scale score $\leq$ 5, and T1/T2-weighted MRI within 12 months and 2 weeks before MEG screening without indication of infection, infarction, or focal lesions (rated by two independent experienced radiologists; Bai et al., 2012). Patients were off those medications that could affect MEG activity, such as cholinesterase inhibitors, 48 h before recordings.

Ethics Statement

Methods were carried out in accordance with the approved guidelines. The study was approved by the Hospital Universitario San Carlos Ethics Committee (Madrid), and all participants signed a written informed consent prior to participation.

MEG Acquisition

Magnetoencephalography signals were measured by a 306 channel Vectorview system (Elekta Neuromag Oy) at the Center for Biomedical Technology (Madrid, Spain), inside a magnetically shielded room (VacuumSchmelze GmbH, Hanau, Germany) within several days after the neuropsychological assessment. Brain magnetic fields were recorded in the morning during a task-free 3 min eyes-closed resting-state condition, while subjects sat comfortably. Participants were instructed to move as little as possible, and were monitored during the recording to ensure that they did not fall asleep.

Sampling frequency was 1000 Hz with an online filter with bandwidth 0.1–300 Hz. The position of the head inside the sensor array was determined using a head-position indicator (HPI) with four coils attached to the scalp (two on the mastoids and two on the forehead). These four coils along with the head shape ($\sim$500 points) of each subject (referenced to three anatomical fiducials: nasion, and left-right preauricular points) were acquired using a three-dimensional Fastrak Polhemus system (manufacturer: Polhemus, Inc., USA). Vertical ocular movements were measured by two bipolar electrodes attached above and below the left eye, and a third one to the earlobe, for electrical grounding.

Maxfilter software (version 2.2, Elekta Neuromag Oy) was used to remove noise from the MEG data using the temporal extension of signal space separation (tSSS) with movement compensation (Taulu and Simola, 2006). Flat channels, or those that contained excessive artifacts, were manually discarded after visual inspection of the data by one of the authors (M. E. López) before estimation of the SSS coefficients. The tSSS filter was subsequently used to remove noise signals that SSS failed to discard, typically from noise sources near the head, using a subspace correlation limit of 0.9 (Medvedovsky et al., 2009) and a sliding window of 10 s.

MRI Acquisition

3D T1 weighted anatomical brain MRI scans were collected with a General Electric 1.5T MRI scanner, using a high resolution antenna and a homogenization PURE filter [Fast Spoiled Gradient Echo (FSPGR) sequence with parameters: TR/TE/TI = 11.2/4.2/450 ms; flip angle 12°; 1 mm slice thickness, a 256 × 256 matrix and FOV 25 cm].

FreeSurfer software (version 5.1.0; Fischl et al., 2002) was used to obtain the hippocampal volumes, which were normalized with the overall intracranial volume (ICV) of each subject.

Co-registration and Beamforming

The outline of the scalp, as obtained from the subject's structural MRI, was used for co-registration with the MEG data using the VUmc Amsterdam co-registration surface matching software, resulting in an estimated co-registration accuracy of approximately 4 mm (Whalen et al., 2008). A single sphere fitted to the scalp surface was used as a volume conductor model for the beamformer analysis. An atlas-based beamformer was used to project the MEG sensor signals to 78 cortical regions-of-interest (ROIs) from the Automatic Anatomical Labeling (AAL) atlas (see Supplementary Material) (Tzourio-Mazoyer et al., 2002; Gong et al., 2009). Based on the broad-band (0.5–48 Hz) beamformer weights, time series of neuronal activity were reconstructed for the voxel with the maximum power within a ROI for each frequency band separately, i.e., a virtual electrode that was representative for that specific ROI was reconstructed. A detailed description of this procedure is given in Hillebrand et al. (2012).

MEG Analysis

Per subject, five artifact free trials of approximately 16.384 s (four times 4096 samples) were selected after careful visual inspection, giving a total of 20 epochs of 4096 samples for further analysis. Time-series of neuronal activation were computed for the six frequency bands: delta (0.5–4 Hz), theta (4–8 Hz), lower alpha (8–10 Hz), upper alpha (10–13 Hz), beta (13–30 Hz), and gamma (30–48 Hz). Selected epochs were converted to ASCII-files and imported into an in-house developed software package BrainWave version 0.9.125, developed by one of the authors (C. J. Stam) and available at: http://home.kpn.nl/stam7883/brainwave.html.

Functional Connectivity

Functional connectivity was assessed with the PLI, which quantifies the consistency of a phase relationship between two signals while zero-lag (mod π) phase differences are ignored (Stam et al., 2007b). Therefore, the PLI is insensitive to spurious interactions caused by the effects of volume conduction and/or field spread (Stam et al., 2007b; Hillebrand et al., 2012). The PLI ranges between 0 and 1 in which 0 represents no consistent coupling or coupling with zero-lag and one represents consistent phase-lagged coupling. First, the instantaneous phase for each time series is computed by taking the argument of the analytic signal (Stam et al., 2007b) as computed using the Hilbert transform. Second, we calculate the asymmetry of the distribution of instantaneous phase differences between two time series:

$$\text{PLI} = |<\text{sign}[\sin(\Delta\Phi_t)]>| \quad (1)$$

where the phase difference $\Delta\Phi_t$ is defined in the interval $[-\pi, \pi]$, $<>$ denotes the mean value, sign stands for signum function, $| |$ indicates the absolute value, and t corresponds to time samples 1, . . ., Ns, where Ns is the number of samples. By calculating the PLI values between all pairs of ROIs, we obtained a 78 × 78 adjacency matrix, which we used for the network analyses (see below).

Small-Worldness

A low characteristic path length (L) and a high clustering coefficient (C) characterize a small-world network (Watts and Strogatz, 1998). In an unweighted network, the C represents the probability that two nodes are connected when they share a neighboring node and the L represents the average of the shortest distance between pairs of nodes, with distance defined by the number of links between nodes. From the weighted graph, the weighted clustering coefficient (Cw) and weighted characteristic path length (Lw) were calculated as described in Stam et al. (2007a). Fifty random control networks were created by randomly shuffling the PLI values in each adjacency matrix while keeping the matrix symmetry intact. For each ensemble of 50 random networks, the average Cw (random) and Lw (random) were computed. The observed network values were divided by the average values obtained for the random networks in order to create normalized values. The resulting normalized clustering coefficient (normalized Cw) and normalized path length (normalized Lw) were used for further analyses. These measures were computed for each epoch, and then averaged over the epochs for each subject.

Minimum Spanning Tree

We constructed the MST from the weighted adjacency matrix containing the PLI values. The MST is a unique subgraph that connects all nodes in the network by the strongest connections (defined as the network links with the highest PLI values) without forming cycles (Stam et al., 2014), and was reconstructed using Kruskal's algorithm (Kruskal, 1956). By using 1/PLI as input to the algorithm, strongest connections are likely to be included in the MST, as long as no cycles are formed. The MST was characterized by the following measures: degree, betweenness centrality (BC), eccentricity, degree distribution (κ), the number of leafs, degree correlation (R), tree hierarchy and diameter. MST measures were computed for each epoch, and then averaged over the epochs for each subject. The degree describes how many links each node has. BC is a measure of the importance of a node within the network. The BC of node i is defined as the number of shortest paths in the network that run through a specific node, divided by the total number of shortest paths from any node to all other nodes in the MST. In our calculations, we used the maximum BC across all nodes as well as per node for further testing. The eccentricity of a node is defined as the longest distance between that node and any other node in the network. The degree distribution is formed by the likelihood (P) that a randomly chosen node of the network will have degree κ (the number of connections of a specific node); it is a plot of P(κ) as a function of κ (Stam and Reijneveld, 2007). The degree correlation is an index of how much the degree of a node is correlated to the degree of nodes it is connected to. The leaf number is the number of nodes that have a degree of 1 representing the "leafs" or "extremities" of the network. Tree hierarchy quantifies the trade-off between large scale integration in the MST and the overload of central nodes. The diameter represents the longest path in the MST. For more information about these measures, we refer to Boersma et al. (2013), Stam et al. (2014), Tewarie et al. (2015).

Statistical Analysis

Subject's characteristics were tested using independent samples t-tests or chi-square tests where appropriate using SPSS (20.0 for windows). For the PLI, permutation testing, based upon t-statistics, was used for each pair of regions [among the 78 studied, (78 × 77)/2 in total], and in each frequency band, with the aim of comparing both groups (Maris and Oostenveld, 2007).

To this end, participants were randomly divided into two sets with the same size as the original groups (29 vs. 29 subjects). This procedure was repeated 2000 times (2000 permutations). A new t-test between each pair of regions [(78 × 77)/2 couples] in each frequency band, was then carried out using these two newly created groups, getting a t-value for each pair of regions and each frequency band. After sorting these 2001 t-test results [2000 corresponding to "randomly divided" groups and another one for the original (MCI vs. Control) subject's distribution], only p-values within the 5% of lower values were considered statistically significant [note that this is for each pair of regions and each frequency band studied: hence it was repeated ((78 × 77)/2) × (number of frequency bands) times]. These analyses were uncorrected for the number of permutations performed and therefore serve as exploratory analyses (see **Figures 1, 2** and **Tables 2, 3**). Afterward, we performed an FDR correction on the data with the goal to examine the statistical significant results that survive a multiple comparison correction. For the network analysis, we focused on those frequency bands in which the connectivity analyses showed (uncorrected) significant differences between the groups. Again, corrected and uncorrected (exploratory) permutation testing was used to compare the groups. All statistical analyses were performed using MATLAB (R2015b, Mathworks).

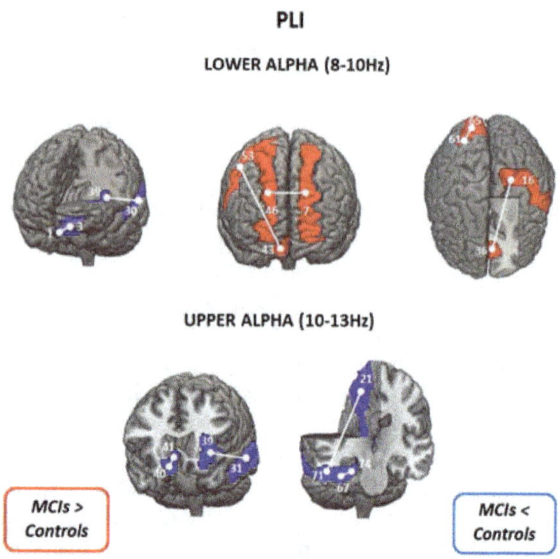

FIGURE 1 | Statistical differences between controls and MCIs in lower alpha (upper panel) and upper alpha (lower panel) bands in PLI values (uncorrected for multiple comparisons). When MCI group show lower connectivity values than the control group is represented in blue: left gyrus rectus (1) – left superior frontal gyrus (3); left superior temporal gyrus (30) – left insula (39) for the lower alpha band; and left insula (39) – left middle temporal gyrus (31); right gyrus rectus (40) – right olfactory cortex (41); left precuneus (21) – right inferior temporal gyrus (71); right fusiform gyrus (67) – right parahippocampal gyrus for the upper alpha band. On the contrary, when MCI group exhibit higher PLI values than the control group is represented in red: left superior frontal gyrus (dorsolateral) (7) – right superior frontal gyrus (dorsolateral) (46); right superior frontal gyrus (medial orbital) (43) – right precentral gyrus (53) – left postcentral gyrus (16) – left anterior cingulate and paracingulate gyri (36) – right superior occipital gyrus (61) – right cuneus (65) for the lower alpha band. AAL numbers appear in parentheses.

RESULTS

Demographics

Subject characteristics are shown in **Table 1**. Controls and MCI patients did not differ in age, gender, or educational level. As expected, the scores of MMSE and two measures of episodic memory (immediate and delayed recall) were both lower in MCI patients compared to controls. Additionally, hippocampal volumes were both lower in the MCI group.

Functional Connectivity

Significant differences between MCI patients and controls in PLI using the uncorrected permutation tests were obtained in the lower (8–10 Hz) and upper (10–13 Hz) alpha band (**Figure 1**). In the lower alpha band, compared to the control group, PLI in the MCI group was lower between left superior frontal gyrus -orbital part- and left gyrus rectus, and between left superior temporal gyrus and left insula ($p < 0.01$). Additionally, in the same frequency band, MCI subjects showed higher PLI values than controls between four regions, namely between right superior frontal gyrus (medial orbital) and right precentral gyrus, right superior frontal gyrus (dorsolateral) and left superior frontal gyrus (dorsolateral), left anterior cingulate and paracingulate gyri and left postcentral gyrus, and between right cuneus and right superior occipital gyrus.

TABLE 1 | Subject's characteristics (Control group, $n = 29$; MCI group, $n = 29$).

	Group	Mean ± SD	p-values
Age (years)	Control	70.62 ± 3.913	0.766*
	MCI	72.55 ± 4.163	
Gender (M/F)	Control	10/19 ± 0.484	0.096**
	MCI	15/14 ± 0.509	
Educational level	Control	3.72 ± 1.162	0.202*
	MCI	2.68 ± 1.362	
MMSE	Control	29.38 ± 0.68	<0.001*
	MCI	27.21 ± 1.75	
Immediate recall	Control	39.14 ± 8.05	<0.001*
	MCI	18.11 ± 10.03	
Delayed recall	Control	24.83 ± 7.18	<0.001*
	MCI	7.59 ± 8.35	
RH_ICV	Control	0.0026 ± 0.0003	0.004*
	MCI	0.0021 ± 0.0006	
LH_ICV	Control	0.0025 ± 0.0003	0.006*
	MCI	0.0022 ± 0.0005	

Mean ± standard deviation (SD) and p-values. The p-values were obtained by two-independent samples t-test (*) or chi-square test (**) where relevant. M, male; F, female; MMSE, Mini Mental State Examination score; RH_ICV and LH_ICV, right and left hippocampal volume normalized with intracranial volume, respectively. Highest education completed, using five levels: (1) Illiterate, (2) Primary studies, (3) Elemental studies, (4) High school studies, and (5) University studies.

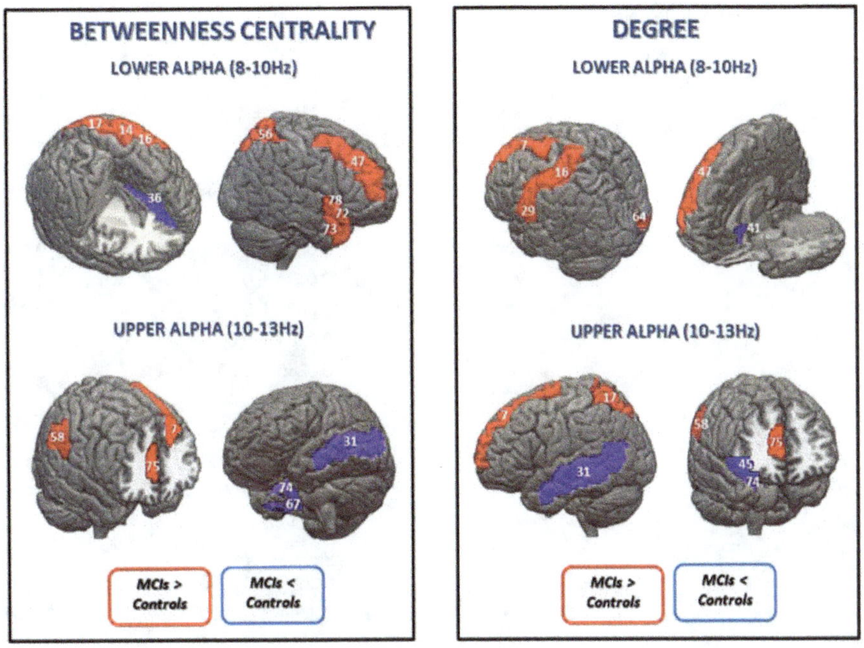

FIGURE 2 | Statistical differences between the control group and the MCI group in betweenness centrality (BC) (Left) and degree (Right) in lower and upper alpha bands (uncorrected for multiple comparisons). Blue is represented when MCIs exhibit lower BC values than the control group in: left anterior cingulate and paracingulate gyri (36) for lower alpha band; left middle temporal gyrus (31), right fusiform gyrus (67) and right parahippocampal gyrus (74) for the upper alpha band; and in degree values in: right olfactory cortex (41) for the lower alpha band; left middle temporal gyrus (31), right inferior frontal gyrus, orbital part (45) and right parahippocampal gyrus (74) for the upper alpha band. Red is represented when the MCI present higher BC values in: left precentral gyrus (14), left postcentral gyrus (16); left superior parietal gyrus (17), right middle frontal gyrus (47), right superior parietal gyrus (56), right temporal pole: superior temporal gyrus (72), right temporal pole: middle temporal gyrus (73) and right Insula for the lower alpha band; left superior frontal gyrus, dorsolateral (7), right supramarginal gyrus (58), and right anterior cingulate and paracingulate gyri (75) for the upper alpha band; and higher degree values in: left superior frontal gyrus, dorsolateral (7), left postcentral gyrus (16), left Heschl gyrus (29) and right middle frontal gyrus (47) for the lower alpha band; left superior frontal gyrus, dorsolateral (7), left superior parietal gyrus (17), right supramarginal gyrus (58) and right anterior cingulate and paracingulate gyri (75) for the upper alpha band. AAL numbers appear in parentheses.

Furthermore, in the upper alpha band, MCI subjects presented lower PLI values than controls between four regions, namely between right gyrus rectus and right olfactory cortex, left insula and left middle temporal gyrus, right parahippocampal gyrus and right fusiform gyrus, and right inferior temporal gyrus and left precuneus.

After FDR-correction for multiple comparisons, none of these significant differences survived.

Small-worldness

We focused the network analysis on those frequency bands in which there were differences in connectivity, namely in lower and upper alpha bands.

Using the uncorrected permutation tests, no differences between controls and MCI subjects were found for normalized Cw and normalized Lw.

Minimum Spanning Tree

We found group differences in BC and degree in lower and upper alpha bands using the uncorrected permutation tests (see below).

Betweenness centrality results are shown in **Figure 2** and **Table 2**. In the lower alpha band, there were no differences between controls and MCI patients in the maximum value of BC globally. However, compared to the healthy controls, the MCI group showed higher BC values in eight brain areas: the left pre- and post-central gyri, the left and right superior parietal gyri, the right middle frontal gyrus, the right superior and middle temporal gyrus (temporal pole) and the right insula; and lower values in one brain area: the left anterior cingulated/paracingulate gyri (see Supplementary Material).

In the upper alpha band, we did not find global differences between the groups, but there were differences in BC for specific brain areas. Compared to controls, MCIs exhibited higher values in three brain areas: the left superior frontal gyrus dorsolateral (lSFGdor), the right supramarginal gyrus (rSMG), and the right anterior cingulate/paracingulate gyri (rACG); and lower BC values in three brain areas: the left middle temporal gyrus (lMTG), the right fusiform gyrus (rFFG) and the right parahippocampal gyrus (rPHG).

Finally, the MCI group showed higher MST degree values than controls in the lower alpha band in five brain areas: the left superior frontal gyrus, dorsolateral, the left postcentral gyrus, the left Heschl gyrus, the right middle frontal gyrus and the right calcarine fissure and surrounding cortex; while they exhibited a lower degree value in one brain area: the right olfactory cortex. In the upper alpha band, MCI subjects exhibited higher degree values in four brain areas: the left superior frontal gyrus, dorsolateral, the left superior parietal gyrus, the rSMG and the

TABLE 2 | Mean ± standard deviation (SD) of the betweenness centrality (BC) in the lower and upper alpha band, *p*-values were obtained using permutation testing without correction for multiple comparisons across regions.

MST BC				
Name of the area	**Group**	**Mean ± *SD***	***p*-values**	**Change**
Lower alpha band				
Left precentral gyrus (lPreCG)	Control	0.0454 ± 0.0039	0.034	↑MCI
	MCI	0.0703 ± 0.0050		
Left postcentral gyrus (lPoCG)	Control	0.0363 ± 0.0016	0.035	↑MCI
	MCI	0.0636 ± 0.0035		
Left superior parietal gyrus (lSPG)	Control	0.0629 ± 0.0043	0.037	↑MCI
	MCI	0.0984 ± 0.0050		
Right middle frontal gyrus (rMFG)	Control	0.0266 ± 0.0013	0.041	↑MCI
	MCI	0.0595 ± 0.0043		
Right superior parietal gyrus (rSPG)	Control	0.2978 ± 0.0097	0.012	↑MCI
	MCI	0.3627 ± 0.0068		
Right temporal pole: superior temporal gyrus (rTPOsup)	Control	0.2673 ± 0.0032	0.012	↑MCI
	MCI	0.3118 ± 0.0041		
Right temporal pole: middle temporal gyrus (rTPOmid)	Control	0.2561 ± 0.0027	0.003	↑MCI
	MCI	0.3019 ± 0.0036		
Right insula (rINS)	Control	0.2644 ± 0.0020	0.032	↑MCI
	MCI	0.3079 ± 0.0067		
Left anterior cingulate and paracingulate gyri (lACG)	Control	0.1077 ± 0.0037	0.002	↓MCI
	MCI	0.0629 ± 0.0034		
Upper alpha band				
Left superior frontal gyrus, dorsolateral (lSFGdor)	Control	0.0443 ± 0.0034	0.018	↑MCI
	MCI	0.0897 ± 0.0079		
Right supramarginal gyrus (rSMG)	Control	0.0593 ± 0.0055	0.012	↑MCI
	MCI	0.0967 ± 0.0059		
Right anterior cingulate and paracingulate gyri (rACG)	Control	0.0320 ± 0.0012	0.014	↑MCI
	MCI	0.0722 ± 0.0040		
Left middle temporal gyrus (lMTG)	Control	0.0998 ± 0.0096	0.014	↓MCI
	MCI	0.0414 ± 0.0017		
Right fusiform gyrus (rFFG)	Control	0.0824 ± 0.0032	0.048	↓MCI
	MCI	0.0586 ± 0.0035		
Right parahippocampal gyrus (rPHG)	Control	0.0904 ± 0.0044	0.004	↓MCI
	MCI	0.0539 ± 0.0057		

Arrows indicate lower or higher values in the MCI group.

right anterior cingulate and paracingulate gyri; and lower degree values in three brain areas: the lMTG, the right inferior frontal gyrus, orbital part and the rPHG. MST degree results are shown in **Figure 2** and **Table 3**.

After FDR-correction for multiple comparisons, none of these significant differences survived. Also, we did not find any differences between the controls and the MCI group for any of the other MST measures in these two frequency bands.

DISCUSSION

With the aim to corroborate our hypothesis about the differences in both functional connectivity and network organization between healthy aging and MCI, we performed a functional connectivity (PLI) and MST analyses in resting state MEG data. The main finding of this study was the detection of differences in both functional connectivity and brain network topology in a group of patients with MCI compared to controls. Note however, that these results are exploratory and the significance between the groups did not survive FDR correction for multiple comparisons. The uncorrected connectivity results showed that the MCI patients exhibited more increases than decreases in PLI values in the lower alpha band, and decreases in the upper alpha band. As differences in connectivity between both groups were found in the alpha band, we examined differences of network's topography in this frequency band by using concepts from graph theory. We did not find any group difference in weighted clustering and path length, but regionally we obtained higher BC and degree values when examining the MST in the MCI group in lower alpha band, and both increases and decreases in the upper alpha band.

Mild cognitive impairment patients demonstrated lower PLI values in the lower alpha band that affected frontal and temporal brain areas within the left hemisphere. Using EEG, an overall decrease in the lower alpha band has been observed in AD

TABLE 3 | Mean ± standard deviation (SD) and *p*-values after a *t*-test without correction for multiple comparisons for degree values in the control group compared with the MCI group in lower and upper alpha bands.

MST DEGREE				
Name of the area	**Group**	**Mean ± *SD***	***p*-values**	**Change**
Lower alpha band				
Left superior frontal gyrus, dorsolateral (lSFGdor)	Control	$0.0221 \pm 8.3 \times 10^{-5}$	0.007	↑MCI
	MCI	$0.0272 \pm 8.5 \times 10^{-5}$		
Left postcentral gyrus (lPoCG)	Control	$0.0204 \pm 3.7 \times 10^{-5}$	0.010	↑MCI
	MCI	$0.0247 \pm 4.8 \times 10^{-5}$		
Left Heschl gyrus (lHES)	Control	$0.0244 \pm 8.2 \times 10^{-5}$	0.038	↑MCI
	MCI	$0.0302 \pm 1.2 \times 10^{-4}$		
Right middle frontal gyrus (rMFG)	Control	$0.0186 \pm 3.3 \times 10^{-5}$	0.008	↑MCI
	MCI	$0.0238 \pm 7.1 \times 10^{-5}$		
Right calcarine fissure and surrounding cortex (rCAL)	Control	0.2559 ± 0.0041	0.022	↑MCI
	MCI	0.2966 ± 0.0052		
Right olfactory cortex (rOLF)	Control	$0.0280 \pm 8.2 \times 10^{-5}$	0.044	↓MCI
	MCI	$0.0230 \pm 5.3 \times 10^{-5}$		
Upper alpha band				
Left superior frontal gyrus, dorsolateral (lSFGdor)	Control	$0.0224 \pm 9.9 \times 10^{-5}$	0.035	↑MCI
	MCI	$0.0278 \pm 1.3 \times 10^{-4}$		
Left superior parietal gyrus (lSPG)	Control	$0.0242 \pm 9.2 \times 10^{-5}$	0.021	↑MCI
	MCI	$0.\ 0320 \pm 2.2 \times 10^{-4}$		
Right supramarginal gyrus (rSMG)	Control	$0.0243 \pm 1.0 \times 10^{-4}$	0.049	↑MCI
	MCI	$0.0291 \pm 9.7 \times 10^{-5}$		
Right anterior cingulate and paracingulate gyri (rACG)	Control	$0.0196 \pm 1.2 \times 10^{-5}$	0.043	↑MCI
	MCI	$0.0241 \pm 7.5 \times 10^{-5}$		
Left middle temporal gyrus (lMTG)	Control	$0.0297 \pm 2 \times 10^{-4}$	0.030	↓MCI
	MCI	$0.0220 \pm 5.6 \times 10^{-5}$		
Right inferior frontal gyrus, orbital part (rORBinf)	Control	$0.0266 \pm 8.5 \times 10^{-5}$	0.023	↓MCI
	MCI	$0.0213 \pm 1.7 \times 10^{-5}$		
Right parahippocampal gyrus (rPHG)	Control	$0.0255 \pm 6.5 \times 10^{-5}$	0.008	↓MCI
	MCI	$0.0211 \pm 9 \times 10^{-5}$		

Arrows indicate lower and higher values in the MCI group.

patients (Stam et al., 2006, 2009), and also in MCI patients (Babiloni et al., 2006). In a recent study performed with EEG data in AD (Engels et al., 2015), the decrease of connectivity in the lower alpha band was related to the severity of the disease, mainly over posterior areas. However, in the present study, MCI patients also showed an increase in connectivity between intra- and inter-hemispheric frontal areas, and in right posterior regions. This intra- and inter-hemispheric increase in connectivity has been usually described in the MCI population while performing a cognitive task. Pijnenburg et al. (2004) found an increase in lower alpha band in MCIs compared to subjects with subjective memory complaints (SMC) during a visual working memory (WM) task. Jiang (2005) and Zheng et al. (2007) obtained higher coherence values in both lower and upper alpha bands during an arithmetic WM paradigm in MCIs compared to healthy controls. In addition, an MEG study performed in progressive MCI patients (pMCI) found a higher synchronization in those patients who finally developed AD, compared with those who remained stable over time (stable MCI, sMCI), in lower alpha and upper alpha bands while performing a memory task (Bajo et al., 2012). In the same vein, a recent resting-state MEG study which did not divide the alpha band into two sub-bands, found that patients with MCI that eventually converted to AD, exhibited a higher connectivity in this frequency range than those MCI patients that remained stable over time, between the right anterior cingulate and temporo-occipital brain regions (López et al., 2014a). Our findings add to the current knowledge that results of functional connectivity in MCI patients are dependent on the region and on the frequency band. However, there is no consistent increase or decrease in connectivity in patients with MCI compared to controls during resting state. Therefore, we conclude that, the increases and decreases of functional connections observed in the MCI population in the lower alpha band may reflect the aberrant functioning until the breakdown of the system, which characterizes AD.

The increase in PLI values found in the lower alpha band in patients with MCI has been commonly considered as a compensatory mechanism. This interpretation was related to the attempt of the brain to overcome the damage caused by the disease in the networks involved in cognitive functioning (see Grady, 2012; Scheller et al., 2014 for reviews). In the case of healthy controls, this mechanism would not be needed while AD patients would not compensate any more due to the severity of the disease. Nonetheless, recent studies postulated that instead of being a compensatory mechanism, it would be a pathological characteristic of MCI patients (de Haan et al., 2012; López et al., 2014a,b). During the course of the disease, there is a loss of GABAergic synapsis caused by the accumulation of β-amyloid (Aβ) plaques (Garcia-Marin et al., 2009), producing an inhibitory deficit. The loss of inhibitory interneurons in the cortex would induce increasing brain activity/connectivity in MCI patients, leading to an aberrant functioning (disinhibition) until the breakdown of the system, which is what occurs in AD.

In agreement with what has previously been described in some AD studies (Stam et al., 2002; Pijnenburg et al., 2004), we obtained lower connectivity values in the MCI group in the upper alpha band mainly concerning temporal and parietal brain areas. As far as we know, no studies have been performed describing this finding in MCI. However, considering the alpha band as one (normally from 8 to 13 Hz), some authors have revealed this decrease in connectivity in MCI patients compared to controls (Koenig et al., 2005; Garcés et al., 2014; Cuesta et al., 2015). Our results point out that networks that are usually implicated in episodic memory, olfactory function, visuospatial processing or executive functioning (previously described in the Results section) are already impaired in MCI patients. These results may indicate that in MCI the disconnection that characterizes AD would have already started, probably contributing to the cognitive deficits observed in this population. According to the increases and decreases obtained in PLI values, which have been also described in previous studies, it might be considered that during the symptomatic pre-dementia phase of AD, two mechanisms could be coexisting in MCI: disconnection and aberrant functioning.

To elucidate about the meaning of this duality of hyper and hypo connectivity we decided to evaluate the functional network organization using the network theory approach. We started with two of the most basic network parameters: the characteristic path length and the clustering coefficient. As firstly described by Watts and Strogatz (1998), these two measures together form the concept of the small-world network topology whereas the network architecture combines an efficient balance between local (short range) and global (long range) connectivity. This small-world configuration is thought to be better suited for information transfer and thus presumably for cognitive processing rather than the topology of random or regular networks (Bassett and Bullmore, 2006; Stam et al., 2007a). We did not find differences in terms of clustering and path length in our MCI cohort. In other studies, however, an increased path length and decreased clustering coefficient in MCI was found (Xiang et al., 2013; Zhang et al., 2015) and therefore MCI mimics results of AD studies (Stam et al., 2007a). MCI has been referred to as an intermediate state between healthy aging and AD in terms of their network topology (Seo et al., 2013). Our cohort did not differ in terms of the small-world parameters clustering coefficient and characteristic path length and therefore the exploration of different network measures is interesting since they may be more sensitive for the subtle changes in MCI.

Studying brain networks using measures like the clustering coefficient and the characteristic path length give useful insights within datasets of similar network sizes and link densities, but cause a comparison problem when these requirements are not met. This problem is thoroughly explained in a paper by van Wijk et al. (2010). It stresses the comparison problem between networks, not only because of the differences in network sizes (number of nodes) and degree but also due to arbitrary choices that have to be made (i.e., the threshold for the link density within a weighted network). This was the main reason for the use of the MST (Stam, 2014). Using MST, no arbitrary choices have to be made in case of unique functional connectivity values: it does not require setting a threshold and the number of nodes and links is fixed. It can be regarded as the backbone of a network (Çiftçi, 2011; Yu et al., 2015). In the present study, we found differences in two measures of centrality when comparing the MST of MCI patients and healthy controls. The MST is regarded as the backbone of a functional network since it merely involves the strongest links of the network (Stam, 2014). The MST-BC as a measure for centrality has previously shown a shifted hub location in patients with AD in high frequency bands (Engels et al., 2015). In our study, we found increased BC values in MCI patients as well as some decreases in lower and upper alpha bands. The degree, also a measure of centrality, was also found to be reduced mainly in the temporal regions. As with the functional connectivity measures, we thus found a dual pattern in the MCI population. These findings may suggest that the loss of BC/degree, mainly in temporal areas, may reflect that these areas are weakened in the brain network while frontal and parietal compensate for this malfunction. It also may reflect that some brain areas lose control within the network while others are functioning in a more aberrant way. In conclusion, although after correcting for multiple comparisons the significant differences in MST disappeared, this study showed that the classical network measures (normalized Lw and Cw) did not distinguish between MCIs and controls during resting state, but MST analysis may be a new and useful procedure to characterize and differentiate both populations. Although the reduction in centrality in temporal regions was not reported in the one study evaluating the MST BC in AD (Engels et al., 2015), this finding can be understood in the light of the disease pathology, which involves the temporal lobe. The differences between these two studies may be explained by differences in age difference (patients in our cohort were older) and therefore parietal pathology may be relatively less present (Adriaanse et al., 2012).

This study has a number of strengths and limitations. A strong point is that we used the PLI as a measure of functional connectivity since it reduces the bias due to volume conduction and/or field spread (Stam et al., 2007b). Another strong point is the use of conventional network measures (i.e., the normalized clustering coefficient and the characteristic path length), which are well described in literature, and MST parameters, that offer an arbitrary-free method for comparing networks with different properties. Our source-space analyses included 78 regions of interest according to the AAL atlas. This is a commonly used atlas, but our approach could be applied to other atlases as well. Besides these advantages, this study has several limitations as well which should be taken into account. Our results may have been influenced by methodological choices such as the selection of artifact-free epochs by one of the authors (M. M. Engels). Epochs with signs of artifacts, drowsiness were discarded. One of the other authors (M. E. López) checked the selected epochs and therefore, we expect that the epochs we have selected for our final analyses are artifact-free. An important consideration for this approach was that we did not want to apply data cleaning approaches (e.g., Delorme et al., 2006) that could modify the connectivity structure of the data, and thereby bias subsequent functional connectivity and network analyses. Consistent with our previous work, we therefore opted to rely on thorough visual inspection for the selection of artifact free data segments.

Finally, it should be pointed that our MCIs were recruited from a clinical context. Several studies have reported that it is easier to find more cases of MCIs within a clinical population and also that the rate of conversion to AD per year is higher in a clinical setting compared to the general population (Farias et al., 2005; Jelic et al., 2006). Although NIA-AA clinical criteria is standard for all subjects (Albert et al., 2011), our findings may be more representative of the clinical than the community population.

Please note that the significant differences described in this study were not corrected for multiple testing. The FDR-corrected results did not show any significant group differences. Therefore, these results are presented as an exploratory study that can be used as a guide for regions and measures that show a trend toward significance between MCI and controls.

Our results revealed differences between MCI patients and controls. These patients did not have dementia yet, although they have an increased risk of developing it. Although these patients only have minor cognitive deficits, the functional connectivity and network differences are striking, suggesting a possible causative role. Therefore, measures of functional connectivity, and the network parameters derived from these inter-areal functional connections, may help to characterize the very early stages of dementia.

AUTHOR CONTRIBUTIONS

ML performed the MEG recordings, wrote the main manuscript, and prepared the figures; ME pre-processed the MEG data, collaborated with the MEG data analysis, and wrote the main manuscript; EvS supervised the study; RB collaborated with the statistical analysis; MD collected the sample; PS supervised the study; AH collaborated with the statistical analysis and supervised the study; CS supervised the study; FM collaborated with the experimental design and supervised the study. All authors reviewed the manuscript.

ACKNOWLEDGMENTS

This study was supported by two projects from the Spanish Ministry of Economy and Competitiveness (PSI2009-14415-C03- 01 and PSI2012-38375-C03-01), and a postdoctoral fellowship to ML (FJCI-2014-22730) from the Spanish Ministry of Economy and Competitiveness.

REFERENCES

Adriaanse, S. M., Sanz-Arigita, E. J., Binnewijzend, M. A. A., Ossenkoppele, R., Tolboom, N., van Assema, D. M. E., et al. (2012). Amyloid and its association with default network integrity in Alzheimer's disease. *Hum. Brain Mapp.* 35, 779–791. doi: 10.1002/hbm.22213

Albert, M. S., DeKosky, S. T., Dickson, D., Dubois, B., Feldman, H. H., Fox, N. C., et al. (2011). The diagnosis of mild cognitive impairment due to Alzheimer's disease: recommendations from the National Institute on Aging-Alzheimer's Association workgroups on diagnostic guidelines for Alzheimer's disease. *Alzheimers Dement.* 7, 270–279. doi: 10.1016/j.jalz.2011.03.008

Alonso, J. F., Poza, J., Mañanas, M. A., Romero, S., Fernández, A., and Hornero, R. (2011). MEG connectivity analysis in patients with Alzheimer's disease using cross mutual information and spectral coherence. *Ann. Biomed. Eng.* 39, 524–536. doi: 10.1007/s10439-010-0155-7

Arendt, T. (2009). Synaptic degeneration in Alzheimer's disease. *Acta Neuropathol.* 118, 167–179. doi: 10.1007/s00401-009-0536-x

Auer, S., and Reisberg, B. (1997). The GDS/FAST staging system. *Int. Psychogeriatr.* 9(Suppl 1), 167–171. doi: 10.1017/S1041610297004869

Babiloni, C., Ferri, R., Binetti, G., Cassarino, A., Dal Forno, G., Ercolani, M., et al. (2006). Fronto-parietal coupling of brain rhythms in mild cognitive impairment: a multicentric EEG study. *Brain Res. Bull.* 69, 63–73. doi: 10.1016/j.brainresbull.2005.10.013

Bai, F., Shu, N., Yuan, Y., Shi, Y., Yu, H., Wu, D., et al. (2012). Topologically convergent and divergent structural connectivity patterns between patients with remitted geriatric depression and amnestic mild cognitive impairment. *J. Neurosci.* 32, 4307–4318. doi: 10.1523/JNEUROSCI.5061-11.2012

Bajo, R., Castellanos, N. P., Cuesta, P., Aurtenetxe, S., Garcia-Prieto, J., Gil-Gregorio, P., et al. (2012). Differential patterns of connectivity in progressive mild cognitive impairment. *Brain Connect.* 2, 21–24. doi: 10.1089/brain.2011.0069

Bassett, D. S., and Bullmore, E. (2006). Small-world brain networks. *Neuroscientist* 12, 512–523. doi: 10.1177/1073858406293182

Benton, A., and Hamsher, K. (1989). *Multilingual Aphasia Examination*, 2nd Edn. Iowa City, IA: University of Iowa.

Blennow, K., Bogdanovic, N., Alafuzoff, I., Ekman, R., and Davidsson, P. (1996). Synaptic pathology in Alzheimer's disease: relation to severity of dementia, but not to senile plaques, neurofibrillary tangles, or the ApoE4 allele. *J. Neural Transm.* 103, 603–618. doi: 10.1007/BF01273157

Boersma, M., Smit, D. J. A., Boomsma, D. I., De Geus, E. J. C., Delemarre-van de Waal, H. A., and Stam, C. J. (2013). Growing trees in child brains: graph theoretical analysis of electroencephalography-derived minimum spanning tree in 5- and 7-year-old children reflects brain maturation. *Brain Connect.* 3, 50–60. doi: 10.1089/brain.2012.0106

Braak, H., and Braak, E. (1991). Neuropathological stageing of Alzheimer-related changes. *Acta Neuropathol.* 82, 239–259.

Buldú, J. M., Bajo, R., Maestú, F., Castellanos, N., Leyva, I., Gil, P., et al. (2011). Reorganization of functional networks in mild cognitive impairment. *PLoS ONE* 6:e19584. doi: 10.1371/journal.pone.0019584

Bullmore, E., and Sporns, O. (2009). Complex brain networks: graph theoretical analysis of structural and functional systems. *Nat. Rev. Neurosci.* 10, 186–198. doi: 10.1038/nrn2575

Canuet, L., Pusil, S., Lopez, M. E., Bajo, R., Pineda-Pardo, J. A., Cuesta, P., et al. (2015). Network disruption and cerebrospinal fluid amyloid-beta and phospho-tau levels in mild cognitive impairment. *J. Neurosci.* 35, 10325–10330. doi: 10.1523/JNEUROSCI.0704-15.2015

Çiftçi, K. (2011). Minimum spanning tree reflects the alterations of the default mode network during Alzheimer's disease. *Ann. Biomed. Eng.* 39, 1493–1504. doi: 10.1007/s10439-011-0258-9

Cuesta, P., Garc, P., Aurtenetxe, S., Bajo, R., Pineda-pardo, A., Bru, R., et al. (2015). Influence of the APOE ε4 allele and mild cognitive impairment diagnosis in the disruption of the MEG resting state functional connectivity in sources space. *J. Alzheimers Dis.* 44, 493–505. doi: 10.3233/JAD-141872

de Haan, W., Mott, K., van Straaten, E. C. W., Scheltens, P., and Stam, C. J. (2012). Activity dependent degeneration explains hub vulnerability in Alzheimer's disease. *PLoS Comput. Biol.* 8:e1002582. doi: 10.1371/journal.pcbi.1002582

Delbeuck, X., Van der Linden, M., and Collette, F. (2003). Alzheimer's disease as a disconnection syndrome? *Neuropsychol. Rev.* 13, 79–92.

Delorme, A., Sejnowski, T., and Makeig, S. (2006). Enhanced detection of artifacts in EEG data using higher-order statistics and independent component analysis. *Neuroimage* 34, 1443–1449.

Engels, M. M., Stam, C. J., van der Flier, W. M., Scheltens, P., de Waal, H., and van Straaten, E. C. (2015). Declining functional connectivity and changing hub locations in Alzheimer's disease: an EEG study. *BMC Neurol.* 15:145. doi: 10.1186/s12883-015-0400-7

Farias, S. T., Mungas, D., and Jagust, W. (2005). Degree of discrepancy between self and other-reported everyday functioning by cognitive status: dementia, mild cognitive impairment, and healthy elders. *Int. J. Geriatr. Psychiatry* 9, 827–834. doi: 10.1002/gps.1367

Fischl, B., Salat, D. H., Busa, E., Albert, M., Dieterich, M., Haselgrove, C., et al. (2002). Whole brain segmentation: automated labeling of neuroanatomical structures in the human brain. *Neuron* 33, 341–355.

Fraschini, M., Demuru, M., Puligheddu, M., Floridia, S., Polizzi, L., Maleci, A., et al. (2014). The re-organization of functional brain networks in pharmaco-resistant epileptic patients who respond to VNS. *Neurosci. Lett.* 580, 153–157. doi: 10.1016/j.neulet.2014.08.010

Friston, K. J. (1994). Functional and effective connectivity in neuroimaging: a synthesis. *Hum. Brain Mapp.* 2, 56–78.

Garcés, P., Ángel Pineda-Pardo, J., Canuet, L., Aurtenetxe, S., López, M. E., Marcos, A., et al. (2014). The Default Mode Network is functionally and structurally disrupted in amnestic mild cognitive impairment — a bimodal MEG–DTI study. *Neuroimage Clin.* 6, 214–221. doi: 10.1016/j.nicl.2014.09.004

Garcia-Marin, V., Blazquez-Llorca, L., Rodriguez, J.-R., Boluda, S., Muntane, G., Ferrer, I., et al. (2009). Diminished perisomatic GABAergic terminals on cortical neurons adjacent to amyloid plaques. *Front. Neuroanat.* 3:28. doi: 10.3389/neuro.05.028.2009

Gómez, C., Stam, C. J., Hornero, R., Fernández, A., and Maestú, F. (2009). Disturbed beta band functional connectivity in patients with mild cognitive impairment: an MEG study. *IEEE Trans. Biomed. Eng.* 56, 1683–1690. doi: 10.1109/TBME.2009.2018454

Gong, G., He, Y., Concha, L., Lebel, C., Gross, D. W., Evans, A. C., et al. (2009). Mapping anatomical connectivity patterns of human cerebral cortex using in vivo diffusion tensor imaging tractography. *Cereb. Cortex* 19, 524–536. doi: 10.1093/cercor/bhn102

Grady, C. (2012). The cognitive neuroscience of ageing. *Nat. Rev. Neurosci.* 13, 491–505. doi: 10.1038/nrn3256

Hillebrand, A., Barnes, G. R., Bosboom, J. L., Berendse, H. W., and Stam, C. J. (2012). Frequency-dependent functional connectivity within resting-state networks: an atlas-based MEG beamformer solution. *Neuroimage* 59, 3909–3921. doi: 10.1016/j.neuroimage.2011.11.005

Jelic, V., Kivipelto, M., and Winblad, B. (2006). Clinical trials in mild cognitive impairment: lessons for the future. *J. Neurol. Neurosurg. Psychiatry* 77, 429–438. doi: 10.1136/jnnp.2005.072926

Jeong, J. (2004). EEG dynamics in patients with Alzheimer's disease. *Clin. Neurophysiol.* 115, 1490–1505. doi: 10.1016/j.clinph.2004.01.001

Jiang, Z. (2005). Study on EEG power and coherence in patients with mild cognitive impairment during working memory task. *J. Zhejiang Univ. Sci. B* 6, 1213–1219. doi: 10.1631/jzus.2005.B1213

Kaplan, E., Goodglass, H., and Weintraub, S. (1983). *The Boston Naming Test.* Philadelphia, PA: Lea and Febiger.

Koenig, T., Prichep, L., Dierks, T., Hubl, D., Wahlund, L. O., John, E. R., et al. (2005). Decreased EEG synchronization in Alzheimer's disease and mild cognitive impairment. *Neurobiol. Aging* 26, 165–171. doi: 10.1016/j.neurobiolaging.2004.03.008

Kruskal, J. B. (1956). On the shortest spanning subtree of a graph and the traveling salesman problem. *Proc. Am. Math. Soc.* 7, 48–50. doi: 10.2307/2033241

Lawton, M. P., and Brody, E. M. (1969). Assessment of older people: self-maintaining and instrumental activities of daily living. *Gerontologist* 9, 179–186. doi: 10.1093/geront/9.3_Part_1.179

Lee, U., Kim, S., and Jung, K.-Y. (2006). Classification of epilepsy types through global network analysis of scalp electroencephalograms. *Phys. Rev. E. Stat. Nonlin. Soft Matter Phys.* 73, 041920.

Lobo, A., Ezquerra, J., Gómez Burgada, F., Sala, J. M., and Seva Díaz, A. (1979). [Cognocitive mini-test (a simple practical test to detect intellectual changes in medical patients)]. *Actas Luso Esp. Neurol. Psiquiatr. Cienc. Afines* 7, 189–202.

López, M. E., Bruna, R., Aurtenetxe, S., Pineda-Pardo, J. A., Marcos, A., Arrazola, J., et al. (2014a). Alpha-band hypersynchronization in progressive mild cognitive impairment: a magnetoencephalography study. *J. Neurosci.* 34, 14551–14559. doi: 10.1523/JNEUROSCI.0964-14.2014

López, M. E., Garcés, P., Cuesta, P., Castellanos, N. P., Aurtenetxe, S., Bajo, R., et al. (2014b). Synchronization during an internally directed cognitive state in healthy aging and mild cognitive impairment: a MEG study. *Age* 36:9643. doi: 10.1007/s11357-014-9643-2

Maestú, F., Peña, J.-M., Garcés, P., González, S., Bajo, R., Bagic, A., et al. (2015). A multicenter study of the early detection of synaptic dysfunction in mild cognitive impairment using Magnetoencephalography-derived functional connectivity. *Neuroimage Clin.* 9, 103–109. doi: 10.1016/j.nicl.2015.07.011

Maris, E., and Oostenveld, R. (2007). Nonparametric statistical testing of EEG- and MEG-data. *J. Neurosci. Methods* 164, 177–190. doi: 10.1016/j.jneumeth.2007.03.024

McKhann, G. M., Knopman, D. S., Chertkow, H., Hyman, B. T., Jack, C. R., Kawas, C. H., et al. (2011). The diagnosis of dementia due to Alzheimer's disease: recommendations from the National Institute on Aging-Alzheimer's Association workgroups on diagnostic guidelines for Alzheimer's disease. *Alzheimers Dement.* 7, 263–269. doi: 10.1016/j.jalz.2011.03.005

Medvedovsky, M., Taulu, S., Bikmullina, R., Ahonen, A., and Paetau, R. (2009). Fine tuning the correlation limit of spatio-temporal signal space separation for magnetoencephalography. *J. Neurosci. Methods* 177, 203–211. doi: 10.1016/j.jneumeth.2008.09.035

Moretti, D. V., Frisoni, G. B., Pievani, M., Rosini, S., Geroldi, C., Binetti, G., et al. (2008). Cerebrovascular disease and hippocampal atrophy are differently linked to functional coupling of brain areas: an EEG coherence study in MCI subjects. *J. Alzheimers Dis.* 14, 285–299.

Olde Dubbelink, K. T. E., Hillebrand, A., Stoffers, D., Deijen, J. B., Twisk, J. W. R., Stam, C. J., et al. (2014). Disrupted brain network topology in Parkinson's disease: a longitudinal magnetoencephalography study. *Brain* 137, 197–207. doi: 10.1093/brain/awt316

Oldfield, R. C. (1971). The assessment and analysis of handedness: the Edinburgh inventory. *Neuropsychologia* 9, 97–113.

Ortega, G. J., Sola, R. G., and Pastor, J. (2008). Complex network analysis of human ECoG data. *Neurosci. Lett.* 447, 129–133. doi: 10.1016/j.neulet.2008.09.080

Otte, W. M., van Diessen, E., Paul, S., Ramaswamy, R., Subramanyam Rallabandi, V. P., Stam, C. J., et al. (2015). Aging alterations in whole-brain networks during adulthood mapped with the minimum spanning tree indices: the interplay of density, connectivity cost and life-time trajectory. *Neuroimage* 109, 171–189. doi: 10.1016/j.neuroimage.2015.01.011

Peña-Casanova, J. (1990). *Programa Integrado de Exploración Neuropsicológica-Test Barcelona. Protocolo.* Barcelona: Masson SA.

Pfeffer, R. I., Kurosaki, T. T., Harrah, C. H. Jr., Chance, J. M., and Filos, S. (1982). Measurement of functional activities in older adults in the community. *J. Gerontol.* 37, 323–329. doi: 10.1093/geronj/37.3.323

Pijnenburg, Y. A., v d Made, Y., Van Cappellen Van Walsum, A. M., Knol, D. L., Scheltens, P., and Stam, C. J. (2004). EEG synchronization likelihood in mild cognitive impairment and Alzheimer's disease during a working memory task. *Clin. Neurophysiol.* 115, 1332–1339.

Pineda-Pardo, J. A., Garcés, P., López, M. E., Aurtenetxe, S., Cuesta, P., Marcos, A., et al. (2014). White matter damage disorganizes brain functional networks in amnestic mild cognitive impairment. *Brain Connect.* 4, 312–322. doi: 10.1089/brain.2013.0208

Reisberg, B., Ferris, S. H., de Leon, M. J., and Crook, T. (1982). The Global Deterioration Scale for assessment of primary degenerative dementia. *Am. J. Psychiatry* 139, 1136–1139. doi: 10.1176/ajp.139.9.1136

Reitan, R. (1958). Validity of the Trail Making test as an indicator of organic brain damage. *Percept. Motor Skill* 8, 271–276.

Rosen, W. G., Terry, R. D., Fuld, P. A., Katzman, R., and Peck, A. (1980). Pathological verification of ischemic score in differentiation of dementias. *Ann. Neurol.* 7, 486–488. doi:10.1002/ana.410070516

Rubinov, M., and Sporns, O. (2010). Complex network measures of brain connectivity: uses and interpretations. *Neuroimage* 52, 1059–1069. doi: 10.1016/j.neuroimage.2009.10.003

Scheller, E., Minkova, L., Leitner, M., and Klöppel, S. (2014). Attempted and successful compensation in preclinical and early manifest neurodegeneration – a review of task fMRI Studies. *Front. Psychiatry* 5:132. doi: 10.3389/fpsyt.2014.00132

Selkoe, D. J. (2002). Alzheimer's disease is a synaptic failure. *Science* 298, 789–791. doi: 10.1126/science.1074069

Seo, E. H., Lee, D. Y., Lee, J.-M., Park, J.-S., Sohn, B. K., Choe, Y. M., et al. (2013). Influence of *APOE* genotype on whole-brain functional networks in cognitively normal elderly. *PLoS ONE* 8:e83205. doi: 10.1371/journal.pone.0083205

Shah, Y., Tangalos, E. G., and Petersen, R. C. (2000). Mild cognitive impairment. When is it a precursor to Alzheimer's disease? *Geriatrics* 55, 62, 65–68.

Stam, C. J. (2014). Modern network science of neurological disorders. *Nat. Rev. Neurosci.* 15, 683–695. doi: 10.1038/nrn3801

Stam, C. J., de Haan, W., Daffertshofer, A., Jones, B. F., Manshanden, I., van Cappellen van Walsum, A. M., et al. (2009). Graph theoretical analysis of magnetoencephalographic functional connectivity in Alzheimer's disease. *Brain* 132, 213–224. doi: 10.1093/brain/awn262

Stam, C. J., Jones, B. F., Manshanden, I., van Cappellen van Walsum, A. M., Montez, T., Verbunt, J. P. A., et al. (2006). Magnetoencephalographic evaluation of resting-state functional connectivity in Alzheimer's disease. *Neuroimage* 32, 1335–1344. doi: 10.1016/j.neuroimage.2006.05.033

Stam, C. J., Jones, B. F., Nolte, G., Breakspear, M., and Scheltens, P. (2007a). Small-world networks and functional connectivity in Alzheimer's disease. *Cereb. Cortex* 17, 92–99. doi: 10.1093/cercor/bhj127

Stam, C. J., Nolte, G., and Daffertshofer, A. (2007b). Phase lag index: assessment of functional connectivity from multi channel EEG and MEG with diminished bias from common sources. *Hum. Brain Mapp.* 28, 1178–1193. doi: 10.1002/hbm.20346

Stam, C. J., and Reijneveld, J. C. (2007). Graph theoretical analysis of complex networks in the brain. *Nonlin. Biomed. Phys.* 1:3. doi: 10.1186/1753-4631-1-3

Stam, C. J., Tewarie, P., Van Dellen, E., van Straaten, E. C. W., Hillebrand, A., and Van Mieghem, P. (2014). The trees and the forest: characterization of complex brain networks with minimum spanning trees. *Int. J. Psychophysiol.* 92, 129–138. doi: 10.1016/j.ijpsycho.2014.04.001

Stam, C. J., van Cappellen van Walsum, A. M., Pijnenburg, Y. A. L., Berendse, H. W., de Munck, J. C., Scheltens, P., et al. (2002). Generalized synchronization of MEG recordings in Alzheimer's disease: evidence for involvement of the gamma band. *J. Clin. Neurophysiol.* 19, 562–574.

Stam, C. J., and van Dijk, B. W. (2002). Synchronization likelihood: an unbiased measure of generalized synchronization in multivariate data sets. *Physica D* 163, 236–251. doi: 10.1016/S0167-2789(01)00386-4

Takahashi, R. H., Capetillo-Zarate, E., Lin, M. T., Milner, T. A., and Gouras, G. K. (2010). Co-occurrence of Alzheimer's disease ß-amyloid and τ pathologies at synapses. *Neurobiol. Aging* 31, 1145–1152. doi: 10.1016/j.neurobiolaging.2008.07.021

Taulu, S., and Simola, J. (2006). Spatiotemporal signal space separation method for rejecting nearby interference in MEG measurements. *Phys. Med. Biol.* 51, 1759–1768. doi: 10.1088/0031-9155/51/7/008

Tewarie, P., van Dellen, E., Hillebrand, A., and Stam, C. J. (2015). The minimum spanning tree: an unbiased method for brain network analysis. *Neuroimage* 104, 177–188. doi: 10.1016/j.neuroimage.2014.10.015

Tijms, B. M., Wink, A. M., de Haan, W., van der Flier, W. M., Stam, C. J., Scheltens, P., et al. (2013). Alzheimer's disease: connecting findings from graph theoretical studies of brain networks. *Neurobiol. Aging* 34, 2023–2036. doi: 10.1016/j.neurobiolaging.2013.02.020

Tzourio-Mazoyer, N., Landeau, B., Papathanassiou, D., Crivello, F., Etard, O., Delcroix, N., et al. (2002). Automated anatomical labeling of activations in SPM using a macroscopic anatomical parcellation of the MNI MRI single-subject brain. *Neuroimage* 15, 273–289. doi: 10.1006/nimg.2001.0978

van Wijk, B. C. M., Stam, C. J., and Daffertshofer, A. (2010). Comparing brain networks of different size and connectivity density using graph theory. *PLoS ONE* 5:e13701. doi: 10.1371/journal.pone.0013701

Wang, J., Zuo, X., Dai, Z., Xia, M., Zhao, Z., Zhao, X., et al. (2013). Disrupted functional brain connectome in individuals at risk for Alzheimer's disease. *Biol. Psychiatry* 73, 472–481. doi: 10.1016/j.biopsych.2012.03.026

Warrington, E., and James, M. (1991). *The Visual Object and Space Perception Battery*. Bury St Edmunds: Thames Valley Test Company.

Watts, D. J., and Strogatz, S. H. (1998). Collective dynamics of "small-world" networks. *Nature* 393, 440–442. doi: 10.1038/30918

Wechsler, D. (1997). *Wechsler Memory Scale—Third Edition Manual*. San Antonio, TX: Psychological Corporation.

Whalen, C., Maclin, E. L., Fabiani, M., and Gratton, G. (2008). Validation of a method for coregistering scalp recording locations with 3D structural MR images. *Hum. Brain Mapp.* 29, 1288–1301. doi: 10.1002/hbm.20465

Xiang, J., Guo, H., Liang, H., and Chen, J. (2013). An abnormal resting- state functional brain network indicates progression towards Alzheimer's disease. *Neural Regen. Res.* 8, 2789–2799.

Yesavage, J. A., Brink, T. L., Rose, T. L., Lum, O., Huang, V., Adey, M., et al. (1982). Development and validation of a geriatric depression screening scale: a preliminary report. *J. Psychiatr. Res.* 17, 37–49. doi: 10.1016/0022-3956(82)90033-4

Yu, M., Hillebrand, A., Tewarie, P., Meier, J., van Dijk, B., Van Mieghem, P., et al. (2015). Hierarchical clustering in minimum spanning trees. *Chaos* 25, 023107. doi: 10.1063/1.4908014

Zhang, B., Zhang, X., Zhang, F., Li, M., Schwarz, C. G., Zhang, J., et al. (2015). Characterizing topological patterns in amnestic mild cognitive impairment by quantitative water diffusivity. *J. Alzheimers Dis.* 43, 687–697. doi: 10.3233/JAD-140882

Zheng, L., Jiang, Z., and Yu, E. (2007). Alpha spectral power and coherence in the patients with mild cognitive impairment during a three-level working memory task. *J. Zhejiang Univ. Sci. B* 8, 584–592. doi: 10.1631/jzus.2007.B0584

18

Does Aerobic Exercise Influence Intrinsic Brain Activity? An Aerobic Exercise Intervention among Healthy Old Adults

Pär Flodin[1,2], Lars S. Jonasson[1,2,3], Katrin Riklund[2,3], Lars Nyberg[2,3,4] and C. J. Boraxbekk[1,2,5]*

[1] Center for Demographic and Aging Research, Umeå University, Umeå, Sweden, [2] Umeå Center for Functional Brain Imaging, Umeå University, Umeå, Sweden, [3] Diagnostic Radiology, Department of Radiation Sciences, Umeå University, Umeå, Sweden, [4] Physiology, Department of Integrative Medical Biology, Umeå University, Umeå, Sweden, [5] Danish Research Centre for Magnetic Resonance, Centre for Functional and Diagnostic Imaging and Research, Copenhagen University Hospital Hvidovre, Copenhagen, Denmark

****Correspondence:***
Pär Flodin
parflodin@gmail.com

Previous studies have indicated that aerobic exercise could reduce age related decline in cognition and brain functioning. Here we investigated the effects of aerobic exercise on intrinsic brain activity. Sixty sedentary healthy males and females (64–78 years) were randomized into either an aerobic exercise group or an active control group. Both groups recieved supervised training, 3 days a week for 6 months. Multimodal brain imaging data was acquired before and after the intervention, including 10 min of resting state brain functional magnetic resonance imaging (rs-fMRI) and arterial spin labeling (ASL). Additionally, a comprehensive battery of cognitive tasks assessing, e.g., executive function and episodic memory was administered. Both the aerobic and the control group improved in aerobic capacity (VO_2-peak) over 6 months, but a significant group by time interaction confirmed that the aerobic group improved more. Contrary to our hypothesis, we did not observe any significant group by time interactions with regard to any measure of intrinsic activity. To further probe putative relationships between fitness and brain activity, we performed *post hoc* analyses disregarding group belongings. At baseline, VO_2-peak was negativly related to BOLD-signal fluctuations ($BOLD_{STD}$) in mid temporal areas. Over 6 months, improvements in aerobic capacity were associated with decreased connectivity between left hippocampus and contralateral precentral gyrus, and positively to connectivity between right mid-temporal areas and frontal and parietal regions. Independent component analysis identified a VO_2-related increase in coupling between the default mode network and left orbitofrontal cortex, as well as a decreased connectivity between the sensorimotor network and thalamus. Extensive exploratory data analyses of global efficiency, connectome wide multivariate pattern analysis (connectome-MVPA), as well as ASL, did not reveal any relationships between aerobic fitness and intrinsic brain activity. Moreover, fitness-predicted changes in functional connectivity did not relate to changes in cognition, which is likely due to absent cross-sectional or longitudinal relationships between VO_2-peak and cognition. We conclude that the aerobic exercise intervention had limited influence on patterns of intrinsic brain activity, although *post hoc* analyses indicated that individual changes in aerobic capacity preferentially influenced mid-temporal brain areas.

Keywords: aerobic exercise, brain plasticity, aging, fMRI, resting-state, ASL

INTRODUCTION

Given the increasing disease burden of age related cognitive problems that comes with an aging world population (Christensen et al., 2009), physical exercise could provide a widely available and cost-effective approach to reduce age related cognitive decline at a large scale (Baker et al., 2010). Prospective studies show that low fitness in early adulthood is associated with increased risk for early onset dementia later in life (Nyberg et al., 2014; Wendell et al., 2014). Moreover, cross-sectional population based studies have confirmed that individuals that stay physically active have an improved brain-behavior relationship (Boraxbekk et al., 2016).

Human intervention studies probing the cognitive effects of exercise have, however, showed mixed findings. Meta-analyses have reported a range of effect sizes on exercise induced improvements of cognition among elderly. Smith et al. (2010) reported modest improvements in attention, processing speed (PS), executive function (EF), and memory. Colcombe and Kramer (2003) report medium improvements (of particularly) EFs, whereas a recent systematic meta-analysis concludes that there is no evidence that aerobic exercise benefit cognition among healthy older adults (Young et al., 2015). Thus, there is a need for further investigations of the extent to which physical exercise interventions among elderly could maintain, or even restore, cognitive function and brain health. For investigations of the neurophysiological mechanisms subserving the neuroprotective effects of aerobic exercise, human brain imaging plays a central role (for a review see, e.g., Stillman et al., 2016).

Evidence suggests that resting state brain activity could be sensitive to also early-stage neuroplastic brain changes (Kelly and Castellanos, 2014). To date, very few studies have investigated changes in intrinsic brain activity following a structured physical exercise intervention among healthy older adults. Voss et al. (2010) investigated longitudinal changes in three age sensitive brain networks, using a region of interested (ROI) based seed correlation analysis (SCA), following 6 and 12 months supervised cardiovascular training. Compared to an active control group, the aerobic (walking) group increased connectivity in parts of the default and frontal executive network after 12 months, although no significant group differences were observed at 6 months.

Among the cross-sectional studies linking fitness to intrinsic brain activity among elderly, a commonly reported finding is reversal of age-related changes. Voss et al. (2016) used network based statistics (NBS) on graphs based on hubs defined in age-sensitive networks. These networks were identified as the default mode- (DMN), dorsal attention-, and executive control-, salience- and sensory related networks. Whereas older subjects displayed enhanced between-network connectivity, younger subjects displayed larger within-network connectivity. They concluded that cardiorespiratory fitness among older was positively associated with connectivity within age-sensitive networks, primarily the DMN, whereas no associations were observed for self-reported physical activity. However, another large scale cross-sectional study, Boraxbekk et al. (2016) found that current and accumulated physical activity was associated with stronger integrity of the DMN in the anterior parts of posterior cingulate cortex (PCC).

In the current study, we wanted to expand on the findings relating aerobic fitness to intrinsic brain activity. In addition to investigate resting-state functional connectivity (i.e., correlations of BOLD-signal time series of distributed brain regions), we also examined fluctuations of BOLD-signal time series ($BOLD_{STD}$). Resting state $BOLD_{STD}$ has previously been used as a proxy measure for vascular flexibility (Burzynska et al., 2015). Moreover, vascular stiffness has in previous studies been linked to aging and cognitive decline (Mitchell et al., 2011; Gauthier et al., 2015), and there is evidence that physical activity counteracts age related vascular stiffness. Burzynska et al. (2015) detected a positive relationship between variability in intrinsic brain activity and physical activity (measured with actigraphs), but not for cardiovascular fitness (VO_2-max). The authors concluded that BOLD-signal fluctuations could provide a putative neural correlate of brain health among elderly, and that "longitudinal and intervention studies will shed more light on the potential of BOLD in detecting changes in brain function as a result of increased physical activity" (Burzynska et al., 2015). Using a more direct MRI based measure of vascular rigidity, aortic pulse wave velocity, Gauthier et al. (2015) reported an increase of vascular rigidity with age, and a negative association to VO_2-max (i.e., maximum rate of oxygen consumption).

Another way to characterize vascular function (which is a likely target for aerobic exercise) is quantification of cerebral blood flow (CBF). Maass et al. (2015) used gadolinium-based perfusion imaging MRI to investigate longitudinal changes among healthy older adults that partook in a 3-months exercise intervention, and found that improvements in aerobic capacity correlated with increases in hippocampal blood flow. In cross-sectional data, Boraxbekk et al. (2016) found a positive relationship between physical activity and CBF (ASL) in PCC.

To our knowledge, the current study is the first to employ pure resting-state functional magnetic resonance imaging (rs-fMRI) scans before and after an actively controlled, long-term physical exercise intervention among healthy elderly. In the current article, we present the resting-state results of the research project "Physical Influences on Brain in Aging" (PHIBRA), for which the design, cognitive performance, and structural MRI-data recently were reported (Jonasson et al., 2017). By using a comprehensive set of analytical approaches of rs-fMRI data, and additional measures of ASL-CBF, we attempted to replicate and extend on previous research that evaluates the impact of aerobic fitness on intrinsic brain activity. Based on previous studies we predicted that analyses of group by time interactions would reveal differential longitudinal changes in (1) hippocampal resting state functional connectivity and betweenness centrality, (2) DMN integrity (3) voxel wise $BOLD_{STD}$ and CBF. Additionally, we aimed to characterize relationships between rs-fMRI and fitness using more exploratory approaches. These included multivariate representations of whole brain connectivity (in the following referred to as multivariate pattern analysis, connectome-MVPA), NBS and graph theoretical measures (global efficiency). In order to investigate the functional significance of any observed fitness-brain relationship stipulated above, we performed *post hoc* analyses relating neurophysiological changes to changes in cognition.

MATERIALS AND METHODS

Subjects

Sixty healthy but sedentary older adults (age 64–78 years) were recruited and randomized into performing either supervised aerobic exercise training, or stretching and toning control training, for 6 months, three times a week (30–60 min per session). In the present analysis, 13 subjects were excluded due to the following reasons: one subject was excluded due to brain abnormalities; two subjects were unable to complete the intervention; one person was excluded since baseline VO_2-peak exceeded the group average by three standard deviations. Another nine persons were excluded due to suprathreshold movement during resting state scans at either pre- or post intervention sessions, see criteria below. Thus, complete data were obtained from 47 subjects, 22 in the aerobic intervention arm and 25 in the active control group. The groups did not significantly differ with respect to age [$t(45) = 0.92$, $p = 0.36$], sex [$\chi 2(1) = 0.045$ $p = 0.83$], education [$t(45) = 0.1$, $p = 0.36$], or BMI [$t(45) = 1.01$, $p = 0.32$], see **Table 1**.

For the ASL analyses, pre- and post intervention data was available from 55 subjects (aerobic group: 30 subjects, 16 females; control group: 25 subjects, 14 females), age 68.7 ± 2.79 years. There were no significant group differences in age, [$t(53) = -1.27$, $p = 0.21$), sex $\chi 2(1) = 0.040$ $p = 0.843$], education [$t(53) = -0.087$, $p = 0.93$], or BMI [$t(53) = -0.98$, $p = 0.33$]. For complete sample characteristics, see Jonasson et al. (2017).

Intervention Procedures and Behavioral Outcome Measures

For detailed descriptions of the intervention, the VO_2-peak assessment, and the cognitive test battery, see Jonasson et al. (2017). In short, the intervention procedure was as follows: Subjects were recruited from local newspaper advertisement. Prior to randomization into either of the two intervention arms, all subjects underwent pre-intervention testing. The testing consisted of visits to the lab at six different days. On the first testing day participants visited the Sports Science Lab, Umeå University, where fitness measures, including VO_2-peak, were assessed using a standardized graded cycle ergometer test. Neuropsychological testing was performed on three separate days. Assessments of cognitive ability included three tests designed to tax (verbal) episodic memory (EM), three test for EF, as well as other tests including assessments of working memory updating (UPD) and PS. A composite score, cognitive score (CS), was computed as a unit-weighted average of EM, EF, UPD, and PS, as a single metric of overall cognition. Finally, MRI-data of different modalities was collected, of which the rs-fMRI and the ASL-CBF data is reported here. Additional questionnaires and dopamine positron emission tomography (PET) imaging were also collected, but will be reported elsewhere. The testing was conducted both before and after the interventions. The cognitive

TABLE 1 | Demographics, and longitudinal changes in VO_2-peak and graph measures.

Measure	Aerobic $n = 22$			Control $n = 25$			Group x time	
	Pre	Post	G	Pre	Post	G	$F(1,43)$	η_p^2
Age	68.41 (2.59)	–	–	69.16 (3.01)	–	–	–	–
Sex (females)	13	–	–	14	–	–	–	–
Education (years)	13.77 (3.74)	–	–	13.84 (5.02)	–	–	–	–
BMI	25.85 (3.52)	–	–	26.92 (3.41)	–	–	–	–
VO_2 peak	21.37 (3.83)	27.87 (6.07)	**1.26 (0.9–61.80)**	19.59 (3.25)	23.56 (5.12)	**0.91 (0.66–1.30)**	**6.20 (0.02)**	**0.12 (0.01–0.33)**
Global efficiency	0.20 (0.01)	0.21 (0.02)	**0.39 (0.05–0.83)**	0.21 (0.02)	0.21 (0.01)	0.18 (−0.17–0.68)	0.7 (0.39)	0.02 (0.00–0.14)
BetweenCent L hippo	293.45 (238.90)	209.45 (110.79)	−0.44 (−0.97–0.12)	300.40 (336.28)	251.52 (289.14)	−0.15 (−0.66–0.36)	0.45 (0.50)	0.01 (0.00–0.14)
BetweenCent R hippo	182.09 (144.63)	143.09 (176.50)	−0.24 (−0.94–0.24)	127.52 (120.91)	173.68 (203.12)	0.27 (−0.22–0.67)	1.35 (0.25)	0.03 (0.00–0.16)

Within group mean values (for pre- and post measures) are reported with SD in parenthesis. Effect sizes for within group longitudinal changes are reported as Hedges G, with lower and upper bound for 95% CI (bootstrapped, n = 10000) in parentheses. Group by time interactions are tested using repeated measure ANOVA, where the F statistics are reported with the significance level in parenthesis. Effect sizes are specified using eta-squared, with the lower and upper bound in parentheses. Significant (unc) effects are in bold. Groups did not significantly differ with regard to age [t(45) = 0.92, p = 0.36] or sex [χ2(1) = 0.045 p = 0.83].

testing, including the tests assessing EM, EF, and CS that are used here, is described in detail in Jonasson et al. (2017).

Acquisition

Brain imaging data was acquired on a 3 T GE scanner equipped with a 32-channel head coil. High-resolution T1-weighted structural images were acquired using the following parameters: 180 slices; 1 mm thickness; repletion time (TR) 8.2 ms; time to echo (TE) 3.2 ms; flip angle 12°; FOV 25 cm × 25 cm. Functional data were acquired with a gradient EPI sequence with the following parameters: 37 transaxial slices, 3.4 mm thickness, 0.5 mm gap, TR 2000 ms, TE 30 ms, flip angle 80°, FOV 25 cm × 25 cm, inplane resolution of 2.6 mm × 2.6 mm. During resting state scan acquisition, subjects were instructed to lie still and keep their eyes on a white fixation cross for 9 min and 40 s, resulting in 290 volumes per subject and session.

Whole brain perfusion was measured with a 3D pseudo-continuous ASL sequence. Labeling time was 1.5 s, post-labeling delay time was 2 s, field of view was 24 cm, slice thickness was 4 mm, number of averages was 3, number of control label pairs was 30, and acquisition resolution was 8 × 512 (arms × data points in spiral scheme). Forty slices covered the whole brain and the reconstructed voxel size was 1.88 mm × 1.88 mm × 4 mm. CBF maps were computed using the standard GE reconstruction, showing tissue CBF in ml/min/100 g.

MRI Data Preprocessing and Denoising

Rs-fMRI data preprocessing was performed in SPM12 using standard preprocessing steps. These included slice time correction, realignment and unwarping using 6th degree B-spline interpolation, and functional to structural coregistration. Structural images were segmented into gray matter, white matter and cerebral spinal fluid images. Coregistered functional and structural images were normalized to standard space using Geodesic Shooting as implemented in the Shoot toolbox in SPM12 (Ashburner and Friston, 2011). In short, a common anatomical group-average 1 mm isotropic template was generated, and subject specific deformation fields were created and used for warping T1- and T2*-weighted images from subject space to group template space. Secondly, non-linear deformation fields pushing images from group space to MNI space were applied. Functional data was then resampled into 2 mm × 2 × 2 mm and finally smoothed using a Gaussian kernel of 8 mm.

Cerebral blood flow data was coregistered to structural data, and normalized using the same normalization procedures as applied to the structural and functional data.

At the subject level, rs-fMRI time series were denoised by controlling for: (1) suprathreshold movement (frame wise displacement >0.25 mm or >3 std change in global signal intensity, similar to, e.g., (Satterthwaite et al., 2013), (2) signals from white matter and cerebrospinal fluid (five most explanatory principal components from each tissue mask), and (3) six movement parameters obtained from spatial realignment plus their time derivatives. Subsequent to nuisance regression, time signals were filtered (band passing 0.008–0.09 Hz). Nine subjects lost >50% of their volumes either at pre- or post intervention sessions (of originally 290 volumes) due to movement censoring, and were therefore excluded from further analysis. Denoising of data was accomplished with the Conn toolbox (version 15.h).

fMRI Analysis

Longitudinal effects of the intervention were evaluated as group by time interactions. Voxel-wise group analyses of functional connectivity were performed using the Conn toolbox, where the two experimental groups were compared in terms of longitudinal changes with regard to the resting state metrics. Likewise, 2-sample *t*-tests of the post minus pre intervention $BOLD_{STD}$ and CBF volumes were analyzed using the 2-sample *t*-test as implemented in SPM12. Group level statistics of graph-theoretical indices (of betweenness centrality and global efficiency) were calculated using repeated measure ANOVA (using MatLab) with group and time as factors.

Post hoc analyses aimed to link individual longitudinal changes in VO_2-peak to changes in brain activity were also conducted, ignoring experimental group-belonging. For these we performed linear regressions, where changes in brain activity were regressed on changes in VO_2-peak. To guide longitudinal analyses, rs-fMRI data were first related to aerobic capacity at baseline. Any obtained significant brain-fitness association at baseline was used to inform subsequent longitudinal analysis (see below).

In all group analyses, we controlled for age and sex (as e.g., done in Maass et al., 2015). For the longitudinal analyses, we also controlled for baseline ratings of VO_2-capacity. Additionally, since the two experiential groups were matched with regard to sex and age, the analyses of group by time interactions were also performed without control for sex, age and VO_2 – peak ratings. In all second-level fMRI analyses, we controlled for mean frame wise displacement (FD).

Seed Based Correlation Analysis

Voxel-wise seed based correlation analyses (SCA) were performed using the Conn toolbox (15.h). For each subject and each seed region, *z*-transformed Pearson correlation maps were brought to second level group analysis. We defined a priori seeds in brain regions that in previous literature have been influenced by aerobic exercise. These included (a) left and right hippocampus obtained from the SPM Wake Forest University (WFU) Pickatlas toolbox (Maldjian et al., 2003), (b) left and right parahippocampus (WFU pickatlas), and (c) PCC, based on a cluster reported by Boraxbekk et al. (2016) (center of gravity MNI coordinates −6, −32, 27; 67 voxels).

BOLD-Signal Fluctuations

Variations in the preprocessed and cleaned resting state BOLD time series were quantified using FSL maths[1], rendering one voxel-wise whole brain map of the standard deviations ($BOLD_{STD}$) for each subject and each session. As a corroborating measure, we also calculated Amplitude of Low Frequency Fluctuations (ALFF) which quantifies the total power within the lower frequency band. ALFF was calculated for the same preprocessed and cleaned volumes as for the $BOLD_{STD}$

[1] http://www.fmrib.ox.ac.uk/fsl

calculations, using the MatLab toolbox DPARSFA[2] (Chao-Gan and Yu-Feng, 2010). Thus, for the examined ALFF calculations, the examined frequency window was essentially the same as the bandpass filter used in the resting state data, i.e., 0.008–0.09 Hz.

Graph Analyses

For the network analyses, we created subject specific weighted graphs based on 264 nodes defined as spherical (4 mm radius) ROIs centered around functionally relevant coordinates (Power et al., 2011; Cole et al., 2013) (see Supplementary Table S1). Edges were defined as Pearson correlation values between each time series of each ROI–ROI pair, where negative correlations were nulled. For measures of hippocampal betweenness centrality, we added two nodes corresponding to the left and right hippocampus (see Seed Based Correlation Analysis) to the original (264 nodes) graph. A high degree of betweenness centrality imply that nodes have central positions, i.e., act as hubs in the given network. Global efficiency is a measure of how efficiently information is exchanged across a network. All graph theoretical measures (i.e., Betweenness Centrality for left and right hippocampus, and global efficiency) were calculated using the brain connectivity toolbox (Rubinov and Sporns, 2010) as implemented in GraphVar1.0 (Kruschwitz et al., 2015).

Independent Component Analyses

Independent component analysis (ICA) was performed using the conn toolbox (v16, Whitfield-Gabrieli and Nieto-Castanon, 2012). Comparable ICA's across subjects were obtained through a dual regression procedure, where we first calculated 20 group level spatial independent components (default value), and subsequently used the time series pertaining to each component to obtain subject-specific spatial components. Longitudinal change in five different networks were analyzed with regard to baseline and change in aerobic capacity, respectively. The ICA components of interest were chosen in an attempt to conceptually replicate the analysis of resting state networks investigated in Voss et al. (2016). Specifically, these included the default mode network (DMN), right and left frontoparietal network (FPN), dorsal attention network (DAN), and Sensorimotor Network (S1M1) (see Supplementary Figure S1).

Network Based Statistics

We also conducted NBS analysis (Zalesky et al., 2010), on the graph consisting of the same 264 nodes as used for graph analysis (see Graph Analyses). NBS allows for identification of group-effects among ROI–ROI connections or subnetworks, while controlling for multiple comparisons. NBS is the conceptual equivalent to cluster statistics for voxel wise whole brain analyses. Analogous to cluster statistics, NBS yields stronger statistical sensitivity for distributed effects, which in turn is traded for spatial resolution which is limited to the size of the identified network (c.f. cluster), rather than individual ROI–ROI connections (c.f. voxels). NBS was used to identify ROI–ROI pairs or subnetworks that revealed group by time interactions, or where connectivity related to aerobic capacity (either at baseline, or in change-change regressions). For this, we employed a typically used network defining ROI–ROI ("primary") connectivity threshold (Zalesky et al., 2010); $p = 0.001$ uncorrected. In order to detect weaker but spatially more distributed sub-graphs for 2nd level contrasts where the original ROI–ROI connectivity threshold did not show any effect, we also investigated fitness-network associations using ROI–ROI connectivity thresholds of $p = 0.01$ and $p = 0.05$ uncorrected (two sided). For NBS (i.e., "network component intensity") threshold, we used the significance level of family-wise error correction (FWE) $p = 0.05$ (1000 permutations).

Whole Brain Pattern of Functional Connectivity

Additionally, we performed a principal component MVPA, or so called "connectome-MVPA," to detect patterns of whole brain connectivity that correlated with aerobic capacity. The MVPA analysis complements the SCA and ICA since the investigated connectivity is not restricted to pre-selected seed regions or independent components, respectively. Instead, it provides a regionally unbiased mapping of brain areas with whole brain connectivity patterns that are predicted by aerobic capacity or longitudinal change thereof. In detail, the MVPA measure was obtained by dimension reduction of the whole brain connectivity matrix of each voxel. The connectivity matrix of each subject was reshaped into a row vector and subsequently concatenated over all participants into a matrix $N \times V$, where N was the number of subjects and V is the number of voxels within the brain mask. The dimensionality of the $N \times V$ group correlation matrix was reduced by principal component analysis (PCA). This yielded an $N \times C$ matrix, where C is the number of maintained principal components. We maintained the first seven principal components that explained the most of the variance of the connectivity matrix ($C = 7$) [according to the rule of thumb to maintain an approximate 1:7 ratio between number of components and subjects, as proposed by the metric implementer Nieto-Castenon (2015)[3]]. In other words, the resulting seven component score volumes best represented the whole brain connectivity pattern for each subject. These volumes were included in an F-test at the 2nd level analysis. Thus, we tested for clusters that were predicted by aerobic capacity with regard to whole brain connectivity.

The reported activation maps (of contrasted regression parameter estimates) in group analyses were considered significant at a cluster-level significance of $p < 0.05$, false-discovery rate (FDR) corrected, and cluster defining voxel threshold of $p < 0.001$, two-sided. Due to unreliable estimations of smoothness of the MVPA rendered PCA maps, we used non-parametric permutation statistics (1000 permutations) as advocated by the implementer of the metric (Alfonso Nieto-Castanon, personal communication, September, 23, 2016). Connectome-MVPA analyses were thresholded using a cluster based significance threshold of $p = 0.05$ (FDR). Un-thresholded statistical maps for all reported results (**Figures 1–3**) are available online at http://neurovault.org/collections/2415/.

[2]http://restfmri.net

[3]http://www.nitrc.org/forum/message.php?msg_id=14332

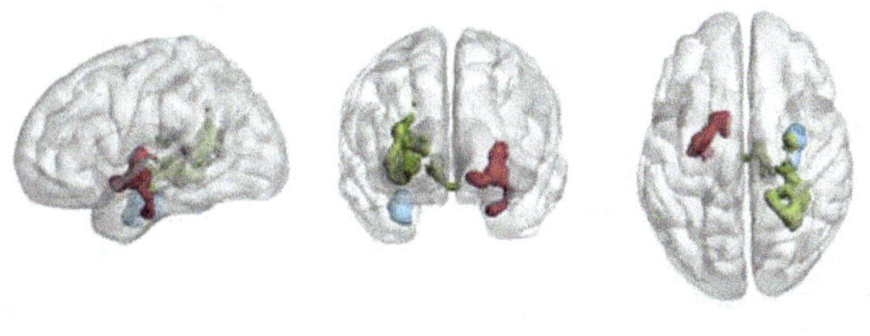

FIGURE 1 | Relationship between aerobic capacity and fluctuations of BOLD signal ($BOLD_{STD}$) at baseline. For three regions in medial temporal areas, we observed a negative relationship between aerobic capacity and $BOLD_{STD}$. Green: a cluster (973 voxels) extending parts of right posterior hippocampus and thalamus. Red: cluster (298 voxels) extending parts of L. Putamen, (l) thalamus and (2) amygdala. Blue: cluster (232 voxels) extending part of right anterior hippocampus and amygdala. Results are visualized using brain net viewer (Xia et al., 2013).

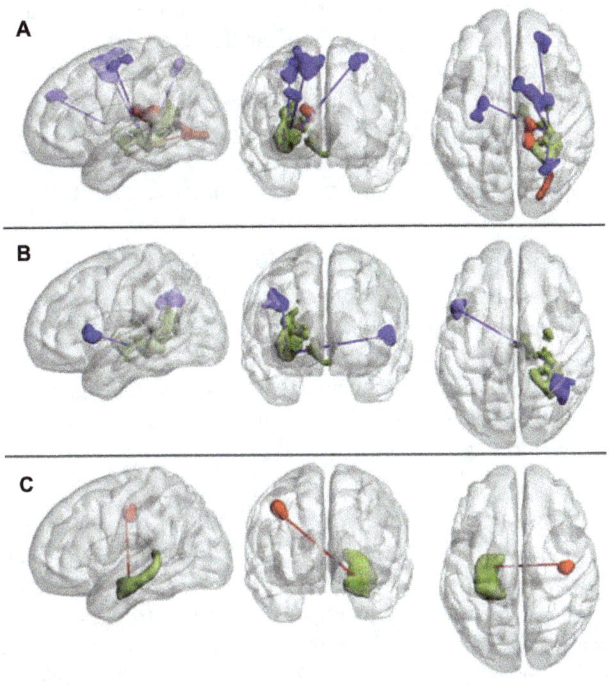

FIGURE 2 | Seed based correlation analysis relating aerobic capacity to resting state functional connectivity. **(A)** At baseline, aerobic capacity (VO_2-peak) was primarily positively (blue) correlated with right medial temporal lobe connectivity to frontal, parietal, and occipital areas. Negative correlations between aerobic capacity and connectivity of the same seed were observed to thalamus and occipital regions. **(B)** Longitudinal gains in aerobic capacity predicted increased functional connectivity between the right medial temporal lobe and frontal and parietal regions. **(C)** Change in aerobic capacity is negatively associated with connectivity between left hippocampus and contralateral precentral gyrus. Green areas indicate seed regions; blue indicate positive associations to (change in) aerobic capacity; red indicates negative associations.

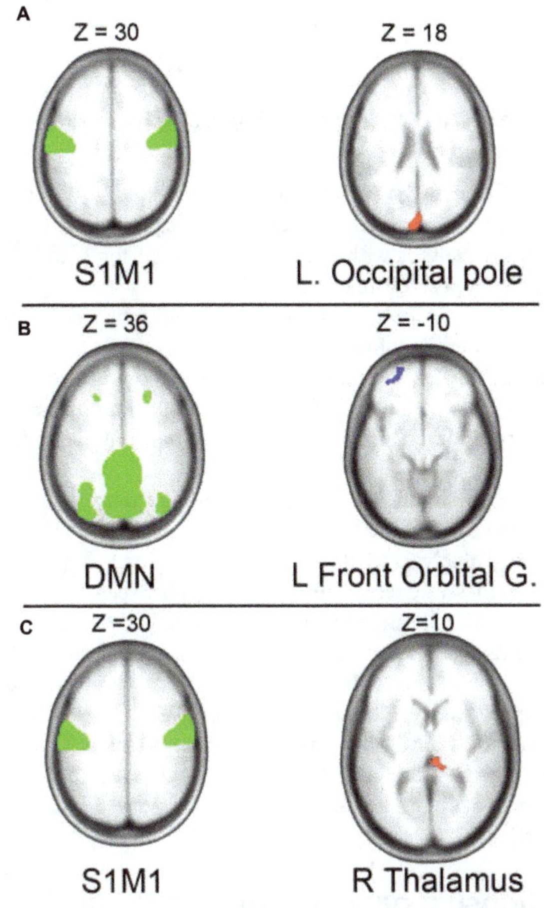

FIGURE 3 | Independent component analysis (ICA). **(A)** ICA revealed a negative association between baseline measures of aerobic capacity and connectivity between the sensorimotor network (left) the occipital pole (right). **(B)** Longitudinal gain in aerobic capacity was associated with increased connectivity between default mode network (DMN) and left prefrontal cortex. **(C)** Change in VO_2-peak was negatively related to change in connectivity of the somatosensory network (S1M1) to right thalamus. Green regions illustrate the independent components (IC) at baseline; red indicates areas experiencing decreased connectivity to the IC with higher (or gain in) VO_2-peak; blue indicates areas with increased fitness predicted connectivity.

For all significant findings of group by time interactions, and associations between intrinsic brain activity either with regard to baseline aerobic capacity or change in aerobic capacity, we further examined the relationships to cognition. More specifically, we defined volumes of interest based on the brain regions that were significantly predicted by aerobic capacity. These volumes were subsequently used as inclusive masks (i.e., small volume correction) within which we investigated effects of either baseline score or longitudinal change in cognition, respectively.

RESULTS

Intervention Induced Gains in Aerobic Capacity

Within the sub-sample used here we observed a significant group by time interaction, with the aerobic group displaying a significantly larger improvement in aerobic capacity compared to the active control group $F(1,43) = 6.20$, $p = 0.02$ (see **Table 1**). This was similar to what Jonasson et al. (2017) reported using the full sample.

Intervention Induced Changes in Intrinsic Brain Activity

None of the analyses (described in the method fMRI Analysis) of intrinsic brain activity reveled significant group by time interactions, neither with nor without control for sex, age and baseline VO_2-peak estimates.

Likewise, the NBS-analysis was non-significant using a range of network defining ROI–ROI thresholds (see Network Based Statistics). Finally, none of the graph theoretical measures (betweenness centrality of left and right hippocampus, or global efficiency) rendered significant group by time interactions, see **Table 1**.

Given non-significant significant group by time interactions with regard to intrinsic brain activity, we conducted additional exploratory analyses that in future may guide confirmatory studies. In these, we tested for relationships between longitudinal change in VO_2-peak and intrinsic brain activity across all participants disregarding group belonging, similar to what has been done previously (Maass et al., 2015; Jonasson et al., 2017). Therefore, we first explored cross-sectional relationships between VO_2-peak and brain activity at baseline. Any relationships observed at baseline data were subsequently used to inform regressions of longitudinal change in VO_2-peak to changes in brain activity.

Relationship between Aerobic Capacity with Resting State Measures at Baseline

BOLD-Signal Fluctuations

Variation of the BOLD signal time series ($BOLD_{STD}$) was negatively correlated with aerobic capacity in three clusters located in midbrain regions at baseline (**Figure 1** and **Table 2**). The largest cluster (973 voxels) extended over right posterior hippocampus and thalamus. A second cluster (298 voxels) covered parts of left pallidum, and to a smaller extent also left thalamus and amygdala. The third cluster (232 voxels) contained right anterior hippocampus and right amygdala. Clusters were anatomically labeled using the WFU pick atlas. $BOLD_{STD}$ were not positively correlated with aerobic capacity in any brain region.

Amplitude of Low Frequency Fluctuations (ALFF), resulted in virtually identical results as $BOLD_{STD}$ (see Supplementary Figure S2), and thus ALFF results are not presented further.

Follow-up analyses that tested for the association between cognitive performance and $BOLD_{STD}$ were restricted to the search volume of regions where aerobic capacity predicted $BOLD_{STD}$ (displayed in **Figure 1**). Given that particularly hippocampal and mid-temporal brain regions displayed fitness related $BOLD_{STD}$, we tested for EM. In addition, a meta-analysis (Colcombe and Kramer, 2003) found the largest association between improved fitness and cognitive performance to be related to EFs. Furthermore, in our previous study, improved fitness was primarily related to improved general cognitive performance (i.e., CS) (Jonasson et al., 2017). Therefore, we also tested the association between EF, CS and $BOLD_{STD}$. Neither EM, EF nor CS were significantly related to $BOLD_{STD}$. (All cognitive outcome measures are presented in detail in Jonasson et al., 2017).

Seed Correlation Analysis (SCA)

None of the *a priori* defined seeds displayed significant VO_2-peak predicted connectivity at baseline. However, connectivity of the *post hoc* seed in the right medial temporal cortex (see BOLD-Signal Fluctuations), to frontal-, parietal-, and occipital regions displayed a positive correlation to aerobic capacity. We also detected a negative association between aerobic capacity and the connectivity between the same seed and right thalamus and right occipital cortex (**Figure 2A** and **Table 3**).

Independent Component Analysis (ICA)

At baseline, among the five investigated ICA-derived networks we observed a negative relationship between VO_2-peak and the connectivity of a sensorimotor network and a brain region extending over calcarine sulcus and precuneus (see **Figure 3A**). No associations between VO_2-peak and connectivity of the other four networks were seen.

Graph Measures, NBS, Connectome-MVPA and ASL

Several measures of intrinsic brain activity turned out not to be significantly related to aerobic capacity. For graph theoretical measures, neither global efficiency [$t(42) = -0.06$, $p = 0.95$] nor left or right hippocampal centrality [L: $t(42) = -0.94$, $p = 0.34$, R: $t(42) = -1.23$, $p = 0.22$] reached significance.

In the NBS analysis, no ROI–ROI connectivities or subnetworks were correlated with aerobic capacity, neither corrected nor uncorrected. Furthermore, the connectome-MVPA did not reveal any significant clusters predicted by baseline VO_2-peak.

Finally, analysis of ASL perfusion data did not reveal any associations between aerobic capacity and CBF from neither whole brain nor small volume voxel based analysis.

TABLE 2 | Significant relationships between $BOLD_{STD}$ and aerobic capacity at baseline.

Contrast	Region (peak co-oridnates)	Cluster size (# voxels)	Cluster p-FDR
Neg pre VO_2-peak	R. Hippocampus (32, −32, −8)	973	<0.000001
	L. Putamen (−22, −2, −6)	298	0.004
	R. Hippocampus (32, −9, 26)	232	0.002

Relationship between Longitudinal Change in Aerobic Capacity and Change in Intrinsic Brain Activity

Seed Correlation Analysis

Longitudinal gain in aerobic capacity was positively associated with changes in functional connectivity between the $BOLD_{STD}$-derived seed region in right medial temporal lobe, and right angular gyrus and left inferior frontal gyrus (**Figure 2B** and **Table 3**). However, change in aerobic capacity was negatively associated with change in connectivity between a priori defined seed regions in the left hippocampus and the right precentral gyrus (**Figure 2C** and **Table 3**). None of the other a priori defined seeds related to change in VO_2-peak.

Behavioral follow-up analyses did not reveal any significant relationships between changes in the fitness related SCA results and EM, EF, or CS.

Independent Component Analysis

Independent component analysis identified two significant associations between changes in VO_2-peak and connectivity. Firstly, there was a positive relationship between gains in VO_2-peak and connectivity between DMN and left frontal pole (see **Figure 3B** and **Table 3**). Secondly, a negative relationship between change in VO_2-peak and the connectivity between the S1M1-network and right hypothalamus was observed (**Figure 3C**). There was no significant relationship to changes in cognition (EM, EF, and CS).

Network Based Statistics

The NBS revealed a subnetwork constituted by connected nodes in the DMN, the frontal parietal-, visual- and ventral attention network (**Figure 4**) in which gains in fitness was related to changes in intra-network connectivity. Since the subgraph detected by NBS does not allow for inferences on individual edges (i.e., ROI–ROI connections), we also correlated change in VO_2-peak to connectivity between all individual ROI–ROI pairs (i.e., 34584 individual connections). In this analysis, no connections were significant (Bonferroni correcting for the edges in the full adjacency matrix).

Graph Measures, $BOLD_{STD}$, Connectome-MVPA and ASL

For the graph analysis, neither global efficiency [$F(1,42) = 0.70$, $p = 0.39$], nor betweenness centrality of hippocampus [left: $F(1,43) = 1.35$, $p = 0.25$; right: $F(1,43) = 0.45$, $p = 0.50$] was significantly related to change in fitness.

None of the other measures of intrinsic brain activity (MVPA, $BOLD_{STD}$,) or ASL yielded significant change-change relationships to fitness.

DISCUSSION

In the current study, we aimed to characterize the effects of exercise induced improvements in aerobic capacity on intrinsic brain activity. To accomplish this, we have employed a wide range of resting-state fMRI metrics as well as measures of CBF using ASL.

No Longitudinal Group Differences in Brain Activity

Based on previous literature, we predicted significant group by time interactions with regard to hippocampal connectivity, DMN integrity and vascular response as revealed by $BOLD_{STD}$ and CBF. In the present study, none of these measures displayed group differences in longitudinal changes.

A possible explanation may be that both groups improved in aerobic capacity. Since we stipulate that gain in VO_2-peak would be the active constituent mediating improvements in cognition and modulations of intrinsic brain activity (in line with the fitness hypothesis of cognition, (North et al., 1990; Kramer et al., 1999)], we reasoned that interindividual change in aerobic capacity across both groups could be a sensitive predictor of brain changes (similar to approaches used in previous studies, e.g., Maass et al., 2015). Thus, we performed *post hoc* analyses

TABLE 3 | Relationships between functional connectivity and aerobic capacity at baseline and change over time.

Contrast	Seed	Target(s) (peak coordinates)	Cluster size (# voxels)	Cluster p-FDR
Pre VO_2-peak	R. Hippocampus*	R. Superior Frontal Gyrus (14, 2, 58)	458	0.000005
		L. Precentral gyrus (−22, −6, 56)	132	0.014
		R. Occipital cortex (28, −62, 58)	116	0.017
		R. Frontal pole (22, 48, 32)	116	0.017
Neg pre VO_2-peak	R. Hippocampus*	R. Thalamus (WM), (12, −28, 18)	178	0.0047
		Occipital (WM) (22, −86, 0)	145	0.012
	ICA S1M1	L. Occipital Pole (2, −92, 18)	133	0.0019
dVO_2-peak	R. Hippocampus*	R. Angular Gyrus (36, −48, 30)	197	0.0013
		L. Inf Frontal Gyrus (−48, 14, 6)	105	0.022
	ICA DMN	L. Front. Orbital (−32, 30, −8)	109	0.019
Neg dVO_2-peak	L. Hippocampus	R. Precentral Gyrus (−36, −12, 36)	139	0.0097
	ICA S1M1	R. Thalamus (−6, −28, 12)	114	0.0043

*Target regions are labeled based on the locations of the largest number of voxels within significant cluster, as identified and labeled within the Conn-toolbox. *Seed region defined post hoc from VO_2-peak predicted $BOLD_{STD}$ effects at baseline.*

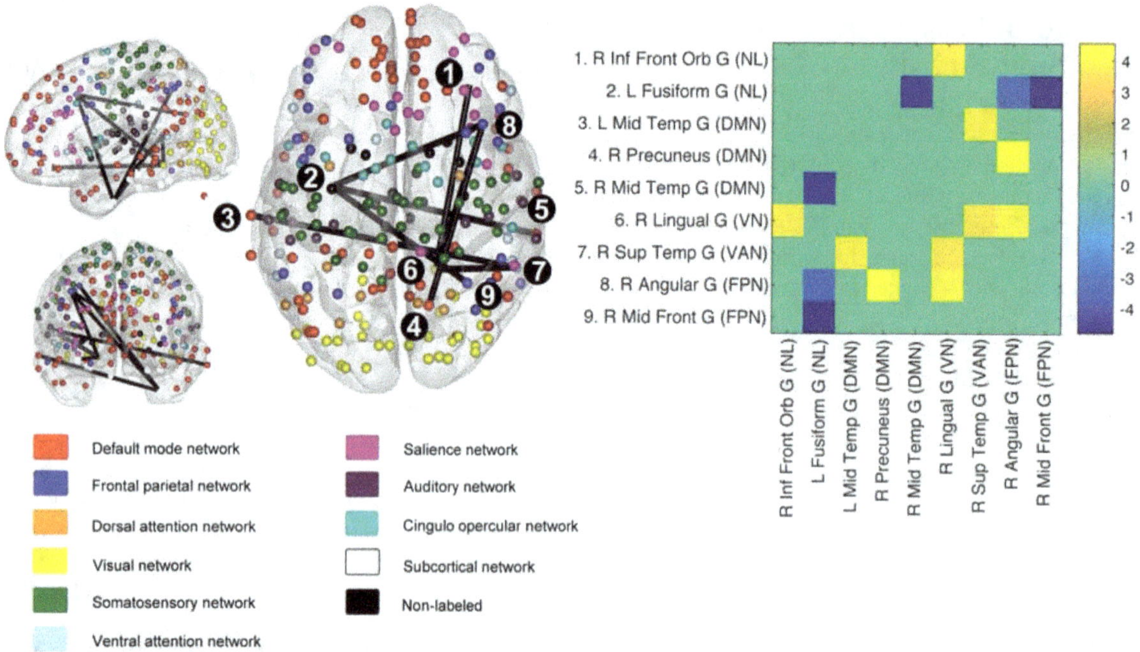

FIGURE 4 | Network based statistics (NBS) derived graph component predicted by change in VO_2-peak. Using change in VO2-peak to predict longitudinal change in the brain graph (264 nodes), we retrieved a subgraph spanning both task-negative and task-positive networks. Edge definition was $p = 0.001$ unc, and network component significance threshold FWE corrected $p < 0.05$. The adjacency matrix (top right) depicts participating nodes, and only significant t-values ($t > 3.54$) are shown. For MNI-coordinates of participating nodes, see Supplementary Table S1.

investigating inter individual change–change relations. The lack of significant effects is discussed in further detail below.

Post hoc Analyses of Fitness-Brain Relationships

Aerobic Capacity and the Medial Temporal Lobe

In the *post hoc* analyses we observed several associations between aerobic fitness and intrinsic brain activity, both at baseline and over time. Longitudinal change in aerobic capacity predicted change in hippocampal connectivity. Whereas left hippocampus displayed a decreased connectivity to precentral gyrus with increasing fitness, the right hippocampus was associated with increased connectivity to frontal and parietal areas. The right hippocampus, similar to baseline, was associated with increased frontal and parietal connectivity. Previously, Voss et al. (2013) reported enhanced connectivity between parahippocampus and bilateral temporal cortex, as well as to occipital and parietal areas following a 12 months aerobic (walking) intervention. Similar to the current findings, they observed reduced connectivity of left hippocampus, although to the right prefrontal cortex rather than to the right precentral gyrus as seen in here. Interestingly, the authors showed that increased connectivity between bilateral parahippocampal gyrus and middle temporal gyri were positively predicted by increases in neurotrophic growth factors, although no direct test of the behavioral significance of any of the connectivity changes was presented.

We detected relationships between $BOLD_{STD}$ and aerobic capacity at baseline, whereas gains in aerobic capacity did not relate to changes in $BOLD_{STD}$ over time. Contrary to what previously has been reported (Burzynska et al., 2015; Gauthier et al., 2015), the relationships between aerobic fitness and $BOLD_{STD}$ were negative and primarily observed in mid-temporal rather than cortical areas. Burzynska et al. (2015) reported cross-sectional associations between $BOLD_{STD}$ and physical activity, suggesting that $BOLD_{STD}$ could reflect a long-term cardiovascular trait, which coheres with the absence of any intervention related changes in current study. Notably, they did not observe relationship between aerobic capacity and $BOLD_{STD}$, but only a positive relationship between $BOLD_{STD}$ and physical activity. Our findings suggest that high aerobic capacity is associated with a more stable BOLD-signal within the temporal medial lobe. Speculative, the high fit subjects would experience relatively lower levels of physical demand, which could reconcile current findings with those reported by Burzynska et al. (2015). However, no on-line monitoring of degree of physical work during scanning was performed. Thus, further studies are required to establish the relationship between gains in aerobic capacity and $BOLD_{STD}$.

Longitudinal changes in intrinsic brain activity that were predicted by change in aerobic fitness did not relate to changes in any of the investigated cognitive domains (EM, EF, and CS). A plausible reason for this is the absent relationships between the cognitive variables and VO_2-peak, both at baseline and in change-change scores (Supplementary Table S2). Unfortunately, this limits the conclusions of the functional meaning of the observed fitness related brain changes. Thus, any functional interpretations of these brain changes are unknown and would have to rely on reverse inference, for which we lack unique cognition-connectivity associations.

Taken together, the findings above support the notion that aerobic fitness primarily affects mid temporal brain regions. In addition to the exercise intervention studies investigating changes in intrinsic brain activity (Voss et al., 2013; Burzynska et al., 2015; Maass et al., 2015; Bär et al., 2016; Tozzi et al., 2016), corroborating evidence of hippocampal involvement is also provided by studies investigating structural changes (e.g., Erickson et al., 2011, for a review, see Erickson et al., 2014; Jonasson et al., 2017). The fact that hippocampus display a high capacity for plastic change in relation to environmental factors (for a review, see Leuner and Gould, 2010), and also undergoes age related resting state connectivity changes (Salami et al., 2016), provides further motivation to specifically probe the intrinsic brain activity in the mid-temporal lobe. By standardizing research protocols and outcome measures, the mechanisms linking hippocampal brain activity, brain structure, vascularity, molecular growth factors and behavior will hopefully be revealed (Duzel et al., 2016; Stillman et al., 2016).

Network Changes

Network based statistics analysis revealed a graph sub-component that was predicted by the longitudinal change in VO_2-peak. Whereas previous cross-sectional reports (Voss et al., 2016) showed a higher within network integrity (particularly in DMN) with higher fitness, our longitudinal findings suggest that increased fitness also modulate between network connectivity. Whether the explanations for the discrepant finding are found in differences in methodological approaches (e.g., graph defining set of nodes) or lack of statistical power remains to be determined.

Resting state networks derived by ICA revealed relationships between fitness and connectivity of both the S1M1 and the DMN. Decreased connectivity between M1S1 and right thalamus was associated with increased aerobic capacity. M1S1 receives input from parts of thalamus, and the decreased connectivity with gains in fitness seems counterintuitive at first. Speculatively, this could reflect enhanced neuronal efficiency, although such a hypothesis should be investigated using methods that complement the correlational fMRI approaches used here. The connectivity between the same S1M1 network and occipital cortex were negatively related to fitness at baseline. In a small exercise intervention among obese children, Krafft et al. (2014) observed that the ICA derived motor network underwent decreased connectivity to visual areas in precuneus in the exercise group, resembling current baseline finding. Although our fitness predicted S1M1 connectivity targeted different regions at baseline compared to over time, it seems that functional segregation of S1M1 reflects better fitness. However, in an aged cohort more similar to ours, Voss et al. (2010) did not see group by time changes in motor connectivity, why this finding would need to be investigated further.

Interestingly, we observed enhanced connectivity between the DMN component and the left orbitofrontal cortex that correlated with gains in fitness. Even though the orbital cluster is localized more laterally than the typical ventromedial frontal DMN hub, the observation bears similarities to previous literature of fitness related connectivity of the posterior anterior midline core of the DMN (Voss et al., 2010, 2016). Both these studies interpret the fitness-related DMN integrity as a rejuvenated connectivity pattern, typical for younger subjects. A similar interpretation could be given here, but the lack of associations between cognition and these fitness-related connectivity patters prevent any firm conclusion of their behavioral significance.

Limited Effects

The *a priori* hypothesized group by time interactions, as well as the majority of the exploratory tests that aimed to relate longitudinal change in VO_2-peak to change in intrinsic brain activity, turned out to be non-significant. Despite drawing on previous literature that have investigated intrinsic capacity in relation to aerobic fitness among elderly, we were largely unable to conceptually replicate these. The replication failures could likely be attributed both to factors pertaining to cognitive brain imaging in general (see below), as well as to factors specific to this study context (e.g., differences in study design, interventions, cohorts and analyses strategies). Another potentially important issue is the fact that the active control group may have exercised more vigorously than in many previous interventions, considering that aerobic capacity increased substantially also for this group. Recent research have shown that resistance and coordination training, part of our active control training regimen, may influence the BOLD-signal during task performance (Voelcker-Rehage et al., 2011; see Voelcker-Rehage and Niemann, 2013, for a review), as well as show similar effects on hippocampus volume as aerobic exercise (Niemann et al., 2014). By comparing two training regimens which both have positive effects on brain and behavior, actual intervention effects may thus have been masked.

The effects of gains in fitness on the exploratory resting-state measures (e.g., global efficiency, connectome-MVPA, $BOLD_{STD}$) of the resting-state brain activity were likely too subtle to be detected in current study. The BOLD signal acquired during resting state fMRI is inherently noisy, and estimations based on high quality fMRI data showed that the variance associated with neuronal activity only constituted around 4% of the total variance of the BOLD-signal time series (Marcus et al., 2013). However, despite the large contribution of non-neuronal noise to the resting state BOLD signal, test–retest reliability of group average of cardinal resting state networks has been reported to be fairly reliable over time (Zuo et al., 2010; Wisner et al., 2013), although the choice of both resting state measures and preprocessing pipeline influence the degree of test–retest reliability (Yan et al., 2013). Not surprisingly, between-group comparisons of brain activity are also typically much smaller than single group averages (for an informative discussion on effect sizes in fMRI, see Poldrack et al., 2017).

Limitations and Future Directions

Current study has several limitations. First, we were unable to selectively induce improvements of VO_2-peak in the aerobic group, although the aerobic group improved more than the control group. This likely decreased any exercise induced group differences of the outcome measures. Although challenging, experimental designs that more efficiently prevent cardiovascular training in the active control group could potentially reveal stronger experimentally induced brain changes.

Furthermore, current study only measured two time points, i.e., before and after the 6-months intervention. Future studies would benefit from sampling data at multiple (>2) time points, for higher temporal resolution of the developmental trajectories. One motive for this is the expansion-partial normalization hypothesis of neuroplasticity (Brehmer et al., 2014), which proposes that longitudinal brain changes commonly follow inverted u-shaped temporal profiles, which could only be detected if data were acquired at multiple time points.

Resting state studies of physical interventions are still sparse. A greater understanding of the mechanisms mediating the neurocognitive effects of aerobic exercise are valuable for optimizing intervention programs to target the relevant neurophysiological processes and cognitive domains with higher precision. To enhance the reliability and replicability of imaging findings, several factors have recently been proposed (Ioannidis et al., 2014; Poldrack et al., 2017). Complete reporting of results (i.e., including null findings), as well as clear declarations of which analyses are *ad hoc* or exploratory and which are hypothesis driven, are both critical when aggregating research findings in meta-analyses, or for informing the design of future studies. Above all, the authors emphasized the importance of attaining proper statistical power, e.g., by enhancing cohort sizes for instance through laudable data sharing initiatives. Moreover, increased statistical power is also obtained by larger effect sizes. Stronger experimental effects could likely be achieved by longer and more intensive interventions. Potentially, longer intervention studies would also enable the observed brain changes to translate into improvements in behavior.

CONCLUSION

We have characterized changes in intrinsic brain activity following a 6-months physical exercise intervention. None of our *a priori* hypothesis of group by time interactions regarding intrinsic brain activity were confirmed. However, when investigating the linear relationships between longitudinal gain in aerobic capacity and changes in functional connectivity we observed exercise modulated hippocampal connectivity. Likewise, gain in aerobic capacity was associated with increased connectivity between the DMN and prefrontal cortex, but negatively related to sensorimotor-thalamic connectivity. However, these changes did not relate to changes in cognition, possibly due to the length of the intervention, or insensitive behavioral measures. The majority of the exploratory analyses did not reveal significant associations between fitness and intrinsic brain activity, although we observed that mid-temporal $BOLD_{STD}$ was negatively associated with fitness at baseline. The current study provides resting-state fMRI evidence that exercise preferentially modulate mid-temporal brain regions and hippocampus. The functional significance of these brain changes should be investigated further, preferably in high powered studies using data acquired at multiple time points.

AUTHOR CONTRIBUTIONS

LJ, LN, KR, and CB designed the study. PF performed the statistical analyses. All authors contributed in revising the work and approved the final version of the manuscript.

FUNDING

The research is part of the programme Paths to Healthy and Active Ageing, funded by the Swedish Research Council for Health, Working Life and Welfare, (Dnr 2013 – 2056). Support was also obtained from the Swedish Research Council (2012-00530), Västerbotten County Council, the Swedish Research Council for Sport Science and Umeå School of Sport Sciences to CB, from the Kamprad Family Foundation to LN and Umeå University.

ACKNOWLEDGMENTS

We thank all participants taking part in this study, the training supervisor Peter Lundström, the staff at Umeå Center for Functional Brain Imaging, University Hospital of Northern Sweden, Umeå, and Sport Science Lab at Umeå School of Sport Sciences Umeå University.

REFERENCES

Ashburner, J., and Friston, K. J. (2011). Diffeomorphic registration using geodesic shooting and Gauss–Newton optimisation. *Neuroimage* 55, 954–967. doi: 10.1016/j.neuroimage.2010.12.049

Baker, L. D., Frank, L. L., Foster-Schubert, K., Green, P. S., Wilkinson, C. W., McTiernan, A., et al. (2010). Effects of aerobic exercise on mild cognitive impairment. *Arch. Neurol.* 67, 71–79. doi: 10.1001/archneurol.2009.307

Bär, K. J., Herbsleb, M., Schumann, A., de la Cruz, F., Gabriel, H. W., and Wagner, G. (2016). Hippocampal-brainstem connectivity associated with vagal modulation after an intense exercise intervention in healthy men. *Front. Neurosci.* 10:145. doi: 10.3389/fnins.2016.00145

Boraxbekk, C.-J., Salami, A., Wåhlin, A., and Nyberg, L. (2016). Physical activity over a decade modifies age-related decline in perfusion, gray matter volume, and functional connectivity of the posterior default-mode network—A multimodal approach. *Neuroimage* 131, 133–141. doi: 10.1016/j.neuroimage.2015.12.010

Brehmer, Y., Kalpouzos, G., Wenger, E., and Lövdén, M. (2014). Plasticity of brain and cognition in older adults. *Psychol. Res.* 78, 790–802. doi: 10.1007/s00426-014-0587-z

Burzynska, A. Z., Wong, C. N., Voss, M. W., Cooke, G. E., Gothe, N. P., Fanning, J., et al. (2015). Physical activity is linked to greater moment-to-moment variability in spontaneous brain activity in older adults. *PLoS ONE* 10:e0134819. doi: 10.1371/journal.pone.0134819

Chao-Gan, Y., and Yu-Feng, Z. (2010). DPARSF: a MATLAB toolbox for "pipeline" data analysis of resting-state fMRI. *Front. Syst. Neurosci.* 4:13. doi: 10.3389/fnsys.2010.00013

Christensen, K., Doblhammer, G., Rau, R., and Vaupel, J. W. (2009). Ageing populations: the challenges ahead. *Lancet* 374, 1196–1208. doi: 10.1016/S0140-6736(09)61460-4

Colcombe, S., and Kramer, A. F. (2003). Fitness effects on the cognitive function of older adults: a meta-analytic study. *Psychol. Sci.* 14, 125–130. doi: 10.1111/1467-9280.t01-1-01430

Cole, M. W., Reynolds, J. R., Power, J. D., Repovs, G., Anticevic, A., and Braver, T. S. (2013). Multi-task connectivity reveals flexible hubs for adaptive task control. *Nat. Neurosci.* 16, 1348–1355. doi: 10.1038/nn.3470

Duzel, E., Van Praag, H., and Sendtner, M. (2016). Can physical exercise in old age improve memory and hippocampal function? *Brain* 139, 662–673. doi: 10.1093/brain/awv407

Erickson, K. I., Leckie, R. L., and Weinstein, A. M. (2014). Physical activity, fitness, and gray matter volume. *Neurobiol. Aging* 35, S20–S28. doi: 10.1016/j.neurobiolaging.2014.03.034

Erickson, K. I., Voss, M. W., Prakash, R. S., Basak, C., Szabo, A., Chaddock, L., et al. (2011). Exercise training increases size of hippocampus and improves memory. *Proc. Natl. Acad. Sci. U.S.A.* 108, 3017–3022. doi: 10.1073/pnas.1015950108

Gauthier, C. J., Lefort, M., Mekary, S., Desjardins-Crépeau, L., Skimminge, A., Iversen, P., et al. (2015). Hearts and minds: linking vascular rigidity and aerobic fitness with cognitive aging. *Neurobiol. Aging* 36, 304–314. doi: 10.1016/j.neurobiolaging.2014.08.018

Ioannidis, J. P. A., Munafò, M. R., Fusar-Poli, P., Nosek, B. A., and David, S. P. (2014). Publication and other reporting biases in cognitive sciences: detection, prevalence, and prevention. *Trends Cogn. Sci.* 18, 235–241. doi: 10.1016/j.tics.2014.02.010

Jonasson, L. S., Nyberg, L., Kramer, A. F., Lundquist, A., Riklund, K., and Boraxbekk, C.-J. (2017). Aerobic exercise intervention, cognitive performance, and brain structure: results from the physical influences on brain in aging (PHIBRA) study. *Front. Aging Neurosci.* 8:336. doi: 10.3389/fnagi.2016.00336

Kelly, C., and Castellanos, F. X. (2014). Strengthening connections: functional connectivity and brain plasticity. *Neuropsychol. Rev.* 24, 63–76. doi: 10.1007/s11065-014-9252-y

Krafft, C. E., Pierce, J. E., Schwarz, N. F., Chi, L., Weinberger, A. L., Schaeffer, D. J., et al. (2014). An eight month randomized controlled exercise intervention alters resting state synchrony in overweight children. *Neuroscience* 256, 445–455. doi: 10.1016/j.neuroscience.2013.09.052

Kramer, A. F., Hahn, S., Cohen, N. J., Banich, M. T., McAuley, E., Harrison, C. R., et al. (1999). Ageing, fitness and neurocognitive function. *Nature* 400, 418–419. doi: 10.1038/22682

Kruschwitz, J. D., List, D., Waller, L., Rubinov, M., and Walter, H. (2015). GraphVar: a user-friendly toolbox for comprehensive graph analyses of functional brain connectivity. *J. Neurosci. Methods* 245, 107–115. doi: 10.1016/j.jneumeth.2015.02.021

Leuner, B., and Gould, E. (2010). Structural plasticity and hippocampal function. *Annu. Rev. Psychol.* 61, C1–C3. doi: 10.1146/annurev.psych.093008.100359

Maass, A., Düzel, S., Goerke, M., Becke, A., Sobieray, U., Neumann, K., et al. (2015). Vascular hippocampal plasticity after aerobic exercise in older adults. *Mol. Psychiatry* 20, 585–593. doi: 10.1038/mp.2014.114

Maldjian, J. A., Laurienti, P. J., Kraft, R. A., and Burdette, J. H. (2003). An automated method for neuroanatomic and cytoarchitectonic atlas-based interrogation of fMRI data sets. *Neuroimage* 19, 1233–1239.

Marcus, D. S., Harms, M. P., Snyder, A. Z., Jenkinson, M., Wilson, J. A., Glasser, M. F., et al. (2013). Human Connectome Project informatics: quality control, database services, and data visualization. *Neuroimage* 80, 202–219. doi: 10.1016/j.neuroimage.2013.05.077

Mitchell, G. F., van Buchem, M. A., Sigurdsson, S., Gotal, J. D., Jonsdottir, M. K., Kjartansson, O., et al. (2011). Arterial stiffness, pressure and flow pulsatility and brain structure and function: the Age, Gene/Environment Susceptibility - Reykjavik study. *Brain* 134, 3398–3407. doi: 10.1093/brain/awr253

Niemann, C., Godde, B., and Voelcker-Rehage, C. (2014). Not only cardiovascular, but also coordinative exercise increases hippocampal volume in older adults. *Front. Aging Neurosci.* 6:170. doi: 10.3389/fnagi.2014.00170

North, T., McCullagh, P., and Tran, Z. (1990). Effect of exercise on depression. *Exerc. Sport Sci.* 18, 379–415.

Nyberg, J., Aberg, M. A. I., Schioler, L., Nilsson, M., Wallin, A., Toren, K., et al. (2014). Cardiovascular and cognitive fitness at age 18 and risk of early-onset dementia. *Brain* 137, 1514–1523. doi: 10.1093/brain/awu041

Poldrack, R. A., Baker, C. I., Durnez, J., Gorgolewski, K. J., Matthews, P. M., Munafò, M. R., et al. (2017). Scanning the horizon: towards transparent and reproducible neuroimaging research. *Nat. Rev. Neurosci.* 18, 115–126. doi: 10.1038/nrn.2016.167

Power, J. D., Cohen, A. L., Nelson, S. M., Wig, G. S., Barnes, K. A., Church, J. A., et al. (2011). Functional network organization of the human brain. *Neuron* 72, 665–678. doi: 10.1016/j.neuron.2011.09.006

Rubinov, M., and Sporns, O. (2010). Complex network measures of brain connectivity: uses and interpretations. *Neuroimage* 52, 1059–1069. doi: 10.1016/j.neuroimage.2009.10.003

Salami, A., Wahlin, A., Kaboodvand, N., Lundquist, A., and Nyberg, L. (2016). Longitudinal evidence for dissociation of anterior and posterior MTL resting-state connectivity in aging: links to perfusion and memory. *Cereb. Cortex* 26, 3953–3963. doi: 10.1093/cercor/bhw233

Satterthwaite, T. D., Elliott, M. A., Gerraty, R. T., Ruparel, K., Loughead, J., Calkins, M. E., et al. (2013). An improved framework for confound regression and filtering for control of motion artifact in the preprocessing of resting-state functional connectivity data. *Neuroimage* 64, 240–256. doi: 10.1016/j.neuroimage.2012.08.052

Smith, P. J., Blumenthal, J. A., Hoffman, B. M., Cooper, H., Strauman, T. A., Welsh-Bohmer, K., et al. (2010). Aerobic exercise and neurocognitive performance: a meta-analytic review of randomized controlled trials. *Psychosom. Med.* 72, 239–252. doi: 10.1097/PSY.0b013e3181d14633

Stillman, C. M., Cohen, J., Lehman, M. E., and Erickson, K. I. (2016). Mediators of physical activity on neurocognitive function: a review at multiple levels of analysis. *Front. Hum. Neurosci.* 10:626. doi: 10.3389/fnhum.2016.00626

Tozzi, L., Carballedo, A., Lavelle, G., Doolin, K., Doyle, M., Amico, F., et al. (2016). Longitudinal functional connectivity changes correlate with mood improvement after regular exercise in a dose-dependent fashion. *Eur. J. Neurosci.* 43, 1089–1096. doi: 10.1111/ejn.13222

Voelcker-Rehage, C., Godde, B., and Staudinger, U. M. (2011). Cardiovascular and coordination training differentially improve cognitive performance and neural processing in older adults. *Front. Hum. Neurosci.* 5:26. doi: 10.3389/fnhum.2011.00026

Voelcker-Rehage, C., and Niemann, C. (2013). Structural and functional brain changes related to different types of physical activity across the life span. *Neurosci. Biobehav. Rev.* 37, 2268–2295. doi: 10.1016/j.neubiorev.2013.01.028

Voss, M. W., Erickson, K. I., Prakash, R. S., Chaddock, L., Kim, J. S., Alves, H., et al. (2013). Neurobiological markers of exercise-related brain plasticity in older adults. *Brain. Behav. Immun.* 28, 90–99. doi: 10.1016/j.bbi.2012.10.021

Voss, M. W., Prakash, R. S., Erickson, K. I., Basak, C., Chaddock, L., Kim, J. S., et al. (2010). Plasticity of brain networks in a randomized intervention trial of exercise training in older adults. *Front. Aging Neurosci.* 2:32. doi: 10.3389/fnagi.2010.00032

Voss, M. W., Weng, T. B., Burzynska, A. Z., Wong, C. N., Cooke, G. E., Clark, R., et al. (2016). Fitness, but not physical activity, is related to functional integrity of brain networks associated with aging. *Neuroimage* 131, 113–125. doi: 10.1016/j.neuroimage.2015.10.044

Wendell, C. R., Gunstad, J., Waldstein, S. R., Wright, J. G., Ferrucci, L., and Zonderman, A. B. (2014). Cardiorespiratory fitness and accelerated cognitive decline with aging. *J. Gerontol. A Biol. Sci. Med. Sci.* 69, 455–462. doi: 10.1093/gerona/glt144

Whitfield-Gabrieli, S., and Nieto-Castanon, A. (2012). Conn: a functional connectivity toolbox for correlated and anticorrelated brain networks. *Brain Connect.* 2, 125–141. doi: 10.1089/brain.2012.0073

Wisner, K. M., Atluri, G., Lim, K. O., and Macdonald, A. W. (2013). Neurometrics of intrinsic connectivity networks at rest using fMRI: retest reliability and cross-validation using a meta-level method. *Neuroimage* 76, 236–251. doi: 10.1016/j.neuroimage.2013.02.066

Xia, M., Wang, J., and He, Y. (2013). BrainNet Viewer: a network visualization tool for human brain connectomics. *PLoS ONE* 8:e68910. doi: 10.1371/journal.pone.0068910

Yan, C.-G., Cheung, B., Kelly, C., Colcombe, S., Craddock, R. C., Di Martino, A., et al. (2013). A comprehensive assessment of regional variation in the impact of head micromovements on functional connectomics. *Neuroimage* 76, 183–201. doi: 10.1016/j.neuroimage.2013.03.004

Young, J., Angevaren, M., Rusted, J., and Tabet, N. (2015). Aerobic exercise to improve cognitive function in older people without known cognitive impairment. *Cochrane Database Syst. Rev.* CD005381. doi: 10.1002/14651858.CD005381.pub4

Zalesky, A., Fornito, A., and Bullmore, E. T. (2010). Network-based statistic: identifying differences in brain networks. *Neuroimage* 53, 1197–1207. doi: 10.1016/j.neuroimage.2010.06.041

Zuo, X.-N., Kelly, C., Adelstein, J. S., Klein, D. F., Castellanos, F. X., and Milham, M. P. (2010). Reliable intrinsic connectivity networks: test-retest evaluation using ICA and dual regression approach. *Neuroimage* 49, 2163–2177. doi: 10.1016/j.neuroimage.2009.10.080

Permissions

All chapters in this book were first published by Frontiers; hereby published with permission under the Creative Commons Attribution License or equivalent. Every chapter published in this book has been scrutinized by our experts. Their significance has been extensively debated. The topics covered herein carry significant findings which will fuel the growth of the discipline. They may even be implemented as practical applications or may be referred to as a beginning point for another development.

The contributors of this book come from diverse backgrounds, making this book a truly international effort. This book will bring forth new frontiers with its revolutionizing research information and detailed analysis of the nascent developments around the world.

We would like to thank all the contributing authors for lending their expertise to make the book truly unique. They have played a crucial role in the development of this book. Without their invaluable contributions this book wouldn't have been possible. They have made vital efforts to compile up to date information on the varied aspects of this subject to make this book a valuable addition to the collection of many professionals and students.

This book was conceptualized with the vision of imparting up-to-date information and advanced data in this field. To ensure the same, a matchless editorial board was set up. Every individual on the board went through rigorous rounds of assessment to prove their worth. After which they invested a large part of their time researching and compiling the most relevant data for our readers.

The editorial board has been involved in producing this book since its inception. They have spent rigorous hours researching and exploring the diverse topics which have resulted in the successful publishing of this book. They have passed on their knowledge of decades through this book. To expedite this challenging task, the publisher supported the team at every step. A small team of assistant editors was also appointed to further simplify the editing procedure and attain best results for the readers.

Apart from the editorial board, the designing team has also invested a significant amount of their time in understanding the subject and creating the most relevant covers. They scrutinized every image to scout for the most suitable representation of the subject and create an appropriate cover for the book.

The publishing team has been an ardent support to the editorial, designing and production team. Their endless efforts to recruit the best for this project, has resulted in the accomplishment of this book. They are a veteran in the field of academics and their pool of knowledge is as vast as their experience in printing. Their expertise and guidance has proved useful at every step. Their uncompromising quality standards have made this book an exceptional effort. Their encouragement from time to time has been an inspiration for everyone.

The publisher and the editorial board hope that this book will prove to be a valuable piece of knowledge for researchers, students, practitioners and scholars across the globe.

List of Contributors

Wen-Cao Liu
Department of Emergency, Shanxi Provincial People's Hospital, Taiyuan, China

Xiaona Wang, Xinyu Zhang and Xinchun Jin
Jiangsu Key Laboratory of Translational Research and Therapy for Neuro-Psycho-Diseases and Institute of Neuroscience, Department of Neurology, the Second Affiliated Hospital of Soochow University, Suzhou, China
School of Pharmacy, Key Laboratory of Molecular Pharmacology and Drug Evaluation (Yantai University), Ministry of Education, Yantai University, Yantai, China

Xi Chen
Department of Core Facility, the People's Hospital of Baoan Shenzhen, Shenzhen, China

Katharina S. Goerlich and Sinika Ellendt
Department of Psychiatry, Psychotherapy and Psychosomatics, Medical Faculty, RWTH Aachen University, Aachen, Germany

Mikhail Votinov
Department of Psychiatry, Psychotherapy and Psychosomatics, Medical Faculty, RWTH Aachen University, Aachen, Germany
Jülich Aachen Research Alliance (JARA) – Translational Brain Medicine, Aachen, Germany
Institute of Neuroscience and Medicine (INM-10), Research Centre Jülich, Jülich, Germany

Ellen Dicks
Department of Psychiatry, Psychotherapy and Psychosomatics, Medical Faculty, RWTH Aachen University, Aachen, Germany
Alzheimer Center and Department of Neurology, Neuroscience Campus Amsterdam, VU University Medical Center, Amsterdam, Netherlands

Gábor Csukly
Department of Psychiatry and Psychotherapy, Semmelweis University, Budapest, Hungary

Ute Habel
Department of Psychiatry, Psychotherapy and Psychosomatics, Medical Faculty, RWTH Aachen University, Aachen, Germany
Jülich Aachen Research Alliance (JARA) – Translational Brain Medicine, Aachen, Germany

Ya-Jing Mi, Na Guo, Zhao-Hua Zhao, Xing-Chun Gao, Xiao-Long Wang and Rui-San Zhang
Institute of Basic and Translational Medicine, and School of Basic Medical Sciences, and Shaanxi Key Laboratory of Brain Disorders, Xi'an Medical University, Xi'an, China

Hai Chen
Institute of Basic and Translational Medicine, and School of Basic Medical Sciences, and Shaanxi Key Laboratory of Brain Disorders, Xi'an Medical University, Xi'an, China
Department of Anesthesiology, Tangdu Hospital, Fourth Military Medical University, Xi'an, China

Xing-Chun Gou
Institute of Basic and Translational Medicine, and School of Basic Medical Sciences, and Shaanxi Key Laboratory of Brain Disorders, Xi'an Medical University, Xi'an, China
Department of Neurosurgery, School of Medicine, Yale University, New Haven, CT, United States

Samir Takillah
Team Neurophysiology and Behavior, Institut de Biologie Paris Seine (IBPS), UMR 8246 Neuroscience Paris Seine (NPS), Sorbonne Universités, Université Pierre et Marie Curie (UPMC), CNRS, INSERM, U1130, Paris, France
Team Brain Development, Repair and Ageing, Institut de Biologie Paris Seine (IBPS), UMR 8256 Biological Adaptation and Ageing (B2A), Sorbonne Universités, Université Pierre et Marie Curie (UPMC), CNRS, Paris, France
APHP Hôpital Charles Foix, DHU Fast, Institut de la Longévité, Ivry-sur-Seine, France
Département Neurosciences et Contraintes Opérationnelles, Institut de Recherche Biomédicale des Armées (IRBA), Unité Fatigue et Vigilance, Brétigny-sur-Orge, France
EA7330 VIFASOM, Université Paris Descartes, Paris, France

Jérémie Naudé, Steve Didienne, Alexandre Mourot and Philippe Faure
Team Neurophysiology and Behavior, Institut de Biologie Paris Seine (IBPS), UMR 8246 Neuroscience Paris Seine (NPS), Sorbonne Universités, Université Pierre et Marie Curie (UPMC), CNRS, INSERM, U1130, Paris, France

Meng-Yi Sun and Jiang-Bing Zhou
Department of Neurosurgery, School of Medicine, Yale University, New Haven, CT, United States

Claude Sebban, Brigitte Decros and Jean Mariani
Team Brain Development, Repair and Ageing, Institut de Biologie Paris Seine (IBPS), UMR 8256 Biological Adaptation and Ageing (B2A), Sorbonne Universités, Université Pierre et Marie Curie (UPMC), CNRS, Paris, France
APHP Hôpital Charles Foix, DHU Fast, Institut de la Longévité, Ivry-sur-Seine, France

Esther Schenker
Neuroscience Drug Discovery Unit, Institut de Recherches Servier, Croissy-sur-Seine, France

Michael Spedding
Spedding Research Solutions SARL, Le Vésinet, France

Pauline L. Baniqued
Helen Wills Neuroscience Institute, University of California, Berkeley, Berkeley, CA, United States
Beckman Institute for Advanced Science and Technology, University of Illinois at Urbana-Champaign, Urbana, IL, United States

Courtney L. Gallen and Mark D'Esposito
Helen Wills Neuroscience Institute, University of California, Berkeley, Berkeley, CA, United States

Michelle W. Voss
Department of Psychological and Brain Sciences, University of Iowa, Iowa City, IA, United States

Agnieszka Z. Burzynska
Department of Human Development and Family Studies, Colorado State University, Fort Collins, CO, United States

Chelsea N. Wong and Kristin Duffy
Beckman Institute for Advanced Science and Technology, University of Illinois at Urbana-Champaign, Urbana, IL, United States

Gillian E. Cooke
Beckman Institute for Advanced Science and Technology, University of Illinois at Urbana-Champaign, Urbana, IL, United States
Interdisciplinary Health Sciences Institute, University of Illinois at Urbana-Champaign, Urbana, IL, United States

Jason Fanning
Department of Kinesiology and Community Health, University of Illinois at Urbana-Champaign, Urbana, IL, United States
Department of Internal Medicine-Gerontology, Wake Forest School of Medicine, Winston-Salem, NC, United States

Diane K. Ehlers, Elizabeth A. Salerno and Susan Aguiñaga
Department of Kinesiology and Community Health, University of Illinois at Urbana-Champaign, Urbana, IL, United States

Edward McAuley
Beckman Institute for Advanced Science and Technology, University of Illinois at Urbana-Champaign, Urbana, IL, United States
Department of Kinesiology and Community Health, University of Illinois at Urbana-Champaign, Urbana, IL, United States

Arthur F. Kramer
Beckman Institute for Advanced Science and Technology, University of Illinois at Urbana-Champaign, Urbana, IL, United States
Psychology Department and Mechanical and Industrial Engineering Department, Northeastern University, Boston, MA, United States

Ganesh B. Chand
Division of General Internal Medicine and Geriatrics, Department of Medicine, Emory University School of Medicine, Atlanta, GA, United States

Junjie Wu
Department of Radiology and Imaging Sciences, Emory University School of Medicine, Atlanta, GA, United States

Deqiang Qiu
Department of Radiology and Imaging Sciences, Emory University School of Medicine, Atlanta, GA, United States
Department of Biomedical Engineering, Georgia Institute of Technology, Emory University, Atlanta, GA, United States

Ihab Hajjar
Division of General Internal Medicine and Geriatrics, Department of Medicine, Emory University School of Medicine, Atlanta, GA, United States
Department of Neurology, Emory Alzheimer's Disease Research Center, Emory University School of Medicine, Atlanta, GA, United States

Vasiliki I. Zilidou
Laboratory of Medical Physics, Medical School, Aristotle University of Thessaloniki, Thessaloniki, Greece
Department of Physical Activity and Recreation, School of Physical Education and Sport Science, Aristotle University of Thessaloniki, Thessaloniki, Greece

Evangelia D. Romanopoulou, Evangelos Paraskevopoulos, Christos A. Frantzidis and Panagiotis D. Bamidis
Laboratory of Medical Physics, Medical School, Aristotle University of Thessaloniki, Thessaloniki, Greece

Styliani Douka
Department of Physical Activity and Recreation, School of Physical Education and Sport Science, Aristotle University of Thessaloniki, Thessaloniki, Greece

Toshikazu Ikuta
Department of Communication Sciences and Disorders, School of Applied Sciences, University of Mississippi, University, MS, United States

Koji Matsuo, Kenichiro Harada, Naoko Higuchi, Fumihiro Higuchi, Koji Otsuki, Toshio Watanuki, Hirotaka Yamagata and Yoshifumi Watanabe
Division of Neuropsychiatry, Department of Neuroscience, Graduate School of Medicine, Yamaguchi University, Ube, Japan

Mami Nakashima
Division of Neuropsychiatry, Department of Neuroscience, Graduate School of Medicine, Yamaguchi University, Ube, Japan
Nagato-Ichinomiya Hospital, Shimonoseki, Japan

Teruyuki Hobara
Division of Neuropsychiatry, Department of Neuroscience, Graduate School of Medicine, Yamaguchi University, Ube, Japan
Department of Psychiatry, Yamaguchi Grand Medical Center, Hofu, Japan

Tomohiko Shibata
Division of Neuropsychiatry, Department of Neuroscience, Graduate School of Medicine, Yamaguchi University, Ube, Japan
Shinwaen Hospital, Onoda, Japan

Toshio Matsubara
Division of Neuropsychiatry, Department of Neuroscience, Graduate School of Medicine, Yamaguchi University, Ube, Japan
Health Administration Center, Yamaguchi University Organization for University Education, Yamaguchi City, Japan

Atsuko Nagano-Saito, Mohamed S. Al-Azzawi, Clotilde Degroot, Béatriz Mejia-Constain and Christophe Bedetti
Centre de Recherche de l'Institut Universitaire de Gériatrie de Montréal, Montréal, QC, Canada

Alexandru Hanganu
Departments of Clinical Neurosciences and Radiology, University of Calgary, Calgary, AB, Canada
Hotchkiss Brain Institute, Calgary, AB, Canada

Anne-Louise Lafontaine
Department of Neurology and Neurosurgery, McGill University, Montreal, QC, Canada

Valérie Soland and Sylvain Chouinard
Centre Hospitalier de l'Université de Montréal, Montréal, QC, Canada

Oury Monchi
Centre de Recherche de l'Institut Universitaire de Gériatrie de Montréal, Montréal, QC, Canada
Departments of Clinical Neurosciences and Radiology, University of Calgary, Calgary, AB, Canada
Hotchkiss Brain Institute, Calgary, AB, Canada
Departments of Clinical Neurosciences and Radiology, University of Calgary, Calgary, AB, Canada
Hotchkiss Brain Institute, Calgary, AB, Canada

Evatte T. Sciberras-Lim and Anthony J. Lambert
Department of Psychology, University of Auckland, Auckland, New Zealand

Jiao Wang, Qian Li, Fangfang Zhou, Jie Li, Weihao Li and Tieqiao Wen
Laboratory of Molecular Neural Biology, School of Life Sciences, Shanghai University, Shanghai, China

Yanyan Kong and Yihui Guan
Position Emission Computed Tomography Center, Huashan Hospital, Fudan University, Shanghai, China

Kai Wang
Shanghai Key Laboratory of Molecular Andrology, Institute of Biochemistry and Cell Biology, Shanghai Institutes for Biological Sciences, Chinese Academy of Sciences, Shanghai, China

Ting Wu
Shanghai Stem Cell Group, Shanghai, China

Jiang Xie
School of Computer Engineering and Science, Shanghai University, Shanghai, China

Ravi Rajmohan
Department of Pharmacology and Neuroscience, Texas Tech University Health Sciences Center, Lubbock, TX, USA

Ronald C. Anderson
Department of Electrical and Computer Engineering, Texas Tech University, Lubbock, TX, USA

Dan Fang
Department of Human Development and Family Studies, Texas Tech University, Lubbock, TX, USA

Austin G. Meyer
School of Medicine, Texas Tech University Health Sciences Center, Lubbock, TX, USA

Pavis Laengvejkal, Parunyou Julayanont and John De Toledo
Department of Neurology, Texas Tech University Health Sciences Center, Lubbock, TX, USA

Greg Hannabas and Hafiz M. R. Khan
Department of Public Health, Texas Tech University Health Sciences Center, Lubbock, TX, USA

Kitten Linton and John Culberson
Department of Family Medicine, Texas Tech University Health Sciences Center, Lubbock, TX, USA

P. Hemachandra Reddy
Department of Pharmacology and Neuroscience, Texas Tech University Health Sciences Center, Lubbock, TX, USA
Garrison Institute on Aging, Texas Tech University Health Sciences Center, Lubbock, TX, USA
Cell Biology and Biochemistry, Texas Tech University Health Sciences Center, Lubbock, TX, USA
Speech, Language and Hearing Sciences, Texas Tech University Health Sciences Center, Lubbock, TX, USA

Michael O'Boyle
Department of Pharmacology and Neuroscience, Texas Tech University Health Sciences Center, Lubbock, TX, USA
Department of Human Development and Family Studies, Texas Tech University, Lubbock, TX, USA

Nicole M. Barcelos, David J. Hayes and Molly Maloney
The Healthy Aging and Neuropsychology Lab, Union College, Schenectady, NY, United States

Earl A. Zimmerman
Alzheimer's Disease Center, Albany Medical Center, Albany, NY, United States

Robert W. Gillen
Sunnyview Rehabilitation Hospital, Schenectady, NY, United States

Mina Dunnam
Stratton VA Medical Center, Albany, NY, United States

Brian D. Cohen
Department of Biology, Union College, Schenectady, NY, United States

Vadim Yerokhin
Biomedical Sciences Department, Oklahoma State University, Tulsa, OK, United States

Kenneth E. Miller
Department of Anatomy and Cell Biology, Oklahoma State University, Tulsa, OK, United States

Paul J. Arciero
Department of Health & Human Physiological Sciences, Skidmore College, Saratoga Springs, NY, United States

Rachel A. Crockett, Chun Liang Hsu, John R. Best and Teresa Liu-Ambrose
Aging, Mobility, and Cognitive Neuroscience Laboratory, Department of Physical Therapy, Djavad Mowafaghian Centre for Brain Health, University of British Columbia, Vancouver, BC, Canada

Chia-Liang Tsai
Institute of Physical Education, Health and Leisure Studies, National Cheng Kung University, Tainan, Taiwan

Chien-Yu Pan and Fu-Chen Chen
Department of Physical Education, National Kaohsiung Normal University, Kaohsiung, Taiwan

Yu-Ting Tseng
Institute of Physical Education, Health and Leisure Studies, National Cheng Kung University, Tainan, Taiwan
School of Kinesiology, University of Minnesota, Minneapolis, MN, United States

Krystallia Pantsiou, Ourania Sfakianaki, Dimitra Savvoulidou and Despina Moraitou
Lab of Psychology, Department of Experimental and Cognitive Psychology, School of Psychology, Aristotle University of Thessaloniki, Thessaloniki, Greece

Vasileios Papaliagkas
Laboratory of Clinical Neurophysiology, Aristotle University of Thessaloniki, Thessaloniki, Greece

Vassiliki Costa
1st Neurology Department, AHEPA Hospital, Aristotle University of Thessaloniki, Thessaloniki, Greece

Georgia Papantoniou
Department of Early Childhood Education, School of Education, University of Ioannina, Ioannina, Greece

Maria E. López
Laboratory of Neuropsychology, Universitat de les Illes Balears, Palma de Mallorca, Spain
Networking Research Center on Bioengineering, Biomaterials and Nanomedicine, Madrid, Spain

Marjolein M. A. Engels and Philip Scheltens
Alzheimer Center and Department of Neurology, Neuroscience Campus Amsterdam, VU University Medical Center, Amsterdam, Netherlands

Elisabeth C. W. van Straaten
Department of Clinical Neurophysiology and MEG Center, Neuroscience Campus Amsterdam, VU University Medical Center, Amsterdam, Netherlands
Nutricia Advanced Medical Nutrition, Nutricia Research, Utrecht, Netherlands

Ricardo Bajo
Laboratory of Cognitive and Computational Neuroscience, Center for Biomedical Technology, Complutense University of Madrid and Technical University of Madrid, Madrid, Spain

María L. Delgado
Seniors Center of the District of Chamartín, Madrid, Spain
Department of Basic Psychology II, Complutense University of Madrid, Madrid, Spain

Arjan Hillebrand and Cornelis J. Stam
Department of Clinical Neurophysiology and MEG Center, Neuroscience Campus Amsterdam, VU University Medical Center, Amsterdam, Netherlands

Fernando Maestú
Networking Research Center on Bioengineering, Biomaterials and Nanomedicine, Madrid, Spain
Laboratory of Cognitive and Computational Neuroscience, Center for Biomedical Technology, Complutense University of Madrid and Technical University of Madrid, Madrid, Spain
Department of Basic Psychology II, Complutense University of Madrid, Madrid, Spain

Pär Flodin
Center for Demographic and Aging Research, Umeå University, Umeå, Sweden
Umeå Center for Functional Brain Imaging, Umeå University, Umeå, Sweden

Lars S. Jonasson
Center for Demographic and Aging Research, Umeå University, Umeå, Sweden
Umeå Center for Functional Brain Imaging, Umeå University, Umeå, Sweden
Diagnostic Radiology, Department of Radiation Sciences, Umeå University, Umeå, Sweden

Katrin Riklund
Umeå Center for Functional Brain Imaging, Umeå University, Umeå, Sweden
Diagnostic Radiology, Department of Radiation Sciences, Umeå University, Umeå, Sweden

Lars Nyberg
Umeå Center for Functional Brain Imaging, Umeå University, Umeå, Sweden
Diagnostic Radiology, Department of Radiation Sciences, Umeå University, Umeå, Sweden
Physiology, Department of Integrative Medical Biology, Umeå University, Umeå, Sweden

C. J. Boraxbekk
Center for Demographic and Aging Research, Umeå University, Umeå, Sweden
Umeå Center for Functional Brain Imaging, Umeå University, Umeå, Sweden
Danish Research Centre for Magnetic Resonance, Centre for Functional and Diagnostic Imaging and Research, Copenhagen University Hospital Hvidovre, Copenhagen, Denmark

Index

www.ingramcontent.com/pod-product-compliance
Lightning Source LLC
LaVergne TN
LVHW081023210926
848485LV00004B/936